The Oxford Handbook of Stress, Health, and Coping

OXFORD LIBRARY OF PSYCHOLOGY

Editor-in-Chief PETER E. NATHAN

The Oxford Handbook of Stress, Health, and Coping

Edited by

Susan Folkman

OXFORD

UNIVERSITY PRESS

2011

OXFORD
UNIVERSITY PRESS

Oxford University Press, Inc., publishes works that further Oxford University's
objective of excellence in research, scholarship, and education.

Oxford New York
Auckland   Cape Town   Dar es Salaam   Hong Kong   Karachi
Kuala Lumpur   Madrid   Melbourne   Mexico City   Nairobi
New Delhi   Shanghai   Taipei   Toronto

With offices in
Argentina   Austria   Brazil   Chile   Czech Republic   France   Greece
Guatemala   Hungary   Italy   Japan   Poland   Portugal   Singapore
South Korea   Switzerland   Thailand   Turkey   Ukraine   Vietnam

Published by Oxford University Press, Inc.
198 Madison Avenue, New York, New York 10016
www.oup.com

Oxford is a registered trademark of Oxford University Press

Library of Congress Cataloging-in-Publication Data

The Oxford handbook of stress, health, and coping / edited by Susan Folkman.
p.; cm. – (Oxford library of psychology)
Other title: Handbook of stress, health, and coping
Includes bibliographical references and index.
ISBN-13: 978-0-19-537534-3
1. Stress management–Handbooks, manuals, etc. I. Folkman, Susan.
II. Title: Handbook of stress, health, and coping. III. Series: Oxford library of psychology.
[DNLM: 1. Stress, Psychological. 2. Adaptation, Psychological. 3. Mental Health.
WM 172 O985 2011]
RA785.O94 2011
155.9'042–dc22
2010007425

9 8 7 6 5 4 3 2

Printed in the United States of America on acid-free paper

To David

SHORT CONTENTS

OXFORD LIBRARY OF PSYCHOLOGY

The *Oxford Library of Psychology*, a landmark series of handbooks, is published by Oxford University Press, one of the world's oldest and most highly respected publishers, with a tradition of publishing significant books in psychology. The ambitious goal of the *Oxford Library of Psychology* is nothing less than to span a vibrant, wide-ranging field and, in so doing, to fill a clear market need.

Encompassing a comprehensive set of handbooks, organized hierarchically, the *Library* incorporates volumes at different levels, each designed to meet a distinct need. At one level are a set of handbooks designed broadly to survey the major subfields of psychology; at another are numerous handbooks that cover important current focal research and scholarly areas of psychology in depth and detail. Planned as a reflection of the dynamism of psychology, the *Library* will grow and expand as psychology itself develops, thereby highlighting significant new research that will impact on the field. Adding to its accessibility and ease of use, the *Library* will be published in print and, later on, electronically.

The *Library* surveys psychology's principal subfields with a set of handbooks that capture the current status and future prospects of those major subdisciplines. This initial set includes handbooks of social and personality psychology, clinical psychology, counseling psychology, school psychology, educational psychology, industrial and organizational psychology, cognitive psychology, cognitive neuroscience, methods and measurements, history, neuropsychology, personality assessment, developmental psychology, and more. Each handbook undertakes to review one of psychology's major subdisciplines with breadth, comprehensiveness, and exemplary scholarship. In addition to these broadly-conceived volumes, the *Library* also includes a large number of handbooks designed to explore in depth more specialized areas of scholarship and research, such as stress, health and coping, anxiety and related disorders, cognitive development, or child and adolescent assessment. In contrast to the broad coverage of the subfield handbooks, each of these latter volumes focuses on an especially productive, more highly focused line of scholarship and research. Whether at the broadest or most specific level, however, all of the *Library* handbooks offer synthetic coverage that reviews and evaluates the relevant past and present research and anticipates research in the future. Each handbook in the *Library* includes introductory and concluding chapters written by its editor to provide a roadmap to the handbook's table of contents and to offer informed anticipations of significant future developments in that field.

An undertaking of this scope calls for handbook editors and chapter authors who are established scholars in the areas about which they write. Many of the nation's and world's most productive and best-respected psychologists have agreed to edit *Library* handbooks or write authoritative chapters in their areas of expertise.

For whom has the *Oxford Library of Psychology* been written? Because of its breadth, depth, and accessibility, the *Library* serves a diverse audience, including graduate students in psychology and their faculty mentors, scholars, researchers, and practitioners in psychology and related fields. Each will find in the *Library* the information they seek on the subfield or focal area of psychology in which they work or are interested.

Befitting its commitment to accessibility, each handbook includes a comprehensive index, as well as extensive references to help guide research. And because the *Library* was designed from its inception as an online as well as a print resource, its structure and contents will be readily and rationally searchable online. Further, once the *Library* is released online, the handbooks will be regularly and thoroughly updated.

In summary, the *Oxford Library of Psychology* will grow organically to provide a thoroughly informed perspective on the field of psychology, one that reflects both psychology's dynamism and its increasing interdisciplinarity. Once published electronically, the *Library* is also destined to become a uniquely valuable interactive tool, with extended search and browsing capabilities. As you begin to consult this handbook, we sincerely hope you will share our enthusiasm for the more than 500-year tradition of Oxford University Press for excellence, innovation, and quality, as exemplified by the *Oxford Library of Psychology.*

Peter E. Nathan
Editor-in-Chief
Oxford Library of Psychology

ABOUT THE EDITOR

Susan Folkman

Susan Folkman is Professor Emeritus at the University of California, San Francisco. She received her Ph.D. in 1979 from the University of California, Berkeley, where with Richard Lazarus she developed a program of research on stress and coping. In 1988 she moved to the University of California, San Francisco, where her research on coping with caregiving and bereavement during the AIDS epidemic led to an interest in the role of positive emotions in the stress process. She is recognized internationally for her theory and research on coping.

CONTRIBUTORS

Glenn Affleck
University of Connecticut Health Center
Farmington, CT

Carolyn Aldwin
Department of Human Development &
Family Sciences
Oregon State University
Corvallis, OR

Michael H. Antoni
Departments of Psychology and
Psychiatry
Biobehavioral Oncology Program,
Sylvester Comprehensive Cancer Center
University of Miami
Coral Gables, FL

Lisa G. Aspinwall
Department of Psychology
University of Utah
Salt Lake City, UT

Anita DeLongis
The Centre for Health and
Coping Studies
Department of Psychology
University of British Columbia
Vancouver, BC

Susan Folkman
Department of Medicine (Emeritus)
University of California, San Francisco
San Francisco, CA

Vicki S. Helgeson
Department of Psychology
Carnegie Mellon University
Pittsburgh, PA

Stevan E. Hobfoll
Department of Behavioral Sciences
Rush Medical College
Chicago, IL

Gail Ironson
Department of Psychology
University of Miami
Coral Gables, FL

Heidemarie Kremer
Department of Psychology
University of Miami
Coral Gables, FL

Mark D. Litt
University of Connecticut Health Center
Farmington, CT

Sonja Lyubomirsky
Department of Psychology
University of California, Riverside
Riverside, CA

Judith Tedlie Moskowitz
Osher Center for Integrative Medicine
University of California, San Francisco
San Francisco, CA

Kenneth I. Pakenham
School of Psychology
University of Queensland
Brisbane, Australia

Kenneth I. Pargament
Department of Psychology
Bowling Green State University
Bowling Green, OH

Crystal L. Park
Department of Psychology
University of Connecticut
Storrs, CT

John W. Reich
Department of Psychology
Arizona State University
Tempe, AZ

Tracey A. Revenson
Department of Psychology
The Graduate Center
City University of New York
New York, NY

Ellen A. Skinner
Psychology Department
Portland State University
Portland, OR

Annette L. Stanton
Department of Psychology
University of California, Los Angeles
Los Angeles, CA

Margaret S. Stroebe
Department of Clinical & Health
Psychology
Utrecht University
Utrecht, The Netherlands

Shelley E. Taylor
Department of Psychology
University of California, Los Angeles
Los Angeles, CA

Howard Tennen
University of Connecticut Health Center
Farmington, CT

Michele M. Tugade
Department of Psychology
Vassar College
Poughkeepsie, NY

Carsten Wrosch
Department of Psychology
Concordia University
Montreal, Quebec

Alex J. Zautra
Department of Psychology
Arizona State University
Tempe, AZ

Melanie J. Zimmer-Gembeck
School of Psychology
Griffith University
Southport, Australia

CONTENTS

PART 1

Overview and Introduction

Stress, Health, and Coping: An Overview

Susan Folkman

Abstract

New technologies, new multidisciplinary approaches, scientific curiosity, and popular demand have all contributed to the growth in the stress, coping, and health research enterprise over the past 30 years. Much of this research originally focused on establishing that stress was in fact harmful to mental and physical health. As these harmful effects became evident, interest grew in coping processes that could mitigate them. Then, in the 1990s, a number of factors converged to generate interest in resilience and well-being in the face of stress. The scope of coping expanded accordingly, and new forms of coping that generated and sustained resilience and well-being were identified and explored. The chapters in this volume are written by leaders in the field who offer authoritative reviews and provocative critiques of where the field is now and exciting previews of new directions in which stress and coping research is headed.

Keywords: Stress, coping, resilience, new directions

The research literature on psychological stress, coping, and health is impressive in its breadth, depth, and complexity. Scientists are exploring the causes and manifestations of stress at every level of analysis, from the micro levels of the genome and cell to the macro levels of culture and society. The continuous and rapid development of new technologies and the concurrent emergence of new multidisciplinary fields of inquiry open the way to new theoretical models, new hypotheses, and new discoveries.

And there is a ready market for these new research findings: a public that has an insatiable appetite for information and advice about how to cope with the stress that pervades daily life. A Google search showed approximately 1.4 million entries for "self-help books on coping." A similar search at Amazon. com showed approximately 2,100 book titles.

Although these self-help books, as well as magazine articles, DVDs, blogs, and other media, are all well intended, many are simplistic and uninformed by science.

Background

Two central themes characterize much of the research literature on psychological stress: (a) the wear and tear of stress on mental and physical health and (b) well-being and resilience in the face of stress. The first theme dominated the field for about 30 years, beginning with the publication of Richard Lazarus' seminal book *Psychological Stress and the Coping Process* (Lazarus, 1966). Research during those years produced substantial evidence of undesirable outcomes associated with stress. The stress of bereavement, for example, was shown to be associated with documented increases in morbidity and mortality (Stroebe & Stroebe, 1987); the stress of caregiving was shown to be associated with deleterious effects on immune functioning (Kiecolt-Glaser et al., 1987); and anger and hostility, emotions often experienced in stressful situations, were shown to have harmful effects on the cardiovascular system (Booth-Kewley & Friedman, 1987). More recently, as several chapters in this volume attest, attention has turned to the genetic, biological, psychological, and social mediating pathways through which stressful life circumstances take their toll on mental, social, and physical functioning.

Interest in how to mitigate the harmful effects of stress, otherwise known as coping, followed quickly. Questions initially dealt with how to conceptualize coping (Coelho, Hamburg, & Adams, 1974). It was viewed as a mature defense mechanism (Vaillant, 1977), as a stable aspect of personality (Miller, 1987), and as a dynamic process shaped by situational demands and the person's resources for coping (Folkman & Lazarus, 1980). Regardless of how coping was conceptualized, these earlier approaches shared a concern with the regulation of negative emotions and distress. The study of well-being and resilience in the face of stress during this period was confined largely to the literature on children (e.g., Murphy, 1974).

The picture changed in the 1990s when a dramatic increase of interest in stress-related resilience signaled a new phase of exploration across the social and behavioral sciences (Bonnano, 2009). Processes that contribute to the maintenance of well-being during stressful situations as well as processes that contribute to recovery in the aftermath became popular topics at conferences and in journals. Ideas came from the emerging area of positive psychology (Seligman & Csikszentmihalyi, 2000), growing recognition of the human capacity to find benefit (Affleck & Tennen, 1996) and grow in the face of stress (Tedeschi, Park, & Calhoun, 1998), and heightened awareness of the benefits of positive emotions (Fredrickson, 1998) and their role in the stress process (Folkman, 1997). As will be evident in the chapters that follow, our understanding of stress and coping processes is broadened significantly by addressing both themes.

Organization
This volume is organized in six sections: developmental perspectives on stress and coping; social aspects of stress and coping; models of stress, coping, and positive and negative outcomes; coping processes and positive and negative outcomes; assessing coping; new technologies and concepts; and coping

interventions. The titles of the sections suggest distinct content, but as will be evident, the discussions in each chapter often cross content areas. The final chapter synthesizes the discussion, offers comments, and suggests directions for future research.

Developmental perspectives on stress and coping
Stress is experienced at every age, and at every age individuals try to cope with it. Developmental perspectives are essential for understanding how stress and coping processes change from childhood through old age.

Carolyn Aldwin (Chapter 2) views stress and coping processes in terms of trajectories over the life span. Aldwin has three goals in her chapter: to examine how stress processes change over the lifespan, how coping processes change, and whether vulnerability to stress varies systematically at different life stages. She points out that stress, coping, and health reflect life-long processes that develop or change through all phases of life as a result of biological factors, individuals' behaviors, and sociocontextual influences. Aldwin's review addresses interesting questions concerning changes in the content and frequency of three categories of stressors—traumas, major life events, and hassles—from early childhood through older ages. These changes, Aldwin argues, reflect the sociocultural and socioenvironmental circumstances of the individual's life. In contrast to changes in stressors, Aldwin believes that changes in coping have to do with changes in the individual's own skills and capacity for learning. Aldwin also provides an overview of the history of stress and coping theory and measurement that serves as a good framework for the chapters in this volume.

Ellen Skinner and *Melanie Zimmer-Gembeck* (Chapter 3) focus on the concept of perceived control. Low perceived control is associated with vulnerability and helpless ways of coping at every age. Young children with low perceived control show less persistence, focus, and concentration on difficult tasks, try out less sophisticated hypothesis testing strategies, and stop working on the tasks as soon as possible and select easier future tasks. Children high in perceived control, in contrast, are oriented towards mastery of difficult tasks, which Skinner and Zimmer-Gembeck refer to as mastery-oriented coping. Skinner and Zimmer-Gembeck discuss how mastery-oriented and helpless ways of coping may change in their form across infancy, childhood, adolescence, adulthood, and old age; how the development of perceived control may contribute to qualitative shifts in how coping is organized as people age; and how coping itself may constitute a proximal process that shapes the development of perceived control. The authors use a multilevel approach and highlight the importance of social contexts, relationships, and partners in shaping both coping and perceived control.

Skinner and Zimmer-Gembeck distinguish three types of control: *regulatory beliefs* that guide actions, including coping; *strategy beliefs*, or generalized expectancies about the effectiveness of certain causes (such as effort, ability, powerful others, luck); and *capacity beliefs*, or generalized expectancies about the extent to which the self possesses or has access to potentially effective causes. The authors discuss the development of these beliefs from childhood to young adulthood. In the final section of their chapter, Skinner and Zimmer-Gembeck discuss the reciprocal relationship between perceived control and coping, noting that the ways people cope "is the grist from which perceptions of control are shaped."

Social aspects of stress and coping

The individual who experiences stress and engages in coping does so within a complex social context. At the macro level, societal factors influence the stress process—for example, by affecting stress exposure or social expectations regarding male and female coping behavior; these gender differences can further be influenced by biology. At the micro level, stress is often interpersonal in its origin, and the subsequent coping processes between or among the involved parties are intricate and highly dynamic.

Vicki Helgeson (Chapter 4) asks a fundamental question: Do the harmful effects of stress differ for men and women, and if so, in what ways? She begins by exploring the sources of observed sex differences in stress, including gender differences in exposure to various types of stressors, differences in gender roles, and gender differences in the encoding and recall of stressful events. Helgeson moves on to explore gender differences in health outcomes and whether they are associated with gender differences in stress exposure or gender differences in vulnerability; she then shifts to gender differences in coping and its relationship to health. The review indicates a number of gender differences in coping, with an overall difference being that women generally report doing more of most types of coping. Helgeson highlights a challenging conundrum, namely that sex differences in coping are inherently confounded with other variables such as status, gender roles, and social

roles, and that these variables also affect the relationship between coping and health.

Shelley Taylor (Chapter 5) explores affiliative responses to threat, which Taylor and her colleagues refer to as Tend and Befriend theory. At the heart of this theory is the assumption of a biological signaling system that is activated when the individual's affiliations fall below an adequate level, a condition that can occur in response to stress.

An appealing characteristic of the Tend and Befriend thesis is its relevance at multiple levels of analysis. For example, affiliating with others serves to calibrate the biological stress systems that regulate responses to stress across the lifespan. It also affects the regulation of the stress response on an acute basis, and serves several practical functions with respect to stress. Taylor discusses the role of brain opioids, including oxytocin and endogenous opioids peptides, in the mitigation of separation distress. Taylor also explores possible genetic pathways that are just now being identified. Taylor returns to the social support literature and uses Tend and Befriend theory to explain the seemingly contradictory finding that having a strong social network appears to be beneficial, whereas actual support transactions are often not. She suggests the interesting hypothesis that the beneficial effects of social networks may be "a basic biopsychosocial process that depends heavily on proximity and/or awareness of others' availability more than on the explicit social support transactions that have been so widely studied."

Tracey Revenson and *Anita DeLongis* (Chapter 6) tackle the complex topic of dyadic coping, highlighting both societal influences and interpersonal processes. They have chosen to examine the chronic physical illness of one partner in order to understand couples coping processes more generally. Revenson and DeLongis state that dyadic coping recognizes mutuality and interdependence in coping responses to a specific shared stressor, such that couples respond to stressors as interpersonal units rather than as individuals in isolation. They review theoretical frameworks of dyadic coping, setting them in their historical context within individual stress and coping models. They turn to the empirical literature on couples coping with illness to examine which models have been supported and where there are gaps. Central to all frameworks is the influence of gender and social role on couples coping. The authors also discuss "relationship-focused coping," cognitive and behavioral efforts to manage and sustain social relationships during stressful episodes.

"Maintaining relatedness with others," argue Revenson and DeLongis, "is a fundamental human need, as fundamental to coping as is emotion or problem management." Relationship-focused coping involves efforts to maintain a balance between self and other, with the goal of maintaining the integrity of the marital relationship above either partner's needs. The chapter concludes with an informative review of the current state of methodology for studying couples coping and challenges for the next generation of research.

Models of stress, coping, and positive and negative outcomes

A fascinating theme in the current literature is how people maintain well-being while they make their way through profoundly stressful situations, coping with intense distress and attending to instrumental demands. Whether early in each chapter's discussion or towards the conclusion, the chapters in this section all call for models that address both aspects of the stress process. The fact that these models are formulated in settings that differ markedly from each other reinforces their relevance to the stress process across settings.

Stevan Hobfoll (Chapter 7) has developed Conservation of Resources (COR) theory, which he describes in this chapter. COR considers both the costs of stress and the processes associated with resilience, described in terms of alternating (and sometimes concurrent) cycles of resource gains and resource losses. *Resources* refer to those things that are universally valued, such as health, well-being, peace, family, self-preservation, and a positive sense of self. Hobfoll places great importance on environmental conditions that foster and protect the resources of individuals, families, and organizations, or that impoverish people's resource reservoirs.

COR theory has been supported in a wide range of studies, including a program of research in Israel on the Al Aqsa Intifada and the effects of terrorism. Hobfoll makes an interesting distinction between *resistance* and *resilience*. A resistance trajectory was defined as having no more than one symptom of depression and no more than one post-traumatic stress (PTS) symptom at either of two time points. A resilience trajectory was defined as having symptoms of depression or PTS at the outset and becoming relatively free of symptoms over the period of study. A sizeable minority of study participants fell in each of these two groups. Hobfoll's discussion of resilience centers on the concept of *engagement*, which is related to discussions of meaning in later

chapters. He and his colleagues found that depression and engagement were not highly related, showing that people can stay committed and involved in life tasks, even in the midst of significant exposure to trauma and stressful environmental conditions. This theme, too, is relevant to discussions in later chapters. Hobfoll also reports finding post-traumatic growth positively correlated with PTS symptoms in several, although not all, studies. Hobfoll's discussion of societal dimensions in relation to these findings is illuminating and provocative.

Margaret Stroebe (Chapter 8) studies bereavement. Stroebe begins by examining bereavement's health consequences, the question of what constitutes adaptive coping, and the links between coping and health. Stroebe's discussion illustrates the importance of critical review. In her discussion of risk factors for morbidity and mortality, she highlights fundamental methodological challenges and quagmires that can lead to erroneous conclusions; she reviews evidence that refutes convictions about desirable responses to bereavement held during the latter part of the 20th century, such as convictions that "grief work," social sharing, emotional disclosure, and the seeking of social support are important for overcoming the impact of bereavement. She also points to evidence that challenges widely held convictions about the detrimental effects of processes such as denial, repression, and avoidance.

Stroebe includes a review of the strengths and weaknesses of theoretical models of bereavement, and concludes with a description of the Dual Process Model (DPM) she developed with her colleague, Henk Schut. The model is organized around two stress and coping themes: "Loss-orientation," which refers to the bereaved person's processing of some aspect of the loss experience itself, and "Restoration-orientation," which refers to the focus on secondary stressors that are also consequences of bereavement. The model allows for full exploration of both past- and future-oriented bereavement-related coping and the processes through which people can address both stress-related harms and the restoration of their well-being. The DPM model has been translated into intervention, and results are promising. Stroebe assigns great importance to coping interventions for bereavement: "even though one cannot change the harrowing reality of the death of a loved one, it is possible to influence the ways that bereaved persons cope with and appraise their loss, and intense suffering can thereby hopefully be lessened." This statement is broadly generalizable, as will be become evident throughout this volume.

Alex Zautra and *John Reich* (Chapter 9) describe a generic model of resilience in the face of stress that takes into account both positive and negative domains of experience. Referring to the recent interest in positive states under conditions of stress, the authors state: "This new paradigm has raised stress and coping approaches into a framework that models the extent to which personal strengths and other psychosocial resources contribute to the prediction of resilience, independent of the catalogue of risks and vulnerabilities identified within the person and his or her social network." Zautra and Reich refer to this as a *resilience model* of well-being. Their model specifies three features of resilience: *recovery* that is swift and thorough; *sustainability* of purpose in the face of adversity; and *growth*, or new learning.

Zautra and Reich argue for the importance of assessing both positive and negative domains of life experience in order to examine the independent effects of positive events over and above the effects of stressful negative events. Zautra and Reich apply the resilience model to organizations and the neighborhood and community, creating a natural complementarity to Hobfoll's perspective.

Michele Tugade (Chapter 10) continues in the dual process mode by distinguishing two distinct though interacting process models of coping. One model focuses on the intersections between positive and negative emotions, and the other model focuses on the interplay between automatic and controlled processes. Both models explore the mechanisms that promote resilience in the midst of short-term and long-term stressors in one's life. Although the issue of automatic versus controlled processes has long been a topic of discussion in the appraisal literature (e.g., Scherer & Ellsworth, 2009), where the issue of the role of subconscious appraisals, or appraisals below the level of awareness, versus appraisals that can be self-reported is often debated, it is not often discussed in relation to coping as Tugade does in this chapter. For example, Tugade points out that positive affect can be activated automatically in the midst of a stressful experience, helping to downregulate the negative experience. She focuses in particular on sensory experiences that can activate positive affect, such as when the feel of warmth from a cup of tea soothes an individual, and interrupt the trajectory of the stressful episode. Tugade reports evidence for the comparative physiological benefits of automatic versus controlled emotion regulation and suggests that with practice, controlled processes can become automatic.

Sonja Lyubomirsky (Chapter 11) concludes this section with a theoretical model of hedonic adaptation that explains the process through which people adapt to the positive as well as negative emotional effects of situations. Lyubomirsky frames her discussion with the Hedonic Adaptation to Positive and Negative Experiences (HAPNE) model developed with her colleague, Ken Sheldon. In the HAPNE model, initial gains in well-being associated with a positive life change or drops in well-being associated with a negative life change erode over time via two separate paths. The first path specifies that the stream of positive or negative emotions resulting from the life change may lessen over time, reverting people's happiness levels back to their baseline. The second path specifies that the stream of positive or negative events resulting from the change may shift people's expectations about the positivity (or negativity) of their lives, such that the individual now takes for granted circumstances that used to produce happiness or is inured to circumstances that used to produce unhappiness.

According to Lyubomirsky, people can control the extent and speed of their hedonic adaptation by developing and practicing relevant skills. Using several "happiness interventions" as illustrations, Lyuobomirsky describes how effortful strategies and practices can instill new ways of thinking and behaving and thereby preserve well-being in the context of stress and trauma, producing potentially lasting increases in well-being in their absence. In an interesting segue to the next section, Lyubomirsky refers to research that shows trying to make sense of a positive event hastens adaptation; the individual can slow down the adaptation process by savoring without trying to explain it. Conversely, it is better to try to make sense out of negative events; it helps cool the negative emotions.

Coping processes and positive and negative outcomes

A logical next step is to learn more about coping processes that sustain well-being and resilience in addition to coping processes that regulate distress. The chapters in this section address both types of coping, but the emphasis is on the more recently defined arena of coping processes that sustain well-being and resilience in the face of stress. Within this arena, meaning-making has emerged as a dominant theme. The discussions review ways of conceptualizing coping in relation to meaning-making.

Crystal Park (Chapter 12) describes meaning in terms of global meaning (what individuals believe and desire) and situational meaning (what is happening in the stressful context). Individuals experience stress when they perceive a discrepancy between the two levels of meaning. The discrepancy motivates individuals to reconcile the discrepancy through coping processes such as modifying the situational meaning through reappraisal processes, social comparisons, goal substitutions, or problem-solving. The meaning-making process should lead to better adjustment to the extent that it produces a satisfactory product, *meaning made.*

Park's review indicates the adjustment of those who try unsuccessfully to make meaning is poor compared with those who are successful in meaning-making and those who do not engage in meaning-making to begin with. However, Park states that more sophisticated research is needed, including better measurement of meaning-related constructs, improved research designs, further specification of the content of global beliefs, interpersonal aspects of meaning-making, and the use of interventions.

Kenneth Pakenham (Chapter 13) provides a comprehensive discussion of benefit-finding and sense-making. Benefit-finding refers to finding benefits in adversity, whereas sense-making involves the development of explanations for adversity. Pakenham's review illustrates the many levels in which each of the meaning-based coping processes must be considered. He begins with theory, moves through measurement, observational research at the individual level, followed by research at social and community levels, and concludes with intervention. Pakenham also reviews theoretical frameworks that have specified roles for benefit-finding and sense-making. The wealth of theories illustrates the many ways in which scholars from diverse perspectives think about these aspects of meaning.

For his own research with multiple sclerosis patients, Pakenham developed theory-based multidimensional scales for sense-making and benefit-finding. While improved measurements appear to resolve certain questions, they also tend to uncover new ones. For example, Pakenham reflects on a question discussed in the literature about how we determine the validity of self-reported benefits: Are they real or are they imagined? These issues notwithstanding, Pakenham provides a highly informative review of the literature on benefit-finding and sense-making and health at the individual level, the interpersonal level, and the community level and in relation interventions.

In his fascinating discussion of religion and coping, *Kenneth Pargament* (Chapter 14) points out that although there are many parallels between the religious and non-religious coping literatures, religious coping has its own special qualities.

Pargament defines religion as "a search for significance in ways related to the sacred," and its role in the stress process is determined by the availability of religion and perceptions that it can offer compelling solutions. Pargament defines these concepts and offers an excellent review of the relevant literatures. Although religion can be involved in every facet of the stress process, it has a particularly powerful role following crises because, Pargament observes, it offers responses to the limits of personal power, or the problem of human insufficiency. But the use of religion for coping does not always lead to improved outcomes. Pargament reviews the conditions under which religion is beneficial and when it is not. The discussion of religious struggle that can ensue when life events challenge or shatter existing beliefs is of special relevance to the whole issue of meaning-making in the face of profound stress. Pargament also includes a section on clinical interventions that integrate spirituality.

Gail Ironson and *Heidemarie Kremer* (Chapter 15) discuss many facets of the coping process within the setting of HIV/AIDS. This setting is of great interest because it represents coping with what is now a chronic, serious illness. They present a Functional Components Approach to stress and coping, which addresses three components of the stress and coping paradigm: the stressor, the self, and the reaction of the self to the stressor. This is followed by a review of the HIV coping literature organized by approach and avoidant coping, cognitive coping, coping styles, social support, and nonspecific stress-reducing activities. In their final section Ironson and Kremer provide an overview of spirituality and coping with HIV in relation to appraisal, coping, physical health, and psychological health, and they also review spiritually oriented coping interventions for people with HIV. They emphasize how spiritual coping gives the individual more options and choices about how to see and deal with stressful situations.

Carsten Wrosch (Chapter 16) focuses on a central aspect of meaning, goals. He notes that "goals are important because they are the building blocks that structure people's lives and imbue life with purpose, both in the short run and on a long-term basis . . . goals motivate adaptive behaviors, direct patterns of life-long development, and contribute to defining a person's identity." But there are times goals cannot be attained, and Wrosch devotes this chapter to the important subject of the self-regulation of unattainable goals.

Wrosch's review of theoretical models on the self-regulation of unattainable goals distinguishes two broad categories of responses: goal engagement processes through which the person continues to invest time and effort in pursuit of a threatened goal, and the exact opposite response—abandoning the threatened goal, managing the emotional consequences of failure, and engaging in other meaningful goals. Overall, the literature shows that goal disengagement and goal reengagement capacities are independent constructs. Goal disengagement capacities are associated with reduced levels of negative aspects of well-being such as negative affect or depressive symptoms, while goal reengagement capacities are more closely associated with positive aspects of subjective well-being such as positive affect or purpose in life. These two processes exemplify the two overarching themes in stress and coping research described earlier: mitigating stress-related harm and sustaining positive well-being.

Lisa Aspinwall (Chapter 17) discusses proactive coping, which refers to anticipating and/or detecting potential stressors and acting in advance either to prevent them altogether or to mute their impact. Proactive coping blends *coping* with *self-regulation*, the processes through which people control, direct, and correct their own actions as they move toward or away from various goals. Aspinwall reviews research in new domains of application for the proactivity concept, such as the management of stigma and discrimination, predictive genetic testing for familial disease, health promotion, and the management of chronic illness. She also describes what is known about those who undertake proactive coping efforts, what determines whether such efforts will be successful and whether and in what ways the potential for proactive coping may differ across different situations. Aspinwall also includes a review of recent developments in the study of future-oriented thinking to help understand whether, how, and with what success proactive coping efforts may be undertaken, as well as the kinds of goals that people seek to manage proactively.

Assessing coping: new technologies and concepts

The coping measures developed during the 1970s and 1980s reflected the diversity of conceptualizations of coping that characterized that period. Vaillant (1977) used qualitative analysis and clinical judgment to evaluate ego processes, with mature

processes defined as coping. Miller (1987) developed a measure of a coping style, monitoring and blunting, that was an aspect of personality. Most of the other new measures approached coping contextually by asking the thoughts and behaviors people used to cope with specific stressful encounters. These measures were multidimensional, the number of dimensions and their content based in part on theory and in part on empirical factor analysis—for example, the COPE (Carver, Scheier, & Weintraub, 1989), the Coping Inventory for Stressful Situations (Endler & Parker, 1990), the Coping Strategies Indicator (Amirkhan, 1990), and the Ways of Coping (Folkman & Lazarus, 1980).

It is probably safe to say that most researchers in the field of stress and coping share a frustration with the vast majority of coping assessment tools that are currently available. The chapters in this section describe advances in assessment that are responses to shortcomings in existing measures. These chapters serve as models for how to develop coping measures that produce interpretable, theoretically relevant data. (See also Pakenham, Chapter 13, for another example.)

Annette Stanton (Chapter 18) observed that many of the earlier measures of emotion-focused coping were seriously flawed because they tended to confound coping with outcomes. Her response was to conceptualize Emotional Approach Coping (EAC), which addressed the confounding problem by focusing on emotion regulation in terms of two dimensions: processing emotion and expressing emotion. Stanton expended great effort in developing a valid and reliable measure of EAC and its two emotion-regulating functions, paying meticulous attention to theoretical relevance and psychometric characteristics.

Stanton used the EAC measure in a number of studies, first testing the direct effects of EAC. She and her colleagues, as well as other researchers, conducted a number of cross-sectional and longitudinal studies that showed beneficial effects of emotion expression in diverse settings. The benefits of emotion processing were less obvious. Stanton then asked about the moderating effects of attributes of the individual and environment, and in a further elaboration of the model, she asked about possible pathways through which EAC might promote positive outcomes. Her chapter thus illustrates the full developmental process, from diagnosis of the weaknesses of available measures, to the careful development and application of a new measure in studies of direct effects, which lead to further elaboration of moderators and mediating pathways of the underlying theoretical model.

Mark Litt, Howard Tennen, and Glenn Affleck (Chapter 19) take on a very different measurement challenge: capturing the dynamic quality of coping. They point out that although coping was initially construed as dynamic and transactional in nature, most models of coping have been unidirectional and have treated coping as a static outcome of the constituent factors. The authors provide an incisive review of diverse approaches to the assessment of coping, distinguishing clearly among methodologies and enumerating their limitations. The review highlights the dearth of attempts to assess the transactional nature of the stress process in which each variable influences the other: appraisal and coping influence outcomes that in turn influence subsequent appraisals and coping. But new technologies for daily and momentary assessment, allied with multilevel statistical techniques, now allow a more detailed understanding of how coping works. The authors describe several promising applications of near-real-time ambulatory assessment and intensive micro-longitudinal study designs, including novel applications in the areas of gene–stress interactions and coping vulnerability and resilience as "behavioral signatures." The authors then move on to discuss the adaptation of intensive measurement of coping to understanding mechanisms of treatment. Drawing on interventions in the contexts of addiction and pain, the authors review studies that test the effects of coping interventions on coping skills and the relationships between coping skills and outcomes. The issues that can be addressed with the methodologies that Litt et al. summarize are at the center of questions about the actual role of coping in the stress process.

Coping interventions

Ultimately, research should lead to clinical interventions that help people manage stress and improve their well-being. The chapters in this section provide examples of theory-based interventions that illustrate the translation from theory and research into practice, and the daunting complexity involved in understanding what transpires during a coping skills intervention and how it affects outcomes.

Judith Tedlie Moskowitz (Chapter 20) offers a comprehensive review of coping interventions that emphasize the regulation of positive affect. The deliberate manipulation through intervention will be key to determining whether positive states actually are protective during periods of stress. This chapter is a valuable resource for researchers who want to pursue this line of inquiry. The substantial array of interventions Moskowitz reviews is evidence of the recent heightened interest in positive states during stress, also reflected in a number of chapters in this volume (e.g., Hobfoll, Chapter 7; Zautra and Reich, Chapter 9; Tugade, Chapter 10; Park, Chapter 12; Pakenham, Chapter 13; Pargament, Chapter 14). Moskowitz discusses single-component and multi-component interventions. Examples of components include positive events and savoring, acts of kindness, positive reappraisal, setting attainable goals, focusing on personal strengths, loving-kindness meditations, forgiveness, and laughter. Moskowitz clarifies issues regarding measurement of affect, with special attention to high- versus low-activation affects, and discusses design issues that need to be addressed in future studies. Overall, it appears that the positive coping interventions do foster well-being and are acceptable to participants.

Michael Antoni (Chapter 21) studies stress, coping, and coping intervention in the context of HIV/AIDS. As noted earlier with respect to the chapter by Ironson and Kremer, stress and coping processes are pertinent throughout the course of HIV disease. For example, the initial transmission of HIV is through behaviors that are often maladaptive responses to stress; stress affects the compromised immune system; stress is caused by treatment side effects; and there is interpersonal stress associated with disclosure of an HIV-positive serostatus. Antoni's group developed CBSM, a 10-week, group-based stress-management program that combines anxiety-reduction techniques with cognitive-behavioral techniques (CBT) to help manage the stress associated with HIV disease. Antoni uses this intervention to examine psychosocial and biobehavioral mechanisms that can explain the effects of stress and coping interventions on health outcomes in persons with HIV. Studies of CBSM, and findings from other CBT-based interventions, show improved mental health outcomes in persons with HIV. Further, participants in CBT-based interventions who show psychological effects also demonstrate changes in endocrine and immunological parameters. Antoni's discussion illustrates the benefits of working with a clinical condition that is well characterized at multiple levels of analysis, and of having a truly interdisciplinary approach to investigating the effects of interventions on diverse pathways through which stress and coping can affect health.

In Chapter 22, I synthesize findings, offer my own opinions, and suggest where researchers might want to focus their attention next.

Conclusion

The chapters in this volume address diverse aspects of the stress process, from antecedents of stress appraisals to the health-related outcomes of coping. The authors are leading researchers in the field, and the perspectives they share are expansive and well informed. The voices of the authors are varied, but the content forms a coherent narrative about stress, health, and coping punctuated with fascinating questions waiting to be addressed.

References

Affleck, G., & Tennen, H. (1996). Construing benefits from adversity: Adaptational significance and dispositional under-pinnings. *Journal of Personality, 64*, 899–922.

Amirkhan, J. H. (1990). A factor analytically derived measure of coping: The coping strategy indicator. *Journal of Personality and Social Psychology, 59*, 1066–74.

Bonnano, G. (2009). *The Other Side of Sadness*. New York: Basic Books.

Booth-Kewley, S., & Friedman, H. S. (1987). Psychological pre-dictors of heart disease: a quantitative review. *Psychological Bulletin, 101*(3), 343–62.

Carver, C. S., Scheier, M. F., & Weintraub, J. K. (1989). Assessing coping strategies: A theoretically based approach. *Journal of Personality and Social Psychology, 56*, 267–83.

Coelho, G. V., Hamburg, D. A., & Adams, J. E. (Eds.). (1974). *Coping and Adaptation*. New York: Basic Books.

Endler, N. S., & Parker, J. D. A. (1990). *Coping Inventory for Stressful Situations*. Toronto: Multi Health Systems.

Folkman, S. (1997). Positive psychological states and coping with severe stress. *Social Science and Medicine, 45*, 1207–21.

Folkman, S., & Lazarus, R. S. (1980). An analysis of coping in a middle-aged community sample. *Journal of Health and Social Behavior, 21*, 219–39.

Fredrickson, B. L. (1998). What good are positive emotions? *Review of General Psychology, 2*, 300–19.

Kiecolt-Glaser, J. K., Glaser, R., Shuttleworth, E. C., Dyer, C. S., Ogrocki, P., & Speicher, C. E. (1987). Chronic stress and immunity in family caregivers of Alzheimer's disease victims. *Psychosomatic Medicine, 49*, 523–35.

Lazarus, R. S. (1966). *Psychological Stress and the Coping Process*. New York: McGraw Hill.

Miller, S. M. (1987). Monitoring and blunting: Validation of a questionnaire to assess styles of information seeking under stress. *Journal of Personality and Social Psychology, 52*, 342–53.

Murphy, L. B. (1974). Coping, vulnerability, and resilience in childhood. In G. V. Coehlo, D. A. Hamburg & J. E. Adams (Eds.), *Coping and Adaption* (pp. 69–100). New York: Basic Books.

Scherer, K. R., & Ellsworth, P. C. (2009). Appraisal theories. In D. Sander & K. R. Scherer (Eds.), *Oxford Companion to Emotion and the Affective Sciences* (pp. 45–49). Oxford: Oxford University Press.

Seligman, M. E. P., & Csikszentmihalyi, M. (2000). Positive psy-chology: An introduction. *American Psychologist, 55*, 5–14.

Stroebe, M., & Stroebe, W. (1987). *Bereavement and Health. The Psychological and Physical Consequences of Partner Loss*. Cambridge, England: Cambridge University Press.

Tedeschi, R. G., Park, C. L., & Calhoun, L. G. (Eds.). (1998). *Posttraumatic Growth*. Mahwah, NJ: Lawrence Erlbaum.

Vaillant, G. E. (1977). *Adaptation to life*. Boston: Little, Brown.

PART 2

Developmental Perspectives on Stress and Coping

Stress and Coping across the Lifespan

Carolyn Aldwin

Abstract

Examination of stress and coping across the lifespan clearly reflects the principles of lifespan development. Stress and coping processes change across the lifespan, require a multidisciplinary perspective to understand that change, are affected by the social context, and demonstrate individual differences in trajectories of change. How stress changes across the lifespan depends upon how stress is defined. For example, stress defined in terms of traumas largely reflects the sociohistorical context, while stress defined in terms of life events and hassles reflects an individual's life stage and social roles. In contrast, coping follows a more developmental progression, especially in childhood. Problem-focused coping in early childhood depends upon the neurological development underlying executive function, and increases in specificity and effectiveness increase with age. Very young children rely primarily on their parents for emotion regulation, and gradually increase their ability to use cognitive strategies and become independent regulators. The developmental progress in adulthood is less clear, but there is some evidence to suggest that older adults use more nuanced coping strategies and may be better at emotion regulation than young or middle-aged adults, especially in interpersonal situations.

Keywords: stress, coping, development, social factors, individual differences, emotion

In the past few decades, the field of stress and coping has seen remarkable growth. In 2007, there were over 186,000 studies of stress and 36,000 studies of coping (Aldwin, 2007). This deluge of scientific research has transformed the way in which we view our health, our understanding of the adaptive abilities not only of humans and animals, but also of plants and microbes, and even how various societal institutions are structured. More importantly, the field has emphasized the importance of the transactional nature of adaptation—that any given outcome is a function not only of the interaction between the person and the environment, but the transaction between the two—that environments influence individuals, but individuals also influence environments (cf., Lazarus & Folkman, 1984). Thus, change, and even development, is at the heart of all stress and coping processes.

This perspective is at marked variance with early, homeostatic ideas of adaptation—that stress resulted in the perturbation of psychological and physical states, and that the purpose of coping was to restore homeostasis (Lazarus, 1966). While this may be true in limited situations, from a developmental perspective, the process of coping generally results in change, whether minor or major, which can be either negative, positive, or, more often, some combination of the two (Aldwin, Sutton, & Lachman, 1996).

For example, encountering stressors may result in an increased sense of vulnerability, changes in coping resources, or changes in values, mastery, relationships with others, and so on. (For a review of the positive aspects of stress and aging, see Park, Mills-Baxter, & Fenster, 2007.)

Spiro (2007) applied a lifespan developmental perspective to health psychology. Originating in adult development and aging (Baltes, 1987; Baltes, Lindenberger, & Staudinger, 2006), this approach is gaining wider acceptance in health-related fields (Kuh & Ben-Shlomo, 2004) and has four key propositions, which are also applicable to the stress and coping process. First, stress, coping, and health reflect *life-long processes* that begin before birth in the intrauterine environment (Barker, 1990) and develop or change through all phases of life as a result of biological factors, individuals' actions, and contextual influences. Second, a *multidisciplinary perspective* is required to understand the development of stress, coping, and health throughout the lifespan, reflecting the various influences on the process, ranging from the cellular (e.g., stress effects at the cellular level), through the organismic (e.g., the hypothalamic-pituitary-adrenal [HPA] axis) and personal (e.g., personality, values, and developmental history) and sociocultural levels (e.g., role constraints, historical circumstances). The latter is especially important because all too often studies of stress and coping are cross-sectional assessments taken only at one time period, and any age differences are imputed to developmental processes when in fact they may be due to cohort (birth year) or period (time of measurement) effects. As we shall see, much stress exposure reflects sociocultural exigencies rather than aging *per se*.

The third proposition emphasizes that *stress, coping, and health* processes reflect current contextual factors, such as socioeconomic status (SES) (e.g., Adler & Snibbe, 2003), or the results of living in impoverished neighborhoods (Evans, 2004). The fourth proposition of the lifespan developmental approach emphasizes individual differences in trajectories across the lifespan, as well as plasticity in developmental processes. Thus, the stress and coping process is plastic and is modulated by a variety of factors, including personal decisions as to how to cope with stress and/or whether or not to expend coping resources. Although there may be normative changes in the stress and coping process with age, there are undoubtedly individual differences in that process.

A developmental perspective addresses not only individual change, but also whether and how social contexts change in a systematic way over the lifespan (Elder & Shanahan, 2006; Ford & Lerner, 1992). In other words, there may be normative changes in the types of stressors that individuals face over the lifespan and/or age-related changes in the impact of stress, as well as cohort-specific stressors, such as wars, famine, and natural disasters.

This chapter will be divided into three major sections: how stress processes change over the lifespan, how coping processes change, and whether vulnerability to stress varies systematically at different life stages. We will argue that stress processes primarily reflect systematic change in the social context across the life course, including factors such as SES, although personality characteristics such as neuroticism also contribute to stress exposure and appraisals. Coping processes also reflect social contexts and are influenced by personal characteristics such as goals in the situation (Carver & Scheier, 1998; Folkman & Moskowitz, 2004; Wrosch, 2011), and sometimes overarching, long-term goals (Park, 2010). However, coping may be more influenced by developmental processes, including increases in coping sophistication and changes in appraisal processes (Boeninger, Shiraishi, Aldwin, & Spiro, 2009). Further, vulnerability to stress must be understood in term of not only the underlying physiology of stress, but also the appraisal and coping strategies that individuals use to protect themselves against vulnerability, especially later in life. Finally, a major purpose of this chapter is to identify gaps in our knowledge, with an eye towards future research.

Stress Across the Lifespan

In order to understand how stress changes across the lifespan, it is first necessary to understand the myriad ways in which stress has been defined and assessed. Thus, this section will first briefly review definitions and types of stress, then examine the types of stressors faced by children and adolescents, and then adults at different life stages.

Definitions of stress

The classical view of stress identified three types of definitions: environmental stress, or stressors; individual stress, or a state of the organism; and stress as resulting from a transaction between the individual and the environment (Mason, 1976). This tripartite definition neatly presaged ensuing decades of debate as to whether stress was largely a function of the subjective personality characteristics, such as neuroticism (McCrae, 1982) or should be perceived as an objective characteristic of the environment

(Dohrenwend, Dohrenwend, Dodson, & Shrout 1984), or if the appraisal of stress resulted from the interaction or transaction between the individual and the environment (Lazarus & Folkman, 1984). This transactional model is currently dominant—namely, that there are individual differences in appraisals of stress that nonetheless reflect environmental contingencies (see Aldwin, 2007, for an explication of these arguments). Thus, appraisals of stress arise when environmental demands exceed the individual's resources, especially in situations that are personally significant (Lazarus & Folkman, 1984).

There are four general types of stress appraisals: a situation may be benign, or it may involve threats of futures stressors, harm or loss, and challenges (Lazarus & Folkman, 1984). Appraisals are important because they are thought to determine how an individual chooses to cope with the stressors, although individuals typically use multiple appraisals (Aldwin, Sutton, Chiara, & Spiro, 1996; Boeninger et al., 2009). Coping with stress is a process that unfolds over time; thus, individuals may alter their initial appraisals of how stressful a situation is based upon an assessment of available coping resources, called secondary appraisal. Secondary appraisals are often cast in terms of controllability or stressfulness of the situation. Some have even begun examining tertiary appraisals, which often occur long after a situation has ended and may involve long-term appraisals of the impact and meaning of the situation (Stanton, Bower, & Low, 2006). For example, individuals in the throes of coping with a life-threatening illness such as cancer often appraise this as an extremely stressful experience with few positive aspects. In remission, however, an individual may be able to look back and identify positive sequelae from this experience, such as clearer values, better relationships with family and friends, and perhaps increased spirituality. This process has been variously called post-traumatic growth (Tedeschi & Calhoun, 2006), stress-related growth (Park, 2011; Park, Cohen, & Murch, 1996) or benefit finding (Pakenham, 2011).

Appraisals are not necessarily a product of conscious, rational processes, but may occur at an unconscious, largely automatic level (Lazarus, 1991; Smith & Kirby, 2004). Nonetheless, they can be reported on after their emergence.

Aldwin et al. (1996) found that the four original appraisals were not always applicable to respondent-identified stressful situations, and added three more categories: hassle (not necessarily a threat, harm, or loss, but just an annoyance), at a loss for what to do next (typically used in situations with great uncertainty), and worry about others—that is, the individual may not be in any difficulty but is concerned over the problems of a friend or family member.

Scherer and Brosch (2009) argued that a more general approach to appraisal should be taken. They posit that there are a number of dimensions on which appraisal can occur, including novelty, agreeable/disagreeable, certainty, predictability, goal conduciveness, agency, controllability, and whether a situation is compatible with internal and/or external standards. To some extent, some of these dimensions are reflective of primary appraisal (agreeable/disagreeable) and others with secondary appraisal (certainty, agency, controllability), yet others, such as goal conduciveness and compatibility with standards, may provide additional insight into why individuals find some situations stressful. Certainly, violation of social norms and expectations can elicit surprising amounts of anger and anxiety, even though there is no clear immediate threat or harm to the individual (e.g., some heterosexuals' reaction to gay marriage).

As will be explored in the section on age and stress vulnerability, appraisals may be the key to understanding the stress, coping, and adaptation process. However, appraisal receives surprisingly little systematic study in the stress and coping literature, and more work is certainly warranted into both the types of appraisals that are relevant to stressful situations and their impact on the adaptive process.

Types of stress

Stress can be further explicated in terms of its severity and duration, reflected in the variety of ways in which stress is measured. Trauma refers to severe stressors that involve the threat of or witnessing deaths or severe bodily injury. In traumatic situations, there may be relatively little or no warning of an impending catastrophe. Traumas can occur within a relatively short period of time, often afford little or no chance of individual control, and may happen to many people simultaneously. Examples of these are natural disasters such as tornadoes or earthquakes; technological disasters such as the Buffalo Creek flood or Chernobyl; and combat and civilian involvement in wars. Wars, especially those of very long duration, tend to have the most widespread results in a population. For example, nearly half of Afghan women show signs of posttraumatic stress disorder, reflecting the devastating effects of over 30 years of nearly constant warfare (Physicians for Human Rights, 1998, http://www.phrusa.org/research/health_effects/exec.html).

Nonetheless, there are also individual traumas such as rape or car accidents. Indeed, Norris-Baker (1992) showed that the most common source of trauma among American adults is car accidents.

Life events are most commonly studied and are generally defined as major events that occur to individuals, such as bereavement, divorce, or job loss. While early views held that any change in the environment, whether positive or negative, was stressful (Holmes & Rahe, 1967), most researchers now recognize that it is primarily negative events that are associated with poor health outcomes (Zautra, 2003).

Chronic stress is generally defined as "an ongoing problem located in the structure of the social environment" (Wheaton, 1996, p. 57), but can also include individual stressors such as chronic illness. These involve several characteristics, including threats of the possibility of harm; long-term, unresolved conflicts; long-term uncertainty; multiple, uncontrollable demands and complexity; underrewards; and structural constraints such as resource deprivation and restriction of choice. Classic examples are poverty, abusive family situations, poor working conditions, and other chronic role strains (Pearlin & Schooler, 1978).

A related construct is daily stressors, or "hassles." These may be minor and of relatively short duration, such as traffic jams or arguments with friends and family, but may also reflect chronic problems, such as ongoing family problems (Conger & Conger, 2002), or living in an impoverished environment (Evans, 2004).

Daily stressors are often assessed at the end of the day using a self-report checklist (e.g., DeLongis, Folkman, & Lazarus, 1988); newer, telephone-based interview schedules have been developed, such as the Daily Inventory of Stressful Events (DISE; Almeida, Wethington, & Kessler, 2002). These types of inventories allow for a closer and theoretically more precise view of stressors. While more commonly used with adult populations, daily stressor inventories are sometimes used with pediatric patients (Walker, Smith, Garber, & Claar, 2007). Others have argued for even more precise measures of daily stressors using Ecological Momentary Assessment (EMA) techniques, which involve current, real-time assessments of everyday experience (for a review see Litt et al., 2011; Shiffman, Stone, & Hufford, 2008). In these types of studies, respondents are provided with a pager or PDA that beeps them at either predetermined or random time points during the day and asks them to fill out simple and usually very brief questionnaires, which can then be transmitted directly to servers and/or downloaded at a later time.

There are positive and negatives with all of these types of stress measurement, involving problems of reliability and validity. Monroe (2008) identified three types of problems in this regard. First, life event measures typically ask for events that occurred over the past year or 18 months, and some have thought that more immediate measures, such as daily stressors, may be more accurate. However, memory for severe stressors is more accurate than that for minor ones. Second, respondents may have a very different interpretation of what a stressful life event means. The same type of event can refer to problems ranging from the trivial to the highly significant, but the outcome of the event may affect whether or not the individual interprets it as stressful. Monroe provides an example of a woman who did not report her husband's heart attack as a stressful health event, because he quit smoking and his health improved. Third, individuals may over- or underreport events, depending upon their interpretation of the purpose of the research.

Which type of stress measure is appropriate depends upon the research question and health outcomes (Aldwin, 2007). More immediate measures such as ECA may be better for assessing very variable health outcomes such as blood pressure or nor adrenaline. However, it is unlikely that a daily stressor by itself is of sufficient magnitude to affect long-term health outcomes, and measures of life events and especially trauma may be more relevant for studies of morbidity and mortality.

Given that stressors often extend across time and social roles (Pearlin, Aneshensel, Mullan, & Whitlatch, 1996), it is unlikely that the occurrences of different types of stressors are orthogonal; rather, they are often linked. Traumas can result in life events, such as divorce or job loss, while life events and ongoing chronic stress may evoke hassles. Nonetheless, these types of stressors, although related, can contribute independent variance to outcomes such as psychological symptoms (Aldwin, Levenson, Spiro, & Bossé, 1989). Thus, they should be viewed as assessing different aspects of the stress experience.

Stress in childhood and adolescence

There is a fairly large literature on stress in children and adolescence. A major focus has been trauma, including child abuse, sexual abuse, domestic violence, and war. Clearly, trauma can have lifelong negative effects on psychological symptoms and physical health (Kendall-Tackett, 2002). There is even some evidence that trauma in children may result in life-long changes in brain structure and function, including hyperreactivity of the HPA axis, mediated via the hippocampus (Jackowski et al., 2009). However, as Finkelhor, Omrod, and Turner (2009a) pointed out, much of this literature is fragmented, and there are relatively few attempts to examine systematic age differences in trauma exposure.

Finkelhor et al. (2009a, 2009b) conducted national surveys of victimization among children and adolescents aged 2 to 17, which included problems such as physical abuse, peer bullying, property crime, and exposure to domestic violence. (For very young children, either parents or caregivers completed the forms.) Surprisingly, 71% to 80% of the samples reported at least one incidence of victimization, although clearly not all of these types of incidents necessarily met the definition of trauma *per se*. Earlier surveys (Finkelhor, Ormrod, Turner, & Hamby, 2005) found that 12% of children experienced abuse, neglect, bullying, or abduction by a caretaker, while 8% experienced sexual victimization. Shockingly, more than a third of children witnessed violence either directly or indirectly (e.g., the murder of a parent).

Finkelhor et al. (2009a, 2009b) found that there were cumulative increases in child victimization with age, which is not surprising. The rates of victimization in past year also increased with age, with adolescents reporting higher levels of victimization than younger children. Further, the mean number of victimizations increased with age, suggesting that older children experience more trauma than do younger ones.

However, the developmental epidemiology of different types of events may not show a linear relationship with age. For example, some studies suggest that bullying is more frequent among middle-schoolers than among high-schoolers (Nansel et al., 2001), while young children may more often be witnesses of domestic abuse than older children (Fantuzzo, Boruch, Beriama, Atkins, & Marcus, 1997). Finkelhor et al. (2009b) found that bullying and chronic victimization were highest in middle childhood but decreased in adolescence, while injuries tended to increase in adolescence, as did sexual abuse, especially for girls. There were also sex differences in child abuse, which increased rapidly for young boys in middle childhood but increased dramatically for girls in adolescence.

Life events may also vary by age. An early study by Coddington (1972) examined events in a sample ranging in age from preschool through high school, examining both the frequency of events (both negative and positive) and their stressfulness, characterized in terms of life change units. Again, parents or caretakers filled out the questionnaires for very young children. Although this was an older scale, Williamson et al. (2003) recently provided strong evidence for its validity and reliability.

For preschoolers, the most frequent life events were entering nursery school and increases in arguments with parents. For elementary school children, the most frequent events were beginning a new school year and an outstanding personal achievement. For junior high school students, the most frequent events were an outstanding personal achievement and breaking up with a girlfriend or boyfriend, while beginning to date and arguments with parents were most frequent for high school students. The content of the forms changed by age, with peer problems emerging in elementary school, problems with drugs or alcohol in middle school, and pregnancy in high school. The most interesting finding from this study was that life events increased slightly from preschool through elementary school, but increased sharply at age 12, peaking around age 15, and declining slightly thereafter. This is very similar to Moffitt's (1993) findings concerning the trajectory of antisocial behavior in youths.

A handful of studies have begun to assess daily stressors (Walker et al., 2007) and ECA of stress in children (Axelson et al., 2003; Helgeson, Lopez, & Karmack, 2009; Simonich et al., 2004). For the most part, these were clinical studies and little or no information on age was provided. One exception was a study by Hema et al. (2007), which examined daily stressors for diabetic children. Younger children reported problems with siblings and peers, while adolescents reported problems with their self, parents, and school. Interestingly, diabetes was not seen as a daily stressor in these children.

The developmental epidemiology of stress is limited in its necessary reliance on parents and caretakers for the reporting of stress in very young children. Both the nature and type of stress change with age in childhood, especially with trauma and life events. Overall, both trauma and life events increase, although the specific type of event and its age trajectory may vary. Thus, it is likely that developmental change in stress exposure varies as a function of the social context for children; the older the child, the greater the exposure to a wider range of social situations, and thus the greater likelihood of exposure to stress. Nonetheless, changes in the social context also influence the types of stressors that children face, with very young children more exposed to domestic violence and those in middle childhood more exposed to bullying (Finkelhor et al., 2009a).

Stress in adulthood

TRAUMA

As Creamer and Parslow (2008) pointed out, there are relatively few studies of trauma exposure in the elderly. Further, most of the extant studies examine cross-sectional data (Norris & Slone, 2007). Nevertheless, there appear to be cohort differences in the prevalence of lifetime trauma. For example, an early study by Norris (1992) showed that younger adults were most likely to report having experienced a traumatic event, including physical and sexual assault, and tragic death. Middle-aged adults were more likely to report other traumas, while the oldest cohort was most likely to report combat exposure. However, the overall rate of trauma exposure was highest in younger adults and lowest in older ones.

Cross-national studies reinforce the suggestion of cohort differences in trauma exposure by age. A comparison of U.S., Mexican, and Polish samples revealed that U.S. elders reported lower trauma levels than young or middle-aged adults, Mexican younger adults reported higher trauma levels than middle-aged or older adults, while no age differences emerged in the Polish sample (Norris, Kaniasty, Conrad, Inman, & Murphy, 2002). In contrast, an Australian study found that middle-aged adults had the highest lifetime exposure to trauma (Creamer & Parslow, 2008). However, there were gender differences. Older women reported lower lifetime rates of trauma exposure, while older men sometimes had higher levels, especially vis-à-vis combat exposure. This reflects earlier observations that combat exposure may be a "hidden variable" in the study of aging (Spiro, Schnurr, & Aldwin, 1994). A life course perspective that takes into account the socio-historical context and an individual's place in it (Elder & Shanahan, 2006) needs to be utilized in studies of trauma exposure.

LIFE EVENTS

Relatively few longitudinal studies have examined age-related changes in the number and type of stressful life events. Early cross-sectional, correlational studies suggested that the number of life events is negatively associated with age, despite the widespread perception that late life is a very stressful time (for reviews see Aldwin, 1990, 1991). However, standard life events inventories are weighted toward events that are more likely to happen to younger individuals, such as graduations, marriages, divorces, beginning new jobs, and having children. Aldwin (1990) developed an inventory, the Elders' Life Stress Inventory (ELSI), specifically designed to tap the types of life events that are more likely to occur to middle-aged and older people, such as death of a parent, divorce of a child, institutionalization of a spouse, and the like. There was no significant correlation with age in a sample ranging from mid-life through late life, although health-related life events did tend to show increased frequency in late life (Aldwin, 1991).

Chiriboga (1997) analyzed data from the San Francisco Transitions Study, a multi-cohort study that followed individuals for 12 years. In preliminary cross-sectional analyses, he found that individuals in mid-life and late life reported similar numbers of life events, but that young adults reported more negative and positive life events, reflecting the acquisition of new roles in their transition to adulthood, such as getting married, having children, graduating, and beginning jobs, as well as being laid off. If the cross-sectional data reflected true age differences, longitudinal analyses should show declines in the reporting of life events with age. However, Chiriboga found that the differences in life event reporting between the cohorts were maintained, suggesting cohort effects, while the number of events fluctuated over time, suggestive of period effects. For example, during economic downturns, individuals may well report an increased incidence of job loss and other forms of economic stress (see Aldwin & Revenson, 1986).

Other longitudinal studies have found more mixed results. In a six-year longitudinal study using the ELSI, Yancura, Aldwin, and Spiro (2000) found a non-linear change over time, with the number of self-reported life events increasing until about age 65, and then decreasing into later life. Ensel and Lin (1996, 2000) had a longer-term (15-year) study, but the 12-year gap between the last two assessments precluded examination of age-related trajectories. Using a life history technique, they did find that distal events had effects on both physical and mental health that weakened over time, especially in older groups, but that distal events also had indirect effects through increasing the number of proximal events. Thus, life events may not be independent episodes, but may alter the frequency of experiencing later events.

A few studies have examined growth curve models of stress in adulthood (George & Lynch, 2003; Lorenz et al., 1997; Lynch & George, 2002). The results were highly varied, depending upon age of the respondents, type of stressor, and the social context. For example, Lorenz et al. found that married women in their thirties showed very little change in stress over a three-year period. In contrast, recently divorced women reported higher levels of stress, which decreased during the ensuing three years. However, divorced women with antisocial behavior showed much less decrease in stress—that is, their stress levels remained high. In contrast, individuals in later life showed increases in loss-related events, especially African Americans (George & Lynch, 2003; Lynch & George, 2002).

Old age is typically characterized as a time of loss, but it is not clear that the incidence of loss necessarily changes with age. For example, older adults often experience the loss of parents, siblings, and friends, but for every adult child who loses a parent, there is often a grandchild who has lost a grandparent. Walter and McCoyd (2009) reviewed studies of grief and loss across the lifespan. They showed that losses occur at every age, and indeed are necessarily part of transitions. For example, a toddler may gain a sibling with the birth of another child in the family, but experiences the loss of caretaker time as the parents of necessity focus more on the infant. Young adults experiencing infertility may experience a profound sense of loss. Walter and McCoyd differentiated between losses due to bereavement and maturational losses, reflecting changes in role expectations and transitions. Older adults may experience more losses due to bereavement of friends and family, but loss *per se* is distributed across the lifespan.

In summary, the type of stressors varies by age and clearly reflects situational demands and life stage. However, the incidence of life events in general may not change very much across the lifespan, except perhaps for a decrease in very late life.

DAILY STRESSORS

This type of stress shows clearer developmental patterns with age (and life stage), and nearly all studies show decreases in most types of daily stressors with age, with the exception of health-related hassles (Aldwin et al., 1996a; Chiriboga, 1997). Stawski, Sliwinski, Almeida, and Smith (2007) contrasted daily stressors among college students with those in a older community sample and also found age-related declines in daily stressors, primarily interpersonal stressors (see also Birditt, Fingerman, & Almeida,

2005). Interestingly, there were no differences in health-related daily stressors. In a national probability sample, Mroczek and Almeida (2004) also found that hassles decreased with age, while Almeida and Horn (2004) also found that adults over the age of 60 reported fewer daily stressors than middle-aged or younger adults. This pattern continues in very late life: an early study by Zautra, Finch, Reich, and Guarnaccia (1991) found age-related declines in "minor life events" assessed on a monthly basis among 60- to 80-year-olds.

Given the difficulties in late life, and the fact that older adults generally report as many life events as do younger adults, it is surprising that hassles decrease. It is likely that this reflects decreases in the number of social roles in late life—that is, retired adults no longer have work roles, and most adults in late life no longer have active parenting roles. Most (but not all) studies find increases in health-related daily stressors. However, the decrease in reported hassles may also reflect changes in coping in later life.

Coping

Coping shows a developmental sequence in childhood, but the developmental change in adulthood is not nearly as clear. Thus, we will address changes in childhood, followed by a discussion of the controversies surrounding coping in adulthood. However, we will first provide a brief primer on basic coping theory and types.

Brief primer on coping

Coping has its roots in several different theoretical traditions. The original psychodynamic approach focused on defense mechanisms, as delineated by Anna Freud (1966), defined as the largely unconscious means by which the ego warded off the anxiety generated by conflicts between the superego and the id. By definition, defense mechanisms distort reality—for example, by denying the existence of problems, projecting them onto others, or transforming them through displacement or reaction formation—and thus are inherently pathological. Vaillant (1977) proposed a hierarchy of defense mechanisms that varied in their degree of pathology, ranging from projective mechanisms such as denial, distortion, and delusional projection, to immature mechanisms, such as projection of passive-aggressive behaviors, through neurotic mechanisms such as repression and intellectualization, to mature mechanisms such as sublimation or altruism.

The extent to which coping is conscious and voluntary versus unconscious and involuntary is still a matter of debate in current coping theory. Lazarus and Folkman (1984) focused on conscious processes, but Compas et al. (1996) pointed out that many coping responses, especially those used with chronic stress, are actually involuntary. Further, strategies can slip back and forth between being voluntary and involuntary, individuals may not always be aware of behaviors they are using to manage stress. Repetti and Wood (1996), for example, found that social withdrawal in the face of stress is fairly common and may not be consciously recognized as a coping attempt. Further, behaviors that were once conscious can become relatively unconscious or reflexive once they become over-learned. For example, contrast initial attempts at driving a car to the smooth, nearly reflexive behaviors used once this skill is mastered. Thus, coping may represent a complex dynamic between unconscious, semi-conscious, and conscious strategies. However, assessing unconscious strategies is problematic, and scales that attempt to do so often have poor psychometric properties (Cramer, 2000).

In contrast, coping styles approaches focus on typical ways of coping with problems with may be rooted in personality (Millon, 1982) or perceptual styles such as repression-sensitization (Byrne, 1964), blunting-monitoring (Miller, 1980), or approach-avoidance (Roth & Cohen 1986). Dichotomizing coping into two or three categories has certain benefits, namely in the good parametric characteristics of coping style scales (e.g., Endler & Parker, 1990). However, they have also been criticized for several shortcomings, including confound with anxiety, poor consistency of coping styles across situations, and their inability to predict situation-specific coping strategies (Cohen & Lazarus, 1973). However, a more recent study confirmed that coping styles are not associated with coping strategies used in any given situation, but studies using daily diary assessments in which coping strategies are aggravated across situations can find that coping styles predict mean levels of coping strategies (Ptacek, Pierce, & Thompson, 2006).

Further, several researchers have argued that individuals may alternate between denial and action (Lazarus, 1983; Pennebaker, Colder, Sharp, 1980). For example, denial may allow a terminally ill individual to maintain hope while simultaneously preparing for funeral arrangements. Stroebe and Schut (1999, 2001; Stroebe, 2011) have proposed a Dual Process model of coping in which individuals are thought to alternate between several dichotomies in a situation, including positive and negative

appraisals, approach and avoidant coping, and so on. Just as with defense mechanisms, coping tends to be a complex of different strategies that may be directed at various facets of the problem and/or show dynamic change over time.

Finally, cognitive or process approaches to coping focus on specific strategies in particular situations (Lazarus & Folkman, 1984). They are thought to be guided by the appraisal of the situation; are conscious, flexible, and responsive to situational contingencies; and include both problem- and emotion-focused strategies—that is, attempts to regulate the situation and one's emotional state. Lazarus and Folkman defined coping as "*constantly changing cognitive and behavioral efforts to manage, [that is master, tolerate, reduce, minimize] specific external and/or internal demands, [and conflicts among them], that are appraised as taxing or exceeding the resources of the person*" (p. 141).

There is a large amount of evidence showing that coping is responsive to situational demands (for a review, see Aldwin, 2007). An elegant series of studies by de Ridder and Kerssens (2003) showed clearly that coping is influenced by both personality and situational characteristics. Further, Folkman and Lazarus (1980) showed that the most people use both problem- and emotion-focused coping in over 80% of situations.

However, there are several problems with this approach (Coyne & Racciopo, 2000; Folkman & Moskowitz, 2004), including the question of the validity of retrospective accounts and the inability of the field to come to a consensus concerning exactly what constitutes a coping strategy and how many there are. A review by Skinner, Edge, Altman, and Sherwood (2003) identified literally hundreds of coping strategies that are currently assessed. They concluded that there were five basic types of strategies: problem solving, support seeking, avoidance, distraction, and positive cognitive restructuring. Problem-solving coping includes not only behavior (instrumental action) but also cognition (e.g., planning) and motivation (perseverance). Support seeking includes reaching out to others for behavioral, cognitive, and emotional support. Avoidance also includes both behavioral and cognitive strategies such as denial. This should not be confused with distraction, which includes positive behaviors and cognitions to minimize stress. Positive cognitive reconstruction involves reinterpreting problematic situations, looking for potential positive facets and outcomes.

Skinner et al. also suggested four additional strong candidates for inclusion in general coping scales: three negative strategies (rumination, help-lessness, and social withdrawal) and one positive one (emotional regulation). Other, more positive, strategies, have recently been proposed, including religious coping such as prayer (Pargament, 2011; Pargament, Koenig, & Perez, 2000) and benefit-finding or meaning-making (Park, 2005; Tennen & Affleck, 2002), as well as emotional processing (Stanton, 2011; Stanton, Danoff-Burg, Cameron, & Ellis, 1994). Others point out that coping does not occur in a vacuum (Hobfoll, 2001; 2011), and that our social context, friends, and family influence not only our appraisals of situations but also our choice of coping strategies (Thoits, 1986). Some researchers have been exploring the phenomenon of dyadic coping, or how couples negotiate problems (DeLongis & Preece, 2002; Revenson & DeLongis, 2011; Revenson & Pranikoff, 2005). Nonetheless, a number of key issues in the field remain unresolved, including how to assess coping efficacy, the stability or change in coping over time, and whether coping has situation-specific effects.

The critical issue in this field that this chapter addresses is the development of coping strategies: How do they arise? What is their developmental course? Are there consistent developmental trajectories across people? The next sections will consider these developmental issues in both childhood and adulthood.

Coping in childhood

Skinner and Zimmer-Gebeck (2009) have proposed the most comprehensive theory of the development of coping strategies in childhood. They propose that coping in infancy, defined as birth to 18 months, initially consists largely of reflexes that form the basis for coordinated action schema. For example, infants (and even fetuses) will engage in self-soothing behaviors such as thumb sucking (Field, 1991; Karraker & Laker, 1991). An early study by Murphy and Moriarty (1976) documented infants' attempts to regulate their environment, using their primitive motor skills to recapture nipples and wriggle out of blankets wrapped too tightly around them. They will turn their heads away or close their eyes to decrease aversive stimulation. Further, they signal their parents by modulating their cries to indicate different types of distress (e.g., hunger or wet diapers). Parents and other caretakers play a major role in helping infants learn to regulate the internal and external environments, and are the primary ways in which infants self-regulate (Eisenberg & Zhou, 2000) and learn to cope (Kliewer, Sandler, & Wolchik, 1994).

Preschoolers (ages 2 to 5) begin to cope using voluntary direct actions (Skinner & Zimmer-Beck, 2009). The ability to regulate internal and external environments reflects the increase in executive function, paralleling the development of the frontal lobes (Lewis, Zimmerman, Hollenstein, & Lamey, 2004; National Research Council, 2000), and promoting better sense of control (Skinner & Zimmer-Beck, 2011). The greater ability of motor skills and language allows for a greater range of coping behaviors (e.g., running away from a frightening dog or protesting parental directives). While many preschoolers still use thumb sucking and rocking to control distress, they may also use transitional objects such as a favorite blanket or stuffed animal and begin rudimentary self-regulation. Wallerstein and Kelly (1980) documented the use of defense mechanisms in young children undergoing the divorce of their parents, including denial and displacement. However, emotion-focused coping strategies are still largely behavioral, and toddlers still turn to adult caregivers for self-regulation.

Cognitive strategies emerge in middle childhood (ages 6 to 9). They are more able to use cognitive distraction and self-reassuring statements (Altschuler & Ruble, 1989), as well as cognitive reframing (Compas, O'Connor-Smith, Saltzman, Thomsen, & Wadsworth, 2001). They more clearly shape their strategies to reflect situational contingencies (Spirito, Stark, Grace, & Stamoulis, 1991), and problem-focused behaviors become more common in interpersonal situations, but may decrease in situations that are recognized as less controllable (Compas, Worsham, & Ey, 1992). They also begin to seek social support outside of their family (Bryant, 1985). More problematically, rumination may also arise in middle childhood (Broderick, 1998), especially among girls (Broderick & Korteland, 2004).

In one of the few longitudinal studies of childhood coping, Eisenberg et al. found that both venting and aggressive coping decreased over time, while avoidant coping increased (for a review see Losoya, Eisenberg, & Fabes, 1998). Both Losoya et al. and Compas et al. found that children in middle school were more able to monitor and inhibit inappropriate action. Nonetheless, Losoya et al. documented considerable inter-individual variability in developmental strategies across a six-year period.

In adolescence, the onset of formal operations can lead to more sophisticated forms of problem-focused coping (Greene & Larson, 1991). Humor may also emerge as an important coping strategy at around age 12 (Führ, 2003), but there may be gender differences, with boys using more aggressive and sexual humor, while girls use humor more to cheer themselves up. In general, girls use more self-soothing strategies than boys, while male adolescents are more likely to use physical and sexual activities (Horton, 2002). While adolescents are more adept than younger children in self-regulation, parents still have a large influence on their use of coping strategies (Seiffge-Krenke, 2004; Wolfradt, Hempel, & Miles, 2003). Nonetheless, adolescents are more likely to turn to siblings and friends for support (Murphy & Moriarty, 1976), especially if there is family discord (Wallerstein & Kelly, 1980), although too much discord may discourage adolescents from turning to siblings (Grych & Fincham, 1997). Adolescents may also rely on romantic partners for social support, although effective dyadic coping strategies may not emerge until late adolescence (Nieder & Seiffge-Krenke, 2001; Seiffge-Krenke, 2006).

Adolescence is also a time for the development of maladaptive coping strategies. They might use external regulators of emotional distress, such as drugs, cigarettes, and alcohol (Wills, Sandy, Yaeger, Cleary, & Shinar, 2001). Social withdrawal as a coping strategy may be particular dangerous for teenagers, as it may be associated with an increased risk of suicide (Spirito, Overholswer, & Stark, 1989).

In sum, coping strategies show clear developmental shifts from early childhood to adolescence. The development of self-regulation follows a particularly clear developmental trajectory, from interpersonal self-regulation (e.g., reliance on parental caregivers) to independent self-regulation in later childhood, concomitant with an increase in cognitive emotion regulation. Problem-focused coping becomes more complex and differentiated, as children recognize that some coping strategies are more effective in some situations than in others. Nonetheless, there are individual differences in coping trajectories, and middle childhood and adolescence constitute a time in which maladaptive strategies such as rumination, substance abuse, risky sexual behavior, and social withdrawal develop, which can have serious long-term consequences (Catanzaro, 2000).

Coping in adulthood

Surprisingly few studies explicitly examine age differences in coping in adulthood, and there has been only one longitudinal study, which focused on defense mechanisms (Vaillant, 1977). This discussion will consider age-related changes in problem- and emotion-focused coping.

The evidence for age differences in problem-focused coping is decidedly mixed, with some studies showing no changes, others suggesting age-related declines, and a few suggesting age-related increases (see Folkman, Lazarus, Pimley, & Novacek, 1987; Blanchard-Fields, Sulsky, & Robinson-Whelen, 1991; Felton & Revenson, 1987; Irion & Blanchard-Fields, 1987). McCrae (1982) argued that age-related differences are largely a function of situational effects: older adults may be coping with more intractable problems such as bereavement, and controlling for the type of problem eliminates age differences in problem-focused coping. In general, however, studies have found that older individuals use fewer strategies, but maintain their self-rated coping effectiveness (Aldwin, 1991; Meeks, Carstensen, Tamsky, Wright, & Pellegrini, 1989).

Aldwin et al. (1996) compared quantitative and qualitative changes in coping among middle-aged and older men. Using the quantitative measure, they found that older men used fewer problem-focused strategies, but no age differences emerged in the qualitative analysis of these strategies. Comparing the two ways of assessing coping yielded some interesting insights into the process. Coping inventories typically assess multiple problem-focused strategies, so simple counts of strategies yield age differences. Qualitative content analysis simply codes whether the individual used a strategy. Older men did use problem-focused strategies, so there were no age differences in the qualitative analysis. However, they used fewer strategies, so they had lower scores on the quantitative measure. Older adults may use fewer strategies in an effort to conserve resources, given their lower levels of energy. For example, when faced with a flooded basement (a common problem in this New England sample), middle-aged men will often attempt to solve the problem themselves, necessitating cognitive plans of action and often multiple types of problem solving. In contrast, older men were more likely to hire plumbers or ask for assistance from their middle-aged sons. Both types of strategies can be effective in solving the problem, but older men used fewer strategies. Thus, one must distinguish between coping effort and coping ability. Older individuals may well use less coping effort in an attempt to conserve resources (Baltes, 1987; Hobfoll, 2001, 2011), but this does not necessarily mean that they are less effective copers. Their greater experience may help them to know which coping strategies work in which particular situations to achieve their goals, and thus older adults may also be more efficient copers (Aldwin et al., 1996). Thus, the use of fewer problem focused strategies in adulthood may reflect more focused and efficient coping, which Skinner and Zimmer-Gembeck (2011) have also noted in the adolescent coping literature.

The problem-focused area in which older adults appear to more consistently cope better than younger adults lies in dyadic coping. In their review, Berg and Upchurch (2007) provide evidence suggesting that older adults are more likely to use collaborative coping than younger adults. In part this is due to the fact that older adults are typically facing problems with chronic illness, which strongly affects both members of the dyad. Thus, collaborative coping not only is an appropriate way to deal with these types of problems, but may also allow for more effective emotion regulation. Coats and Blanchard-Fields (2008) also suggested that middle-aged adults may be more effective than younger ones with interpersonal stressors, in part because older adults are more focused on emotion regulation and are less likely to become angry (Blanchard-Fields & Coats, 2008). Older adults also have more generative goals when coping (Hoppman, Coats, & Blanchard-Fields, 2008).

The evidence for improved emotion regulation with age is more consistent. Older adults use fewer escapist, hostile, and avoidant strategies (Aldwin, 1991; Aldwin et al., 1996; McCrae, 1989), as well as less rumination, emotional numbing, escape, and wishful thinking and more positive reappraisal (Wadsworth et al., 2004). Both cross-sectional and longitudinal studies suggest that the use of mature defense mechanisms increase with age (Bond et al., 1983; Diehl, Coyle, & Labouvie-Vief, 1996; Vaillant, 1977, 1993). Further, they may also be more reliant on religious coping (Krause, 2006), especially in situations involving health-related disabilities (Ai & Branco, 2008).

There is also some suggestion that coping in later life may become more nuanced. For example, there may be few differences in the amount of social support that older individuals use as a coping strategy, but they may have different motivations. Labouvie-Vief et al. (1987) found that younger adults used social support primarily as a means of self-validation, but older adults were more likely to seek information about the effectiveness of their coping strategies. In contrast, Carstensen, Mikels, and Mather (2006) suggested that younger adults were more likely to use social support as ways of obtaining more information, while older adults were more likely to seek emotion regulation.

Older adults may also be more differentiated in their coping strategies. Coats and Blanchard-Fields (2008) found that older adults used more problem-focused coping for financial problems than did younger adults, but were more likely to use avoidant coping for interpersonal problems. Avoidant coping in interpersonal situations, however, does not necessarily mean passivity. A woman I interviewed as part of a project on wisdom and coping related a good example of this. She was eagerly anticipating the birth of her grandchild, attending her daughter-in-law in the delivery room. Her daughter-in-law became very upset and ordered her out of the room. The woman bit her tongue and left. On a standard coping checklist, this would be seen as avoidant coping (left the situation). However, the interview provided greater insight. The woman said that when she was younger, she probably would have gotten very hurt and angry and argued with the other woman. But she realized that the situation wasn't about her, it was about her daughter-in-law. Further, she recognized that birthing is a very difficult emotional process, and remarked that it wasn't really her daughter-in-law, but just the "hormones talking." Further, she felt that maintaining good relations with her daughter-in-law, a long-term goal, was more important that her short-term goal of witnessing the birth of her grandchild. Thus, she was using very mature coping strategies, which typically are not included in standard coping inventories. These included *decentering*, understanding that another person's needs were greater than her own. She also avoided blaming her daughter-in-law by attributing her behavior to a temporary state rather than a long-term trait (being difficult). She also kept in mind her long-term goal, and sacrificed her short-term goal for it. Labouvie-Vief et al. (1987) argued that our current coping inventories do not include the more sophisticated strategies that may emerge in late life.

In summary, it appears likely that coping does change with age in adulthood. Simple mean differences may not reveal some of the more subtle changes. Older adults may conserve resources, by using both more efficient and more nuanced strategies. With experience, older adults may also develop better emotion regulation strategies and may learn more collaborative coping skills. They may learn to relinquish unattainable goals (Wrosch, 2011) and learn to cope in ways that are more accommodative of the situation in which they find themselves (Rothermund & Brandstädter, 2003). They may also learn to downplay the stressfulness of situations and are less likely to appraise them as stressful (Aldwin et al., 1996). This may explain why neuroticism appears to decrease with age (Mroczek & Spiro, 2007) and why older adults are more able to focus on positive emotions (Carstensen et al., 2006). This process is sometimes mistaken for passivity, but deeper examination suggests that these are highly adaptive strategies that allow individuals to maintain emotional equilibrium in the face of the declines and losses common in later life.

Age Differences in Stress Vulnerability

The question of whether or not there are age differences in stress vulnerability needs to take into account the type of stress. Specifically, age differences in vulnerability may vary depending upon whether the individual is facing a physical stressor or a psychosocial one.

Vulnerability to physical stressors

There is little doubt that both the very young and the very old are more vulnerable to physical stressors. In natural disasters, it is the very young and the very old who are most likely to die, albeit for different reasons. Infants are small and have a greater surface to body ratio. This, combined with relatively low levels of body fat, makes it more difficult for them to regulate their temperature, and thus they are more vulnerable to both heat and cold. Older adults also experience difficulty in regulating body temperature, but this may be due more to neurological and cardiovascular causes. The recent tragedies in which thousands of older adults died in the recent heat waves underline their vulnerability to this type of physical stressor. For example, nearly 30,000 senior citizens died in the heat waves in Europe in 2003 (Haines, Kovats, Campbell-Lendrum, & Corvalan, 2006).

The immune systems of the very young and the very old also make them more susceptible to pathogens, but again for different reasons. The very young tend to use more innate immunity, which involves defenses such as fevers, vomiting, and diarrhea, which is very costly to the body, and risk death from very high fevers and dehydration. Older adults rely on learned immunity and have a good "memory bank" for pathogens to which they have been previously exposed but are less adept at mounting defenses for new pathogens (see Gruenewald & Kemeny, 2007; Miller, 1996).

Chronic illnesses play the largest role in the greater susceptibility of older adults to natural disasters and other physical stressors. Chronic illnesses such as diabetes and cardiovascular disease can rapidly turn into acute illnesses in the absence of medications, food, water, proper sanitation, and so forth (Mokdad et al., 2005). Older adults with mobility problems may be unable to flee impending disasters, which is one reason why the mortality rate among elders caught in Hurricane Katrina was so high. Similarly, young children may simply not have the physical strength and mobility to escape from the more devastating consequences of natural disasters, so both groups are highly vulnerable to physical stressors.

Vulnerability to psychosocial stressors

It is by no means certain that there are age differences in vulnerability to psychosocial stressors, as studies on age-related vulnerability are scarce. One type of stressor for which this issue has been well researched is parental divorce. Early studies suggested that children in middle childhood are more susceptible to adverse effects from parental divorce. Younger children were thought to be more oblivious to parental discord, and adolescents had greater ability to withdraw from familial distress than children in middle childhood, who are often acutely aware of parental discord but are unable to do much to affect the situation. However, reviews by Amato (2001) and Wolfinger (2005) found no consistent age differences in children's vulnerability to parental divorce.

In some ways, the timing of the event may be more important than an individual's age. As we have seen, events are often linked to particular life stages and can be thought of as normative or even "on-time." Off-time events—those that occur before or after the normative time—may be more stressful than on-time events (for a review, see Elder & Shanahan, 2006). For example, having a first child in early adolescence or in one's forties may prove more challenging than having one at a more normative time (e.g., mid-twenties).

There are several examples of this in the literature. For example, Ge, Conger, and Elder (1996) found that girls, but not boys, experience more distress from early puberty than those who experience on-time onset of menses. Younger soldiers may be more vulnerable to post-traumatic stress disorder (PTSD) and older ones to career disruptions than those who enter the military in their early twenties (Elder & Clipp, 1989). Further, those experiencing widowhood in mid-life may have higher mortality rates than those in late life (Johnson, Backlund, Sorlie, & Loveless, 2000).

Nonetheless, it is widely assumed that older adults are more vulnerable to psychosocial stressors, especially those with chronic illnesses. Yet the literature is decidedly mixed, with some studies finding that vulnerability increases with age, others that vulnerability decreases, and yet others finding no age differences (for a review, see Aldwin, Park, & Spiro, 2007a). For example, there is little evidence to suggest that older adults differ from younger adults in the development of PTSD following traumatic events (Weintraub & Ruskin, 1999), although Creamer and Parslow (2008) suggest that older cohorts may have lower rates. Williams (2000) argued that older adults are *less* vulnerable to psychosocial stress due to survivor effects: presumably individuals who survive to late life are fairly resilient.

Aldwin, Park, and Spiro (2007b) recently edited a handbook in which the authors were asked to explicitly examine whether old adults were more vulnerable to psychosocial stress. Most chapters concluded that the evidence was extremely mixed and that there were many gaps in the literature that precluded a definitive answer. Nonetheless, we were able to draw some preliminary conclusions (Aldwin, Park, & Spiro, 2007c). First, it was clear that the immune (Grunewald & Kemeny, 2007) and neuroendocrine systems (Epel, Burke, & Wolkowitz, 2007), as well as the ability of the cardiovascular system to respond to demands (cardiovascular reactivity; Cooper, Katzel, & Waldstein, 2007), demonstrate increasing dysregulation with age, creating greater susceptibility to the adverse effects of psychosocial stress. However, there are many psychosocial moderators of the stress responses, including appraisal and coping processes, social support, multidimensional aspects of control, religiosity, and certain personality traits such as conscientiousness and emotional stability, which in many instances served to protect older individuals from the adverse effects of psychosocial stress.

For example, Boeninger et al. (2009) found that older individuals were less likely to appraise events as problems, and had lower stress ratings and fewer stress appraisals for those events that were perceived as problems. They examined both the type of problem and personality characteristics and found that age was the most consistent predictor of the number of stress appraisals. They interpreted this as reflecting a developmental process: with age comes greater experience with a variety of problems, which can provide greater perspective on the seriousness of current difficulties. Older adults may understand that they are more vulnerable to stress and thus use appraisal processes to forestall interpreting situations as problems—or at least as serious problems. For example, one older man I interviewed stated that he used to get very upset when he was younger, but once he was diagnosed with hypertension, he learned not to get upset about minor problems (Aldwin et al., 1996b).

An early study found that older adults were not only less likely to appraise problems as stressful, but they were also less likely to perceive responsibility for either the occurrence of the event or its solution. Nonetheless, they were just as likely as younger adults to use problem-focused coping (Aldwin, 1991). Perhaps not accepting responsibility was a way of distancing themselves from the problems and avoiding self-blame and rumination, thereby avoiding attendant emotional distress. Further, all of the (negative) relationship between age and depressive symptoms was accounted for by stress, appraisal, and coping processes. If older individuals do exhibit better emotion regulation or control over internal states than younger adults (Davis, Zautra, Johnson, Murray, & Okvat, 2007; Skaff, 2007), then this may also prove to be a powerful protective factor.

There are individual differences in stress vulnerability in later life. Cognitive impairment may erode both problem-solving abilities and emotion regulation (Coats & Blanchard-Fields, 2008). Further, older individuals who are high in neuroticism show the greatest reactivity to stress of any age group, while those low in neuroticism reported the lowest negative affect in response to stress of any age group (Mroczek, Spiro, Griffin, & Neupert, 2006).

In summary, both the very young and the very old are most susceptible to physical stressors. Chronic illness, cognitive impairment, and neuroticism may increase susceptibility to psychosocial stress in late life. However, there are tantalizing hints in the literature that older adults recognize this vulnerability and use a variety of appraisal and coping processes to better regulate their emotional responses to stress. Nonetheless, there are clear individual differences in vulnerability to psychosocial stress in later life, supporting the lifespan developmental perspective that, in general, individual differences increase across the lifespan.

Summary and Conclusions

This chapter addressed three major questions: how stress changes across the lifespan, whether coping changes consistently with age, and whether there are age effects on stress vulnerability. The relationships between age and stress and coping processes are highly complex, reflecting a combination of age, cohort, and period effects. The literature reviewed here supports a lifespan developmental approach. First, it is clear that these processes change over the lifespan, influenced by biological and social contexts, as well as individual motivation and behaviors. Second, a multidisciplinary approach, including biology, psychology, sociology, and anthropology, is necessary to understand how these myriad influences combine to affect individuals' exposure to and experience of stress, as well as how they cope with problems (see Aldwin, 2007). Third, the immediate context also has large influences on stress exposure, its interpretation or appraisal, and how individuals cope. Finally, there are also clear differences in individual trajectories of stress and coping processes.

How and why stress changes across the lifespan depends upon the level at which stress is assessed. Traumatic events are clearly most influenced by the sociohistorical context, and even lifetime exposure shows little consistent relationship with age in adults (Norris & Slone, 2007). In children, levels of trauma/victimization are surprisingly high, and, to a certain extent, the type of trauma appears to reflect life stage, with adolescents reporting higher levels of victimization (Finkelhor et al., 2009a, 2009b). The type of life events also varies by life stage, but there is less evidence for age-related differences in the number of life events (Coddington, 1972). In adulthood, life events appear to reflect both cohort influences and life stage (Chiriboga, 1997), with young adults reporting more life events, as they acquire new roles such as work and parenting that expose them to stresses. However, life events clearly reflect the influence of historical periods: during times of economic downturn, for example, individuals are more likely to experience job loss and other types of economic distress (Aldwin & Revenson, 1987).

Daily stressors undoubtedly reflect the same dynamics but do show more consistent age-related effects. Children's daily stressors also appear to reflect their life stage (Hema et al., 2007), but there are as yet relatively few studies and it is not clear whether the amount of daily stress increases in childhood and adolescence. In adulthood, younger adults report the largest numbers of daily stressors, more than middle-aged adults, despite the latter's great responsibility both for their adolescent children and aging parents, as well as the managerial duties at work common in mid-life. Aldwin et al. (1996) speculated that middle-aged individuals have developed better coping skills (and perhaps anticipatory coping strategies) that allow them to avoid some of the more routine stresses that young adults who are just beginning to manage their own lives are facing. Surprisingly, older adults report the fewest daily stressors, despite the increases in chronic illnesses in late life. While health-related hassles do appear to increase, this is not enough to offset the decrease in other domains, reflecting the relinquishment of parenting and work roles. Boeninger et al. (2009) suggest that this decrease in stress appraisals reflects not only contextual changes, but also a developmental change in perspective: a lifetime of exposure to major stressors may render more minor ones as less important. As one older man remarked, watching a daughter die of cancer makes little else seem stressful (Aldwin et al., 1996).

Coping in children most clearly demonstrates a developmental progression. Very young children have only rudimentary problem-solving skills, and emotion regulation largely depends upon parental/caregiver efforts. Neurological maturation underlies increases in executive skills, which in turn are reflected in more sophisticated problem-focused coping strategies. Cognitive emotion-focused coping strategies emerge in middle childhood, and adolescents show increasingly independent and sophisticated problem- and emotion-focused coping. However, maladaptive coping strategies such as substance abuse and risky sexual behavior also arise in middle childhood and adolescence, with the potential for life-long difficulties (Catanzaro, 2000; Wills et al., 2001).

There is less evidence for a developmental progression in adulthood, although the bulk of the evidence suggests an increase in coping abilities with age. Studies that examine age differences in quantitative measures suggest older adults are less likely to use negative strategies such as wishful thinking and avoidance, and may exhibit better emotion regulation. They also are more likely to use collaborative coping (Berg & Upchurch, 1987) and in general may show more nuanced strategies (Coates & Blanchard-Fields, 2009). While there is some evidence to suggest that problem-focused coping may decrease, Aldwin et al. (1996) suggests that this may be in the service of conservation of resources, as no age differences in coping efficacy are seen.

Both the very young and the very old show heightened vulnerability to physical stressors, but many questions remain as to whether physiological vulnerability to psychosocial stressors changes across the lifespan. Again, there is some suggestion that the increased dysregulation in a number of regulatory systems in late life increases vulnerability to stress, but older adults appear to be able to make good use of emotion regulation strategies to moderate this increased vulnerability, except for those high in neuroticism (Mroczek et al., 2006) or those who are cognitively impaired (Coats & Blanchard-Fields, 2008).

Future Directions

Despite the extensive amount of work in this area, a number of questions remain. There is by and large a dearth of quantitative longitudinal studies of stress and coping processes, without which it is difficult to disentangle age, cohort, and period effects. While stress is clearly influenced by the sociohistorical context, there is less evidence for this type of influence on coping strategies. However, this may reflect the state of the field, and it is likely that preferred coping measures also may change across cohorts (Aldwin, 2007). Further, it is clear that better coping strategies are needed to assess the more nuanced strategies that older adults may be more likely to use. In particular, we need to understand how individuals are able to maintain an awareness of long-term goals in stressful situations, how they can relinquish unattainable goals, how they imbue meaning to everyday encounters, and how they are able to better use collaborative strategies. Further, it is important not to confuse better emotion regulation with passivity, especially if it involves choosing to withhold or delay action.

Finally, coping research needs to be more fully embedded within developmental frameworks. We need to place more emphasis on the role of positive coping strategies in optimal aging. Golub and Langer (2007) argue that we need a better understanding of what is gained in late life as well as what is lost. In particular, the relationship between coping and positive outcomes such as wisdom needs to be better understood. Aldwin, Levenson, and Kelly (2009) have suggested that there are conceptual similarities among emotional maturity, stress-related growth, and wisdom. How individuals learn to cope with stress may play a large role in the development of these positive resources, and more research is needed on precisely how this occurs, preferably using longitudinal studies with multiple cohorts.

References

Adler, N. E., & Snibbe, A.C. (2003). The role of psychosocial processes in explaining the gradient between SES and health. *Current Directions in Psychological Science, 12,* 119–23.

Ai, A. L., & Branco, K. (2008). Faith, function, and well-being in coping with aging: An interdisciplinary inquiry. *Journal of Religion, Spirituality & Aging, 20,* 247–8.

Aldwin, C. (1990). The Elders Life Stress Inventory (ELSI): Egocentric and nonegocentric stress. In M. A. P. Stephens, S. E. Hobfoll, J. H. Crowther, & D. L. Tennenbaum (Eds.), *Stress and coping in late life families* (pp. 49–69). New York: Hemisphere.

Aldwin, C. (1991). Does age affect the stress and coping process? Implications of age differences in perceived control. *Journal of Gerontology, 46,* 174–80.

Aldwin, C. M. (2007). *Stress, coping, and development* (2nd ed.). New York: Guilford.

Aldwin, C. M., Levenson, M. R., & Kelly, L. L. (2009). Lifespan developmental perspectives on stress-related growth. In C. L. Park, S. Lechner, A. Stanton, & M. Antoni (Eds.), *Positive life changes in the context of medical illness* (pp. 87–104). Washington, DC: APA Press.

Aldwin, C., Levenson, M.R., Spiro, A. III, & Bosse, R. (1989). Does emotionality predict stress? Findings from the Normative Aging Study. *Journal of Personality and Social Psychology, 56,* 618–24.

Aldwin, C. M., Park, C. L. & Spiro, A. III (2007a). Health psychology and aging: An introduction. In C. M. Aldwin, C. L. Park, & A. Spiro III (Eds.), *Handbook of health psychology & aging* (pp. 3–8). New York: Guilford.

Aldwin, C. M., Park, C. L., & Spiro, A.III (Eds.) (2007b). *Handbook of health psychology & aging* (pp. 3–8). New York: Guilford.

Aldwin, C. M., Park, C. L., & Spiro, A.III (2007c). Health psychology and aging: Moving to the next generation of research. In C. M. Aldwin, C. L. Park, & A. Spiro III (Eds.), *Handbook of health psychology & aging* (pp. 413–26). New York: Guilford.

Aldwin, C., & Revenson, T. (1986). Vulnerability to economic stress. *American Journal of Community Psychology, 14,* 161–75.

Aldwin, C. M., Sutton, K. J., Chiara, G., & Spiro, A. III (1996). Age differences in stress, coping, and appraisal: Findings from the Normative Aging Study. *Journals of Gerontology: Psychological Sciences, 51B,* P179.

Aldwin, C. M., Sutton, K., & Lachman, M. (1996). The development of coping resources in adulthood. *Journal of Personality, 64,* 91–113.

Almeida, D. M., Wethington, E., & Kessler, R. C. (2002). The daily inventory of stressful events: An interview-based approach for measuring daily stressors. *Assessment, 9,* 41–55.

Almeida, D. M., & Horn, M. C. (2004). Is daily life more stressful during middle adulthood? In O. G. Brim, C. D. Ryff, & R. C. Kessler (Eds.), *How healthy are we? A national study of well-being at midlife* (pp. 425–51). Chicago: University of Chicago Press.

Altschuler, J. A., & Ruble, D. N. (1989). Developmental changes in children's awareness of strategies for coping with uncontrollable stress. *Child Development, 60,* 1337–49.

Amato, P. R. (2001). Children of divorce in the 1990s: An update of the Amato and Keith (1991) meta-analysis. *Journal of Family Psychology, 15,* 355–71.

Axelson, D. A., Bertocci, M. A., Lewin, D. S., Trubnick, L.S, Birmaher, B., Williamson, D. E., Ryan, N.D., Dahl, R. E. (2003). Measuring mood and complex behavior in natural environments: Use of ecological momentary assessment in pediatric affective disorders. *Journal of Child and Adolescent Psychopharmacology, 13,* 253–66.

Baltes, P. B. (1987). Theoretical propositions of life-span developmental psychology: On the dynamics between growth and decline. *Developmental Psychology, 24,* 611–26.

Baltes, P. B., Lindenberger, U., & Staudinger, U. M. (2006). Life span theory in developmental psychology. In W. Damon & R. M. Lerner (Vol. Ed.), *Handbook of child psychology* (6th ed., Vol. 1). New York: Wiley.

Barker, D. J. (1990). The fetal and infant origins of adult disease. *British Medical Journal, 301,* 1111.

Berg, C. A., & Upchurch, R. (2007). A developmental-contextual model of couples coping with chronic illness across the adult life span. *Psychological Bulletin, 133,* 920–54.

Birditt, K. S., Fingerman, K. L., & Almeida, D. M. (2005). Age differences in exposure and reactions to interpersonal tensions: A daily diary study. *Psychology and Aging, 20,* 330–40.

Blanchard-Fields, F., Sulsky, L., & Robinson-Whelen, S. (1991). Moderating effects of age and context on the relationship between gender, sex role differences, and coping. *Sex Roles, 25,* 645–60.

Boeninger, D. K., Shiraishi, R. W., Aldwin, C. M. & Spiro, A. III. (2009). Why do older men report lower stress ratings? Findings from the Normative Aging Study. *International Journal of Aging & Human Development, 68*(2), 149–70.

Bond, M., Gardiner, S. T., Christian, J., & Sigel, J. J. (1983). An empirical examination of defense mechanisms. *Archives of General Psychiatry, 40,* 33–8.

Broderick, P. C. (1998). Early adolescent gender differences in the use of ruminative and distracting coping strategies. *Journal of Early Adolescence, 18,* 173–91.

Broderick, P. C., & Korteland, C. (2004). A prospective study of rumination and depression in early adolescence. *Clinical Child Psychology & Psychiatry, 9,* 383–94.

Bryant, B. K. (1985). The neighborhood walk: Sources of support in middle childhood. *Monographs of the Society for Research in Child Development, 50*(3, Serial No. 210).

Byrne, D. (1964). Repression-sensitization as a dimension of personality. In B. A. Maher (Ed.), *Progress in experimental personality research* (Vol. 1, pp. 169–220). New York: Academic Press.

Carstensen, L. L., Mikels, J. A., & Mather, M. (2006). Aging and the intersection of cognition, motivation and emotion. In J. Birren & K. W. Schaie (Eds.), *Handbook of the psychology of aging,* 6th ed. (pp. 343–62). San Diego: Academic Press.

Carver, C. S., & Scheier, M. F. (1998). *On the self-regulation of behavior.* New York: Cambridge University Press.

Catanzaro, S. (2000). Mood regulation and suicidal behavior. In T. Joiner & M. D. Rudd (Eds.), *Suicide science: Expanding the boundaries* (pp. 81–103). New York: Kluwer/Plenum.

Chiriboga, D. A. (1997). Crisis, challenge, and stability in the middle years. In M. E. Lachman & J. B. James (Eds.), *Multiple paths of midlife development* (pp. 293–343). Chicago: University of Chicago.

Coats, A. H., & Blanchard-Fields, F. (2008). Emotion regulation in interpersonal problems: The role of cognitive-emotional complexity, emotion regulation goals, and expressivity. *Psychology and Aging, 23,* 39–51.

Coddington, R. D. (1972). The significance of life events as etiologic factors in the diseases of children—II. A study of a normal population. *Journal of Psychosomatic Research, 16,* 205–13.

Cohen, F., & Lazarus, R. S. (1973). Active coping processes, coping dispositions, and recovery from surgery. *Psychosomatic Medicine, 35,* 375–89.

Compas, B. E., Worsham, N. L., & Ey, S. (1992). Conceptual and developmental issues in children's coping with stress. In A. M. La Greca, L. J. Siegel, J. L. Wallander, & C. E. Walker (Eds.), *Stress and coping in child health* (pp. 7–24). New York: Guilford Press.

Compas, B. E., Connor, J., Osowiecki, D., & Welch, A. (1996). Effortful and involuntary responses to stress: Implications for coping with chronic illness. In B. H. Gottlieb (Ed.), *Coping with chronic stress* (pp. 107–132). New York: Plenum.

Compas, B., O'Connor-Smith, J. K., Saltzman, S., Thomsen, A. H., & Wadsworth, M. E. (2001). Coping with stress during childhood and adolescence: Problems, progress, and potential in theory and research. *Psychological Bulletin, 127,* 87–127.

Conger, R. D., & Conger, K. J. (2002). Resilience in midwestern families: Selected findings from the first decade of a prospective, longitudinal study. *Journal of Marriage & Family, 64,* 361–373.

Cooper, D. C., Katzel, L. I., & Waldstein, S. R. (2007). Cardiovascular reactivity in older adults. In C. M. Aldwin, C. L. Park, & A. Spiro III (Eds.), *Handbook of health psychology & aging* (pp. 142–66). New York: Guilford.

Coyne, J. C., & Racioppo, M. (2000). Never the twain shall meet? Closing the gap between coping research and clinical intervention research. *American Psychologist, 55,* 655–64.

Cramer, P. (2000). Defense mechanisms in psychology today: Further processes for adaptation. *American Psychologist, 55,* 637–46.

Creamer, M., & Parslow, R. (2008). Trauma exposure and post-traumatic stress disorder in the elderly: A community prevalence study. *American Journal of Geriatric Psychiatry, 16,* 853–6.

de Ridder, D., & Kerssens, J. (2003). Owing to the force of circumstances? The impact of situational features and personal characteristics on coping patterns across situations. *Psychology & Health, 18,* 217–36.

Davis, M., C., Zautra, A. J., Johnson, L. M., Murray, K. E., & Okvat, H. A. (2007). Psychosocial stress, emotion regulation, and resilience among older adults. In C. M. Aldwin, C. L. Park, & A. Spiro III (Eds.), *Handbook of health psychology & aging* (pp. 250–66). New York: Guilford.

DeLongis, A., & Preece, M. (2002). Emotional and relational consequences of coping in stepfamilies. *Marriage & Family Review, 34,* 115–38.

DeLongis, A., Folkman, S., & Lazarus, R. S. (1988). The impact of daily stress on health and mood: Psychology and social resources as mediators. *Journal of Personality and Social Psychology, 54,* 486–95.

Diehl, M., Coyle, N., & Labouvie-Vief, G. (1996). Age and sex differences in strategies of coping and defense across the life span. *Psychology and Aging, 11,* 127–39.

Dohrenwend, B. S., Dohrenwend, B. P., Dodson, M., & Shrout, P. E. (1984). Symptoms, hassles, social supports, and life events: Problem of confounded measures. *Journal of Abnormal Psychology, 93,* 222–30.

Eisenberg, N., & Zhou, Q. (2000). Regulation from a developmental perspective. *Psychological Inquiry, 11,* 167–71.

Elder, G., & Clipp, E. (1989). Combat experience and emotional health: Impairment and resilience in later life. *Journal of Personality, 57,* 311–41.

Elder, G. H., Jr., & Shanahan, M. J. (2006). The life course and human development. In R. M Lerner (Ed.), *Handbook of child psychology (Vol. 1, 6th ed.): Theoretical models of human development* (pp. 665–715). New York: Wiley & Sons.

Endler, N., & Parker, J. D. A. (1990). Multidimensional assessment of coping: A critical evaluation. *Journal of Personality and Social Psychology, 58,* 844–854.

Ensel, W. M., & Lin, N. (1996). Distal stressors and the life stress process. *Journal of Community Psychology, 24,* 66–82.

Ensel, W. M., & Lin, N. (2000). Age, the stress process, and physical distress: The role of distal stressors. *Journal of Aging & Health, 12,* 139–68.

Epel, E. S, Burke, H. M., & Wolkowitz, O. M. (2007). The psychoneuroendocrinology of aging: Anabolic and catabolic hormones. In C. M. Aldwin, C. L. Park, & A. Spiro III (Eds.), *Handbook of health psychology & aging* (pp. 119–41). New York: Guilford.

Evans, G. W (2004). The environment of childhood poverty. *American Psychologist,* 59, 77–92.

Fantuzzo, J., Boruch, R., Beriama, A., Atkins, M., & Marcus, S. (1997). Domestic violence and children: Prevalence and risk in five major U.S. cities. *Journal of the American Academy of Child and Adolescent Psychiatry, 36,* 116–22.

Felton, B. J., & Revenson, T. A. (1987). Age differences in coping with chronic illness. *Psychology and Aging, 2,* 164–70.

Field, T. (1991). Stress and coping from pregnancy through the postnatal period. In E. M. Cummings, A. L. Greene, & K. H. Karraker (Eds.), *Life-span developmental psychology: Perspectives on stress and coping* (pp. 45–59). Hillsdale, NJ: Erlbaum.

Finkelhor, D., Ormrod, R. K., & Turner, H. A. (2009a). The developmental epidemiology of childhood victimization. *Journal of Interpersonal Violence, 24,* 711–31.

Finkelhor, D., Ormrod, R. K., & Turner, H. A. (2009b). Lifetime assessment of poly-victimization in a national sample of children and youth. *Child Abuse & Neglect, 33,* 403–11.

Finkelhor, D., Ormrod, R., Turner, H., & Hamby, SL. (2005). The victimization of children and youth: a comprehensive, national survey. *Child Maltreatment, 10,* 5–25.

Folkman, S., & Lazarus, R. S. (1980). An analysis of coping in a middle-aged community sample. *Journal of Health and Social Behavior, 21,* 219–39.

Folkman, S., & Moskowitz, J. T. (2004). Coping: Pitfalls and promise. *Annual Review of Psychology, 55,* 745–74.

Folkman, S., Lazarus, R. S., Pimley, S., & Novacek, J. (1987). Age differences in stress and coping processes. *Psychology and Aging, 2,* 171–84.

Ford, D. H., & Lerner, R. M. (1992). *Developmental systems theory: An integrative approach.* Newbury Park, CA: Sage.

Freud, A. (1966). *The ego and the mechanisms of defense* (rev. ed.). New York: International Universities Press.

Führ, M. (2002). Coping humor in early adolescence. *Humor: International Journal of Humor Research, 15,* 283–304.

Ge, X., Conger, R. D., & Elder, G. H. Jr. (1996). Coming of age too early: pubertal influences on girls' vulnerability to psychological distress. *Child Development, 67,* 3386–400.

George, L. K., & Lynch, S. M. (2003). Race differences in depressive symptoms: A dynamic perspective on stress exposure and vulnerability. *Journal of Health & Social Behavior, 44,* 353–69.

Golub, S., & Langer, E. (2007). Challenging assumptions about adult development: implications for the health of older adults. In C. M. Aldwin, C. L. Park, & A. Spiro III (Eds.), *Handbook of health psychology & aging* (pp. 9–29). New York: Guilford.

Greene, A. L., & Larson, R. W. (1991). Variation in stress reactivity during adolescence. In E. M. Cummings, A. L. Greene, & K. H. Karraker (Eds.) *Life-span developmental psychology: Perspectives on stress and coping* (pp. 195–209). Hillsdale, NJ: Erlbaum.

Gruenewald, T. L., & Kemeny, M. E. (2007). Aging and health: Psychoneuroimmunological processes. In C. M. Aldwin, C. L. Park, & A. Spiro III (Eds.), *Handbook of health psychology & aging* (pp. 97–118). New York: Guilford.

Grych, J. H., & Fincham, F. D. (1997). Children of depressed parents: The stress context. In S. A. Wolchik and I. N. Sandler (Eds.), *Handbook of children's coping: Linking theory and intervention* (pp. 159–194). New York: Plenum Press.

Haines, A., Kovats, R. S., Campbell-Lendrum, D., & Corvalan, C. (2006) Climate change and human health: Impacts, vulnerability and public health. *Public Health, 120,* 585–96.

Helgeson, V., Lopez, L. C., & Kamarck, T. (2009). Peer relationships and diabetes: Retrospective and ecological momentary assessment approaches. *Health Psychology, 28,* 273–82.

Hema, D. A., Roper, S. O., Nehring, J. W., Call, A., Mandleco, B. L., & Dyches, T. T. (2009). Daily stressors and coping responses of children and adolescents with type 1 diabetes. *Child Development: Care, Health, & Developmen, 35,* 330–9.

Hobfoll, S. E. (2001). The influence of culture, community, and the nested-self in the stress process: Advancing conservation of resources theory. *Applied Psychology: An International Review, 50,* 337–70.

Hobfoll, S. E. (2011). Conservation of resources theory: Its implication for stress, health, and resilience. In S. Folkman (Ed.), *Oxford handbook of stress, health, and coping.* New York: Oxford University Press.

Holmes, D., & Rahe, R. (1967). The Social Readjustment Rating Scale. *Journal of Psychosomatic Research, 11,* 213–8.

Hoppmann, C. A., Coats, A. H., & Blanchard-Fields, F. (2008). Goals and everyday problem solving: Examining the link between age-related goals and problem-solving strategy use. *Aging, Neuropsychology, and Cognition, 15,* 401–23.

Horton, P. C. (2002). Self-comforting strategies used by adolescents. *Bulletin of the Menninger Clinic, 66,* 259–72.

Irion, J. C., & Blanchard-Fields, F. (1987). A cross-sectional comparison of adaptive coping in adulthood. *Journal of Gerontology, 42,* 502–4.

Jackowski, A. P., de Araújo, C. M., de Lacerda, A. L. T., de Jesus Mari, J. & Kaufman, J. (2009). Neurostructural imaging findings in children with post-traumatic stress disorder: Brief review. *Psychiatry and Clinical Neurosciences, 63,* 1–8.

Johnson, N. J., Backlund, E., Sorlie, P. D., & Loveless, C. A. (2000). Marital status and mortality: The Longitudinal Mortality Study. *Annals of Epidemiology, 19*(4), 224–38.

Karraker, K. H., & Lake, M. (1991). Normative stress and coping processes in infancy. In E. M. Cummings, A. L. Greene, & K. H. Karraker (Eds.), *Life-span developmental psychology: Perspectives on stress and coping* (pp. 85–108). Hillsdale, NJ: Erlbaum.

Kendall-Tackett, K. (2002). The health effects of childhood abuse: four pathways by which abuse can influence health. *Child Abuse and Neglect, 6/7,* 715–30.

Kliewer, W., Sandler, I. N., & Wolchik, S. (1994). Family socialization of threat appraisal and coping: Coaching, modeling, and family context. In K. Hurrelmann & F. Festmann (Eds.), *Social networks and social support in childhood and adolescence* (pp. 271–91). Berlin: Walter de Gruyter.

Krause, N. (2006). Religion and health in late life. In J. E. Birren, & K. W. Schaie (Eds.), *Handbook of the psychology of aging* (6th ed., pp. 499–518). Amsterdam, Netherlands: Elsevier.

Kuh, D. & Ben-Shlomo, Y. (Eds.). (2004). *A life course approach to chronic disease epidemiology* (2nd ed.). New York: Oxford University Press.

Labouvie-Vief, G., Hakim-Larson, J., & Hobart, C. (1987). Age, ego level, and the life-span development of coping and defense processes. *Psychology and Aging, 2,* 286–93.

Lazarus, R. S. (1966). *Psychological stress and the coping process.* New York: McGraw-Hill.

Lazarus, R. S. (1983). The costs and benefits of denial. In S. Breznitz (Ed.), *The denial of stress* (pp. 1–30). New York: International Universities Press.

Lazarus, R. S. (1991). *Emotion and adaptation.* New York: Oxford University Press.

Lazarus, R. S., & Folkman, S. (1984). *Stress, appraisal, and coping.* New York: Springer.

Lewis, M. D., Zimmerman, S., Hollenstein, T., & Lamey, A. V. (2004). Reorganization in coping behavior at 1½ years: Dynamic systems and normative change. *Developmental Science, 7,* 56–73.

Litt, M. D., Tennen, H., & Affleck, G. (2011). The dynamics of health: assessing coping processes in near real time. In S. Folkman (Ed.), *Oxford handbook of stress, health, and coping.* New York: Oxford University Press.

Lorenz, F. O., Simons, R. L., Conger, R. D., Elder, G. H., Jr., Johnson, C., & Chao, W. (1997). Married and recently divorced mothers' stressful events and distress: Tracing change over time. *Journal of Marriage & the Family, 59,* 219–32.

Losoya, S., Eisenberg, N., & Fabes, R. A. (1998). Developmental issues in the study of coping. *International Journal of Behavioral Development, 22,* 287–313.

Lynch, S. M., & George, L. K. (2002). Interlocking trajectories of loss-related events and depressive symptoms among elders. *Journals of Gerontology: Social Sciences, 57B,* S117–S125.

Mason, J. W. (1975). A historical view of the stress field. *Journal of Human Stress, 1,* 6–27.

McCrae, R. R. (1982). Age differences in the use of coping mechanisms. *Journal of Gerontology, 37,* 454–60.

McCrae, R. R. (1989). Age differences and changes in the use of coping mechanisms. *Journals of Gerontology: Psychological Sciences, 44,* 161–9.

Meeks, S., Carstensen, L., Tamsky, B., Wright, T., & Pellegrini, D. (1989). Age differences in coping: Does less mean worse? *International Journal of Aging and Human Development, 28,* 127–40.

Miller, S. (1980). When is a little information a dangerous thing? Coping with stressful events by monitoring vs. blunting. In S. Levine & H. Ursin (Eds.), *Coping and health* (pp. 145–70). New York: Plenum.

Miller, R. A. (1996). The aging immune system: Primer and prospectus. *Science, 273,* 70–4.

Millon, T. (1982). On the nature of clinical health psychology. In T. Millon, C. Green, & R. Meagher (Eds.), *Handbook of clinical health psychology* (pp. 1–28). New York: Plenum.

Moffitt, T. E. (1993). Adolescent-limited and life-course-persistent antisocial behavior: A developmental taxonomy. *Psychological Bulletin, 100,* 674–701.

Mokdad, A. H., Mensah, G. A., Posner, S. F., Reed, E., Simoes, E.J., Engelgau, M. M., and the Chronic Diseases and Vulnerable Populations in Natural Disasters Working Group. (2005). When chronic conditions become acute: Prevention and control of chronic diseases and adverse health outcomes during natural disasters. *Prevention of Chronic Disease* [serial online]. Available from: URL: http://www.cdc.gov/pcd/issues/2005/nov/05_0201.htm.

Monroe, S. M. (2008). Modern approaches to conceptualizing and measuring human life stress. *Annual Review of Clinical Psychology, 4,* 33–52.

Mroczek, D. K., & Almeida, D. (2004). The effect of daily stress, personality, and age on daily negative affect. *Journal of Personality, 72,* 355–78.

Mroczek, D. K., & Spiro, A. (2007). Personality change influences mortality in older men. *Psychological Science, 18,* 371–6.

Mroczek, D. K., Spiro, A. III, Griffin, P., & Neupert, S. D. (2006). Social influences on adult personality, self-regulation, and health. In K. W. Schaie & L. Carstensen (Eds.), *Social structures, aging and self-regulation* (pp. 69–84). New York: Springer.

Murphy, L. B., & Moriarty, A. E. (1976). *Vulnerability, coping and growth from infancy to adolescence.* Oxford, England: Yale University Press.

Nansel, T. R., Overpeck, M., Pilla, R. S., Ruan, W. J., Simons-Morton, B., & Scheidt, P. C. (2001). Bullying behaviors among US youth: Prevalence and association with psychosocial adjustment. *Journal of the American Medical Association, 285,* 2094–100.

National Research Council (2000). *From neurons to neighborhoods* (J.P. Shonkoff & D. Phillips, Eds.). Washington, DC: National Academies Press.

Nieder, T., & Seiffge-Krenke, I. (2001). Coping with stress in different phases of romantic development. *Journal of Adolescence, 24,* 297–311.

Norris, F. H. (1992). Epidemiology of trauma: Frequency and impact of different potentially traumatic events on different demographic groups. *Journal of Consulting and Clinical Psychology, 60,* 409–18.

Norris, F. H., Kaniasty, K., Conrad, M. L., Inman, G. L., & Murphy, A. D. (2002). Placing age differences in cultural context: A comparison of the effects of age on PTSD after disasters in the United States, Mexico, and Poland. *Journal of Clinical Geropsychology, 8,* 153–73.

Norris, F. H., & Slone, L. B. (2007). The epidemiology of trauma and PTSD. In M. J. Friedman, T. M. Keane, & P. A. Resick (Eds.), *Handbook of PTSD: Science and practice* (pp. 78–98). New York: Guilford Press.

Pakenham, K. (2011). Benefit-finding and sense-making in chronic illness. In S. Folkman (Ed.), *Oxford handbook of stress, health, and coping.* New York: Oxford University Press.

Pargament, K. I. (2011). The spiritual dimension of coping: implications for health and well-being. In S. Folkman (Ed.), *Oxford handbook of stress, health, and coping.* New York: Oxford University Press.

Pargament, K. I., Koenig, H. G., & Perez, L. M. (2000). The many methods of religious coping: development and initial validation of the RCOPE. *Journal of Clinical Psychology, 56,* 519–43.

Park, C. L. (2005). Religion as a meaning-making framework in coping with life stress. *Journal of Social Issues, 61,* 707–29.

Park, C. L. (2011). Meaning, coping, and health. In S. Folkman (Ed.), *Oxford handbook of stress, health, and coping.* New York: Oxford University Press.

Park, C. L., Cohen, L., & Murch, R. (1996). Assessment and prediction of stress-related growth. *Journal of Personality, 64,* 71–105.

Park, C. L., Mills-Baxter, M. A., & Fenster, J. R. (2005). Posttraumatic growth from life's most traumatic event: Influences on elders' current coping and adjustment. *Traumatology, 11,* 297–306.

Pearlin, L. I., Aneshensel, C. S., Mullan, J. T., & Whitlatch, C. J. (1996). Caregiving and its social support. In R. H. Binstock & L. K. George (Eds.), *Handbook of aging and the social sciences* (4th ed., pp. 283–302). San Diego, CA: Academic Press.

Pearlin, L., & Schooler, C. (1978). The structure of coping. *Journal of Health and Social Behavior, 19,* 2–21.

Pennebaker, J. W., Colder, M., & Sharp, L. K. (1990). Accelerating the coping process. *Journal of Personality and Social Psychology, 58,* 528–37.

Physicians for Human Rights (1998). *Afghanistan campaign. The Taliban's war on women: A health and human rights crisis in Afghanistan.* Available at: http://www.phrusa.org/research/health_effects/exec.html.

Ptacek, J. T., Pierce, G. R., & Thompson, E. L. (2006). Finding evidence of dispositional coping. *Journal of Research in Personality, 40*(6), 1137–51.

Rabkin, J., & Streuning, E. (1976). Life events, stress, and illness. *Science, 194,* 1013–20.

Repetti, R. L., & Wood, J. (1996). Families accommodating to chronic stress: Unintended and unnoticed processes. In B. Gottlieb (Ed.), *Coping with chronic stress* (pp. 191–220). New York: Plenum.

Revenson, T. A., & DeLongis, A. (2011). Couples coping with chronic illness. In S. Folkman (Ed.), *Oxford handbook of stress, health, and coping.* New York: Oxford University Press.

Revenson, T. A., & Pranikoff, J. R. (2005). A contextual approach to treatment decision making among breast cancer survivors. *Health Psychology, 24,* S93–S98.

Roth, S., & Cohen, L. J. (1986). Approach, avoidance, and coping with stress. *American Psychologist, 41,* 813–9.

Rothermund, K., & Brandstädter, J. (2003). Coping with deficits and losses in later life: From compensatory action to accommodation. *Psychology & Aging, 18,* 896–905.

Scherer, K. R., & Brosch, T. (2009). Culture-specific appraisal biases contribute to emotion dispositions. *European Journal of Personality, 23,* 265–88.

Seiffge-Krenke, I. (2004). The long-term impact of functional and dysfunctional coping styles for predicting attachment representation. *Zeitschrift für Medizinische Psychologie, 13,* 37–45.

Seiffge-Krenke, I. (2006). Coping with relationship stressors: the impact of different working models of attachment and links to adaptation. *Journal of Youth and Adolescence, 35,* 25–39.

Shiffman, S., Stone, A. A., & Hufford, M. R. (2008). Ecological momentary assessment. *Annual Review of Clinical Psychology, 4,* 1–32.

Skaff, M. (2007). Sense of control and health: A dynamic duo in the aging process. In C. M. Aldwin, C. L. Park, & A. Spiro III (Eds.), *Handbook of health psychology & aging* (pp. 186–209). New York: Guilford.

Simonich, H., Wonderlich, S., Crosby, R., Smyth, J. M., Thompson, K., Redlin, J., et al. (2004). The use of Ecological Momentary Assessment approaches in the study of sexually abused children. *Child Abuse & Neglect, 28,* 803–9.

Skinner, E. A., Edge, K., Altman, J., & Sherwood, H. (2003). Searching for the structure of coping: A review and critique of category systems for classifying ways of coping. *Psychological Bulletin, 129,* 216–69.

Skinner, E. A., & Zimmer-Gembeck (2009). Challenges to the developmental study of coping. In E. A. Skinner, & M. J. Zimmer-Gembeck, M. J. (Eds.). *Coping and the development of regulation* (pp. 1–17). R. W. Larson & L. A. Jensen (Eds.-in-Chief), *New directions in child and adolescent development.* San Francisco: Jossey-Bass.

Skinner, E. A., & Zimmer-Gembeck, M. J. (2011). Perceived control and the development of coping. In S. Folkman (Ed.), *Oxford handbook of stress, health, and coping.* New York: Oxford University Press.

Smith, C. A., & Kirby, L. D. (2004). Appraisal as a pervasive determinant of anger. *Emotion, 4,* 133–8.

Spirito, A., Stark, L. J., Grace, N., & Stamoulis, D. (1991). Common problems and coping strategies reported in childhood and early adolescence. *Journal of Youth and Adolescence, 20,* 531–44.

Spiro, A. III. (2007). The relevance of a lifespan developmental approach to health. In C. M. Aldwin, C. L. Park, & A. Spiro III (Eds.), *Handbook of health psychology & aging* (pp. 75–93). New York: Guilford.

Spiro, A. III, Schnurr, P., & Aldwin, C. M. (1994). Combat-related PTSD in older men. *Psychology and Aging, 9,* 17–26.

Stanton, A. L. (2011). Regulating emotions during stressful experiences: The adaptive utility of coping through emotional approach. In S. Folkman (Ed.), *Oxford handbook of stress, health, and coping.* New York: Oxford University Press.

Stanton, A. L., Bower, J. E., &. Low, C. A. (2006). Posttraumatic growth after cancer. In L. G. Calhoun & R. G. Tedeschi (Eds.), *Handbook of posttraumatic growth: Research and practice* (pp. 138–75). Mahwah, NJ: Lawrence Erlbaum.

Stanton, A. L., Danoff-Burg, S., Cameron, C.L., & Ellis, A. P. (1994). Coping through emotional approach: Problems of conceptualization and confounding. *Journal of Personality & Social Psychology, 66,* 350–62.

Stawski, R. S., Sliwinski, M. J., Almeida, D. M., & Smyth, J. M. (2008). Reported exposure and emotional reactivity to daily stressors: The roles of adult age and global perceived stress. *Psychology and Aging, 23,* 52–61.

Stroebe, M. (2011). Coping with bereavement. In S. Folkman (Ed.), *Oxford handbook of stress, health, and coping.* New York: Oxford University Press.

Stroebe, M., & Schut, H. (1999). The dual process model of coping with bereavement: rationale and description. *Death Studies, 23,* 197–224.

Stroebe, M. S., & Schut, H. (2001). Meaning making in the Dual Process model of coping with bereavement. In R. A. Neimeyer (Ed.), *Meaning reconstruction & the experience of loss* (pp. 55–73). Washington, DC: American Psychological Association.

Tennen, H., & Affleck, G. (2002). Benefit-finding and benefit-reminding. In C. R. Synder & S. J. Lopes (Eds.), *The handbook of positive psychology* (pp. 584–97). New York: Oxford University Press.

Thoits, P. A. (1986). Social support as coping assistance. *Journal of Consulting and Clinical Psychology, 54,* 416–23.

Vaillant, G. (1977). *Adaptation to life: How the best and the brightest came of age.* Boston: Little Brown.

Vaillant, G. E. (1993). *The wisdom of the ego.* Cambridge, MA: Harvard University Press.

Wadsworth, M. E., Gudmundsen, G. R., Raviv, T., Ahlkvist, J. A., McIntosh, D. N., Kline, G. H., et al. (2004). Coping with terrorism: Age and gender differences in effortful and involuntary responses to September 11th. *Applied Developmental Science, 8,* 143–57.

Walker, L. S., Smith, C. A., Garber, J., & Claar, R. L. (2007). Appraisal and coping with daily stressors by pediatric patients with chronic abdominal pain. *Journal of Pediatric Psychology, 32,* 206–16.

Wallerstein, J. S., & Kelly, J. B. (1980). *Surviving the breakup: How children and parents cope with divorce.* New York: Basic Books.

Walter, C. A., & McCoyd, J. L. M. (2009). *Grief and loss across the lifespan: A biopsychosocial perspective.* New York: Springer Publishing.

Weinstein, S. M., Mermelstein, R. J., Hankin, B. L., Flay, B. R., & Hedeker, D. (2007). Longitudinal patterns of daily affect and global mood during adolescence. *Journal of Research on Adolescence, 17,* 587–600.

Weintraub, D., & Ruskin, P. E. (1999). Posttraumatic stress disorder in the elderly: A review. *Harvard Review of Psychiatry, 7*(3), 144–52.

Wheaton, B. (1996). The nature of chronic stress. In B. H. Gottlieb (Ed.), *Coping with chronic stress* (pp. 343–74). New York: Plenum.

Williams, R. B. (2000). Psychological factors, health, and disease: The impact of aging and the life cycle. In S. B. Manuck, R. Jennings, B. S Rabin, & A. Baum (Eds.), *Behavior, health, and aging* (pp. 135–51). Mahwah, NJ: Lawrence Erlbaum.

Williamson, D. E., Birmaher, B., Ryan, N. D. Shiffrin, T. P., Lusky, J. A., Protopapa, J., et al. (2003). The Stressful Life Events Schedule for children and adolescents: Development and validation. *Psychiatry Research, 119,* 225–41.

Wills, T. A., Sandy, J. M., Yaeger, A. M., Cleary, S. D., & Shinar, O. (2001). Coping dimensions, life stress, and adolescent substance use: A latent growth analysis. *Journal of Abnormal Psychology, 110,* 309–23.

Wolfinger, N. H. (2005). *Understanding the divorce cycle: The children of divorce in their own marriages.* Cambridge, UK: Cambridge University Press.

Wolfradt, U., Hempel, S., & Miles, J. N. V. (2003). Perceived parenting styles, depersonalisation, anxiety and coping behavior in adolescents. *Personality & Individual Differences, 34,* 521–32.

Wrosch, C. (2011). Self-regulation of unattainable goals and pathways to quality of life. In S. Folkman (Ed.), *Oxford handbook of stress, health, & coping.* New York: Oxford University Press.

Yancura, L. A., Aldwin, C. M., & Spiro, A. III. (August 2000). *A longitudinal examination of life events in the Normative Aging Study.* Paper presented at the annual meeting of the American Psychological Association, Washington, DC.

Zautra, A. J. (2003). *Emotions, stress, and health.* Oxford, New York: Oxford University Press, 2003.

Zautra, A. J., Finch, J. F., Reich, J. W., & Guarnaccia, C. A. (1991). Predicting the everyday life events of older adults. *Journal of Personality, 59,* 507–38.

Perceived Control and the Development of Coping

Ellen A. Skinner *and* Melanie J. Zimmer-Gembeck

Abstract

Perceived control is a powerful resource when dealing with stressful life events. Research on perceived control (in all its guises, including locus of control, self-efficacy, causal attributions, confidence, and perceived competence) documents its role in supporting constructive mastery-oriented coping at all points in the lifespan. Likewise, research at every age reveals the vulnerabilities induced by a sense of helplessness and loss of control, and documents their effects in undermining how people deal with difficulties and failures. This chapter uses work on the development of perceived control to help guide the developmental study of coping, examining (1) how mastery-oriented and helpless ways of coping may change in their form across infancy, childhood, adolescence, adulthood, and old age; (2) how the development of perceived control may contribute to qualitative shifts in how coping is organized as people age; and (3) how coping itself may constitute a proximal process that shapes the development of perceived control. Throughout the chapter, a multi-level systems view on the development of coping is highlighted, with a strong emphasis on the role of social partners, relationships, and contexts in shaping both coping and perceived control.

Keywords: perceived control, self-efficacy, coping, aging, social factors

The controllability of stress appears to be information that may be processed at an automatic and a conscious level and serves to shape and organize the ways that individuals mobilize their responses. However, changes in the nature of perceptions of control and the ways in which the objective and perceived controllability shape coping responses across development is not known and is an important agenda for future research.

(Compas, 2009, p. 96)

Fifty years of research have documented the crucial role played by control, both objective and subjective, when people are faced with challenges and difficulties (Bandura, 1997; Dweck, 1999; Folkman, 1984; Lefcourt, 1992; Peterson, Maier, & Seligman, 1993; Seligman, 1975; Skinner, 1995; Taylor & Stanton, 2007; Weiner, 1986). For example, degree of objective controllability is considered a defining characteristic of negative life events, with loss of control one of the few events that researchers acknowledge as universally stressful (Miller, 1979; Thompson, 1981). Even more extensively studied, however, is *perceived* or subjective control, one of the most powerful personal resources that can be called upon in dealing with obstacles or failures (Folkman, 1984; Taylor, 2007). Its salutary effects have been demonstrated across domains and age groups from earliest infancy (Watson, 1966) to oldest age

(Baltes & Baltes, 1986). Multiple programs of research have traced the many pathways by which a sense of control influences reactions to stress, including through physiology, behavior, emotions, energy, attention, motivation, volition, and cognition.

The vast majority of research has focused on individual differences, examining how people who experience differing levels of objective or perceived control behave differently during stressful encounters. This focus meshes well with the majority of research on coping, which also examines individual differences: how people who possess different levels of personal and social resources (e.g., perceived control or social support) show different kinds of coping, and how different kinds of coping contribute to aspects of individual physical, psychological, and social functioning (Aldwin, 2007; Compas et al., 2001; Folkman & Moskowitz, 2004). Many fewer studies have considered the development of either control or coping, at least partly because the work on individual differences seems so unequivocal: The benefits of perceived control when dealing with stress are found at all ages.

However, at a general level, researchers also agree that every aspect of how individuals detect and respond to stress is shaped by their developmental level (Aldwin, 2007; Compas, 1998; Garmezy & Rutter, 1983; Murphy & Moriarity, 1976; Skinner & Zimmer-Gembeck, 2007). For example, infants, children, adolescents, adults, and the elderly differ in the kinds of encounters they experience as stressful, in the nature of their appraisals, in their repertoires of potential coping responses, and in the role played by social partners. All these processes should show age-graded shifts, at least up until early adulthood, and potentially across the lifespan (Aldwin, 2007). At the same time, however, researchers have noted the difficulty of realizing a developmental agenda for the study of coping (Compas, 1998, 2009; Coping Consortium, 1998, 2001; Fields & Prinz, 1997; Skinner & Edge, 1998; Skinner & Zimmer-Gembeck, 2007, 2009), precisely because coping reflects a higher-order construct, integrating work on a variety of processes involved in detecting and responding to challenges, threats, and losses.

The goal of this chapter is to use research on the development of perceived control to serve as a scaffold for work on the development of coping. Although most studies of control, like most studies of coping, have focused on individual differences, pockets of research have examined age-graded shifts in many of the processes used for perceiving and interpreting control experiences (e.g., Flammer,

1995; Gurin & Brim, 1984; Heckhausen, 1982, 1984; Skinner & Connell, 1986; Skinner, Zimmer-Gembeck, & Connell, 1998; Wang & Pomerantz, 2009; Weisz, 1980, 1986; Wigfield et al., 2006; Wigfield & Eccles, 2002). Taken together, they suggest fundamental and systematic shifts at many ages, for example, in the kinds of information used to infer control, in the strategies used to exert control, in the understanding of the causes of control (e.g., effort, task difficulty, luck, ability), and even in the nature of the self to which control is attributed (Flammer, 1995; Skinner, 1995; Weisz, 1986). Hence, a careful consideration of developmental shifts in control, which is a reliably robust contributor to coping, might help map out some key developmental landmarks in coping processes.

This chapter is organized in four sections. After providing an overview of current multi-level systems conceptualizations of coping and a brief summary of the nature and terminology of control, we use research on the development of control to explore three issues: (1) how mastery-oriented and helpless ways of coping change in their form across infancy, childhood, adolescence, adulthood, and old age; (2) how the development of perceived control contributes to qualitative shifts in organization of coping as people age; and (3) how coping itself may constitute a proximal process that shapes the development of perceived control. Running throughout the chapter is a strong emphasis on the role of social partners, relationships, and contexts in shaping both coping and perceived control.

Multi-level Systems Views of Coping

At the core of the study of coping are the ways that people actually react to and deal with real stressors in their daily lives. As a result, the building blocks of the area are "ways of coping," including constructive responses, such as problem-solving, effort exertion, help-seeking, distraction, or accommodation, as well as maladaptive responses, such as helplessness, escape, opposition, social isolation, or rumination. A focus on actual stressful interactions means that the study of coping has the potential to add value to work on risk and resilience by investigating how overarching risk factors may (or may not) produce daily encounters with stress, and how individuals' everyday dealings with stress may (or may not) contribute cumulatively to lasting resources and vulnerabilities (Coping Consortium, 1998, 2001). Moreover, because coping entails a repertoire of responses, its study has the potential to integrate research across a range of individual responses to stress, such as help-seeking or rumination, which typically have been studied in relative isolation from each other (Coping Consortium, 1998, 2001).

Although ways of coping are a defining feature of research in the area, systems conceptualizations point out that these ways, even though expressed by individuals, are actually a function of the entire transactional "coping system" in which the individual is embedded. A schematic of the coping system can be seen in the middle portion of Figure 3.1. This system includes many interacting components, such as the nature of the stressor itself (e.g., its actual severity and controllability), the context in which the encounter takes place, the appraisal of what is at stake, and the personal and social resources available to the individual when dealing with the event (Lazarus & Folkman, 1984). In addition, coping episodes unfold over time, so previous encounters and ongoing iterations influence how people deal with both novel and recurrent stressors (Folkman & Lazarus, 1985).

At the same time, as also depicted in Figure 3.1, coping can be considered part of a multi-level process that extends from conditions of risk and resilience at the highest level to individual moment-to-moment transactions with stressors at the lowest level (Coping Consortium, 1998, 2001). As shown in the top portion of Figure 3.1, coping can be viewed as an adaptive process that potentially mediates the effects of risk or adversity on the development of competence. So within the larger frame of work on risk and resilience, coping can be considered a "proximal process" or driver of development under conditions of adversity (Bronfenbrenner & Morris, 1998). At the same time, as shown in the bottom portion of Figure 3.1, coping episodes can be decomposed into individual stressful encounters that take place in real time and are shaped by the actions of particular social partners as well as by the subsystems that give rise to specific individual reactions, such as physiology, emotion, attention, cognition, motivation, and behavior. At this level, coping overlaps with work on regulation, specifically the study of regulation under stressful conditions (Compas, 2009; Eisenberg, Fabes, & Guthrie, 1997; Eisenberg, Valiente, & Sulik, 2009; Skinner & Zimmer-Gembeck, 2009).

Such a multi-level view has been used by theorists to describe the place and purpose of research on coping with respect to work on resilience (which takes place at a higher level) and work on regulation (which takes place at a lower level) (Skinner, 1999). Researchers point out the requirements that such a task places on conceptualizations of coping, but also highlight the potential of coping to contribute to the integration of a range of theories, methodologies, and findings relevant to understanding how individual development is shaped by stress and adversity, work that currently inhabits a variety of niches distributed across all of psychology (Coping Consortium, 1998, 2001).

Nature of Control and Control Constructs

In attempting to use research on the development of control to inform work on coping, it is important to be clear about the nature and functioning of control. Because the area of control is so fertile, it has supported research on a variety of constructs, including locus of control (Lefcourt, 1992; Rotter, 1966; Strickland, 1989), expectancies of success (Wigfield & Eccles, 2000), causal attributions (Weiner, 2005), learned helplessness (Seligman, 1975), self-efficacy (Bandura, 1997), mastery (Dweck, 1999), and perceived competence (Harter, 2006). (See Heckhausen, 1991; Stipek, 2002; or Wigfield et al., 2006, for more details.) On the one hand, the simultaneous investigation of these overlapping processes has produced a mature understanding of the antecedents, consequences, and mechanisms of control across multiple domains and age groups. On the other hand, the profusion of constructs has made it difficult to judge the validity of competing claims or even to discern the boundaries of the field of control itself (Skinner, 1996).

The nature of control

Although consensus is not complete, a generally accepted assumption in the area is that the power of control to organize human behavior is based on the fact that all people (and many other species) come with a fundamental psychological need to be effective in their interactions with the environment (Connell & Wellborn, 1990; Deci & Ryan, 1985; Elliot & Dweck, 2005; Elliot, McGregor, & Thrash, 2002; Harter, 1978; Koestner & McClelland, 1990; Skinner, 1995). Referred to as the need for effectance, competence, or control, this idea was first articulated in the psychological literature in 1959 by Robert White, who assembled a wide range of observations and research suggesting humans possess an intrinsic desire to create effects in the environment, apparent, for example, in infants' delight in making things rattle and fall. White's insight—that this motive offers an adaptive edge because people are naturally motivated to discover how the world works and how their actions can be effective—has proven durable. Successive generations

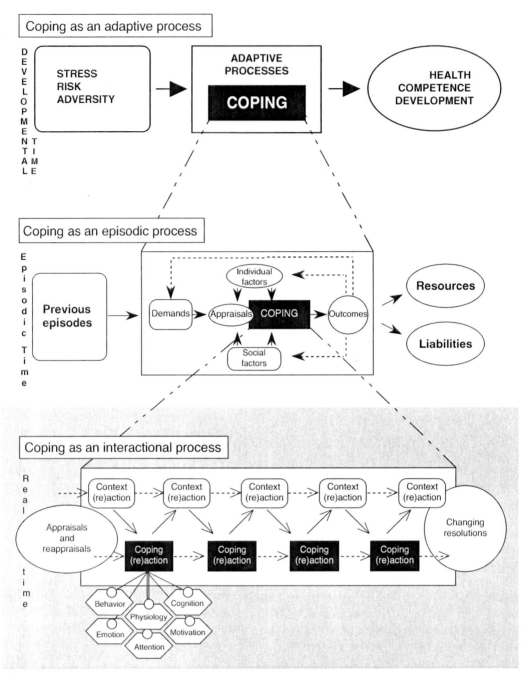

Fig. 3.1 A model of coping as a multi-level adaptive system operating (top) as an adaptive process across developmental time, (middle) as an episodic process across episodic time, and (bottom) as an interactional process across real time. (Reprinted, with permission, from the *Annual Review of Psychology*, Vol. 58, 2007.)

of researchers have shown how species-wide human neurophysiology supports this motivation, providing energy and effort focused on producing desired and preventing undesired outcomes, and leading to joy upon creating effects and dejection at non-contingency and loss of control (e.g., Amat et al., 2007; Gunnar & Quevado, 2007; Watson & Ramey, 1972).

Terminology of control

Hence, at the core of control is the experience of exerting effort that produces a desired outcome (Skinner, 1996). Also referred to as *generative transmission* or *personal force*, these *experiences of control* or *mastery* can be distinguished from objective and subjective control. *Objective control conditions* refer to the actual controllability of outcomes, usually depicted by the objective contingencies in the environment (the conditional probability of an outcome given action compared to the probability of an outcome given no action) and the actual competencies of the actor (Seligman, 1977). Careful experimental studies of objective non-contingency have been able to uncover the neurological and hormonal pathways by which it shapes stress responses, and have shown that its deleterious effects can be found across a range of mammalian species (Maier & Watkins, 2005).

Subjective control refers to perceived control or the actor's estimations of the control available to him or her. Most theories in the area are focused on perceived control, and so their names refer to facets of subjective control: an overall sense of control (e.g., expectancies of success, control beliefs), beliefs about available contingencies (e.g., locus of control, causal attributions, learned helplessness, strategy beliefs), or beliefs about one's access to effective means (e.g., self-efficacy, perceived competence, perceived ability, capacity beliefs). In discussions of whether more control is better, these different kinds of control are often confused. Mastery experiences have consistently been found to result in a range of physiological and psychological benefits. However, although objective control and subjective control usually produce positive effects, they do not always. For example, sometimes the availability of control can prove to be coercive—pressuring people to exert effort or to engage with stressors when they might prefer not to.

Individual Differences in Control and Coping

All three kinds of control, that is, objective, subjective, and experiences of control—shape coping (Folkman, 1984). *Objective* controllability is a defining feature of the stressors to which individuals are exposed (Seligman, 1975). When examining coping, researchers are usually careful to distinguish situations that are objectively uncontrollable from those that are open to influence (Compas et al., 1991). Controllability matters, whether the event is relatively trivial and short-lived (e.g., going to the dentist or giving a report in front of the class) or more chronic and potentially life-changing (e.g., parents' divorce or life-threatening illness). In fact, a key difference between stressors appraised as challenge, threat, or loss is the degree of controllability, with loss events by definition offering no possibility of reversing the outcome (Lazarus & Folkman, 1984).

Subjective control describes an important personal resource individuals draw upon in forming appraisals and planning actions (Dweck, 1999; Folkman, 1984). It is the conduit by which objective control conditions shape coping (Abramson, Seligman, & Teasdale, 1978). In contrast to objective and subjective control, *experiences* of control describe the coping process itself: Mastery refers to coping episodes in which problem-solving efforts are deployed, and in which, over time, desired outcomes are produced and undesired ones are prevented or terminated. In the same vein, helplessness describes coping experiences in which attempts to influence the outcome do not produce their desired effects.

Control and the dynamics of coping

The effects of control are apparent at every point in the coping process (Dweck, 1999; Folkman, 1984; Skinner, 1995; Wigfield et al., 2006). When events are objectively controllable or when individuals have high confidence and efficacy, they are more likely to expect to be effective in stressful situations and so to appraise negative events as challenges rather than threats. They approach tasks with concentration and vigor, break them into manageable sequential parts, and employ a variety of alternative strategies. They look for action opportunities as events unfold, and remain focused on problem solutions. They maintain access to their cognitive resources and so perform close to the ceiling of their capacity. They show flexible and creative problem-solving, and seek help when needed. Regulation is constructive—that is, focused on generating strategies and shaping actions to be effective. People collect information about potential contingencies, viewing even failed attempts as instructive. They show more planning and proactive coping, taking preemptive actions. This pattern of coping is likely to be more successful in actually dealing with stressful situations, and even when problems are not immediately solvable, produces gains in knowledge and skills. Over time, these coping episodes augment actual competence and may even reduce the likelihood of subsequent encounters with stressful events, both of which in the long run bolster a sense of control (e.g., Schmitz & Skinner, 1993).

Processes of helplessness have also been studied in detail (Dweck, 1999; Peterson et al., 1993). People who are exposed to uncontrollable events, who feel incompetent, or who believe that events are contingent on unknown or uncontrollable causes (like powerful others, chance, luck, or fate) seem to be debilitated by obstacles or failures. They are more upset and show greater involuntary stress reactions. They appraise events as more threatening and tend to procrastinate or give up quickly. They lose focus and concentration, becoming distracted by self-doubt, rumination about failure, and worries about lack of ability. These preoccupations rob them of their previous skills at hypothesis-testing and strategizing (Dweck, 1999), resulting in more rigid problem-solving, passivity, confusion, escape, or help avoidance. This pattern of coping is not effective in dealing with stressors or learning from mistakes, and interferes with the development of actual skills and competencies, even making future stressors more likely (Downey, Freitas, Michaelis, & Khouri, 1998). In the long run, such experiences cement pessimism and expectations of future helplessness (e.g., Nolen-Hoeksma, Girgus, & Seligman, 1986).

As can be seen, these dynamics are amplifying. Individuals who are initially high on perceived control, through the ways they engage with problems, become even more competent and efficacious, whereas individuals who initially doubt their capacity to influence events, through their ineffectual handling of challenges, become even less competent and more helpless. Such cycles, if they iterate over time, can magnify initial individual differences, making the rich richer and the poor even poorer, and transforming subjective control to objective control. Taken together with information about objective control conditions (actual stressors and difficulties) and social supports, these dynamics can provide one account of the development of individual differences in perceived control, competence, and patterns of coping with stress (Seligman, 1975; Skinner et al., 1998).

Developmental Conceptualizations of Coping

It has proven surprisingly difficult to move beyond research on individual differences in coping in order to focus on the study of its development. A developmental agenda calls for research that identifies age-graded shifts in how infants, children, youth, adults, and the elderly detect, appraise, and respond to actual stressful events in their everyday lives, and would depict the underlying developments responsible for these changes (Compas, 1998, 2009; Murphy & Moriarity, 1976; Skinner & Edge, 1998; Skinner & Zimmer-Gembeck, 2007). In making progress on this agenda, researchers have had to construct "developmentally friendly" conceptualiza-

tions that link coping to basic adaptive processes. An important step in this regard has been consensus that coping can be considered "regulation under stress" (Compas et al., 2001; Eisenberg et al., 1997, 2009; Skinner & Zimmer-Gembeck, 2007). From this perspective, coping refers to how people mobilize, coordinate, manage, and direct their actions (including behavior, emotion, attention, cognition, and physiology) under conditions of challenge, threat, or loss. This definition establishes links between coping and the normative development of emotional, attentional, and behavioral regulation as well as the underlying constitutional and social factors that shape their development.

A second important step has been the use of overarching families to help organize the seemingly endless lists of ways of coping that have been studied to date (Skinner, Edge, Altman, & Sherwood, 2003). It has proven impossible to integrate studies of coping across (or even within) age groups because assessments utilize a wide variety of disparate and partially overlapping categories of coping (Compas et al., 2001; Zimmer-Gembeck & Skinner, in press). Analyses of their multiple functions allow ways of coping to be classified into about a dozen families that serve three major adaptive functions (Table 3.1). The major adaptive function of the ways of coping organized around control is to find actions that are effective in operating contingencies in the environment. The four families that serve this function are: (1) *problem-solving*, which allows people to generate and adjust their actions so that they are effective; (2) *information-seeking*, which allows people to discover new contingencies in the environment; (3) *helplessness*, which identifies the limits of effective action; and (4) *escape*, which is an extreme form of avoidance that allows people to leave, distance themselves from, or deny non-contingent environments.

Each of these families contains many ways of coping in addition to the one used as its label. For example, "problem-solving" includes all ways of coping that serve the function of adjusting actions to be more effective, such as effort exertion, persistence, instrumental action, strategizing, planning, active attempts, and so on. Likewise, "information-seeking" includes many ways of collecting knowledge about how to produce desired and prevent undesired events, including asking others, looking up information in reference sources, direct observation of others' performances, reading, experimentation, and so on. These four families of coping have been the subject of intense scrutiny: Within research on coping, they are some of the most common ways

Table 3.1 A hierarchical model of adaptive processes and families of coping

Adaptive Process #1: Coordinate Actions and Contingencies in the Environment

Family of Coping	1. Problem-solving	2. Information-Seeking	3. Helplessness	4. Escape
Family Function in Adaptive Process	Adjust actions to be effective	Find additional contingencies	Find limits of actions	Escape non-contingent environments
Ways of Coping	Strategizing Instrumental action Planning Mastery	Reading Observation Asking others	Confusion Cognitive interference Cognitive exhaustion Passivity	Behavioral avoidance Mental withdrawal Flight Denial Wishful thinking

Adaptive Process #2: Coordinate Reliance and Social Resources Available

Family of Coping	5. Self-reliance	6. Support-Seeking	7. Delegation	8. Social Isolation
Family Function in Adaptive Process	Protect available social resources	Use available social resources	Find limits of resources	Withdraw from unsupportive contexts
Ways of Coping	Emotion regulation Behavior regulation Emotional expression Emotion approach	Contact-seeking Comfort-seeking Instrumental aid Social referencing	Maladaptive help-seeking Complaining Whining Self-pity	Social withdrawal Concealment Avoiding others Freeze

Adaptive Process #3: Coordinate Preferences and Available Options

Family of Coping	9. Accommodation	10. Negotiation	11. Submission	12. Opposition
Family Function in Adaptive Process	Flexibly adjust preferences to options	Find new options	Give up preferences	Remove constraints
Ways of Coping	Distraction Cognitive restructuring Minimization Acceptance	Bargaining Persuasion Priority-setting	Rumination Rigid perseveration Intrusive thoughts	Other-blame Projection Aggression Defiance

studied and some of the most common reactions to stress (Skinner et al., 2003). Within the area of control, they are the operational definitions of mastery and helplessness. These families represent complete overlap between the areas of coping and control and so are the primary ways of coping considered in this chapter.

Perceived Control and the Development of Ways of Coping

The first way that research on perceived control may be able to contribute to developmental studies of coping is to reveal how mastery-oriented and helpless ways of coping change in their form across infancy, childhood, adolescence, adulthood, and old age. The analysis of overarching functions of coping families marks the beginning of such a catalog. Functions can be used to identify corresponding lower-order ways of coping that, despite their apparent topological differences, are developmentally graded members of the same family. Functional analyses have been used in work on emotion and attachment to show that a variety of forms of action (such as crying, calling, and crawling to a caregiver) fall within the same category because they serve the same function (in this case, proximity-seeking) (Cassidy, 1994; Cassidy & Shaver, 1999). The identification of functionally analogous categories allows a phenomenon to be followed across developmental periods even if it changes its form. A consideration of the action outcomes of perceived control at successive ages may be helpful in identifying functionally analogous ways of coping for the families of problem-solving, information-seeking, helplessness, and escape.

Perceived control and coping during infancy

Newborns react to stressors based on their species' general stress physiology and their temperamental characteristics (Derryberry et al., 2003; Gunnar & Quevado, 2007). Generally, infants come with the capacity to detect action-outcome contingencies and to respond to them with interest and energy (Papousek & Papousek, 1979; Watson, 1966). At the same time, there also seem to be inborn individual differences in sensitivity to contingencies, interest in creating effects, focus of attention, and intensity of emotional responsiveness to contingent stimulation. Studied individually as dimensions of temperament or collectively as mastery motivation (Morgan & Harmon, 1984), such differences have been documented in the first months of life (Rueda & Rothbart, 2009).

Critical to understanding perceived control in infancy is the recognition that the earliest experiences of control are created by caregivers when they show sensitive responsiveness to infants' signals (Davidov & Grusec, 2006; Lamb & Easterbrooks, 1981; Landry, Smith, & Swank, 2006; Papousek & Papousek, 1980). Social partners can provide contingency long before infants have the motor coordination to create effects in the physical world. Control experiences (and early coping) for infants consist of sending out distress signals, and gaining confidence that caregivers will soon respond with appropriate comforting actions. The same experiences that promote a sense of control also promote a secure attachment, and such attachments have been shown to buffer stress and shape the development of stress reactions, including physiological ones, starting at birth (Nachmias, Gunnar, Mangelsdorf, Parritz, & Buss, 1996).

The earliest forms of stress reactions are based on reflexes and temperament, but they are soon supplemented by action schemes, such as directing bids or shaping the distress signals sent to caregivers (Barrett & Campos, 1991; Kopp, 1989). If caregiver reactions are not forthcoming, efforts are normally intensified (Goldstein, Bornstein, & Schwade, 2009). In terms of creating contingencies in the physical world, early object play involves repetition and "practice" creating desired effects, such as shaking rattles or hitting dangling toys (Piaget, 1976). Early forms of information-seeking may include social referencing, in which infants study their caregivers for signs communicating the severity and emotional significance of novel or stressful events (Diamond & Aspinwall, 2003; Hornik, Risenhoover, & Gunnar, 1987; Lewis & Ramsay, 1999; Sorce et al., 1985). Infants use this information to guide their actions, deciding, for example, whether to continue into a potentially dangerous situation or to scoot back to the caregiver. Other early forms of information-seeking may include object play, in which the various potentials of an object are explored, and "learning by doing," in which infants successively try out multiple variants on an action, such as banging a spoon with varying amounts of force (Piaget, 1976).

The earliest forms of helplessness usually involve passivity in the face of objectively controllable events, and may also involve protest and other forms of emotional distress (Watson & Ramey, 1972). When infants are passive, they create fewer action-event contingencies. Moreover, learned helplessness implies that they also pay less attention to effects that are created, and so are less sensitive to detecting existing contingencies. In terms of escape, its prototypical expression involves leaving the stressful situation, and so is most obvious after an infant can locomote. Nevertheless, prior to independent locomotion, infants can express the desire to escape by reaching for the caregiver (Robinson & Acevedo, 2001) or leaning/looking away from an event (Gianino & Tronick, 1988). They may also escape through gaze aversion, head turning, or sleep (Kopp, 1989; Kopp & Neufeld, 2003; Mangelsdorf, Shapiro, & Marzolf, 1995).

Perceived control and coping during preschool age

Ages 2 to 5 bring a major shift in children's action potential. For the first time, they become able to intentionally direct their own behaviors, stopping themselves from doing things they spontaneously want to do and making themselves do things they do not really want to (Kochanska, Coy, & Murray, 2005). This expands their repertoire of effective actions and allows them to be more self-reliant in producing desired effects. Temperament continues to play a role, with children higher in emotional reactivity less able to regulate and children higher in effortful control more able to regulate their behaviors of their own accord (Kochanska, Aksan, & Carlson, 2005). Information-seeking can also become more intentional. Preschool-age children can pose explicit requests to adults and peers, asking for information about what to do when faced with obstacles and difficulties (Kerns et al., 2006).

Young children still rely on caregivers and adults in stressful situations, but with enough support they are often able to carry out effective actions on their own (Bronson, 2000). At the same time, however, the severity of the stressful event and the quality of adult participation determine whether children will be able to act effectively in a given situation (Kopp, 2009). Joint problem-solving with caring adults likely represents the kind of coping episodes out of which a repertoire of adaptive strategies, as well as confidence and actual competence, emerge (Kopp, 2009).

At this age, helplessness and escape take on their prototypical forms (Burhans & Dweck, 1995). Compared to mastery-oriented children, young children with low perceived control show less persistence, focus, and concentration on difficult tasks, and try out less sophisticated hypothesis-testing strategies. In terms of escape, they stop working as soon as possible and select easier future tasks. Although there was initially some speculation that young children might be less vulnerable to helplessness than older children, subsequent research has demonstrated that preschool-age children, given appropriate tasks and concrete evidence of failure, show full-blown helplessness effects, including behavioral, emotional, and self-derogatory components (e.g., Boggiano et al., 1993).

It is important to note that the development of coping strategies seems to be cumulative (Zimmer-Gembeck & Skinner, in press)—that is, there is no evidence that, as new ways of coping emerge, old strategies disappear. For example, as young children become able to intentionally deploy actions and explicitly request information, they nevertheless continue to have access to action schema that served them as infants, such as direct action, effort exertion, expressions of distress, direct observation of others, and social referencing. In this way, coping repertoires are expanded and may become more organized and integrated, although few studies of coping have empirically examined this possibility (Zimmer-Gembeck & Skinner, in press).

Perceived control and coping during childhood

A major shift taking place between ages 5 and 7 is the development of problem-solving that is largely cognitive in nature (Sameroff & Haith, 1996)—that is, children are better able to imagine the effects of different strategies, and then select the one they think is most likely to be effective, without needing to actually try them out on the plane of action (Piaget, 1976). This expands coping possibilities, saving children a great deal of time and energy, by bringing strategies forward from previous episodes and by avoiding potential failures and negative social reactions. Children are also increasingly able to use cognitive means of information-seeking, for example reading, even though social means of information-seeking are still preferred, including going to adults for advice and, for specific issues, turning to peers (Zimmer-Gembeck & Skinner, 2008, in press).

The use of cognition to organize coping responses opens the way for adaptive strategies, but it can also play a role in the creation of helplessness. During middle childhood, children's cognitive expectancies become important and stubborn drivers of action (Dweck, 1999). If children believe they have little or no control (Carpenter, 1992) or are given less objective control over a stressor (Manne et al., 1992), they manage stressful events less competently (see Miller et al., 1999, for a review). As a result, children's cognitions interfere with the production of evidence that would disconfirm their expectations of helplessness. Escape can also take cognitive forms. In addition to physically escaping situations in which they do not expect to succeed, children increasingly escape via cognitive means, such as daydreaming or withdrawal of mental effort (Zimmer-Gembeck & Skinner, in press). These forms of escape may be less disruptive than physical attempts to leave (in the classroom, for example), but they are also harder to detect, which means that they can impede teachers' and other adults' attempts to remedy them.

Perceived control and coping during adolescence

A major shift during adolescence is the potential for youth to use meta-cognitive strategies when dealing with challenges and failures (Kuhn & Franklin, 2006; see Compas et al., 2001, for a review). Meta-cognition, or the capacity to reflect on one's own cognitive processes, emotions, and actions, provides at least two advantages to coping. First, it allows a teenager to use information about the long-term effects of a course of action in making local decisions about which strategy to use in solving a problem. The capacity to imagine future emotional and social consequences of an action extends the potential effectiveness of coping beyond the current episode (Aspinwall & Taylor, 1997). Second, meta-cognition allows adolescents to coordinate multiple perspectives and alternative pathways in deciding how to deal with a challenge or setback. They can comfort themselves using largely cognitive means—such as telling themselves that a depressed mood is only temporary—and can coordinate their own wishes and desires with those of others in their problem-solving (e.g., Band & Weisz, 1990). Although representations of attachment figures play a role in stress reactions beginning in infancy (Lewis & Ramsay, 1999; Nachmias et al., 1996; Urban, Carlson, Egeland, & Sroufe, 1991), adolescents have the potential to construct even more advanced and coherent representations of others as available and secure sources of comfort and aid. Hence, adolescents' cognitive representations can serve as stronger and more durable sources of support when others are not physically present, alleviating distress and allowing adolescents to better focus their coping actions (Seiffge-Krenke, 2004; Shaver, Belsky, & Brennan, 2000).

Consistent with growth in meta-cognitive strategies, adolescents experience other cognitive advances that expand their capacity to manage daily stressors and major life events. These include abstract rather than concrete representations, improvements in working memory capacity, the ability to engage in multidimensional thinking, and a greater capacity for self-reflection (Keating, 1999). Moreover, based on practical experiences, adolescents also gain knowledge in a range of content areas, including knowledge about stressful events, controllability, and coping, which assists them to automatize their responses or to more easily recognize the most salient cues and draw upon their knowledge of relevant and useful responses. By having the background knowledge and the capacity to think about multiple dimensions and self-reflect, adolescents often show signs of broader conceptual reorganizations (Case, 1985; Case, Hayward, Lewis, & Hurst, 1988), and they are more likely to use their new abilities to adopt the perspectives of others, to negotiate and accommodate, and to consider multiple solutions to their problems (Seiffge-Krenke, 2004).

The use of meta-cognitive strategies and other advances in thinking can have drawbacks, too. The same skills that permit adolescents to imagine long-term consequences and think about multiple aspects of phenomena also permit them to worry about the future and imagine negative outcomes and failures. They are more likely than children to ruminate and worry excessively (Zimmer-Gembeck & Skinner, in press). The inferential power of adolescents also allows them to become stuck within a mindset of helplessness (Dweck, 2002). Once an adolescent views himself or herself as incompetent, even multiple experiences of success can be discounted using inferential tactics—deciding that high performance is due to luck, easy tasks, or the favor of powerful others. The capacity to take multiple perspectives can also be deployed to evade detection when escaping, whether that be via actual physical escape (like skipping school) or procrastination (like delaying household chores). Adolescents also have greater access to and participate in some potentially detrimental escape coping behaviors, such as binge drinking, other drug use, or risky sexual behavior, and they report that they do so in order to cope with stress (Frydenberg & Lewis, 2000).

Perceived control and coping during adulthood

Compared with childhood and adolescence, age-graded shifts in the means of exerting control are not as well documented during adulthood (Baltes & Baltes, 1986; Lachman & Prenda-Firth, 2004;

Wolinsky et al., 2003; Zarit, Pearlin, & Schaie, 2003). However, it is assumed that as adults develop domain-specific expertise, they will be more effective in problem-solving and strategizing. One possible new skill is the capacity to integrate and prioritize competing demands (Deci & Ryan, 1985). This would allow people to recognize situations in which different facets of themselves are pulling for different strategies, and to use their genuine priorities to sort out the right course of action for themselves to use in dealing with challenges or failures. This might help explain individuals' increasing capacity to decline to employ the most effective strategy for producing a given outcome, if the strategy has negative side effects, for example, if it violates their own moral code or inflicts harm on someone else (Deci & Ryan, 1985, 2000).

During adulthood and old age, changes in how control is exerted seem to be less a function of age and more a function of social structure and the nature of events that are encountered (Aldwin, Sutton, Chiara, & Spiro, 1996; Heckhausen & Schulz, 1998; Zarit et al., 2003). So, for example, social and biological timelines seem to shape individuals' control efforts, with increased activity immediately prior to a developmental deadline (such as childbearing age) and activities focused on devaluing the outcome once the deadline has passed (Schulz, Wrosch, & Heckhausen, 2003). Despite researchers' assumptions that biological and cognitive declines in old age should result in more helplessness and maladaptive coping, empirical evidence contradicts this idea, leading researchers to focus on the capacities of the elderly to deal with objective losses without falling into helplessness (Aldwin, 2007). Moreover, although so far no evidence suggests that it is age-graded, the emergence of wisdom and spiritual developments during adulthood and old age would be likely to reorganize people's coping strategies (Baltes & Staudinger, 1995), including problem-solving and information-seeking, as well as potentially reducing helplessness and the desire for escape.

Summary of developmentally graded ways of coping organized around control

Development decisively constrains the expression of the four families of coping organized around adjusting actions to be effective in producing desired outcomes. The limited repertoire of infants involves reflexes, temperamental preferences, and action schema. However, if infants have responsive caregivers, their joint coping repertoire is expanded greatly.

Infants learn in the first days of life whether their expressed desires create changes in the world. This discovery, the origins of a sense of control, can provide motivation for efforts to deploy increasingly more differentiated and appropriate signals when distressed (Holodynski & Friedlmeier, 2006). Such experiences actually reduce reactivity in stress physiology and prepare the infant to be more curious and active in subsequent interactions with the social and physical world.

Consistent with research on regulation, research on control suggests that general mechanisms of coping accumulate developmentally, for example, adding regulation via *action schemes* during infancy, supplemented by coping through *direct action* during preschool age, coping using *cognitive means* during middle childhood, and coping using *metacognitive means* during adolescence (Table 3.2; Skinner & Zimmer-Gembeck, 2007). Perhaps these means of coping continue to be integrated and elaborated during adulthood, becoming more selective and flexible, at the same time that the development of domain-specific expertise enriches coping capacity in selected areas. The entire repertoire will be needed to deal adaptively with the normative challenges of aging (Aldwin, 2007).

These developmental phases are accompanied by different kinds of participation by social partners. During infancy, caregivers carry out coping actions based on the expressed intentions of their infants. During toddlerhood and preschool age, children directly enlist the participation of social partners. During middle childhood, children are increasingly able to coordinate their coping efforts with those of others, consulting both peers and adults. By adolescence, social partners are a backup system, with much of their functioning expressed through the internalization of values and guides by the adolescent. During adulthood, individuals create their own dyadic and family-level coping systems to which they contribute and that shape their own stress reactions and coping (Berg et al., 1998). During later life, the loss of social partners and roles requires significant adjustment to maintain high-quality coping, and constructive help from social partners (e.g., an aging spouse, siblings, or adult children) is an important interpersonal resource for coping (Aldwin et al., 2009; Zarit et al., 2003). Throughout the lifespan, reliance on others when dealing with stressful life events is both normative and adaptive (Newman, 2000). In fact, learning to "cope well with others" is an important developmental task at every age (Berg et al., 1998).

Table 3.2   Broad outlines of possible developmental shifts in means of coping

Developmental Period	Approximate Ages	Nature of Coping	Role of Social Partners	Nature of Regulation
Infancy	Birth to 18 months	From reflexes to coordinated *action schema*	Carry out coping actions based on infant's expressed intentions	Interpersonal co-regulation
Preschool age	Ages 2 to 5	Coping using voluntary *direct actions*	Available for direct help and participation	Intrapersonal self-regulation
Middle childhood	Ages 6 to 8	Coping using *cognitive means*	Cooperate with and support child's coping efforts	Coordinated self-regulation
Early adolescence	Ages 10 to 12	Coping using *meta-cognitive means*	Reminder coping	Proactive self-regulation
Middle adolescence	Ages 14 to 16	Coping based on *personal values*	Backup coping	Identified self-regulation
Late adolescence	Ages 18 to 22	Coping based on *long-term goals*	Monitoring coping	Integrated self-regulation

Development of Perceived Control and Age-Graded Shifts in Coping

The second way that work on perceived control may be able guide the developmental study of coping is to use research on age changes in the processes of perceiving and interpreting control experiences to identify developmental periods marked by qualitative changes, and to explore whether they correspond to landmark shifts in processes of coping. In examining the development of perceived control, researchers find it useful to organize the variety of constructs populating the area according to the functions they serve in an action sequence, such as a coping transaction (Heckhausen, 1991; Skinner, 1995). Beliefs that come into play *prior* to the initiation of action can be thought of as regulatory beliefs; beliefs that make sense of action sequences *after* they have occurred can be referred to as interpretative beliefs. Regulatory beliefs launch and guide coping; they shape whether and how people approach and engage in a stressful transaction. The beliefs that regulate action are *control beliefs* or the sense that "I can do it." Variously labeled as perceived control, sense of control, expectancies of success, and self-efficacy, these constructs refer to generalized expectations that the self can produce desired and prevent undesired outcomes.

After performance outcomes, individuals employ interpretative beliefs to translate the causal meaning of the action episode. These include people's explanations about the likely causes of desired and unde-sired events (also called *strategy* beliefs), as well as people's explanations about their own role in producing success or failure (also known as *capacity* beliefs). Strategy beliefs refer to generalized expectancies about the effectiveness of certain causes (such as effort, ability, powerful others, luck, and unknown); they are similar to locus of control, causal attributions, explanatory style, or response-outcome expectancies. Capacity beliefs refer to generalized expectancies about the extent to which the self possesses or has access to potentially effective causes; they are similar to self-efficacy, perceived competence, or perceived ability (Connell, 1985; Skinner, 1995, 1996; Weisz, 1986). Both strategy and capacity beliefs are important in interpreting the meaning of a causal episode. For example, individuals may believe that effort is a good *strategy* for success, but doubt that they have the personal *capacity* to exert effort. Unknown strategy beliefs, or the conviction that one has no idea how to succeed, are some of the most pernicious and maladaptive beliefs people can hold and, developmentally, some of the earliest predictors of helplessness (Connell, 1985).

Profiles of control

Patterns of perceived control can be identified that are powerful predictors of motivation, performance, and coping. Optimal profiles include high control expectancies, high beliefs in effort as a strategy, and high confidence in one's own capacities, combined with low dependence on uncontrollable strategies (such as ability, powerful others, luck, and unknown). In contrast, the most maladaptive profile incorporates a low generalized sense of control, low beliefs in effort as an effective strategy, and low confidence in one's own capacities, combined with high reliance on uncontrollable strategies. Aggregate scores created to reflect these profiles in the academic domain are strong predictors of engagement, achievement, and eventually retention or dropout, all the way from elementary to high school (e.g., Connell et al., 1994, 1996; Skinner et al., 1998).

Developmental course of perceived control

Distinguishing among these different kinds of beliefs has been important for research on development because different aspects of perceived control show different patterns of age-graded change[1] (Skinner et al., 1988). In general, young children's beliefs start out optimistic, undifferentiated, and unrealistic, in that their outcome expectations are much higher than their actual levels of performance would warrant (Stipek et al., 1992). It is as if young children have an amalgamated sense of personal force, which incorporates not only actual effectiveness but also the intensity of their wishes and desires. At the most general level, normative development involves successively differentiating other important causes from this amalgam, coming to recognize, for example, the roles played by other people, task difficulty, luck, and ability (Weisz, 1980, 1981, 1986). Children become more effective agents as they increasingly understand how outcomes are shaped by the interplay among multiple necessary and sufficient causes. In this sense, normative change is a series of developments leading toward more realistic and complex causal schema as children grow older (Sedlak & Kurtz, 1981; Weisz, 1983, 1984).

At the same time, however, an increasingly realistic understanding of how to exert control comes with a potential downside. As children become more clear about the important role played by causes other than personal force, their sense of their own competence (which relies on the strength of personal force) is naturally diminished. This general pattern can be discerned in research on the development of children's causal conceptions and perceived competence in the academic domain (Skinner et al., 1998; Weisz, 1986). As causal schema develop that allow children to successively differentiate conceptions of effort from the contributions of other people, from their own desires and wishes, from task difficulty, from luck, and from ability, a steady decline in children's sense of their own competence can be detected (Stipek & Daniels, 1988), accompanied by evidence that these perceptions come to be calibrated to their actual levels of performance (e.g., Stipek, 1984).

In integrating work on development with research on individual differences, the key question for control theorists becomes: How can children's generalized sense of control, which ideally would remain strong, weather the successive developments needed to produce a more realistic understanding of the complexity (and potential uncontrollability) of causes? In other words, how can children construct a successively more complex and veridical picture of causal phenomena without exerting so much downward pressure on their control expectancies that it undermines their motivation, engagement, and coping? We consider these questions briefly for three well-documented developmental shifts that take place during early childhood, middle childhood, and early adolescence. We also speculate about some less well-studied shifts during adulthood and aging. In keeping with a multi-level developmental framework, the answers to these questions include a consideration of what the individual brings from previous developmental periods, as well as the nature of the current shift (typically based on underlying cognitive developments), and the demands and supports provided by social partners in the current context.

Differentiating self and other as causes of outcomes

Sometime during the second year, children come to appreciate the difference between the actions of the self and those of other people as causal factors in producing task outcomes (Heckhausen, 1982, 1984). In the parlance of control, conceptions of personal force no longer include concrete instrumental help from others. Hence, to feel efficacious, a toddler needs to "Do it myself!" (Geppert & Kuster, 1983). This development may be one factor underlying the emergence of the desire for autonomous action, which is a marked characteristic of 2-year-olds (Heckhausen, 1988). In terms of coping, such a development suggests that caregivers may need to take a step back from directly carrying out coping actions for children or risk undermining their sense of control. However, despite the fact that it reflects a cognitive advance and may contribute to gains in self-reliance, the loss of direct physical assistance from caregivers seriously limits what children are able to achieve, and so creates its own corresponding risk of helplessness.

To negotiate this transition in ways that support independence and still preserve a sense of efficacy, caregivers are required to show careful developmental attunement during coping episodes (Kliewer, Sandler, & Wolchik, 1994). Caregivers can gently move to more distal forms of support, scaffolding toddlers' performance with suggestions, ideas, and encouragement. Patience is also required, as children's initial struggles take longer than caregivers' solutions, and children's frustration and discouragement may be difficult for caregivers to tolerate. In a sense, caregivers now move to standby alert, so they are available if children ask for direct help, to respond with a teaching attitude, suggesting to the child "I'll show you how, so you can do it yourself."

The transition in modes of coping is smoother if, prior to toddlers' demands for independence, caregivers have a history of actively promoting children's skill acquisition and independent coping. This increases the likelihood that toddlers have more actual competence at their disposal when attempting to be self-reliant. Moreover, the handoff to more independent coping is facilitated by a secure attachment, based on a previous history of sensitive cooperation between caregiver and child. This results in more flexibility on the child's part in relying on and welcoming appropriate forms of participation from caregivers. It also supports the development of a child's sense that he or she has access to powerful others during coping episodes. In contrast, when caregivers are intrusive and continue to insert themselves into children's coping episodes when help is not needed or over children's protests, children can become helpless, passive, resistant, or angry (Pomeranz & Eaton, 2000, 2001). In a similar vein, when children try to cope by themselves with events that overwhelm them, such as often occurs with neglectful parenting, children can become discouraged, confused, or anxious. Both intrusive and neglectful parenting undermine the development of self-reliant strategies for dealing with challenges and threats, as well as interfering with a sense of control (Flammer, 1995; Skinner, 1995).

No wonder this transition can feel like a balancing act, in which caregivers are continually gauging whether children are competent enough to handle certain tasks on their own and how to provide the minimum support necessary to allow toddlers to eventually achieve success through their own sustained efforts (Heckhausen, 1988; Skinner & Edge, 1998). Ensuring that the challenges toddlers face are developmentally appropriate, in turn, depends not only on whether caregivers can show the kind of authoritative parenting that sets firm limits on the everyday tasks toddlers are allowed to tackle, but also on whether caregivers have the higher-order resources they need to keep overwhelming stressors out of their children's lives (Tolan & Grant, 2009).

Throughout coping episodes, of critical importance are the explanations that caregivers offer children for their successes and failures (Dweck & Molden, 2005). The most beneficent attributions are ones that direct children's causal interpretations toward their efforts and strategies, and away from their permanent characteristics and abilities. Perhaps surprisingly, even praise for *positive* traits, such as goodness and smartness, focuses children's attention on the causal force of immutable entities, which are by definition uncontrollable (Kamins & Dweck, 1999). Of course, when children do not succeed and adult help is needed, caregivers can assure children that they will be successful at more difficult tasks by themselves when they are older and have more practice.

Social comparison, perceived control, and coping

Starting in about fifth grade, children become more interested and able to use the performances of peers as a standard against which to measure their own levels of performance (Ruble, 1983). This new skill reflects a gain in the accuracy of control beliefs in that normative performance information allows children to distinguish task difficulty (when everyone performs poorly) as a cause of performance outcomes. It also allows children to recognize when it is something about their own action that is contributing to performance, namely, when their own level of performance differs from the norm (i.e., when they perform better or worse than everyone else) (Weiner, 1986). Social comparison can be seen in many domains in middle childhood, but it is most obvious in areas that are highly valued by the social context, and in which outcomes are directly compared and evaluated, such as in school, sports, physical appearance, and popularity.

Social comparison can serve useful purposes when coping. An accurate estimate of difficulty can be used to gather the resources and allow the time needed to be effective. If one is performing poorly on tasks while others are succeeding, it can also be interpreted as information that one needs to apply more effort or try different strategies. In fact, downward social comparison seems to be an important mechanism for dealing with losses during old age, when the elderly compare their well-being and performance with other people their own age, and note that they themselves are better off in comparison (e.g., Heckhausen & Krueger, 1993).

However, despite the fact that better estimates of task difficulty represent a cognitive advance, they also create a potential vulnerability for coping and a sense of control. When dealing with difficulties and setbacks, they can add the burden of self-evaluation, of "looking over one's shoulder" at how everyone else is doing. For children who are lagging behind their age-mates, it is easy to become discouraged and to denigrate their own potential. Such a mind-set adds stress to already demanding situations and subtracts resources that could be used for coping. It can even be a basis for devaluing whole areas of activity, namely, those in which one is behind or in which one needs to exert much more effort compared to others. It is a sad irony that such decisions can steer children away from precisely those activities where more experience and practice could lead to improvement.

This transition is easier for children who have developed adequate levels of social, academic, and physical competence *before* social comparison comes online. Social partners, both adults and peers, can also ease the transition if they encourage children to use normative comparisons as information about task difficulty and effort, but not about capacity (Dweck, 1999). At the level above individual partners, social contexts communicate key messages about the centrality and meaning of performance comparisons (Elliot, 1999). For example, work on achievement goals shows that explicit rankings and competition, which characterize many schools, sports teams, and peer groups, exacerbate the potential negative impact of social comparison, leading children to focus on their relatively stable attributes as causes of performance and to avoid participation in areas where their rankings are low (Anderman et al., 2002).

In contrast, social groups or classrooms with a "learning" orientation lead children to concentrate on effort and improvement, emphasizing intra-individual comparisons in which children track their own past performance to mark progress. Participation in activities in which sustained practice results in obvious improvements, such as sports or the creative arts, is a concrete operational way to demonstrate to children that sustained effort has the power to lift their level of performance. Of course, high-quality teaching or tutoring (which transmits effective strategies) as well as consistent practice are necessary if children's efforts are to be effective in boosting their performance outcomes.

Conceptions of ability, perceived control, and coping

In late middle childhood or early adolescence (between the ages of 10 and 12), children come to understand the cognitively complex notion of ability (Nicholls, 1978). "Ability" is an inferential concept; it represents an invisible capacity that can only be inferred from a pattern of performance outcomes: success on normatively hard tasks with little effort. To make such inferences, children must be cognitively capable of understanding inverse compensatory relations between effort and ability (Miller, 1985; Nicholls, 1984). This means children understand that to produce the same outcome, smart children do not need to try as hard. With this cognitive advance, however, comes the vulnerability described as "the double-edged sword of effort" (Covington & Omelich, 1979), in which children come to see that high exertion that ends in failure can imply low ability, thus making all-out effort a potentially risky proposition. At this age, the aspects of perceived control that best predict engagement (and that are best predicted by performance) change from those focused on the capacity to exert effort to those focused on one's own level of ability (Skinner et al., 1998).

In early studies of the development of learned helplessness, researchers hypothesized that young children, because they did not have the cognitive capacity to infer ability, would be shielded from the effects of non-contingency, and that all children, once they acquired "mature" conceptions of ability during early adolescence, would be more vulnerable to helplessness. However, both these hypotheses turned out to be incorrect. For younger children, research shows that there is no age at which they are free from the effects of repeated failure (Burhans & Dweck, 1995). Instead, the experiences that produce helplessness are different for younger children. In early elementary school, more concrete tasks and more directly observable outcomes exacerbate the effects of repeated failure (e.g., Boggiano et al., 1993). Moreover, although young children are not able to make complex inferences about the relations of patterns of outcomes to levels of ability, they can construct conceptions of their traits (e.g., goodness and badness) as fixed and immutable (Dweck, 1999). These are the experiences and belief systems that make young children more vulnerable to helplessness.

For older children and young adolescents, it turns out that the effects of cognitive advances on control and coping depend completely on the social context, both local and cultural. When children acquire the cognitive capacity to understand inverse compensatory relations among causes, they will apply these schema to effort and ability *only* in cultures (such as the United States) that endorse conceptions of ability as a fixed entity that can be diagnosed from levels of performance (Nicholls, 1984; Rosenholtz & Simpson, 1984). Moreover, these cultural conceptions must be communicated to children, for example, by teachers who respond to children's failures by doubting their capacities (Graham, 1990). Finally, these messages must be internalized by children, so that they are convinced that their own ability is a fixed immutable entity that is demonstrated by every performance (Dweck, 1999). In contrast, if children operate in classrooms and cultures that allow them to continue to see ability or competence as a flexible, incremental attribute, open to cultivation through effort and practice, young adolescents (despite cognitive advances) will maintain a high sense of control and high levels of effort and engagement in the face of obstacles and setbacks (Mueller & Dweck, 1998).

Adulthood and aging

Work during adulthood and old age has not been able to identify specific age-graded changes in perceived control (Aldwin, 2007; Baltes & Baltes, 1986; Lachman & Prenda-Firth, 2004; Wolinsky et., 2003; Zarit, Pearlin, & Schaie, 2003). However, lifespan theories have suggested that a general shift from primary to secondary control takes place across later life (Heckhausen & Schulz, 1995). In this context, primary control refers to reliance on prototypical control strategies, such as effort and instrumental action, aimed at bringing the external world in line with one's own preferences, whereas secondary control refers to effort that "targets the self and attempts to achieve changes directly within the individual" (1995, p. 285).

The basic idea is that, due to societal constraints and biological declines, people are not as able to exercise primary control as they age, so they come to rely more and more on secondary control. Two main kinds of secondary control can be distinguished. The first refers to secondary control as a backup system: After initial attempts have failed, people can shift resources from other endeavors to the implementation of the blocked goal (Thompson

et al., 1998). This kind of control, sometimes referred to as compensatory secondary control, includes processes like increased efforts or the construction of new strategies. Especially important during aging, secondary control increasingly involves having access to the resources of others (such as doctors or one's adult children) through "proxy" control (Bandura, 1997; Brandtstädter & Renner, 1990; Heckhausen & Schulz, 1995).

The second kind of secondary control refers to a hierarchy of outcomes. From this perspective, when it is no longer possible to "fix" the primary outcome of choice, people can shift their focus toward "secondary" targets that are more amenable to control. For example, in the face of a chronic medical condition, elderly people can shift their focus from finding a cure to having an impact on the daily symptoms or treatment of the condition, and minimizing its effects on others (Thompson et al., 1993). This kind of secondary control can also include attempts to influence one's own internal states (such as emotional reactions or attitudes) (Heckhausen & Schulz, 1995); these are also studied as emotion regulation (Gross, 1998).

Many of these "secondary control strategies" have already been studied in research on coping, which is the more common term used to describe how people deal with losses, failures, and difficulties that threaten control (Folkman, 1984; Lockenhoff & Carstensen, 2003). Both coping and secondary control can serve to create control experiences even in "low control" circumstances (Thompson et al., 1993). In fact, people's ingenuity in finding secondary outcomes they can influence, even in "uncontrollable circumstances," has compelled researchers to rename such real-life situations as "low control" circumstances. Outside of the laboratory, researchers have not been able to identify any situations in which people cannot find something of value to influence. Hence, it is possible that these ways of coping, or secondary control strategies, are elaborated and consolidated as people age, perhaps resulting in increased confidence in one's capacity to enact them (also called coping self-efficacy), despite normative declines in primary control.

Coping as a Process that Shapes the Development of Perceived Control and Competence

The third and final goal of this chapter is to highlight the reciprocal dynamics that exist between control and coping. If coping describes how people deal with ongoing challenges, difficulties, and failures, then it becomes clear that coping transactions are an important form of control experiences. That is, the ways in which people actually approach and engage with real-life stressors, how they cope, is the grist from which perceptions of control are shaped. All of the basic elements of the coping process can be found in theories about the construction of control, namely, the actual stressor and its objective controllability, the individual's personal resources (including previous perceived control and actual competence), and the participation of social contexts (e.g., the availability and responsiveness of social partners). Hence, one important resource that can be influenced by coping is an individual's sense of control, with adaptive coping promoting confidence, perceived competence, and a focus on mastery, and maladaptive coping contributing to helplessness.

Failure experiences and perceived control

One situation in which coping can have a decisive effect on a sense of control is when individuals are dealing with objectively uncontrollable events and losses. As mentioned previously, the notion of secondary control has been useful in understanding how people can deal adaptively with situations where primary control is not working, and has helped explain how people, when they do succumb to experiences of non-contingency and loss, can navigate their way back from helplessness. Control-related conceptions of secondary control focus on strategies that increase effort and concentration, access supplementary social resources, and locate sub-goals where control can be effectively enacted. These coping strategies create a feedback loop back toward a sense of renewed efficacy and control.

Equally important in dealing with uncontrollable events and failures are coping *appraisals*. Decades of research on causal attributions and explanations have demonstrated that, although unsuccessful attempts to produce a desired or prevent an undesired outcome are a risk factor for becoming helpless, it is the *interpretation* of the experience that mediates its effects on subsequent control expectations (e.g., Abramson et al., 1978; Weiner, 2005). Work on control paints a clear picture of the kinds of appraisals that support adaptation in the face of failures, as well as the important roles played by social partners in shaping those appraisals.

Although some theories emphasize the importance of attributions of failure to unstable and controllable causes (most notably lack of effort), the overarching mindset that seems to promote a sense of control is the conviction that all transactions contain important information about how to produce outcomes, that is, how to exert control. Failures and mistakes can be "our friends" in that they tell us what isn't working "yet." They can imply that more effort, time, or concentration is needed, that different actions or better strategies are required, and that the task is harder than expected (Dweck, 1999). Interestingly enough, such a mindset even allows people to discover more quickly that tasks are objectively unsolvable and so to stop working on them sooner (Janoff-Bulman & Brickman, 1982).

It turns out that social factors are critical to the development of this mindset. Parents, teachers, and friends who view mistakes and "failures," not as embarrassing and shameful events to be hidden, but as fascinating learning opportunities will invite children to see them the same way (Dweck & Molden, 2005). Although studied most often during childhood and in the academic domain, there is no reason to think that the same principles would not apply at other points in the lifespan and in other arenas. For example, during old age, when elderly people make mistakes or can no longer perform at previous levels, it is easy for them and their social partners to see these "failures" as signs of irreversible losses of aging. Alternatively, they can be viewed as temporary setbacks that can be worked around or compensated for by various coping strategies, such as increased practice, external aids, or social supports. This mindset facilitates the types of coping that maintain a sense of control late into old age.

Beyond control in processes of coping and resilience

At the same time, the picture painted in the control area is incomplete. Recovery from setbacks, losses, and helplessness can be conceived more broadly as issues of resilience, and there can be no question that true resilience relies on other adaptive processes in addition to control (Brandtstädter & Rothermund, 2002). The analyses of coping families can immediately suggest two additional fundamental processes by which coping contributes to resilience: one organized around *relatedness* and one around *autonomy* (Baumeister & Leary, 1995; Connell & Wellborn, 1989; Deci & Ryan, 1985; Skinner & Wellborn, 1994). The primary ways of coping that follow from relatedness are part of the family of *seeking social support* (see Table 3.1).

Support-seeking seems to be a general all-purpose strategy that is extremely common at every age (Skinner et al., 2003; Zimmer-Gembeck & Skinner, in press). It can include contacts that directly support control—for example, asking for advice about effective strategies or requesting direct help. However, support-seeking adds value to resilience beyond its instrumental potential. Processes of relatedness can add perspective to issues of control (e.g., "I love you whether or not you get that outcome"), failure (e.g., "You did everything you could"), and disappointment ("Well, we still have each other, so it's really not so bad"). And when it really is so bad, such as dealing with the death of a loved one, the presence and support of caring others can provide comfort, distraction, and healing, even when there is nothing to be done (Stroebe et al., 1996).

The adaptive function of autonomy is to coordinate preferences with available options, and the adaptive families of coping organized around autonomy are negotiation and accommodation (see Table 3.1). *Negotiation*, of course, refers to attempts to locate or create desirable options, and so clears the way for control efforts aimed at securing those options. However, in the control area, much more interest has been focused on processes of *accommodation*, which allow people to actually adjust their preferences to fit within existing constraints (Brandtstädter & Renner, 1990). Once considered part of secondary control, researchers now view it as a distinguishable set of processes that involve fit, "going with the flow," willing acceptance, acquiescence, adjustment, and "getting into it" (Morling & Evered, 2006, 2007; Rothbaum et al., 1983; Skinner, 2007). As opposed to control-related processes of secondary control, which involve adding instrumental resources or changing the self to be more effective, accommodation has nothing to do with control: it is about letting go of desired outcomes and previously held goals (Brandtstädter & Rothermund, 2002; Skinner, 2007). Researchers emphasize that accommodation can be adaptive when primary control is not available. However, it can also be used as a *first* line of defense, with primary control engaged only if accommodation proves impossible. In many cases, accommodation can replace primary control all together from the outset, for example, in situations where people feel that pursuing control (even successfully) would use too many resources, upset relationships, or interfere with other more important commitments.

The opposite of accommodation is not control, it is "rigid perseveration," in which an outcome is inflexibly pursued no matter what the cost (Brandtstädter & Renner, 1990). No complete analysis has been made of the processes that defuse rigid perseveration and allow accommodation to occur when coping with stressful life events (Brandtstädter & Rothermund, 2002). However, it is likely that strategies will include cognitive restructuring and focusing on the positive aspects of the current situation, making meaning and finding benefits in adversity, distraction with genuinely pleasurable alternative activities (Folkman & Moskowitz, 2000; Thompson, 1985), and intentionally seeking downward social comparisons. Broadening the study of resilience to include not only strategies of control but also ways of coping organized around relatedness and autonomy will provide a more complete picture of the processes needed to deal constructively with stress and adversity.

Implications for Research on the Development of Coping

The central implication of a developmental analysis of perceived control is that the study of coping as it develops can be organized around specific ages during which children's understanding of control undergoes qualitative shifts, likely based on underlying temperamental traits, as well as physiological, neurological, and cognitive developments, and changes in the environmental challenges and supports available to children. These shifts produce changes in the strategies individuals use to coordinate actions with contingencies in the environment and in the causal schema they use to predict and process causal experiences. Both of these changes shape the ways people cope, and so can be used to focus the developmental study of coping on specific age windows during which corresponding qualitative shifts in coping may be found.

Developmentally graded ways of coping

An analysis of age-graded changes in the means for exerting mastery and becoming helpless has important implications for the measurement of coping. First, assessments of coping should include developmentally appropriate markers of all four coping families organized around control (i.e., problem-solving, information-seeking, helplessness, and escape) at every age. Second, when studies seek to examine age differences or changes, they should be sure that assessments distinguish each of the means hypothesized to characterize coping at different ages, for example, both behavioral and cognitive means of problem-solving and escape (Zimmer-Gembeck & Skinner, 2009).

This analysis also suggests that developmental studies should examine qualitative changes in coping as a supplement to the typical focus on quantitative changes. For example, an important empirical question would be whether one developmentally graded form of coping predicts the subsequent use of a different, but functionally analogous, way of coping at later ages; and whether during transitions when both forms should be readily accessible, the two forms of coping are tightly coupled. Research could also examine whether developmentally-graded members of the same family become hierarchically organized as new forms are added, and could investigate the factors that determine which of the strategies from a person's repertoire will be deployed in a given transaction. For example, do children and youth fall back on earlier forms of coping as stress levels rise, and do they return to more mature forms as social supports increase? Such studies will add to our understanding of the "building blocks" of the area, namely, ways of coping—and should help to move dominant conceptualizations in the field beyond an age-delimited focus on individual differences and toward a view of coping as an increasingly elaborated and flexible repertoire of developmentally ordered responses.

Qualitative shifts in the understanding of control

The development of perceived control includes the construction of increasingly complex schema for analyzing multiple causes of success and failure as well as increasingly veridical analyses of individuals' own roles in producing desired and preventing undesired outcomes. These qualitative shifts represent progress toward more accurate prediction and analysis of causal experience. However, each transition also represents a potential turning point during which vulnerabilities can be introduced that will undermine subsequent confidence, engagement, and coping. Future research can focus short-term longitudinal studies on these normative shifts as time windows that may be critical to the development of coping. Explanatory studies can locate normative shifts by focusing on the cognitive developments that likely underlie qualitative changes (Band & Weisz, 1990). Such studies should incorporate important predictors of how the transition will be negotiated, including the individual's previous level of functioning and the nature of the demands in the current situation, especially their severity and objective controllability.

Theories of control also highlight the importance of mapping the roles of social partners, especially caregivers, in shaping the development of coping. They are critical in helping children achieve normative developments in causal understanding without undercutting their initially high sense of efficacy. At the same time, studies should include information from multiple levels of the social context, not only about immediate social partners who participate in coping transactions but also about the social climates and societal assumptions that frame these transactions. Pivotal in this regard are societal and individual mindsets about the nature of personal force, whether it is a stable immutable entity that is displayed by every performance or, instead, is a dynamic plastic capacity that can be improved through sustained effort and practice (Dweck, 1999).

Studies can include key markers of how the developmental shift is progressing, such as individuals' appraisals and reappraisals of the transaction as well as the strategies that people are actually using to cope with real-life demands—the balance of constructive (e.g., problem-solving, information-seeking) and maladaptive (e.g., helplessness, escape) ways of coping, and the general reliance on immature, age-appropriate, or mature strategies. Research can also trace the emergence of new and adaptive ways of dealing with stress and follow their integration into an increasingly dependable yet flexible repertoire of coping strategies. Critical in this regard would be the identification of factors that allow people to maintain access to the most constructive ways of coping in their current repertoire.

Especially important to assess across these transitions would be the individual's sense of control and efficacy, which can survive normative improvements in causal understanding only if children and youth (and adults) repeatedly experience transactions with the environment in which outcomes of value can be achieved through sustained effort. Such experiences require objective control conditions characterized by contingency, responsiveness, and manageable levels of difficulty, which remain attuned to the person as he or she develops. They also require judicious social support and the development of increasing levels of actual competence in the person. Such a view makes clear the interlocking dynamics of perceived control and coping, and how previous coping episodes are carried forward in individuals' own characteristics and in their social relationships. From this perspective, adaptive coping is the grist from which a sense of control is won just as control, strategy, and capacity beliefs permeate stress appraisals and coping responses.

Conclusion

Both perceived control and coping have largely been conceptualized and studied as individual differences phenomena. We hope that by focusing on what is known about the development of perceived control, and highlighting its connections to coping, this chapter may contribute to progress in realizing a developmental agenda for the study of coping. This agenda will conceive of coping as an organizational construct that has the potential to provide an integrative link across multiple levels—from the physiological processes of individual stress reactions to the sociocultural forces that determine the stressors societies allow into people's lives.

Note

1. Since the most detailed research on development has been conducted in the achievement domain, many of the findings about age changes cannot yet be generalized to other domains of functioning during childhood (for example, peers, or physical or artistic endeavors) or during adulthood (for example, work, romantic relationships, or health).

References

Abramson, L. Y., Seligman, M. E. P., & Teasdale, J. D. (1978). Learned helplessness in humans. *Journal of Abnormal Psychology, 87*, 49–74.

Aldwin, C. M. (2007). *Stress, coping, and development: An integrative perspective, 2nd ed.* New York: Guilford Press.

Aldwin, C. M., Sutton, K. J., Chiara, G., & Spiro, A. (1996). Age differences in stress, coping, and appraisal: Findings from The Normative Aging Study. *Journal of Gerontology, 51*, 179–88.

Amat, J., Paul, E., Zarza, C., Watkins, L.R., & Maier, S.F. (2007). Previous experience with behavioral control over stress blocks the behavioral and dorsal raphe nucleus activating effects of later uncontrollable stress: Role of the ventral medial prefrontal cortex. *The Journal of Neuroscience, 26*, 13264–72.

Anderman, E. M., Austin, C. C., & Johnson, D. M. (2002). The development of goal orientation. In A. Wigfield & J. S. Eccles (Eds.), *Development of achievement motivation* (pp. 197–220). San Diego: Academic Press.

Anderman, E. M., Maehr, M. L., & Midgley, C. (1999). Declining motivation after the transition to middle school: Schools can make a difference. *Journal of Research and Development in Education, 32*, 131–47.

Anderman, L. H. (1999). Classroom goal orientation, school belonging, and social goals as predictors of students' positive and negative affect following transition to middle school. *Journal of Research and Development in Education, 32*(2), 89–103.

Anderman, L. H., & Anderman, E. M. (1999). Social predictors of changes in students' achievement goal orientations. *Contemporary Educational Psychology, 25*, 21–37.

Anderman, L. H., & Anderman, E. M. (Eds.) (2000). The role of social context in educational psychology: Substantive and methodological issues. Special issue of *Educational Psychologist*, 35 (2).

Aspinwall, L. G., & Taylor, S. E. (1997). A stitch in time: Self-regulation and proactive coping. *Psychological Bulletin, 121*, 417–36.

Baltes, M. M., & Baltes, P. B. (Eds.). (1986). *The psychology of control and aging*. Hillsdale, NJ: Lawrence Erlbaum Associates.

Baltes, P. B., & Staudinger, U. M. (1995). Wisdom. In G. Maddox (Ed.), *Encyclopedia of aging* (2nd ed., pp. 971–4). New York: Springer.

Band, E. B., & Weisz, J. R. (1990). Developmental differences in primary and secondary control coping and adjustment to juvenile diabetes. *Journal of Clinical Child Psychology, 19*, 150–8.

Bandura, A. (1997). *Self-efficacy: The exercise of control*. New York: W. H. Freeman.

Barrett, K. C., & Campos, J. J. (1991). A diacritical function approach to emotions and coping. In E. M. Cummings, A. L. Greene, & K. H. Karraker (Eds.), *Life-span developmental psychology: Perspectives on stress and coping* (pp. 21–41). Hillsdale, NJ: Erlbaum.

Baumeister, R. F., & Leary, M. R. (1995). The need to belong: Desire for interpersonal attachments as a fundamental human motivation. *Psychological Bulletin, 117*, 497–529.

Berg, C., Meegan, S., & Deviney, F. (1998). A social-contextual model of coping with everyday problems across the life span. *International Journal of Behavioral Development, 22*, 239–61.

Boggiano, A. K., Barrett, M., & Kellam, T. (1993). Competing theoretical analyses of helplessness: A social-developmental analysis. *Journal of Experimental Child Psychology, 55*, 194–207.

Brandtstädter, J., & Renner, G. (1990). Tenacious goal pursuit and flexible goal adjustment: Explication and age-related analysis of assimilative and accommodative strategies of coping. *Psychology and Aging, 5*(1), 58–67.

Brandtstädter, J., & Rothermund, K. (2002). The life-course dynamics of goal pursuit and goal adjustment: A two-process framework. *Developmental Review, 22*, 117–50.

Brim, O. G. (1992). *Ambition: How we manage success and failure throughout our lives*. New York: Basic Books.

Bronfenbrenner, U., & Morris, P. A. (1998). The ecology of developmental processes. In W. Damon (Series Ed.) & R. M. Lerner (Vol. Ed.), *Handbook of child psychology: Vol. 1. Theoretical models of human development* (5th ed., pp. 993–1028). New York: Wiley.

Bronson, M. B. (2000). *Self-regulation in early childhood: Nature and nurture*. New York: Guilford Press.

Burhans, K. K., & Dweck, C. S. (1995). Helplessness in early childhood: The role of contingent worth. *Child Development, 66*, 1719–38.

Carpenter, P. J. (1992). Perceived control as a predictor of distress in children undergoing invasive medical procedures. *Journal of Pediatric Psychology, 17*, 757–73.

Case, R. (1985). *Intellectual development: Birth to adulthood*. New York: Academic Press.

Case, R., Hayward, S., Lewis, M., & Hurst, P. (1988). Toward a neo-Piagetian theory of cognitive and emotional development. *Developmental Review, 8*, 1–51.

Cassidy, J., (1994). Emotion regulation: Influences of attachment relationships. *Monographs of the Society for Research in Child Development, 59* (2/3, Serial No. 240), 228–49.

Cassidy, J., & Shaver, P. R. (Eds.) (1999). *Handbook of attachment*. New York: Guilford Press.

Compas, B. E. (1998). An agenda for coping research and theory: Basic and applied developmental issues. *International Journal of Behavioral Development, 22*, 231–7.

Compas, B. E. (2006). Psychobiological processes of stress and coping: Implications for resilience in childhood and adolescence. *Annals of the New York Academy of Sciences, 1094*, 226–34.

Compas, B. E. (2009). Coping, regulation, and development during childhood and adolescence. In E. A. Skinner & M. J. Zimmer-Gembeck (Eds.), *Coping and the development of regulation*. A volume for the series, R. W. Larson & L. A. Jensen (Eds.-in-Chief), *New Directions in Child and Adolescent Development*, San Francisco: Jossey-Bass.

Compas, B. E., Banez, G. A., Malcarne, V., & Worsham, N. (1991). Perceived control and coping with stress: A developmental perspective. *Journal of Social Issues, 47*(4), 23–34.

Compas, B. E., Connor-Smith, J. K., Saltzman, H., Thomsen, A. H., & Wadsworth, M. E. (2001). Coping with stress during childhood and adolescence: Problems, progress, and potential in theory and research. *Psychological Bulletin, 127*, 87–127.

Compas, B. E., Connor, J. K., Saltzman, H., Thomsen, A. H., & Wadsworth, M. (1999). Getting specific about coping: Effortful and involuntary responses to stress in development. In M. Lewis & D. Ramsay (Eds.), *Soothing and stress* (pp. 229–56). Mahwah, NJ: Erlbaum.

Connell, J. P. (1985). A new multidimensional measure of children's perceptions of control. *Child Development, 56*, 1011–8.

Connell, J. P., & Wellborn, J. G. (1991). Competence, autonomy and relatedness: A motivational analysis of self-system processes. In M. Gunnar & L. A. Sroufe (Eds.), *Minnesota Symposium on Child Psychology: Vol. 23. Self processes in development* (pp. 43–77). Chicago: University of Chicago Press.

Coping Consortium (I. Sandler, B. Compas, T. Ayers, N. Eisenberg, E. Skinner, & P. Tolan) (Organizers) (1998, 2001). *New Conceptualizations of Coping*. Workshop sponsored by the Arizona State University Prevention Research Center, Tempe, AZ.

Covington, M. V., & Omelich, C. L. (1979). Effort: The double-edged sword in school achievement. *Journal of Educational Psychology, 71*, 169–82.

Davidov, M., & Grusec, J. E. (2006). Untangling the links of parental responsiveness to distress and warmth to child outcomes. *Child Development, 77*, 44–58.

Deci, E. L., & Ryan, R. M. (1985). *Intrinsic motivation and self-determination in human behavior*. New York: Plenum Press.

Deci, E. L., & Ryan, R. M. (2000). The "what" and "why" of goal pursuits: Human needs and the self-determination of behavior. *Psychological Inquiry, 11*, 227–68.

Derryberry, D., Reed, M. A., & Pilkenton-Taylor, C. (2003). Temperament and coping: Advantages of an individual differences perspective. *Development and Psychopathology, 15*, 1049–66.

Diamond, L. M., & Aspinwall, L. G. (2003). Emotion regulation across the life span; An integrative perspective emphasizing self-regulation, positive affect, and dyadic processes. *Motivation and Emotion, 27*, 125–56.

Downey, G., Freitas, A. L., Michaelis, B., & Khouri, H. (1998). The self-fulfilling prophecy in close relationships: Rejection sensitivity and rejection by romantic partners. *Journal of Personality and Social Psychology, 75*, 545–60.

Dweck, C. S. (1999). *Self-theories: Their role in motivation, personality, and development*. Philadelphia: Psychology Press.

Dweck, C. S. (2002). The development of ability conceptions. In A. Wigfield & J. S. Eccles (Eds.), *Development of achievement motivation* (pp. 57–88). San Diego: Academic Press.

Dweck, C. S., & Molden, D. C. (2005). Self-theories: Their impact on competence motivation and acquisition. In A. J. Elliot & C. S. Dweck (Eds.), *Handbook of competence and motivation* (pp. 12–140). New York: Guilford.

Eccles, J. S., & Wigfield, A. (2002). Motivational beliefs, values, and goals. *Annual Review of Psychology, 53*, 109–32.

Eisenberg, N., Valiente, C., & Sulik, M. (2009). How the study of regulation can inform the study of coping. In E. A. Skinner & M. J. Zimmer-Gembeck (Eds.). *Coping and the development of regulation. A volume for the series*, R. W. Larson & L. A. Jensen (Eds.-in-Chief), *New Directions in Child and Adolescent Development*, San Francisco: Jossey-Bass.

Eisenberg, N., Fabes, R. A., & Guthrie, I. K. (1997). Coping with stress: The roles of regulation and development. In S. A. Wolchik & I. N. Sandler (Eds.), *Handbook of children's coping: Linking theory and intervention* (pp. 41–70). New York: Plenum Press.

Elliot, A. J. (1999). Approach and avoidance motivation and achievement goals. *Educational Psychologist, 34*, 169–89.

Elliot, A. J., & Dweck, C. S. (Eds.). (2005). *Handbook of competence and motivation*. New York: Guilford.

Elliot, A. J., McGregor, H. A., & Thrash, T. M. (2002). The need for competence. In E. L. Deci & R. M. Ryan (Eds.), *Handbook of self-determination theory research* (pp. 361–87). Rochester, NY: University of Rochester Press.

Fields, L., & Prinz, R. J. (1997). Coping and adjustment during childhood and adolescence. *Clinical Psychology Review, 17*, 937–76.

Flammer, A. (1995). Developmental analysis of control beliefs. In A. Bandura (Ed.), *Self-efficacy in changing societies* (pp. 69–113). New York: Cambridge University Press.

Folkman, S. (1984). Personal control and stress and coping processes: A theoretical analysis. *Journal of Personality and Social Psychology, 46*(4), 839–52.

Folkman, S., & Lazarus, R. S. (1985). If it changes it must be a process: Study of emotion and coping during three stages of a college examination. *Journal of Personality and Social Psychology, 48*, 150–70.

Folkman, S., & Moskowitz, J. T. (2000). Positive affect and the other side of coping. *American Psychologist, 55*, 647–54.

Folkman, S., & Moskowitz, J. T. (2004). Coping: Pitfalls and promise. *Annual Review of Psychology, 55*, 745–74.

Folkman, S., Lazarus, R., Pimley, S., & Novacek, J. (1987). Age differences and coping processes. *Journal of Personality and Social Psychology, 2*, 171–84.

Frydenberg, E., & Lewis, R. (2000). Teaching coping to adolescents: When and to whom? *American Educational Research Journal, 37*, 727–45.

Garmezy, N., & Rutter, M. (Eds.). (1983). *Stress, coping and development in children*. New York: McGraw-Hill.

Geppert, U., & Kuster, U. (1983). The emergence of "wanting to do it oneself": A precursor of achievement motivation. *International Journal of Behavioral Development, 6*, 355–69.

Gianino, A., & Tronick, E. Z. (1988). The mutual regulation model: The infant's self and interactive regulation, coping and defensive capacities. In T. Field, P. McCabe, & N. Schneiderman (Eds.), *Stress and coping across development* (pp. 47–68). Hillsdale, NJ: Erlbaum.

Goldstein, M. H., Bornstein, M. H., & Schwade, J. A. (2009). The value of vocalizing: Five-month-old infants associate their own non-cry vocalizations with responses from caregivers. *Child Development, 80*, 636–44.

Graham, S. (1990). Communicating low ability in the classroom: Bad things good teachers sometimes do. In S. Graham & V. S. Folkes (Eds.), *Attribution theory: Applications to achievement, mental health, and interpersonal conflict* (pp. 17–36). Hillsdale, NJ: Erlbaum.

Gross, J. (1998). The emerging field of emotion regulation: An integrative review. *Review of General Psychology, 2*, 271–99.

Gunnar, M. R., & Quevedo, K. (2007). The neurobiology of stress and development. *Annual Review of Psychology, 58*, 11.1–11.29.

Gurin, P., & Brim, O. G. (1984). Change in self in adulthood: The example of sense of control. In P. B. Baltes & O. G. Brim (Eds.), *Life-span development and behavior* (pp. 282–334). New York: Academic Press.

Harter, S. (1978). Effectance motivation reconsidered: Toward a developmental model. *Human Development, 21*, 36–64.

Harter, S. (2006). The self. In W. Damon (Series Ed.) & N. Eisenberg (Volume Ed.), *Handbook of child psychology, 6th Ed. Vol. 3. Social, emotional, and personality development* (pp. 505–70). New York: John Wiley.

Heckhausen, H. (1982). The development of achievement motivation. In W. W. Hartup (Ed.), *Review of child development research, Vol. 6* (pp. 600–68). Chicago: University of Chicago Press.

Heckhausen, H. (1984). Emergent achievement behavior: Some early developments. In M. Haehr (Ed.), *Advances in motivation and achievement* (pp. 1–32). Greenwich, CT: JAI Press.

Heckhausen, H. (1991). *Motivation and action* (P. K. Leppmann, Trans.). Berlin: Springer-Verlag.

Heckhausen, J. (1988). Becoming aware of one's competence in the second year: Developmental progression within the mother-child dyad. *International Journal of Behavioral Development, 11*, 305–26.

Heckhausen, J. (1997). Developmental regulation across adulthood: Primary and secondary control of age-related challenges. *Developmental Psychology, 33*, 176–87.

Heckhausen, J., & Krueger, J. (1993). Developmental expectations for the self and 'most other people': Age grading in three functions of social comparison. *Developmental Psychology, 29*, 539–48.

Heckhausen, J., & Schulz, R. (1995). A life-span theory of control. *Psychological Review, 102*, 284–304.

Heckhausen, J., & Schulz, R. (1998). Developmental regulation in adulthood: Selection and compensation in primary and secondary control. In J. Heckhausen & C. S. Dweck (Eds.), *Motivation and self-regulation across the life span* (pp. 50–77). Cambridge, UK: Cambridge University Press.

Holodynski, M., & Friedlmeier, W. (2006). *Development of emotions and emotion regulation*. New York: Springer.

Hornik, R., Risenhoover, N., & Gunnar, M. (1987). The effects of maternal positive, neutral, and negative affective communications on infant responses to new toys. *Child Development, 58*, 937–44.

Janoff-Bulman, R., & Brickman, P. (1982). Expectations and what people learn from failure. In N. T. Feather (Eds.), *Expectations and actions: Expectancy-value models in psychology* (pp. 207–37). Hillsdale, NJ: Erlbaum.

Kamins, M. L., & Dweck, C. S. (1999). Person versus process praise and criticism: Implications for contingent self-worth and coping. *Developmental Psychology, 35*, 835–47.

Keating, D. (1999). Adolescent thinking. In S. S. Feldman & G. R. Elliott (Eds.), *At the threshold: The developing adolescent* (pp. 54–90). Cambridge, MA: Harvard University Press.

Kerns, K. A., Tomich, P. L., & Kim, P. (2006). Normative trends in children's perceptions of availability and utilization of attachment figures in middle childhood. *Social Development, 15*, 1–22.

Kliewer, W., Sandler, I., & Wolchik, S. (1994). Family socialization of threat appraisal and coping: Coaching, modeling, and family context. In K. Hurrelman & F. Nestmann (Eds.), *Social networks and social support in childhood and adolescence* (pp. 271–91). Berlin: Walter de Gruyter.

Kochanska, G., Aksan, N., & Carlson (2005). Temperament, relationships, and young children's receptive cooperation with their parents. *Developmental Psychology, 41*, 648–60.

Kochanska, G., Coy, K. T., & Murray, K. T. (2005). The development of self-regulation in the first four years of life. *Child Development, 72*, 1091–111.

Koestner, R., & McClelland, D. C. (1990). Perspectives on competence motivation. In L. A. Pervin (Ed.), *Handbook of personality: Theory and research* (pp. 527–48). New York: Guilford Press.

Kopp, C. B. (1989). Regulation of distress and negative emotions: A developmental view. *Developmental Psychology, 25*, 343–54.

Kopp, C. B. (2009). Emotion-focused coping in young children: Self and self-regulatory processes. In E. A. Skinner & M. J. Zimmer-Gembeck (Eds.). *Coping and the development of regulation*. A volume for the series, R. W. Larson & L. A. Jensen (Eds.-in-Chief), *New Directions in Child and Adolescent Development*, San Francisco: Jossey-Bass.

Kopp, C. B., & Neufeld, S. J. (2003) Emotional development during infancy. In R. J. Davidson, K. R. Scherer, & H. H. Goldsmith (Eds.), *Handbook of affective sciences* (pp. 347–74). New York: Oxford University Press.

Kuhl, J. (1984). Volitional aspects of achievement motivation and learned helplessness: Toward a comprehensive theory of action control. In B. A. Maher & W. A. Maher (Eds.), *Progress in experimental personality research* (pp. 99–171). New York: Academic Press.

Kuhn, D., & Franklin, S. (2006). The second decade: What develops (and how)? In W. Damon & R. Lerner (Eds.). *Handbook of child psychology* (6th ed.). New York: Wiley.

Lachman, M. E., & Prenda-Firth, K. M. (2004). The adaptive value of feeling in control during midlife. In O. G. Brim, Jr., C. D. Ryff & R. C. Kessler (Eds.), *How healthy are we? A national study of well-being at midlife* (pp. 320–49). Chicago: The University of Chicago Press.

Lamb, M. E., & Easterbrooks, M. A. (1981). Individual differences in parental sensitivity: Some thoughts about origins, components, and consequences. In M. E. Lamb & L. R. Sherrod (Eds.), *Infant social cognition: Empirical and theoretical considerations* (pp. 127–53). Hillsdale, NJ: Erlbaum.

Landry, S. H., Smith, K. E., & Swank, P. R. (2006). Responsive parenting: Establishing early foundations for social, communication, and independent problem-solving skills. *Developmental Psychology, 42*, 627–42.

Lazarus, R. S., & Folkman, S. (1984). *Stress, appraisal, and coping*. New York: Springer.

Lefcourt, H. M. (1992). Durability and impact of the locus of control construct. *Psychological Bulletin, 112*(3), 411–4.

Lewis, M., & Ramsay, D. (1999). Environments and stress reduction. In M. Lewis & D. Ramsay (Eds.), *Soothing and stress* (pp. 171–92). Mahwah, NJ: Erlbaum.

Lockenhoff, C. E., & Carstensen, L. L. (2003). Is the life span theory of control a theory of development or a theory of coping. In S. H. Zarit, L. I. Pearlin & K. W. Schaie (Eds.), *Personal control in social and life course contexts* (pp. 263–80). New York: Springer.

Maier, S. F., & Watkins, L. R. (2005). Stressor controllability and learned helplessness: The roles of the dorsal raphe nucleus, serotonin, and corticotropin-releasing factor. *Neuroscience and Behavioral Reviews, 29,* 829–41.

Mangelsdorf, S. C., Shapiro, J. R., & Marzolf, D. (1995). Developmental and temperamental differences in emotion regulation in infancy. *Child Development, 66,* 1817–28.

Manne, S. L., Bakeman, R., Jacobsen, P. B., Gorfinkle, K., Bernstein, D., & Redd, W. H. (1992). Adult-child interaction during invasive medical procedures. *Health Psychology, 11,* 241–9.

Miller, A. (1985). A developmental study of the cognitive basis of performance impairment after failure. *Journal of Personality and Social Psychology, 49,* 529–38.

Miller, S. M. (1979). Controllability and human stress: Method, evidence and theory. *Behavior Research and Theory, 17,* 287–304.

Miller, S. M., Green, V. A., & Bales, C. B. (1999). What you don't know can hurt you: A cognitive-social framework for understanding children's responses to stress. In M. Lewis & D. Ramsay (Eds.), *Soothing and stress* (pp. 257–92). Mahwah, NJ: Erlbaum.

Morling, B., & Evered, S. (2006). Secondary control reviewed and defined. *Psychological Bulletin, 132,* 269–96.

Mueller, C. M., & Dweck, C. S. (1998). Praise for intelligence can undermine children's motivation and performance. *Journal of Personality and Social Psychology, 75,* 33–52.

Murphy, L., & Moriarity, A. (1976). *Vulnerability, coping, and growth: From infancy to adolescence.* New Haven: Yale University Press.

Nachmias, M., Gunnar, M., Mangelsdorf, S., Parritz, R. H., & Buss, K. (1996). Behavioral inhibition and stress reactivity: The moderating role of attachment security. *Child Development, 67,* 508–22.

Newman, R. S. (2000). Social influences on the development of children's adaptive help seeking: The role of parents, teachers, and peers. *Developmental Review, 20* (3), 350–404.

Nicholls, J. G. (1978). The development of the concepts of effort and ability, perceptions of academic attainment, and the understanding that difficult tasks require more ability. *Child Development, 49,* 800–14.

Nicholls, J. G. (1984). Achievement motivation: Conceptions of ability, subjective experience, task choice, and performance. *Psychological Review, 91,* 328–46.

Nolen-Hoeksema, S., Girgus, J. S., & Seligman, M. E. P. (1986). Learned helplessness in children: A longitudinal study of depression, achievement, and explanatory style. *Journal of Personality and Social Psychology, 51,* 435–42.

Papousek, H., & Papousek, M. (1979). The infant's fundamental adaptive response system in social interaction. In E. B. Thoman (Ed.), *Origins of the infant's social responsiveness.* Hillsdale, NJ: Erlbaum.

Papousek, H., & Papousek, M. (1980). Early ontogeny of human social interaction: Its biological roots and social dimensions. In M. von Cranach, K. Foppa, W. Lepenies, & D. Ploog (Eds.), *Human ethology: Claims and limits of a new discipline.* Cambridge: Cambridge University Press.

Peterson, C., Maier, S. F., & Seligman, M. E. P. (1993). *Learned helplessness: A theory for the age of personal control.* New York: Oxford University Press.

Piaget, J. (1976). *The grasp of consciousness: Action and concept in the young child.* Cambridge, MA: Harvard University Press.

Pomerantz, E. M., & Eaton, M. M. (2000). Developmental differences in children's conceptions of parental control: "They love me, but they make me feel incompetent." *Merrill-Palmer Quarterly, 46,* 140–67.

Pomerantz, E. M., & Eaton, M. M. (2001). Maternal intrusive support in the academic context: Transactional socialization processes. *Developmental Psychology, 37,* 174–86.

Pomerantz, E. M., & Ruble, D. N. (1997). Distinguishing multiple dimensions of conceptions of ability: Implications for self-evaluation. *Child Development, 68,* 1165–80.

Pomerantz, E. M., & Saxon, J. L. (2001). Conceptions of ability as stable and self-evaluative processes: A longitudinal examination. *Child Development, 72,* 152–73.

Robinson, J. L., & Acevedo, M. C. (2001). Infant reactivity and reliance on mother during emotion challenges: Prediction of cognition and language skills in a low-income sample. *Child Development, 72,* 402–15.

Rosenholtz, S. J., & Simpson, C. (1984). The formation of ability conceptions: Developmental trend or social construction? *Review of Educational Research, 54,* 31–63.

Rothbaum, F., Weisz, J. R., & Snyder, S. S. (1982). Changing the world and changing the self: A two-process model of perceived control. *Journal of Personality and Social Psychology, 42,* 5–37.

Rotter, B. (1966). Generalized expectancies for internal versus external control of reinforcement. *Psychological Monographs, 80* (Whole No. 609).

Ruble, D. (1983). The development of social comparison processes and their role in achievement-related self-socialization. In E. T. Higgins, D. N. Ruble, and W. W. Hartup (Eds.*), Social cognition and social development: A sociocultural perspective* (pp. 134–57). New York: Cambridge University Press.

Rueda, M. R., & Rothbart, M. K. (2009). Temperament, coping, and development. In E. A. Skinner & M. J. Zimmer-Gembeck (Eds.), *Perspective on children's coping with stress as regulation of emotion, cognition and behavior. New directions in child and adolescent development series.* San Francisco: Jossey-Bass.

Sameroff, A. J., & Haith, M. M. (1996). *The five to seven year shift: The age of reason and responsibility.* Chicago: University of Chicago Press.

Schmitz, B., & Skinner, E. (1993). Perceived control, effort, and academic performance: Interindividual, intraindividual, and multivariate time-series analyses. *Journal of Personality and Social Psychology, 64*(6), 1010–28.

Schulz, R., Wrosch, C., & Heckhausen, J. (2003). The life-span theory of control: Issues and evidence. In S. H. Zarit, L. I. Pearlin, & K. W. Schaie (Eds.), *Personal control in social and life course contexts* (pp. 233–62). New York: Springer.

Sedlak, A. J., & Kurtz, S. T. (1981). A review of children's use of causal inference principles. *Child Development, 57,* 759–84.

Seiffge-Krenke, I. (2004). Adaptive and maladaptive coping styles: Does intervention change anything? *European Journal of Developmental Psychology, 1,* 367–82.

Seligman, M. E. P. (1975). *Helplessness: On depression, development, and death.* San Francisco: Freeman.

Shaver, P. P., Belsky, J., & Brennan, K. (2000). The adult attachment interview and self-reports of romantic attachment:

Associations across domains and methods. *Personal Relationships, 7*, 25–43.

Skinner, E. A. (1995). *Perceived control, motivation, and coping.* Newbury Park, CA: Sage Publications.

Skinner, E. A. (1996). A guide to constructs of control. *Journal of Personality and Social Psychology, 71*, 549–70.

Skinner, E. A. (1999, April). The place and the purpose of coping theory and research. In I. N. Sandler & B. Compas (Co-chairs), *Beyond simple models of coping: Advances in theory and research.* Symposium conducted at the biennial meetings of the Society for Research in Child Development, Albuquerque, NM.

Skinner, E. A. (2007). Secondary control critiqued: Is it secondary? Is it control? (Commentary on Morling and Evered, 2006). *Psychological Bulletin, 133*(6), 911–6.

Skinner, E. A., & Connell, J. P. (1986). Control understanding: Suggestions for a developmental framework. In M. M. Baltes & P. B. Baltes (Eds.), *The psychology of control and aging* (pp. 35–69). Hillsdale, NJ: Erlbaum.

Skinner, E. A., & Edge, K. (1998). Reflections on coping and development across the lifespan. *International Journal of Behavioral Development, 22*, 357–66.

Skinner, E. A., & Wellborn, J. G. (1994). Coping during childhood and adolescence: A motivational perspective. In D. Featherman, R. Lerner, & M. Perlmutter (Eds.), *Life-span development and behavior* (Vol. 12, pp. 91–133). Hillsdale, NJ: Erlbaum.

Skinner, E. A., & Zimmer-Gembeck, M. J. (2007). The development of coping. *Annual Review of Psychology, 58,* 119–44.

Skinner, E. A., Chapman, M., & Baltes, P. B. (1988). Beliefs about control, means-ends, and agency: Developmental differences during middle childhood. *International Journal of Behavioural Development, 11*, 369–88.

Skinner, E. A., Edge, K., Altman, J., & Sherwood, H. (2003). Searching for the structure of coping: A review and critique of category systems for classifying ways of coping. *Psychological Bulletin, 129*, 216–69.

Skinner, E. A., Zimmer-Gembeck, M. J., & Connell, J. P. (1998). Individual differences and the development of perceived control. *Monographs of the Society for Research in Child Development, 63* (nos. 2 and 3), whole no. 254.

Sorce, J. F., Emde, R. N., Campos, J.,& Klinnert, M. D. (1985). Maternal emotional signaling: Its effect on the visual cliff behavior of 1-year-olds. *Developmental Psychology, 21*, 195–200.

Stipek, D. J. (1984a). The development of achievement motivation. In C. Ames & R. Ames (Eds.), *Research on motivation and education. Student motivation* (Vol. 1, pp. 145–74). San Diego, CA: Academic Press.

Stipek, D. J. (1984b). Young children's performance expectations: Logical analysis or wishful thinking? In M. Haehr (Ed.), *Advances in motivation and achievement* (pp. 33–56). Greenwich, CT: JAI Press.

Stipek, D. J. (2002). *Motivation to learn: From theory to practice* (4th ed.). Needham Heights, MA: Allyn & Bacon.

Stipek, D. J., & Daniels, D. H. (1988). Declining perceptions of competence: A consequence of changes in the child or in the educational environment? *Journal of Educational Psychology, 80*, 352–6.

Stipek, D. J., & Mac Iver, D. (1989). Developmental change in children's assessment of intellectual competence. *Child Development, 60*, 521–38.

Stipek, D. J., Recchia, S., & McClintic, S. M. (1992). Self-evaluation in young children. *Monographs of the Society for Research in Child Development, 57* (2, Serial No. 226).

Strickland, B. R. (1989). Internal-external control expectancies: From contingency to creativity. *American Psychologist, 44*(1), 1–12.

Stroebe, W., Stroebe, M., Abakoumkin, G., & Schut, H. (1996). The role of loneliness and social support in adjustment to loss: A test of attachment versus stress theory. *Journal of Personality and Social Psychology, 70*, 1241–9.

Taylor, S. E., & Stanton, A. L. (2007). Coping resources, coping processes, and mental health. *Annual Review of Clinical Psychology, 3*, 377–401.

Thompson, S. C. (1981). Will it hurt less if I can control it? A complex answer to a simple question. *Psychological Bulletin, 90*(1), 89–101.

Thompson, S. C. (1985). Finding positive meaning in a stressful event and coping. *Basic and Applied Social Psychology, 6*, 279–95.

Thompson, S. C., Sobolew-Shubin, A., Galbraith, M. E., Schwankovsky, L., & Cruzen, D. (1993). Maintaining perceptions of control: Finding perceived control in low-control circumstances. *Journal of Personality and Social Psychology, 64*(2), 293–304.

Urban, J., Carlson, E., Egeland, N., & Sroufe, L. (1991). Patterns of individual adaptation across childhood. *Development and Psychopathology, 3*, 445–60.

Wang, Q., & Pomerantz, E. M. (2009). The motivational landscape of early adolescence in the United States and China: A longitudinal investigation. *Child Development, 80*, 1272–87.

Watson, J. S. (1966). The development and generalization of "contingency awareness" in early infancy: Some hypotheses. *Merrill-Palmer Quarterly, 12*, 123–35.

Watson, J. S., & Ramey, C. T. (1972). Reactions to response-contingent stimulation in early infancy. *Merrill–Palmer Quarterly, 18*, 219–27.

Weiner, B. (1986). *An attributional theory of motivation and emotion.* New York: Springer.

Weiner, B. (2005). Motivation from an attributional perspective and the social psychology of perceived competence. In A. J. Elliot & C. S. Dweck (Eds.), *Handbook of competence and motivation* (pp. 73–84). New York: Guilford.

Weisz, J. R. (1980). Developmental change in perceived control: Recognizing noncontingency in the laboratory and perceiving it in the world. *Developmental Psychology, 16*, 385–90.

Weisz, J. R. (1981). Illusory contingency in children at the state fair. *Developmental Psychology, 17*, 481–9.

Weisz, J. R. (1983). Can I control it? The pursuit of veridical answers across the life span. In P. B. Baltes & O. G. Brim, Jr. (Eds.), *Life-span development and behavior* (pp. 233–300). New York: Academic Press.

Weisz, J. R. (1984). Contingency judgments and achievement behavior: Deciding what is controllable and when to try. In M. Haehr (Ed.), *Advances in motivation and achievement* (vol. 3, pp. 107–36). Greenwich, CT: JAI Press.

Weisz, J. R. (1986). Understanding the developing understanding of control. In M. Perlmutter (Ed.), *Minnesota Symposium on Child Psychology: Vol. 18. Social cognition* (pp. 219–78).

White, R. W. (1959). Motivation reconsidered: The concept of competence. *Psychological Review, 66*, 297–333.

Wigfield, A., & Eccles, J. S. (2000). Expectancy-value theory of motivation. *Contemporary Educational Psychology, 25,* 68–81.

Wigfield, A., & Eccles, J. S. (2002). *Development of achievement motivation.* San Diego: Academic Press.

Wigfield, A., Eccles, J. S., Schiefele, U., Roeser, R., & Davis-Kean, P. (2006). Development of achievement motivation. In W. Damon (Series Ed.) & N. Eisenberg (Volume Ed.), *Handbook of child psychology, 6th Ed. Vol. 3. Social, emotional, and personality development* (pp. 933–1002). New York: Wiley.

Wolchik, S. A., & Sandler, I. N. (Eds.). (1997). *Handbook of children's coping: Linking theory and intervention.* New York: Plenum Press.

Wolinsky, F. D., Wyrwich, K. W., Babu, A. N., Kroenke, K., & Tierny, W. M. (2003). Age, aging, and the sense of control among older adults: A longitudinal reconsideration. *Journal of Gerontology: Social Sciences, 58B*(4), S212–20.

Zarit, S. H., Pearlin, L. I., & Schaie, K. W. (Eds.) (2003). *Personal control in social and life course contexts.* New York: Springer.

Zimmer-Gembeck, M. J., & Skinner, E. A. (2008). Adolescents' coping with stress: Development and diversity. *Prevention Researcher, 15,* 3–7.

Zimmer-Gembeck, M. J., & Skinner, E. A. (in press). The development of coping across childhood and adolescence: An integrative review and critique of research, *International Journal of Behavioral Development.*

PART 3

Social Aspects of Stress and Coping

Gender, Stress, and Coping

Vicki S. Helgeson

Abstract

In this chapter, I discuss how sex is empirically and conceptually related to the experience of stressful life events and coping with stressful life events. I also review the literature that has attempted to link these sex differences to social or psychological gender role characteristics. Sex not only may influence the stressors one faces and how one copes with stressors but also may influence the relation of stressful life events and coping to health. Thus, I address sex as a moderator variable. The section on stressful life events distinguishes between the experience and impact of stressful events as well as the different kinds of stressful events men and women face. The section on coping reflects the traditional ways of coping as well as work on specific aspects of coping, such as rumination and benefit-finding. The research reviewed spans childhood, adolescence, and early and later adulthood. The chapter concludes with an outline of directions for future research.

Keywords: gender, stress, coping

The first section of the chapter is devoted to stressful life events and the second section of the chapter is devoted to coping. To understand the implications of sex (or gender) for each, one can ask two questions. First, do men and women differ in these domains? In other words, are there sex differences in stressful life events, and are there sex differences in coping? The second question is whether the health implications of stressful life events and coping strategies are the same for men and women—that is, does sex moderate the relation of stressful life events and coping to health? Within the two sections of the chapter (stressful life events, coping), I first review the literature that has compared men and women. Following these sex-specific comparisons, I examine whether sex is a moderator of the relation of stressful life events and coping to health.

The chapter concludes with a discussion of future research directions.

Stressful Life Events: Exposure

It would be a gross oversimplification to state that one sex experiences more stress than the other sex. One needs to distinguish between traumatic life events, more common stressful events, daily hassles, and perceptions of stress. When traumatic events have been examined, a meta-analytic review of the literature concluded that men experienced more trauma than women (Tolin & Foa, 2006). However, this sex difference greatly depended on the nature of the trauma. Men were 3.5 times as likely as women to experience combat/war/terrorism and over 1.5 times as likely as women to experience nonsexual assault, whereas women were 6 times as likely as men to report adult sexual assault and 2.5 times as likely as men to report child sexual assault. The incidence of post-traumatic stress disorder (PTSD) is higher among women than men (Olff, Langeland, Draijer, & Gersons, 2007), possibly because the traumas that women experience occur at younger ages (e.g., sexual abuse) or because the traumas that women experience are interpersonal in nature.

There are certain classes of stressors that men are more likely to experience and certain classes of stressors that women are more likely to experience because of their social roles (i.e., male role is agentic; female role is communal) and/or their relative status to one another (Nolen-Hoeksema, 2001). Men are more likely than women to experience unemployment and to be victims of physical violence, each of which has been linked to mental and physical health problems. By contrast, women are more likely to experience chronic sources of strain such as poverty, sexual harassment, discrimination, and caregiving for young children and the elderly. Each of these sources of strain has been strongly linked to mental health problems in women, including depression and PTSD. Below we briefly review the research on some of these major classes of stressors that differentially affect men and women.

Unemployment

Whereas women's labor force participation increased during the last half of the 20th century, men's labor force participation decreased (Toossi, 2006). The primary reason is unemployment. During the 1970s and 1980s, the unemployment rate was higher for women than men (Bureau of Labor Statistics, 2009), but since the year 2000, the rate has been higher for men than women. The recent economic downturn has had a disproportionate effect on the unemployment rate of men: Of job losses over the past year, 82% have occurred to men (Rampell, 2009).

Not surprisingly, unemployment is associated with mental health problems (Artazcoz, Benach, Borrell, & Cortes, 2004; Murphy & Athanasou, 1999), not only from financial strains but also due to an increase in other stressors, a decrease in social support, a loss of social status, and a loss of self-esteem (Bartley, 1994). Unemployment seems to have more hazardous effects on mental health for men than women—especially married men (Artazcoz et al., 2004). Whereas marriage seems to buffer women from the negative effects of unemployment on mental health, marriage exacerbates the adverse effects of unemployment on mental health among

men. This is most likely because unemployment undermines the traditional family role for men but not women. Unemployment also may lead to physical health problems, in part because prolonged unemployment has lasting negative effects on health behaviors, such as diet, exercise, and smoking (Wadsworth, Montgomery, & Bartley, 1999), and in part because unemployment leads to physiological changes such as increased cholesterol and decreases in immune function (Bartley, 1994).

Physical violence

We easily recollect that men are more likely than women to be perpetrators of aggression, but we often lose sight of the fact that men are also more likely than women to be victims of aggression. Men are more likely than women to be assaulted, robbed, threatened with violence, and killed. In the year 2007, men were almost four times as likely as women to be killed (U.S. Department of Justice, 2008). Among Black persons, men were almost six times as likely as women to be killed. In a study of college students, men were twice as likely to report having been kicked, bitten, hit by a fist, and hit by another object (Harris, 1996). Men were three times as likely to report being threatened with a gun or a knife. In a survey over 15,000 sixth- through tenth-graders, more boys than girls reported being bullied in school (Nansel et al., 2003).

By contrast, women are more likely than men to be victims of intimate violence. Women are more likely than men to be killed by someone they know than a stranger (Bureau of Justice Statistics, 2009). However, keep in mind that men are much more likely than women to be killed, so the actual number of men and women killed by someone they know is more similar. It seems that men and women are equally likely to be victims of domestic abuse (Currie, 1998), but women experience more severe violence compared to men (Archer, 2000). In addition, violence is associated with greater distress among women than men (Williams & Frieze, 2005). Intimate violence has been related to depression and PTSD in women (Golding, 1999; Koss, Bailey, Yuan, Herrera, & Lichter, 2003).

One source of physical violence that men face more than women is war. Although the number of women serving in the military has increased over the past few decades, men remain far more likely than women to serve in the military. In 2008, men represented 86% of active duty military (U.S. Coast Guard and Departments of Defense and Veteran Affairs, 2008).

Although women suffer higher rates of PTSD in the general population compared to men, this is not necessarily the case for war veterans. In a study of Vietnam veterans, men had higher rates of PTSD than women (Turner, Turse, & Dohrenwend, 2007). Reasons for this included demographic differences between the two groups (i.e., men were younger and less educated than the women who served) and the fact that men were more likely than women to be exposed to combat-related atrocities. A study of veterans from Gulf War I also showed that men were more likely than women to face combat (Vogt, Pless, King, & King, 2005).

Poverty

Poverty is a stressor that more women than men face and is a particularly potent source of distress for women for several reasons. First, poverty interferes with women being able to purchase goods and services that might be useful in coping with stressors. Second, one of the primary ways in which women cope with stressors is by drawing upon social networks (as will be discussed later in the chapter), but the network members of women in poverty are often too burdened with their own stressors (e.g., financial, drugs/alcohol) to be of assistance. Thus, the social networks of women in poverty often consist of people who utilize rather than provide resources. Among men and women in poverty, women report more economic strain than men (e.g., Siddiqui & Pandey, 2006). Poverty has been strongly linked to depression (Belle & Doucet, 2003).

Sexual harassment

Sexual harassment is a stressor faced by more women than men. However, sex differences in sexual harassment are somewhat controversial because the pervasiveness of sexual harassment depends on how sexual harassment is defined. If one considers sexual harassment charges filed with the EEOC, far more women than men report sexual harassment. In 2006, 12,025 charges of sexual harassment were filed (EEOC, 2007). Of those, 15% were filed by men and 85% were filed by women. However, the rate of men's reports has increased, as only 9% of charges were filed by men in 1992. In survey studies of adults, women report more sexual harassment than men (Newell, Rosenfeld, & Culbertson, 1995), but sex differences are most apparent for the more severe forms of harassment, such as requiring a worker to have sex with someone at work as part of the job. Men and women are equally likely to report the milder forms of harassment (Gutek, 1985).

The majority of harassment incidents consist of verbal behaviors, such as lewd comments, jokes, sexual innuendoes, and remarks about body parts. However, men themselves do not necessarily define the milder forms of harassment as sexual harassment (Gutek, 1985).

Regardless of the prevalence of sexual harassment, especially the milder forms, it is clear that sexual harassment is more strongly linked to adverse health outcomes among women than men. For example, one study of college students found that male and female students were equally likely to report harassment but that females were more bothered by it compared to males (Huerta, Cortina, Pang, Torges, & Magley, 2006).

Caregiving

Women are more likely than men to be found in the caregiver role. Women are more likely than men to be the primary caretakers of children and to take care of elderly parents, including in-laws (Cancian & Oliker, 2000). Caregiving also is more likely to lead to distress in women than in men. A longitudinal study of dual-earner couples who transitioned into caregiving showed that the transition led to an increase in distress among women but not men (Chesley & Moen, 2006). Instead, men who transitioned into caregiving experienced increases in personal growth. One reason that caregiving may be associated with greater distress among women is that some women decrease or cease employment when they become caregivers (Pavalko & Woodbury, 2000), whereas men are more likely to obtain assistance with caregiving (Yee & Schulz, 2000).

In a meta-analytic review of the caregiving literature, women reported greater burden than men, greater depression than men, and a greater number of caregiving tasks than men (Pinquart & Sorensen, 2006). However, a meta-analysis on the effects of caregiving on physical health found mixed results for gender (Vitaliano, Zhang, & Scanlan, 2003). For some physical health outcomes, effects were stronger for female than male caregivers, but the authors were unable to distinguish whether these sex differences were unique to caregiving. A recent study examined the effects of caregiving on men's and women's health and found that the effects depended on the specific health outcome. Partially consistent with the two previous meta-analyses, caregiving in women was associated with greater psychological distress and worse physical health (e.g., self-report, doctor visits), whereas caregiving in men was associated with greater physiological effects (e.g., body mass index, insulin, glucose; Zhang, Vitaliano, & Lin, 2006).

The effects of caregiving on men and women may depend in part on their relationship to the person needing care. One study found that female caregivers of spouses, children, or parents were more likely to be distressed than female non-caregivers, but male caregivers were more distressed than male non-caregivers only when the person they were taking care of was a spouse (Marks, 1998).

Other major stressors

We have reviewed several major stressors that differentially affect men and women. In addition to these stressors, research also has examined more common stressful events that people experience, including job loss, divorce, relationship problems, and financial difficulties—often summarizing across these events to derive an index of stressful life events. A meta-analytic review of such studies conducted between 1960 and 1996 revealed a small tendency for females to report more stressful events than males (Davis, Matthews, & Twamley, 1999). The size of this effect was extremely small ($d = .12$), and a number of variables, such as measure employed, nature of the stressor, and age of the sample, influenced the size of the relation, as will be described below.

EXPOSURE VERSUS IMPACT

One factor that influenced the effect size in the meta-analysis of stressful life events was how stress was measured (Davis et al., 1999). Researchers typically present respondents with a list of life events and ask them to indicate whether each event has happened within a certain period of time. Researchers also may ask respondents to indicate how strongly they were affected by each event. In other words, ratings are made of stress exposure and stress impact. When these two kinds of ratings were distinguished from one another in the meta-analysis, the sex difference in exposure was smaller than the sex difference in impact ($d = +.08$ vs. $d = +.18$). Thus, the evidence that women appraise stressors as more severe than men is stronger than the evidence that women experience more stressors than men.

NATURE OF STRESSOR

Just as men and women experience major stressors in different domains, they also experience more ordinary stressors in different domains. The meta-analysis revealed that the sex difference for interpersonal stressors was larger than the sex difference for non-interpersonal stressors ($d = +.17$ vs. $d = +.07$; Davis et al., 1999). There was no category of stressor for which men scored higher than women.

AGE OF SAMPLE

The meta-analytic review of the literature on sex differences in stress also showed that the age of the sample influenced the size of the relation (Davis et al., 1999). Sex differences were larger for adolescent samples than younger or older groups, supporting Nolen-Hoeksema's (1994) claim that adolescent females face more stress than adolescent males. This may be due, in part, to the fact that boys and girls begin to experience different kinds of stressors during adolescence—that is, the age effect might be partly driven by the nature of stressor effect. Adolescence is a time of gender intensification (Hill & Lynch, 1983), when gender-role norms become salient. For girls, this means an increasing focus on relationships (Larson & Richards, 1989; 1991). The increase in affiliation may present women with more opportunities to experience interpersonal stressors.

There are numerous studies of adolescents that show that girls experience more interpersonal stressors than boys. For example, a study of preadolescent (ages 8 to 12) and adolescent (ages 13 to 18) boys and girls showed that there was no sex difference in the total number of stressful events reported, but that girls reported greater interpersonal stress and boys reported greater non-interpersonal stress (Rudolph & Hammen, 1999). However, age moderated this effect. Among preadolescents, there were no sex differences in interpersonal or non-interpersonal stressors. Among adolescents, girls reported more interpersonal stressors compared to boys, and boys reported more non-interpersonal stressors compared to girls (Figure 4.1). Other studies of adolescents have shown that girls report more relationship stressors than boys (Hampel & Petermann, 2006; Murberg & Bru, 2004), and boys report more of some categories of personal stressors than girls (Murberg & Bru, 2004; Shih, Eberhart, Hammen, & Brennan, 2006).

One study proposed that the increase in depression among adolescent females is due to a specific interpersonal stressor—involvement in romantic relationships. The study showed that both boys and girls who became involved in romantic relationships over the course of a year showed a larger increase in depression, but the effect was stronger among girls (Joyner & Udry, 2000). The stronger effect among girls was partly due to the deterioration in

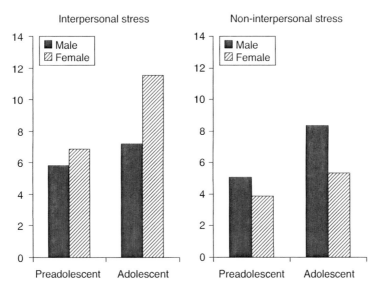

Fig. 4.1 Sex comparisons of interpersonal and non-interpersonal stress among preadolescents and adolescents. Adolescent girls reported higher levels of interpersonal stress compared to adolescent boys and either group of preadolescents. Adolescent boys reported higher non-interpersonal stress compared to adolescent girls and either group of preadolescents. (Reprinted with permission from John Wiley and Sons.)

relationships with parents over the course of the year. Time spent with romantic partners might have detracted from time spent with family, or girls' involvement in romantic relationships could have become a subject of conflict with parents. Other research with freshmen college students has shown that females who are involved in romantic relationships are more distressed than males who are involved in romantic relationships, whereas there is no sex difference in distress among those not involved in romantic relationships (Helgeson, 1994). Thus, involvement in romantic relationships may be a specific domain of interpersonal vulnerability for adolescent females.

Others' stressful events
Another kind of event that women appear to experience more frequently than men is events experienced by others. For example, a study of physically disabled people found no sex difference in the number of stressful events that happened to the self, but found that women were more likely than men to report events that occurred to others (Turner & Avison, 1989). One possibility is that women were more likely than men to remember events that occurred to others. However, when the authors examined the timeframe during which life events occurred, men and women reported similar numbers of events occurring to others in more recent months, but women reported significantly more

events that occurred to others compared to men in more distant months. Thus, the authors concluded that men were more likely than women to forget others' events. However, the authors also argued that this memory bias could not fully account for the findings. Women cast a wider network of caring than men, potentially making them more aware of events that occur to others.

Explanations for sex differences in stressful life events
There are a variety of explanations for the sex differences in traumatic and stressful life events. Men experience more aggression than women because the male role is associated with dominance, and it is more acceptable to behave aggressively toward a dominant person. Women experience greater poverty, sexual harassment, and discrimination than men due to their lower status. Women experience more strain related to caregiving due to the relationship orientation of the female social role. Below we examine specific aspects of gender roles that may explain why women report more stressors than men. Then, we examine a more cognitive explanation for sex differences in stressful life events that is linked to gender roles.

GENDER ROLES
The female gender role is a communal role that involves connections to others. There are at least

two aspects of that role that have been distinguished from one another—communion and unmitigated communion. Whereas communion represents a healthy focus on others and is related to good relationship outcomes, unmitigated communion represents a focus on others to the exclusion of the self that is related to poor relationship and poor health outcomes (Helgeson, 1994; Helgeson & Fritz, 1998). Unmitigated communion consists of overinvolvement with others and self-neglect. The two are undoubtedly related; overinvolvement with others leads to self-neglect. Adolescents who score high on unmitigated communion report more interpersonal stressors than those who score low on unmitigated communion (Helgeson & Fritz, 1996). In a study of adults in which events that happened to the self were distinguished from events that happened to others, unmitigated communion was related to the latter but not the former (Fritz & Helgeson, 1998). Recall that women are more likely than men to report stressful events that occurred to others. Unmitigated communion may provide one explanation for this sex difference.

Unmitigated communion is related to reports of others' stressors for at least two reasons. First, unmitigated communion may be associated with exposure to others' problems because such individuals seek out others to help. The self-esteem of the unmitigated communion individual rests upon being the support provider (Helgeson & Fritz, 1998). Second, the person who scores high on unmitigated communion may be more likely than others to interpret another person's problem as his or her own. For example, two people may be exposed to a neighbor going through a divorce, but only the unmitigated communion person defines this stressful event as his or her own personal stressor.

ENCODING
Another explanation for women reporting more life events than men has to do with differential encoding and recall of those events. In other words, men and women may experience the same number of stressful life events, but women may be more likely than men to recall those events. There is a literature on autobiographical memory that is consistent with this possibility. The literature shows that females—both children and adults—are more likely than males to recall both positive and negative events from their childhood (Davis, 1999). Interestingly, it appears that this bias may be limited to events that are associated with emotion.

This differential recall is *not* due to affect intensity; that is, it is not that women simply experience more intense emotion during life events than men, which facilitates better recall. Instead, it seems that women encode emotional events in more detail than men. These ideas were supported by a daily diary study in which college students recorded their best and worst events and rated the intensity of those events each day over a period of 43 days (Seidlitz & Diener, 1998). At the end of the study, participants were asked to recall as many of these events as possible using words as similar as possible to their original reports. Women recalled more events than men. Recalled events were not rated as more intense than events that were not recalled—for either men or women. Instead, recalled events were described in greater detail by women than men. This conclusion fits with other research that shows women have more detailed and complex representations of emotion than men (Feldman-Barrett, Lane, Sechrest, & Schwartz, 2000).

Why might women have more elaborate representations of emotion and emotional events than men? Women are socialized from an early age to focus on others and their environment. Because women have a more interdependent sense of self (Cross & Madson, 1997), they may pay closer attention to the environment, leading them to encode events that involve others in greater detail. It also is the case that women have a lower status then men, which implies that the environment has greater effects on the lives of women than the lives of men. It is to the low status person's advantage to be aware of all aspects of the environment that may affect her.

Thus, it appears that the link of gender to trauma and stress has more to do with men and women experiencing different kinds of traumas and stressors rather than one sex experiencing more trauma or stress than the other. Women are more likely than men to report stressful events that involve relationships and that actually occur to others. Although both of these events are sometimes referred to as relationship stressors, there is a difference. In the first case, investigators are finding that women are more likely to report problems within relationships, such as conflicts, breakups, or losses. In the second case, research is showing that women are more likely than men to perceive stressful events that occur to others as their own personal stressors. Reasons for these differences may have to do with the different social roles or the different statuses that men and women hold. Now, we turn to the question of whether men or women are more strongly affected by stressful life events.

Stressful Life Events: Implications for Health

Do stressful life events show the same relation to health for men and women? This question is similar to the distinction that we made between stress exposure and stress impact, but the question here is addressed in a statistical or experimental fashion rather than relying on individuals' reports of the effects of stressful life events. Survey studies have examined whether the relation of stressors to outcomes is statistically stronger in one sex than the other, whereas laboratory experiments have manipulated stressors and determined whether physiological responses are the same for males and females.

Survey studies

Investigators have asked whether sex differences in some health outcomes, such as depression, are due to differential exposure to stressful events or differential vulnerability to stressful events. Differential exposure suggests that women are more depressed than men because they experience more of a certain kind of stressful event. In fact, some of the major stressors that women experience more than men, such as poverty and sexual abuse, are associated with depression (Nolen-Hoeksema & Keita, 2003). Although controlling for these events reduces the sex difference in depression, it does not eliminate it (Kessler, 2000). In fact, if all the stressful events were statistically controlled (not just the ones that affect women more than men), the sex difference in depression would be unchanged. Thus, women are not more depressed than men because they simply experience more stressful events. By contrast, differential vulnerability implies that certain stressful events are more strongly associated with distress among women than men. For example, one study showed that conflict with friends was a stronger predictor of alcohol consumption, alcohol problems, and depression over the course of a year for women than men (Skaff, Finney, & Moos, 1999). The distinction between differential exposure and differential vulnerability, as it pertains to depression, has been summed up nicely by Turner and Avison (1989): "Women may care about more people or care more about the people they know, or both" (p. 450). The first part of the sentence pertains to exposure, and the second part pertains to vulnerability.

INTERPERSONAL STRESSORS

Studies that have compared the differential exposure and differential vulnerability hypotheses largely conclude that there is more evidence for differential vulnerability in the domain of interpersonal stressors. A review of five epidemiological studies showed that men and women were exposed to different kinds of stressors, but stress exposure did not explain sex differences in depression to the extent that sex differences in vulnerability did (Kessler & McLeod, 1984). Men reported more life events in the categories of income loss and ill health, and women reported more life events in the categories of death of a loved one and other network events. Events that involved social networks were more strongly related to depression for women than men. When the effect of women's exposure to network events was compared to the effect of women's vulnerability to network events, vulnerability appeared to account for more of women's depression.

Three more recent studies have supported this conclusion. A study of couples showed that network-related stressors were more strongly related to depression in women than men (Nazroo, Edwards, & Brown, 1997). A study of adults from the community showed that women were three times as likely as men to experience depression in response to stressful events, especially when the events involved network members (Maciejewski, Prigerson, & Mazure, 2001). Another study showed that women were more adversely affected by life events that occurred to others compared to men, but were not more adversely affected by life events that occurred to the self (Turner & Avison, 1989).

COUPLES WITH CHRONIC ILLNESS

Another area of research that supports the differential vulnerability hypothesis with respect to interpersonal stressors is research on couples in which one member has a chronic illness. To the extent that females are socialized to be more oriented toward others, one would predict that females will be more reactive to the distress of their partner compared to males. Indeed, there are some data to support this hypothesis. Several studies have shown that female spouses are more distressed than male spouses when their partner has a chronic illness (Rohrbaugh et al., 2002; Tuinstra et al., 2004). Because women are more distressed than men in general, however, those studies do not necessarily convey whether there is something unique about being a spouse of an ill patient that exacerbates women's distress. Indeed, a meta-analytic review of the literature on distress among couples coping with cancer showed that women are more distressed than men, regardless of whether they are the patient or the spouse (Hagedoorn, Sanderman, Bolks, Tuinstra, & Coyne, 2008).

Several studies have attempted to determine whether there is something unique about being a spouse of a chronically ill patient that poses an added burden for women. One study compared couples in which one person had cancer to couples in which both persons were healthy (Hagedoorn, Buunk, Kuijer, Wobbes, & Sanderman, 2000). They found that both female patients and female spouses were more distressed than healthy women, but that only male patients were more distressed than male spouses or healthy men. This study demonstrated that there was psychological distress unique to being a female spouse. Two other studies compared wives of husbands who did and did not have a chronic illness. In a study of elderly couples, wives' psychological distress was affected by whether spouses had a health condition, but husbands' psychological distress was not (Hagedoorn et al., 2001). An older study showed that wives' marital satisfaction was influenced by whether or not their husband had a chronic illness but was not influenced by whether they had the chronic illness themselves (Hafstrom & Schram, 1984). These kinds of studies suggest that female spouses are more strongly affected than male spouses by their partner's illness.

One reason for these findings is that women are socialized to focus on others and others' feelings more so than men are. Thus, husbands' emotions may affect wives more than wives' emotions affect husbands. One study showed that husbands' depression was associated with wives' depression, but wives' depression was not associated with husbands' depression (Whiffen & Gotlib, 1989). There seems to be more evidence for **emotional transmission** from husbands to wives than from wives to husbands (Larson & Almeida 1999).

ADOLESCENTS
Studies of adolescents also have supported the differential vulnerability hypothesis. In a 4-year longitudinal study of 9- to 17-year-olds, boys reported more stressful life events than girls before age 12, but girls reported more stressful life events than boys after age 12 (Ge, Lorenz, Conger, Elder, & Simons, 1994). The change in stressful life events paralleled the change in depressive symptoms, and the increase in stressful life events was associated with an increase in depression—but only for girls.

The authors concluded that girls were more depressed than boys not only because they experienced more stressful events but also because they were more vulnerable to them. More recently, a study of over 2,000 adolescents from the Netherlands showed that stressful life events were more strongly related to an increase in depression over 2 years among females than males (Bouma, Ormel, Verhulst, & Oldehinkel, 2008). Finally, another study of adolescents showed that interpersonal stressors were more strongly associated with depression in females than males, whereas non-interpersonal stressors had similar effects on males and females (Shih et al., 2006).

WORK AND FINANCIAL STRESSORS
While the evidence among adolescents and adults suggests that females are more vulnerable than males to a particular category of stressor—interpersonal—there is some evidence that men are differentially more vulnerable to stressors that involve work and finances. In a study of married couples, men reported greater distress than women in response to work and financial stressors (Conger, Lorenz, Elder, Simons, & Ge, 1993). Anecdotally, one can think of several noteworthy cases in which men committed suicide in the wake of recent financial crises, including a former executive of Enron and a French investment manager who lost substantial sums of money in the Madoff scandal. Suicide rates are more strongly tied to unemployment rates among men than among women (Lester & Yang, 1998).

A poignant example of men's vulnerability to economic stressors is the aftermath of the breakup of the Soviet Union. The subsequent economic and social instability following the breakup was associated with stronger adverse health consequences for the men than the women of the country. Between 1990 and 1994, the life expectancy for men declined by 6 years, whereas the life expectancy for women declined by 3 years. Even today, the sex difference in life expectancy in Russia (men 60; women 74) is the largest among industrialized nations (World Factbook, 2007). The decline in life expectancy in the early 1990s was due in large part to the increase in death from heart disease, injuries, suicide, and homicide among people ages 25 to 64. Deaths from these causes can be directly linked to the increase in poverty, increase in stress, and rise in alcohol intake that occurred during this time period. All of these factors seem to have had a greater impact on men's than women's mortality rates. Loss of jobs and loss of income are more threatening to the traditional male gender role than the traditional female gender role. In interviews with men and women from Russia following the fall of communism, the majority of both men and women said that they thought the economic changes were much harder on the men than the women in the country (Pietila & Rytkonen, 2008).

GENDER-RELATED TRAITS

There also is evidence that gender-related traits are associated with differential vulnerability to stress in survey studies. One study of adolescents showed that it was not just being female that was associated with being reactive to interpersonal stressors, but also that those with an interpersonal orientation were more reactive to interpersonal stressors (Gore, Aseltine, & Colten, 1993). Two studies have shown that people who score high on unmitigated communion are more reactive to interpersonal stress than people who score low on unmitigated communion. In a study of adolescents with diabetes, relationship stressors were more strongly related to psychological distress for those who scored high than low on unmitigated communion (Helgeson & Fritz, 1996). In a study of college students that involved nightly phone interviews for 7 consecutive days, daily interpersonal conflict was associated with daily distress for individuals both high and low in unmitigated communion (Reynolds et al., 2006). However, interpersonal conflict was associated with distress the following day only for individuals high in unmitigated communion. These findings suggest that unmitigated communion individuals' reaction to interpersonal stress is more prolonged. Similar findings appeared in a study that measured a construct related to unmitigated communion, interpersonal sensitivity (i.e., how much feelings and behavior of others affect the self). In a study that involved 12 weekly phone calls with adult women who had osteoarthritis or rheumatoid arthritis, the relation of interpersonal stress to negative affect was stronger for those who scored high on interpersonal sensitivity (Smith & Zautra, 2002).

Laboratory studies

The differential vulnerability issue also has been addressed in the laboratory. There is a great deal of research that shows men and women respond differently to laboratory stressors in terms of cardiovascular reactivity. The first studies in this area consistently showed that men exhibited greater cardiovascular reactivity than women (Matthews, Gump, & Owens, 2001). However, researchers soon realized that men

may have shown greater reactivity than women because the laboratory tasks used were more relevant to men than women. Subsequent work showed that women exhibit greater reactivity than men when the domain is made to be more relevant to women, such as a discussion of a relationship conflict. In fact, the marital interaction literature has shown that wives are more physiologically reactive to conflict discussions than husbands in terms of cardiovascular, immune, and endocrine parameters (Ewart, Taylor, Kraemer, & Agras, 1991; Gottman & Levenson, 1992; Kiecolt-Glaser et al., 1993). In addition, husbands' behaviors during these interactions, as coded by observers, are more strongly linked to women's physiological reactivity than wives' behaviors are to men's reactivity (Kiecolt-Glaser et al., 1996).

To test the idea that men and women are differentially vulnerable to stressors that are linked to the male and female gender roles, research has compared men's and women's reactivity to a series of stressors in the laboratory, varying relevance to gender roles. One study showed that men were more reactive than women to two masculine tasks, serial subtraction and a handgrip squeeze, whereas women were more reactive than men to a feminine task, giving a speech on likes and dislikes about one's physical appearance (Stroud, Niaura, & Salovey, 2001). In another study, college males showed greater cortisol increases in response to achievement stressors (math, verbal memorization), and college females showed greater cortisol increases in response to an interpersonal stressor (rejection; Stroud, Salovey, & Epel, 2002; Figure 4.2). A stronger test of this hypothesis was made when studies employed a single gender-neutral task and manipulated its relevance to gender. Two studies employed this approach with the cold pressor test and found that men were more reactive when the task was described as masculine and women were more reactive when the task was described as feminine (Lash, Eisler, & Southard, 1995; Lash, Gillespie, Eisler, & Southard, 1991).

Researchers also have moved beyond sex to explore the effects of psychological gender roles on reactivity to laboratory stressors. Part of the reason that females are more strongly affected by interpersonal events than males is that being female is associated with a communal or relationship orientation in our culture. Part of the reason that males are more strongly affected by achievement events than females is that being male is associated with an agentic or instrumental orientation. Thus, one would expect more communally oriented people to

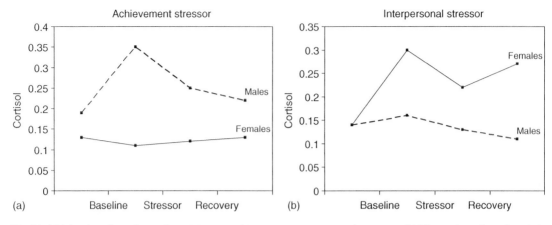

Fig. 4.2 (a) Men show elevated cortisol reactivity to an achievement stressor compared to women. (b) Women show elevated cortisol reactivity to an interpersonal stressor compared to men.
(Reprinted from *Biological Psychiatry*, 52, Stroud, L. R., Salovey, P., & Epel, E. S., Sex differences in stress responses: Social rejection versus achievement stress, pp. 318–327. Copyright 2002, reprinted with permission from Elsevier.)

be more reactive to interpersonal stressors and more agentic people to be more reactive to achievement stressors. Few studies, however, have tested this possibility. One study manipulated the relevance of a cognitive task to the male gender role and found that men who scored higher on a measure of male gender role stress (i.e., viewed threats to the male gender role as stressful) showed greater cardiovascular reactivity as well as poorer performance when the task was described as relevant to the male gender role than when it was not relevant to the male gender role (Cosenzo, Franchina, Eisler, & Krebs, 2004). Men who scored low on gender role stress did not behave differently in the two conditions. Another study examined achievement motivation in the context of a naturally occurring stressor—taking an exam—and found that achievement motivation was associated with physiological reactivity to the exam in males but not females (Rauste-von Wright, von Wright, & Frankenhaeuser, 1981; van Doornen, 1986).

A more complicated association of gender-related traits to cardiovascular reactivity to stress was examined in one study that involved pairs of college friends discussing a problem. The investigators did not examine whether gender-related traits were directly associated with cardiovascular reactivity but tested whether they moderated the effects of social interaction variables on cardiovascular reactivity (Fritz, Nagurney, & Helgeson, 2003). One gender-related trait that was examined was unmitigated agency, which involves an excessive self-focus and a cynical mistrust of others. It appeared to be an important moderator of the effects of emotional

support on reactivity. Partner emotional support was associated with reduced reactivity only when it was provided by a partner who was low on unmitigated agency. It might be that emotional support provided by a high unmitigated agency person was viewed as less genuine or was conveyed in a less caring manner. The second gender-related trait that was examined was communion—the healthy focus on others that involves warmth and caring. Instead of moderating the effects of emotional support, communion moderated the effects of negative interactions on cardiovascular recovery to the stressor. Negative interactions were associated with delayed recovery when provided by partners who were high in communion, perhaps because such social exchanges are unexpected.

All of the studies conducted to date have suggested that men or masculine people are more reactive to stressors that threaten the male role and women or feminine people are more reactive to stressors that threaten the female role. One study showed just the opposite—that men and women are more reactive to tasks that are *incongruent* with their gender or gender role. In other words, masculine people were more reactive to a feminine stressor, and feminine people were more reactive to a masculine stressor (Davis & Matthews, 1996). In this study, participants who scored high on masculinity or femininity were randomly assigned to either persuade or empathize with their partner. Masculine people were more reactive when they had to empathize with rather than persuade their partner, whereas feminine people were more reactive when they had to persuade rather than empathize with their partner. The authors suggested that gender-role incongruent tasks are more challenging or stressful.

The disparate findings were reconciled by Wright, Murray, Storey, and Williams' (1997) suggestion that the difficulty of the task must be taken into consideration when trying to understand which tasks will arouse the most reactivity in men and women. They argued that task difficulty influences whether a task is perceived as a challenge or a threat. When difficulty is high, the thought of not performing well on a task consistent with one's gender role is perceived as a threat. Thus, when faced with a difficult task, women should show greater reactivity than men to a feminine task, and men should show greater reactivity than women to a masculine task. By contrast, in the context of an easy task, people whose gender role is congruent with the task expect to perform well and are not threatened by the task. People whose gender role is incongruent with the task are likely to perceive the task as more of a challenge—in a sense, a higher difficulty level. These people feel less capable and expend more effort. Thus, when faced with an easy task, women should show greater reactivity than men to the masculine task, and men should show greater reactivity than women to the feminine task. In sum, the difficulty of a gender-role congruent task determines whether the person feels comfortable and competent or threatened by the possibility of failure. The study Wright et al. (1997) conducted supported these ideas.

These ideas also were extended beyond sex to gender role. In a replication study, masculine and feminine people were more reactive to the gender congruent task when the task was more difficult, but masculine and feminine people were more reactive to the gender-incongruent task when the task was easier (van Well, Kolk, & Klugkist, 2008).

Taken collectively, the weight of the evidence in the area of gender and stress supports differential vulnerability rather than differential exposure. For example, differential vulnerability rather than differential exposure accounts for more of the sex difference in depression. Women are more strongly affected than men by stressors that involve others. This finding is robust across studies of adolescents, adults, and the elderly. By contrast, men are more strongly affected by work and financial stressors than women, which could be implicated in some of the health outcomes for which men are more vulnerable (e.g., heart disease, suicide, accidents). Laboratory research has demonstrated that men and women are differentially responsive to different classes of stressors that can be divided along gender-role lines. There also may be biological differences in the way men and women respond to stress, but those differences are beyond the scope of this chapter (Dedovic, Wadiwalla, Engert, & Pruessner, 2009).

Gender and Coping
Sex differences in coping strategies
Coping refers to the different strategies that we use to manage stressful events and the accompanying distress associated with them. A major distinction that has been made in the coping literature is between problem-focused and emotion-focused (Lazarus & Folkman, 1984). **Problem-focused coping** refers to attempts to alter the stressor itself, such as finding a solution to the problem, seeking the advice of others, and developing a plan to approach the problem. **Emotion-focused coping** refers to ways in which we accommodate ourselves to the stressor. Emotion-focused coping strategies are quite varied, ranging from distraction, avoidance, and denial to talking about the problem, accepting the problem, and focusing on the positive. Investigators frequently suggest that women are more likely to engage in emotion-focused coping and men are more likely to engage in problem-focused coping. However, this kind of summary statement is too simplistic. The broad categories of emotion-focused coping and problem-focused coping include distinct coping strategies, only some of which may show sex differences. For example, researchers often hypothesize that men are more likely than women to engage in problem-focused coping. Yet one primary problem-focused coping strategy is to seek the advice of others, a behavior that we typically ascribe to women. Emotion-focused coping includes discussing one's feelings about the problem, a behavior we typically attribute to women, but also avoidance and distraction, behaviors we typically attribute to men.

To address these issues, my colleagues and I conducted a meta-analytic review of the literature on sex comparisons in coping (Tamres, Janicki, & Helgeson, 2002). The largest sex differences appeared for positive self-talk (i.e., encouraging oneself), seeking support, and rumination—all in the direction of women utilizing the strategies more than men. Interestingly, all three coping differences involved the expression of feelings, either to oneself or to someone else. More recent studies of coping among children have confirmed these findings. For example, a study of adolescents in Austria showed that girls were more likely than boys to use social support and to engage in rumination (Hampel & Petermann, 2006). A study of children and adolescents with chronic pain (ages 8 to 18) found that girls were more likely than boys to seek social support, and boys were more likely than girls to engage in behavioral distraction, (Lynch, Kashikar-Zuck, Goldschneider, & Jones, 2007).

There are conceptual frameworks for the coping domains that revealed the largest sex differences. For example, the sex difference in seeking support is consistent with Shelley Taylor and colleagues' (2000) theory that women respond to stress with a "tend and befriend" strategy as opposed to the more typically studied "fight or flight" response. The sex difference in rumination is consistent with a large literature established by Susan Nolen-Hoeksema that shows women are more likely to ruminate in response to stressful life events, while men are more likely to distract themselves. This literature is reviewed below.

The meta-analysis also showed that women engaged in more of nearly all the coping strategies than men, those that were problem-focused and emotion-focused. Although the sex differences were often small in magnitude, the direction was consistent across the wide range of coping strategies examined. In an earlier review of the literature, Peggy Thoits (1991) reached a similar conclusion—that women engage in more of all kinds of coping strategies than men. There are a variety of reasons for this sex difference. One possibility is that women are more flexible than men in their approach to coping. It also is possible that women are more distressed than men, which requires them to use a variety of approaches to coping. This possibility was tested in the meta-analytic review of sex differences in coping by examining stressor appraisal as a moderator of sex differences (Tamres et al., 2002). If women are engaging in more coping strategies than men because they are more distressed than men, sex differences in coping should be limited to studies in which there are sex differences in distress or sex differences in stressor appraisal. For several coping strategies, sex differences in usage appeared only in studies in which women appraised the stressor as more severe then men. There were two exceptions—rumination and seeking support. Women appeared to engage in more rumination and more support-seeking than men even when they did not appraise the stressor as more severe. Thus, it appears that part of the reason that women engage in more coping strategies than men is that women are more distressed than men. However, it also is the case that there are some sex differences in coping that exist regardless of the level of distress experienced.

Another way to examine sex differences in coping that avoids the confounding factor of differential levels of distress is to examine **relative coping**. Instead of comparing the frequency with which men and women engage in a specific kind of coping, one compares the frequency with which men engage in one coping strategy compared to another strategy and the frequency with which women engage in one coping strategy compared to another strategy, or relative coping (Vitaliano, Maiuro, Russo, & Becker, 1987). In two studies, one of college students coping with an achievement stressor and an interpersonal stressor and one of people with coronary heart disease coping with their health, we compared relative coping to absolute coping (Tamres et al., 2002). For each of the three stressors, absolute coping scores showed that women engaged in more coping than men. There was not a single coping strategy in which men engaged in more than women. However, when relative coping scores were examined, men engaged in *relatively* more active coping strategies, men engaged in *relatively* more distraction, and women engaged in *relatively* more support-seeking.

We now turn to research that has examined specific kinds of coping that may have implications for gender: rumination, co-rumination, primary versus secondary control, and stress-related growth.

RUMINATION

One of the more sizeable sex differences to emerge from the meta-analysis was that women ruminate more than men. This finding is not surprising as there is a large literature on rumination, largely concluding that rumination is an antecedent to depression and explains part of why women are more depressed than men. Susan Nolen-Hoeksema (1987, 1994) has argued that women are more depressed than men because women ruminate about their feelings after negative events and men distract themselves. However, the sex difference in rumination is more consistent than the sex difference in distraction (Nolen-Hoeksema & Davis, 1999; Strauss, Muday, McNall, & Wong, 1997). For example, in a 1-year longitudinal study of over 1,000 community residents (Nolen-Hoeksema, Larson, & Grayson, 1999), women reported a greater tendency than men to ruminate, and rumination explained the greater increase in depression over the year among women compared to men.

There is a great deal of evidence that rumination leads to depression. Numerous studies have shown that people who tend to ruminate in response to a stressful event end up more distressed. Nolen-Hoeksema (2006) argues that individuals get involved in a cycle of rumination and depression. Rumination increases depression, which then increases rumination. The reciprocal relation between rumination and depression has been demonstrated in longitudinal studies of bereaved adults (Nolen-Hoeksema Parker, & Larson, 1994) and community residents (Nolen-Hoeksema et al., 1999). Rumination increases depression (a) by interfering with instrumental behavior, which might alleviate depression; (b) by making other negative feelings and negative memories more salient, which reinforces depression; and (c) by leading people to make pessimistic explanations for negative events. Rumination has been linked to pessimistic thinking (Nolen-Hoeksema, Parker, & Larson, 1994) and cognitive inflexibility (i.e., perseverance of thought, inability to respond to feedback; Davis & Nolen-Hoeksema, 2000). This explains why the cycle of rumination and depression is so difficult to break.

More recently, researchers have examined the content of the rumination scale in more depth and noted that some of the items are confounded with depression (e.g., think about how sad you feel; Treynor, Gonzalez, & Nolen-Hoeksema, 2003). After removing these confounding items, a factor analysis of the remaining items revealed two kinds of rumination: (1) reflective pondering (e.g., go away by yourself and think about why you feel this way; write down what you are thinking about and analyze it) and (2) brooding (Think "Why do I have problems other people don't have?"; Think "Why do I always react this way?"). Although women score higher than men on both, the brooding items are more predictive of depression than the reflective items and account for the sex difference in depression.

Why are women more likely than men to ruminate in response to stressful events? One possibility is that people encourage women to ruminate more than men. One study showed that college students gave more ruminative advice (i.e., figure out why you are depressed) to women than to men (Ali & Toner, 1996). Students were equally likely to give distracting advice to men and women. In another study, sixth-, seventh-, and eighth-graders responded to vignettes of men and women ruminating or distracting (Broderick & Korteland, 2002). Distraction was viewed as more appropriate for males than females, and rumination was viewed as more appropriate for females than males. People might encourage women to ruminate because they do not believe

it is maladaptive—at least for women. In fact, college students perceive rumination strategies (e.g., talking with someone, determining the cause of one's feelings) as more effective in alleviating depression than distraction strategies (Strauss et al., 1997).

CO-RUMINATION

Females also are more likely than males to engage in a behavior referred to as **co-rumination** (Rose, 2002). Co-rumination involves repeatedly discussing problems with a friend, including the causes, the consequences, and the negative feelings associated with those problems. Co-rumination is similar to self-disclosure in that it involves sharing thoughts and feelings, but co-rumination also is similar to rumination in that it involves an excessive focus on problems and negative affect (Rose, Carlson, & Waller, 2007). Paradoxically, co-rumination is linked to both higher friendship quality and higher depression (Calmes & Roberts, 2008; Rose, 2002; Rose et al., 2007). Negative effects of co-rumination have been demonstrated in a laboratory study in which college women were randomly assigned to talk to a friend about one another's problems or about a neutral topic (Byrd-Craven, Geary, Rose, & Ponzi, 2008). Women who talked about mutual problems with a friend showed a greater increase in salivary cortisol than women who talked about a neutral topic. In addition, the amount of co-rumination in the problem discussion condition, as identified by coders, was positively associated with cortisol increases. Coders identified four aspects of co-rumination: mutual encouragement of problem talk, rehashing, examining causes and consequences of problems, and dwelling on negative affect. Among the different aspects of co-rumination, the strongest adverse effects occurred for dwelling on negative affect.

What is the difference between co-rumination and the previously described self-focused rumination? Calmes and Roberts (2008) demonstrated that the two were distinct via factor analysis. In their study of college students, they found that the detrimental effects of co-rumination were limited to close friendships. When co-rumination was assessed with a close friend, parents, roommates, and romantic partners, only co-rumination with a best friend predicted depression and accounted for the sex difference in depression. However, when self-focused rumination was statistically controlled, the effects of co-rumination on depression disappeared, suggesting that co-rumination's maladaptive effects operate via self-focused rumination. Not surprisingly, self-focused rumination did not account for the relation of co-rumination to friendship satisfaction. Thus, the maladaptive aspect of co-rumination is linked to self-focused rumination, whereas the adaptive aspect of co-rumination that fosters connection is independent of self-focused rumination.

PRIMARY VERSUS SECONDARY CONTROL

There are a variety of ways in which feelings of control have been conceptualized as coping strategies. One important distinction that has been made is that between primary control and secondary control (Rothbaum, Weisz, & Snyder, 1982). Paralleling the distinction between problem-focused coping and emotion-focused coping, primary control strategies are control strategies that alter the environment, whereas secondary control strategies are control strategies that alter the self to accommodate to the environment. Primary control strategies are often preferred in Western cultures, but it is not always the case that primary control is possible. There are constraints in the extent to which the environment can be altered.

The distinction between primary and secondary control has been particularly useful in helping to understand how control strategies are affected by aging. Heckhausen and Schulz (1995) have outlined a lifespan theory of control, in which the early stages of development are characterized by increased capacities and opportunities for the exertion of primary control and the very late stages of life are characterized by physical, financial, and cognitive limitations that reduce opportunities for primary control. Thus, later in life, secondary control processes can compensate for primary control losses.

There is some suggestion that women may use more secondary control strategies than men. A study of elderly men and women (ages 73 to 98) who had health restrictions showed no sex difference in the use of primary control but showed that women used a more diverse set of secondary control strategies than men (Chippenfield, Perry, Bailis, Ruthig, & Loring, 2007). In addition, the occurrence of an acute health event was associated with lower primary control strategies for women but not men—men continued to use primary control regardless of whether they had experienced an acute health event. The authors concluded that women adjust their use of primary control strategies when they experience a threat to health.

STRESS-RELATED GROWTH

Stress-related growth or benefit-finding is a term that reflects the positive changes that occur in one's life following a stressful or traumatic life event. The term stress-related growth has been used to reflect both an outcome and a process—or way of coping. As an outcome, the growth literature addresses the possibility that there might be positive effects of trauma. As a process, the growth literature addresses the way in which people try to make sense of or derive meaning from trauma. Common areas of stress-related growth are reassessment of priorities, increased spirituality, improvement in relationships, enhanced appreciation of life, and increased personal strength.

In response to relationship stressors, several studies have shown that women construe more benefits than men. For example, women find more benefits than men following the breakup of a romantic relationship (Sprecher, 1994; Tashiro & Frazier, 2003), regardless of who initiated it (Helgeson, 1994). One might argue that women derive more benefits than men in this context because relationships are more central to the female than the male gender role—leading women to reflect more generally on the meaning of a relationship event.

However, a meta-analytic review of the literature on stress-related growth across an array of stressors found that women were more likely than men to engage in benefit-finding in general (Helgeson, Reynolds, & Tomich, 2006)—although the effect size was small. More recently, this sex difference has been confirmed in a study of men and women with cancer (Park, Edmondson, Fenster, & Blank, 2008), a study of men and women with HIV (Littlewood, Vanable, Carey, & Blair, 2008), and a study of therapists responding to their occupations (Linley & Joseph, 2007). The sex difference in benefit-finding is consistent with the finding from the previous meta-analysis on gender and coping—that women are more likely than men to engage in positive reappraisal (Tamres et al., 2002).

Explanations for sex differences in coping
STATUS

One limitation of the gender and coping literature is that sex is inherently confounded with a number of other variables, such as status. Thus, some of the sex differences in coping may be status differences in coping. Thoits (2006) argues that women's greater distress compared to men has to do with the fact that women have a lower status than men and, thus, fewer resources to engage in effective coping efforts. People who are of lower status may be less likely to engage in problem-focused coping because they have fewer resources at their disposal to alter the problem. People who are of lower status also might engage in more emotion-focused coping strategies because they are more likely to face uncontrollable stressors and emotion-focused strategies are more adaptive in the face of less controllable stressors. Some support for this theory comes from a study of men and women in India who were living in poverty (Siddiqui & Pandey, 2006). Although both men and women lived in poverty, women had a lower status than men, were less educated than men, and perceived greater economic strain compared to men. Women also were more likely than men to use coping styles that could be characterized as helpless and fatalistic—coping styles reflective of a lower status.

GENDER ROLES

Sex also is confounded with gender roles, which could explain some of the links of sex to coping. Aspects of both the male and female social roles have been linked (in opposite directions) to rumination. In a study of children (fourth through sixth grade), psychological femininity, an aspect of the female gender role, was related to more rumination (Broderick & Korteland, 2004). In another study, instrumentality, an aspect of the male gender role, was associated with lower levels of rumination (Wupperman & Neumann, 2005), independent of sex. In both studies, gender roles were stronger predictors of rumination than sex.

We introduced the concept of the gender-related trait "unmitigated communion" earlier in the chapter. Unmitigated communion is associated with worrying about other people's problems. Thus, not surprisingly, in a community sample, unmitigated communion was related to rumination and partly explained the sex difference in rumination (Nolen-Hoeksema & Jackson, 2001). However, unmitigated communion should be related to a specific kind of rumination: rumination about others' problems. Two laboratory studies showed that people high in unmitigated communion ruminate about others' problems (Fritz & Helgeson, 1998). In the first study, a stranger (a confederate) disclosed a problem to the participant; in the second study, a friend disclosed a problem. Participants who scored high on unmitigated communion reported more intrusive thoughts about the discloser's problem

2 days later, whether the discloser was a friend or a stranger.

CONTEXT

Some have argued that context is more important than gender in influencing coping. Rosario, Shinn, Morch, and Huckabee (1988) stated that men and women occupy different social roles and that these roles are associated with different kinds of stressors that require different coping responses. According to this **role constraint theory**, social roles influence the stressors that one faces and the nature of the stressor drives the coping response rather than biological sex. For example, men's social role is to be part of the paid workforce. Problems that arise at work might best be addressed by active coping. Thus, it is not so much that men engage in more active coping as it is that paid employment is associated with problems that might best be dealt with via active coping. By contrast, women's social role is to take care of the home and the children. The stressors faced in this environment might be more likely to be interpersonal and require emotion-focused coping.

In support of this theory, Rosario et al. (1988) found no sex differences in coping among undergraduates (who at this point in time occupy similar social roles) but found that the nature of the stressor influenced coping. Relationship problems were associated with emotion-focused coping among both men and women, and problems with school were associated with problem-focused coping among both men and women. When men and women who occupied similar roles (e.g., human service workers; child-care workers) were studied, there were no sex differences in coping (Rosario et al., 1988). The authors concluded that sex differences in coping are diminished when men and women occupy the same social roles.

Sex Differences in Relation of Coping to Health

The question that we address in the final section of the chapter is whether there are coping strategies that are more or less effective for men compared to women. A recent meta-analysis of coping among people with HIV found that gender was not a significant moderator of the relation of any of 18 coping variables to health (Moskowitz, Hult, Bussolari, & Acree, 2009). However, there is other evidence that the implications of coping styles for health are consistent with gendered expectations. There is some suggestive evidence that problem-focused coping is more effective for men than women and seeking social support is more effective for women than men (see Tamres et al., 2002, for a review); however, few studies in this area explicitly test whether the relation of a specific coping strategy to a health outcome significantly differs for men and women. In one exception, a study of employees of a financial organization in Spain showed that support-seeking coping was associated with less distress among women but more distress among men (González-Morales, Peiró, Rodríguez, & Greenglass, 2006). In addition, direct action coping was related to reduced distress among both men and women, but the relations were statistically stronger for men.

Why would active coping be more beneficial for men and support seeking be more beneficial for women? One explanation has to do with skill strengths and deficits (Gonzalez-Morales et al., 2006). Women might lack skills in direct action coping, and men might lack skills in seeking support—possibly because they have fewer opportunities to enact these strategies. The second explanation has to do with the social environments in which men and women are embedded (Gonzalez-Morales et al., 2006). People may not respond favorably to men and women engaging in gender-role inconsistent behavior (men asking for support and women engaging in direct action), which then makes the outcome less successful.

However, it also is possible that men and women would benefit more from engaging in a coping strategy that is not typical of their gender role. Perhaps women would benefit from the opportunity to engage in active coping and men would benefit from the opportunity to seek support because they would be able to add these strategies to their coping repertoire. There is evidence to support this possibility from the literature on written emotional expression. Numerous studies have shown that expressing one's thoughts about a traumatic event through writing is related to good health outcomes (see Smyth, 1998, for a review). Gender appears to be a significant moderator variable, in the direction of men accruing more benefits than women (Smyth, 1998). Writing may benefit men more than women because men do not have the same opportunities as women to engage in emotional expression in their naturally occurring social network. The traditional male role discourages the expression of thoughts and feelings.

Evidence from two bereavement coping interventions, one problem-focused and one emotion-focused, is consistent with this possibility (Schut,

Stroebe, Van den Bout, & De Keijser, 1997). Men and women who had reported medium to high levels of distress 11 months following the loss of their spouse were randomly assigned to either a problem-focusing coping intervention that was directed toward changing behaviors that might exacerbate grief or an emotion-focused coping intervention that was directed toward the expression and acceptance of emotions. As shown in Figure 4.3, men benefited more from the emotion-focused coping intervention, whereas women benefitted more from the problem-focused coping intervention both at post-treatment and then 7 months later. The authors suggested that men and women benefited from coping strategies that were less familiar to them because their typical coping strategies may not have worked. The findings from this study should be interpreted with caution, however, due to the small sample sizes (n = 23 women, 23 men).

We now turn to the literature on specific kinds of coping to determine whether they have been shown to be more strongly related to health for one sex than the other.

Rumination and health

We know that women are more likely than men to ruminate, but is rumination more maladaptive for women than men? Nolen-Hoeksema (1994) partly addressed this issue when she explained why sex differences in depression emerge during adolescence. She suggests that females are more likely than males to ruminate even before adolescence, but the negative events that occur to females during adolescence (i.e., body changes, relationship difficulties) make the ruminative response more detrimental for females. Thus, it is the interaction between the ruminative response to stress and the uncontrollable stressors of adolescence that lead to the increase in depression among girls during adolescence. This theory was put to the test in a study of over 1,200 adolescents aged 10 through 17 who were followed over time (Jose & Brown, 2008). Sex differences in rumination appeared at age 12, and sex differences in stressful life events and depression appeared 1 year later at age 13. The emergent sex difference in depression was explained by rumination. In addition, the link between rumination and depression was stronger for girls than boys. Thus, not only did the sex difference in rumination precede the sex difference in depression, but the link of rumination to depression was also stronger for girls than boys. Consistent with these findings, research on a related

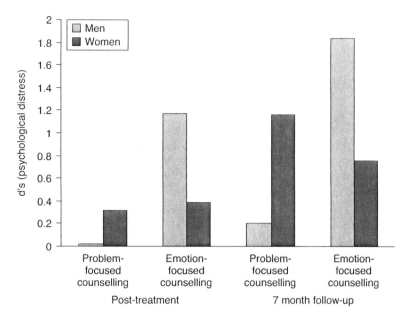

Fig. 4.3 Among the bereaved, men benefitted more from the emotion-focused coping intervention and women benefitted more from the problem-focused coping intervention post-intervention and 7 months later. The figure displays the *d's* (effect sizes) for psychological distress.

construct—catastrophizing—has found that girls and boys with chronic pain were equally likely to engage in catastrophizing, but that catastrophizing was related to poor outcomes (lower pain-coping efficacy) only for girls (Lynch et al., 2007). However, studies of adults have rarely examined whether gender moderates the relation of rumination to distress. One study of adults that tested the interactive effects of gender with rumination did not find any support for moderation (Nolen-Hoeksema, Parker, & Larson, 1994).

Co-rumination and health

The effects of co-rumination on health and on friendship may differ for males and females. In a longitudinal study of children in grades three, five, seven, and nine, co-rumination predicted increases in anxiety and depression over 6 months for girls but not boys (Rose et al., 2007). By contrast, co-rumination predicted increases in friendship quality for both males and females. Thus, it appears that boys obtain the relationship benefits of co-rumination without the psychological costs. Future research should explore the nature of boys' and girls' co-ruminations to see if the content of these dialogs differs in some way.

The results for co-rumination might explain some of the more mixed findings regarding the effects of social networks on women's health. On the one hand, social networks provide women with more

resources (i.e., social support) than they do men. On the other hand, being embedded in social networks has more costs to women than to men, as women are often the care providers of network members. This explains why one study showed that the number of social roles was related in a linear way to fewer mental health problems among men but showed a curvilinear relation to mental health problems among women (Weich, Sloggett, & Lewis, 1998). Among women, having too few or too many social roles was associated with mental health problems. That a large number of social roles has negative health consequences for women but not men could be due to the double-edged sword relationships pose for women—more support to receive and more support to provide.

Primary versus secondary control

Some investigators have suggested that secondary control strategies might be more adaptive for women than men—at least later in life, when opportunities for control are diminished. In a study of people with coronary heart disease, a type of secondary control referred to as vicarious control (i.e., belief that others have influence over your outcomes) was related to positive adjustment among women but not men (Taylor, Helgeson, Reed, & Skokan, 1991). In a prospective study of the elderly (age 60 and older), secondary control was examined in terms of folk beliefs (e.g., "every cloud has a silver lining"; Swift, Bailis, Chipperfield, Ruthig, & Newall, 2008). All of the folk beliefs reflected an emphasis on the positive. Although there were no sex differences in the endorsement of folk beliefs, coping via the use of folk beliefs was more strongly related to higher life satisfaction and more positive emotions 7 years later for women compared to men—specifically women with health problems.

There is other evidence that secondary control might be most beneficial to women with health problems. In a community study of the elderly (ages 73 to 98) who were suffering from health-related restrictions, the investigators hypothesized that secondary control strategies would be more effective for women than men because women were more likely than men to be functionally and physically limited in later life (Chipperfield & Perry, 2006). In this study, participants were asked how they coped with an activity or task in which they were restricted. Primary control strategies, such as trying to alter the task and task persistence, were more strongly related to fewer hospital admissions for men than women, whereas some secondary control strategies, such as positive reappraisal and optimistic social comparisons, were related to shorter hospital stays for women than men. These findings held even when controlling for health status, functional limitations, and income. Because all of these studies involved older adults, it is not clear whether secondary control strategies are more adaptive for women than men always or only during the later years when opportunities for primary control are diminished. Because women have more non-fatal chronic illnesses than men later in life, women also might be less able to enact primary control than men. Future studies should control for physical health when examining the relation of primary and secondary control to health.

Future Directions

There are several directions that future researchers should pursue. Researchers should start by moving beyond the examination of sex differences in stress and coping and focus on explicating the reasons for those differences. The two most common categories of explanations have to do with status and gender roles, as sex is confounded with both. Although researchers have acknowledged the role of status and social roles, little research has explicitly examined whether sex differences in stress and coping are due to these variables. Some studies have examined the implications of gender roles or gender-related traits

for stress and coping, but there are many more studies that examine sex rather than the psychological roles or traits that accompany sex in our culture. The studies that do examine gender roles often find that they are better predictors of stress and coping than biological sex. The similarities between men and women far outweigh their differences. Because our explanations for why men and women are differentially vulnerable to different classes of stressors or utilize different coping strategies often have to do with differential socialization, more research ought to test which aspects of the male and female gender roles are most predictive of stress and coping. Having identified gender roles or social roles as important contributors to the area of stress and coping, researchers also should focus more in depth on the precise mechanisms by which these characteristics affect stress and coping. The literature on encoding is a good example of this kind of effort.

When examining sex differences in the experience of stressful events, researchers need to be aware that there are often sex differences in stressor appraisal, meaning that women report being more strongly affected by a given stressor than men. The experience of stressful life events is not the same as the effects of those events, and researchers should be careful not to confuse the two.

In the area of gender and coping, researchers should consider adopting the relative coping approach. If the goal of the research is simply to understand whether one sex uses a coping strategy more than the other sex, an examination of absolute coping scores might suffice. However, if one is truly interested in understanding which coping strategies men use more and which coping strategies women use more, it might be more informative to examine relative coping. To the extent that women are more distressed than men, women might engage in more coping in general. Thus, a simple comparison of men and women on a certain coping strategy is not necessarily informative with respect to gender.

When sex comparisons are made in the area of stress and coping, researchers need to take into consideration the fact that there are a multitude of sex differences in health. For example, women are more depressed than men, women have more non-fatal chronic illnesses than men, and women perceive their health as generally worse than men. Thus, one cannot compare the effects of stressful life events on men and women without some kind of a comparison group of men and women who are not facing the stressor. Otherwise, it is easy to conclude that women are more distressed than men in the aftermath of an acute or chronic stressor when actually women might have been more distressed than men prior to the stressor.

Within the gender and coping domain, research that has examined whether there are specific coping strategies that are more adaptive for men or women has not been conclusive. Simply testing whether sex moderates the relation of coping to health does not seem to be a fruitful avenue of research. Once again, the problem-focused versus emotion-focused dichotomy is probably too simplistic of a framework to use to examine this issue. It is intriguing that the expressive writing studies show stronger effects for men than for women, given that one would expect this coping style to be more consistent with the expressiveness of the female gender role. The lack of clear findings in this area probably suggests that there are other variables that are more important than gender—or other variables that need to be considered in the context of gender— that predict coping. The nature of the stressor is a good candidate, but even that could be influenced by gender. For example, both men and women may face the death of a spouse, but the challenges that follow are not necessarily the same. The question is whether men and women employ different coping strategies when they are faced with similar stressors that have similar demands.

Finally, one gender-related theme that appears throughout the area of gender, stress, and coping has to do with whether men's and women's behavior is accentuated or diminished in the face of gender-consistent stimuli/events. Research in the area of stress reactivity shows that under some conditions men and women are more physiologically reactive to stressors that are relevant to their gender roles and at other times less physiologically reactive to stressors that are relevant to their gender roles. Whether a stressor is appraised as a threat or a challenge is one potential framework for resolving these inconsistencies. Research in the area of coping shows that at times men and women benefit from coping styles that are consistent with their gender roles and at times benefit from coping styles that are inconsistent with their gender roles. Thus, there seem to be two opposing forces at work: (1) an enhancement model in which men and women thrive or are less stressed when faced with gender-role consistent stimuli that augment their traditional gender roles, and (2) a deficit model in which men and women thrive or are less stressed when presented with gender-role inconsistent stimuli that force them to expand beyond traditional gender roles. Future research should more closely examine the conditions under which these two models operate. To more fully understand how gender roles affect the relation of stress and coping to health, one likely has to consider the relevance of gender roles to the individual—perhaps harking back to Sandra Bem's (1981) work on gender schematicity. Not only do people differ in the extent to which they adhere to gender roles, people also differ in the extent to which they encode the world in terms of gender.

References

Ali, A., & Toner, B. B. (1996). Gender differences in depressive response: The role of social support. *Sex Roles, 35*, 281–93.

Archer, J. (2000). Sex differences in aggression between heterosexual partners: A meta-analytic review. *Psychological Bulletin, 126*, 651–80.

Artazcoz, L., Benach, J., Borrell, C., & Cortes, I. (2004). Unemployment and mental health: Understanding the interactions among gender, family roles, and social class. *American Journal of Public Health, 94*, 82–8.

Bartley, M. (1994). Unemployment and ill health: Understanding the relationship. *Journal of Epidemiology and Community Health, 48*, 333–7.

Belle, D., & Doucet, J. (2003). Poverty, inequality, and discrimination as sources of depression among U.S. women. *Psychology of Women Quarterly, 27*, 101–13.

Bem, S. L. (1981). Gender schema theory: A cognitive account of sex typing. *Psychological Review, 88*, 354–64.

Bouma, E. M. C., Ormel, J., Verhulst, F. C., & Oldehinkel, A. J. (2008). Stressful life events and depressive problems in early adolescent boys and girls: The influence of parental depression, temperament and family environment. *Journal of Affective Disorders, 105*, 185–93.

Broderick, P. C., & Korteland, C. (2002). A prospective study of rumination and depression in early adolescence. *Clinical Child Psychology and Psychiatry, 9*, 383–94.

Bureau of Justice Statistics (July 11, 2007). Homicide trends in the U.S.: Gender Retrieved July 7, 2009, from http://www.ojp.usdoj.gov/bjs/homicide/gender.htm

Bureau of Labor Statistics (2009). Employment status of the civilian noninstitutional population 16 years and over by sex, 1973 to date, from http://www.bls.gov/cps/cpsaat2.pdf

Byrd-Craven, J., Geary, D. C., Rose, A. J., & Ponzi, D. (2008). Co-ruminating increases stress hormone levels in women. *Hormones and Behavior, 53*, 489–92.

Calmes, C. A., & Roberts, J. E. (2008). Rumination in interpersonal relationships: Does co-rumination explain gender differences in emotional distress and relationship satisfaction among college students? *Cognitive Therapy and Research, 32*, 577–90.

Cancian, F. M., & Oliker, S. J. (2000). *Caring and gender.* Walnut Creek, CA: AltaMira Press.

Chesley, N., & Moen, P. (2006). When workers care: Dual-earner couples' caregiving strategies benefit use, and psychological well-being. *American Behavioral Scientist, 49*, 1248–69.

Chipperfield, J., & Perry, R. P. (2006). Primary and secondary control strategies in later life: Predicting hospital outcomes in men and women. *Health Psychology, 25*, 226–36.

Chipperfield, J., Perry, R. P., Bailis, D., Ruthig, J., & Loring, P. (2007). Gender differences in use of primary and secondary control strategies in older adults with major health problems. *Psychology and Health, 22*, 83–105.

Conger, R. D., Lorenz, F. O., Elder, G. H., Simons, R. L., & Ge, X. (1993). Husband and wife differences in response to undesirable life events. *Journal of Health and Social Behavior, 34*, 71–88.

Cosenzo, K. A., Franchina, J. J., Eisler, R. M., & Krebs, D. (2004). Effects of masculine gender-relevant task instructions on men's cardiovascular reactivity and mental arithmetic performance. *Psychology of Men and Masculinity, 5*, 103–11.

Cross, S. E., & Madison, L. (1997). Models of the self: Self-construals and gender. *Psychological Bulletin, 122*, 5–37.

Currie, D. H. (1998). Violent men or violent women? Whose definition counts? In R. K. Bergen (Ed.), *Issues in intimate violence* (pp. 97–111). Thousand Oaks, CA: Sage.

Davis, M. C., & Matthews, K. A. (1996). Do gender-relevant characteristics determine cardiovascular reactivity? Match versus mismatch of traits and situation. *Journal of Personality and Social Psychology, 71*, 527–35.

Davis, M. C., Matthews, K. A., & Twamley, E. W. (1999). Is life more difficult on Mars or Venus? A meta-analytic review of sex differences in major and minor life events. *Annals of Behavioral Medicine, 21*, 83–97.

Davis, P. (1999). Gender differences in autobiographical memory for childhood emotional experiences. *Journal of Personality and Social Psychology, 76*, 498–510.

Davis, R. N., & Nolen-Hoeksema, S. (2000). Cognitive inflexibility among ruminators and nonruminators. *Cognitive Therapy and Research, 24*, 699–711.

Dedovic, K., Wadiwalla, M., Engert, V., & Pruessner, J. C. (2009). The role of sex and gender socialization in stress reactivity. *Developmental Psychology, 45*, 45–55.

Equal Employment Opportunity Commission (2007). Sexual harassment charges. *EEOC & FEPAs combined (FY1997-FY2006)* Retrieved July 10, 2007, from www.eeoc.gov/stats/harass.html

Ewart, C. K., Taylor, C. B., Kraemer, H. C., & Agras, W. S. (1991). High blood pressure and marital discord: Not being nasty matters more than being nice. *Health Psychology, 10*, 155–63.

Feldman-Barrett, L., Lane, R. D., Sechrest, L., & Schwartz, G. E. (2000). Sex differences in emotional awareness. *Personality and Social Psychology Bulletin, 26*, 1027–35.

Fritz, H. L., & Helgeson, V. S. (1998). Distinctions of unmitigated communion from communion: Self neglect and over-involvement with others. *Journal of Personality and Social Psychology, 75*, 121–40.

Fritz, H. L., Nagurney, A. J., & Helgeson, V. S. (2003). Social interactions and cardiovascular reactivity during problem disclosure among friends. *Personality and Social Psychology Bulletin, 29*, 713–25.

Ge, X., Lorenz, F. O., Conger, R. D., Elder, G. H., & Simons, R. L. (1994). Trajectories of stressful life events and depressive symptoms during adolescence. *Developmental Psychology, 30*, 467–83.

Golding, J. M. (1999). Intimate partner violence as a risk factor for mental disorders: A meta-analysis. *Journal of Family Violence, 14*, 99–132.

Gonzalez-Morales, M. G., Peiro, J. M., Rodriguez, I., & Greenglass, E. R. (2006). Coping and distress in organizations: The role of gender in work stress. *International Journal of Stress Management, 13*, 228–48.

Gore, S., Aseltine, R. H., & Colten, M. E. (1993). Gender, social-relational involvement, and depression. *Journal of Research on Adolescence, 3*, 101–25.

Gottman, J. M., & Levenson, R. W. (1992). Marital process predictive of later dissolution: Behavior, physiology, and health. *Journal of Personality and Social Psychology, 63*, 221–33.

Gutek, B. A. (1985). *Sex and the workplace*. San Francisco: Jossey-Bass.

Hafstrom, J. L., & Schram, V. R. (1984). Chronic illness in couples: Selected characteristics, including wife's satisfaction with and perception of marital relationships. *Family Relations, 33*, 195–203.

Hagedoorn, M., Buunk, B. P., Kuijer, R. G., Wobbes, T., & Sanderman, R. (2000). Couples dealing with cancer: Role and gender difference regarding psychological distress and quality of life. *Psycho-oncology, 9*, 232–42.

Hagedoorn, M., Sanderman, R., Bolks, H. N., Tuinstra, J., & Coyne, J. C. (2008). Distress in couples coping with cancer: A meta-analysis and critical review of role and gender effects. *Psychological Bulletin, 134*, 1–30.

Hagedoorn, M., Sanderman, R., Ranchor, A., Brilman, E. I., Kempen, G. I. J. M., & Ormel, J. (2001). Chronic disease in elderly couples: Are women more responsive to their spouses' health condition than men? *Journal of Psychosomatic Research, 51*, 693–6.

Hampel, P., & Petermann, F. (2006). Perceived stress, coping, and adjustment in adolescents. *Journal of Adolescent Heath, 38*, 409–15.

Harris, M. B. (1996). Aggressive experiences and aggressiveness: Relationship to ethnicity, gender, and age. *Journal of Applied Social Psychology, 26*, 843–70.

Heckhausen, J., & Schulz, R. (1995). A life-span theory of control. *Psychological Review, 102*, 284–304.

Helgeson, V. S. (1994). Long-distance romantic relationships: Sex differences in adjustment and breakup. *Personality and Social Psychology Bulletin, 20*, 254–65.

Helgeson, V. S., & Fritz, H. L. (1996). Implications of communion and unmitigated communion for adolescent adjustment to Type 1 diabetes. *Women's Health: Research on Gender, Behavior, and Policy, 2*(3), 169–94.

Helgeson, V. S., & Fritz, H. L. (1998). A theory of unmitigated communion. *Personality and Social Psychology Review, 2*, 173–83.

Helgeson, V. S., Reynolds, K., & Tomich, P. (2006). A meta-analytic review of benefit finding and growth. *Journal of Consulting and Clinical Psychology, 74*, 980–7.

Hill, J. P., & Lynch, M. E. (1983). The intensification of gender-related role expectations during early adolescence. In J. Brooks-Gunn & A. C. Petersen (Eds.), *Girls at puberty* (pp. 201–28). New York: Plenum Press.

Huerta, M., Cortina, L. M., Pang, J. S., Torges, C. M., & Magley, V. J. (2006). Sex and power in the academy: Modeling sexual harassment in the lives of college women. *Personality and Social Psychology Bulletin, 32*, 616–28.

Jose, P. E., & Brown, I. (2008). When does the gender difference in rumination begin? Gender and age differences in the use of rumination by adolescents. *Journal of Youth and Adolescence, 37*, 180–92.

Joyner, K., & Urdy, J. R. (2000). You don't bring me anything but down: Adolescent romance and depression. *Journal of Health and Social Behavior, 41*, 369–91.

Kessler, R. C. (2000). Gender differences in major depression. In E. Frank (Ed.), *Gender and its effects on psychopathology* (pp. 61–84). Washington, DC: American Psychiatric Press, Inc.

Kessler, R. C., & McLeod, J. (1984). Sex differences in vulnerability to undesirable life events. *American Sociological Review, 49*, 620–31.

Kiecolt-Glaser, J. K., Malarkey, W. B., Chee, M., Newton, T., Cacioppo, J. T., Mao, H.-Y., et al. (1993). Negative behavior during marital conflict is associated with immunological down-regulation. *Psychosomatic Medicine, 55*, 395–409.

Kiecolt-Glaser, J. K., Newton, T., Cacioppo, J. T., MacCallum, R. C., Glaser, R., & Malarkey, W. B. (1996). Marital conflict and endocrine function: Are men really more physiologically affected than women? *Journal of Consulting and Clinical Psychology, 64*, 324–32.

Koss, M. P., Bailey, J. A., Yuan, N. P., Herrera, V. M., & Lichter, E. L. (2003). Depression and PTSD in survivors of male violence: research and training initiatives to facilitate recovery. *Psychology of Women Quarterly, 27*, 130–42.

Larson, R., & Almeida, D. M. (1999). Emotional transmission in the daily lives of families: A new paradigm for studying the family process. *Journal of Marriage and the Family, 61*, 5–20.

Larson, R., & Richards, M. (1989). The changing life space of early adolescence. *Journal of Youth and Adolescence, 16*, 561–78.

Larson, R., & Richards, M. (1991). Daily companionship in late childhood and early adolescence: Changing developmental contexts. *Child Development, 62*, 284–300.

Lash, S. J., Eisler, R. M., & Southard, D. (1995). Sex differences in cardiovascular reactivity as a function of the appraised gender relevance of the stressor. *Behavioral Medicine, 21*, 86–94.

Lash, S. J., Gillespie, B., Eisler, R. M., & Southard, D. (1991). Sex differences in cardiovascular reactivity: Effects of the gender relevance of the stressor. *Health Psychology, 10*, 392–8.

Lazarus, R. S., & Folkman, S. (1984). *Stress, appraisal, and coping*. New York: Springer.

Lester, D., & Yang, B. (1998). *Suicide and homicide in the twentieth century: Changes over time*. Commack, AL: Nova Science.

Linley, P. A., & Joseph, S. (2007). Therapy work and therapists' positive and negative well-being. *Journal of Social and Clinical Psychology, 26*, 385–403.

Littlewood, R. A., Vanable, P. A., Carey, M. P., & Blair, D. C. (2008). The association of benefit finding to psychosocial and health behavior adaptation among HIV+ men and women. *Journal of Behavioral Medicine, 31*, 145–55.

Lynch, A. M., Kashikar-Zuck, S., Goldschneider, K. R., & Jones, B. A. (2007). Sex and age differences in coping styles among children with chronic pain. *Journal of Pain and Symptom Management, 33*, 208–16.

Maciejewski, P. K., Prigerson, H. G., & Mazure, C. M. (2001). Sex differences in event-related risk for major depression. *Psychological Medicine, 31*, 593–604.

Marks, N. F. (1998). Does it hurt to care? Caregiving, work-family conflict, and midlife well-being. *Journal of Marriage and the Family, 60*, 951–66.

Matthews, K. A., Gump, B. B., & Owens, J. F. (2001). Chronic stress influences cardiovascular and neuroendocrine responses during acute stress and recovery, especially in men. *Health Psychology, 20*, 403–10.

Moskowitz, J. T., Hult, J. R., Bussolari, C., & Acree, M. (2009). What works in coping with HIV? A meta-analysis with implications for coping with serious illness. *Psychological Bulletin, 135*, 121–41.

Murberg, T. A., & Bru, E. (2004). Social support, negative life events and emotional problems among Norwegian adolescents. *Social Psychology International, 25*, 387–403.

Murphy, G. C., & Athanasou, J. A. (1999). The effect of unemployment on mental health. *Journal of Occupational and Organizational Psychology, 72*, 83–99.

Nansel, T. R., Overpeck, M. D., Haynie, D. L., Ruan, W. J., & Scheidt, P. C. (2003). Relationships between bullying and violence among U.S. youth. *Archives of Pediatrics and Adolescent Medicine, 157*, 348–52.

Nazroo, J. Y., Edwards, A. C., & Brown, G. W. (1997). Gender differences in the onset of depression following a shared life event: A study of couples. *Psychological Medicine, 27*, 9–19.

Newell, C. E., Rosenfeld, P., & Culbertson, A. L. (1995). Sexual harassment experiences and equal opportunity perceptions of Navy women. *Sex Roles, 32*, 159–68.

Nolen-Hoeksema, S. (1987). Sex differences in unipolar depression: Evidence and theory. *Psychological Bulletin, 101*, 259–82.

Nolen-Hoeksema, S. (1994). An interactive model for the emergence of gender differences in depression in adolescence. *Journal of Research on Adolescence, 4*, 519–34.

Nolen-Hoeksema, S. (2001). Gender differences in depression. *Current Directions in Psychological Science, 10*, 173–6.

Nolen-Hoeksema, S. (2006). The etiology of gender: Differences in depression. In C. M. Mazure & G. Puryear (Eds.), *Understanding depression in women: Applying empirical research to practice and policy* (pp. 9–43). Washington, DC: American Psychological Association.

Nolen-Hoeksema, S., & Davis, C. G. (1999). "Thanks for sharing that": Ruminators and their social support network. *Journal of Personality and Social Psychology, 77*, 801–14.

Nolen-Hoeksema, S., & Jackson, B. (2001). Mediators of the gender difference in rumination. *Psychology of Women Quarterly, 25*, 37–47.

Nolen-Hoeksema, S., & Keita, G. P. (2003). Women and depression: Introduction. *Psychology of Women Quarterly, 27*, 89–90.

Nolen-Hoeksema, S., Larson, J., & Grayson, C. (1999). Explaining the gender difference in depressive symptoms. *Journal of Personality and Social Psychology, 77*, 1061–72.

Nolen-Hoeksema, S., Parker, L. E., & Larson, J. (1994). Personality processes and individual differences: Ruminative coping with depressed mood following loss. *Journal of Personality and Social Psychology, 67*, 92–104.

Olff, M., Langelande, W., Draijer, N., & Gersons, B. P. R. (2007). Gender difference in posttraumatic stress disorder. *Psychological Bulletin, 133*, 183–204.

Park, C. L., Edmondson, D., Fenster, J. R., & Blank, T. O. (2008). Meaning making and psychological adjustment following cancer: The mediating roles of growth, life meaning, and restored just-world beliefs. *Journal of Consulting and Clinical Psychology, 76*, 863–75.

Pavalko, E. K., & Woodbury, S. (2000). Social roles as process: Caregiving careers and women's health. *Journal of Health and Social Behavior, 41*, 91–105.

Pietila, I., & Rytkonen, M. (2008). Coping with stress and by stress: Russian men and women talking about transition, stress, and health. *Social Science and Medicine, 66*, 327–38.

Pinquart, M., & Sorensen, S. (2006). Gender differences in caregiver stressors, social resources, and health: An updated meta-analysis. *Journal of Gerontology, 61B*, 33–45.

Rampell, C. (2009). As layoffs surge, women may pass men in job force. *The New York Times*, from http://www.nytimes.com/2009/02/06/business/06women.html

Rauste-von Wright, M., von Wright, J., & Frankenhaeuser, M. (1981). Relationships between sex-related psychological characteristics during adolescent and catecholamine excretion during achievement stress. *Psychophysiology, 18*, 362–70.

Reynolds, K. A., Helgeson, V. S., Seltman, H., Janicki, D., Page-Gould, E., & Wardle, M. (2006). Impact of interpersonal conflict on individuals high in unmitigated communion. *Journal of Applied Social Psychology, 36*, 1595–616.

Rohrbaugh, M. J., Cranford, J. A., Shoham, V., Nicklas, J. M., Sonnega, J. S., & Coyne, J. C. (2002). Couples coping with congestive heart failure: Role and gender differences in psychological distress. *Journal of Family Psychology, 16*, 3–13.

Rosario, M., Shinn, M., Morch, H., & Huckabee, C. B. (1988). Gender differences in coping and social supports: Testing socialization and role constraints theories. *Journal of Community Psychology, 16*, 55–69.

Rose, A. J. (2002). Co-rumination in the friendships of girls and boys. *Child Development, 73*, 1830–43.

Rose, A. J., Carlson, W., & Waller, E. M. (2007). Prospective associations of co-rumination with friendship and emotional adjustment: Considering the socioemotional trade-offs of co-rumination. *Developmental Psychology, 43*, 1019–31.

Rothbaum, F., Weisz, J. R., & Snyder, S. S. (1982). Changing the world and changing the self: A two-process model of perceived control. *Journal of Personality and Social Psychology, 42*, 1162–72.

Rudolph, K., & Hammen, C. (1999). Age and gender as determinants of stress exposure, generation, and reactions in youngsters: A transactional perspective. *Child Development, 70*, 660–77.

Schut, H. A. W., Stroebe, M. S., Van den Bout, J., & de Keijser, J. (1997). Intervention for the bereaved: Gender differences in the efficacy of two counseling programmes. *British Journal of Clinical Psychology, 36*, 63–72.

Seidlitz, L., & Diener, E. (1998). Sex differences in the recall of affective experiences. *Journal of Personality and Social Psychology, 74*, 262–71.

Shih, J. H., Eberhart, N. K., Hammen, C., & Brennan, P. A. (2006). Differential exposure and reactivity to interpersonal stress predict sex differences in adolescent depression. *Journal of Clinical Child and Adolescent Psychology, 35*, 103–15.

Siddiqui, R. N., & Pandey, J. (2006). Gender differences in coping with economic stressors and health consequences. *Psychological Studies, 51*, 152–60.

Skaff, M. M., Finney, J. W., & Moos, R. H. (1999). Gender differences in problem drinking and depression: Different "vulnerabilities"? *American Journal of Community Psychology, 27*, 25–54.

Smith, B. W., & Zautra, A. J. (2002). The role of personality in exposure and reactivity to interpersonal stress in relation to arthritis disease activity and negative affect in women. *Health Psychology, 21*, 81–8.

Smyth, J. (1998). Written emotional expression: Effect sizes, outcome types, and moderating variables. *Journal of Consulting and Clinical Psychology, 66*, 174–84.

Sprecher, S. (1994). Two sides to the breakup of dating relationships. *Personal Relationships, 1*, 199–222.

Strauss, J., Muday, T., McNall, K., & Wong, M. (1997). Response style theory revisited: Gender differences and stereotypes in rumination and distraction. *Sex Roles, 36*, 771–92.

Stroud, L. R., Niaura, R. S., & Stoney, C. M. (2001). Sex differences in cardiovascular reactivity to physical appearance and performance challenges. *International Journal of Behavioral Medicine, 8*, 240–50.

Stroud, L. R., Salovey, P., & Epel, E. S. (2002). Sex differences in stress responses: Social rejection versus achievement stress. *Biological Psychiatry, 52*, 318–27.

Swift, A., Bailis, D., Chipperfield, J., Ruthig, J., & Newall, N. (2008). Gender differences in the adaptive influence of folk beliefs: A longitudinal study of life satisfaction in aging. *Canadian Journal of Behavioural Science, 40*, 104–12.

Tamres, L. K., Janicki, D., & Helgeson, V. S. (2002). Sex differences in coping behavior: A meta-analytic review. *Personality and Social Psychology Review, 6*, 2–30.

Tashiro, T., & Frazier, P. (2003). "I'll never be in a relationship like that again": Personal growth following romantic relationship breakups. *Personal Relationships, 10*, 113–28.

Taylor, S. E., Helgeson, V. S., Reed, G. M., & Skokan, L. A. (1991). Self-generated feelings of control and adjustment to physical illness. *Journal of Social Issues, 47*, 91–109.

Taylor, S. E., Klein, L. C., Lewis, B. P., Gruenewald, T. L., Gurung, R. A. R., & Updegraff, J. A. (2000). Biobehavioral responses to stress in females: Tend-and-befriend, not fight-or-flight. *Psychological Review, 107*, 411–29.

Thoits, P. A. (1991). Gender differences in coping with emotional distress. In J. Eckenrode (Ed.), *The social context of coping* (pp. 107–38). New York: Plenum Press.

Thoits, P. A. (2006). Personal agency in the stress process. *Journal of Health and Social Behavior, 47*, 309–23.

Tolin, D. F., & Foa, E. B. (2006). Sex differences in trauma and posttraumatic stress disorder: A quantitative review of 25 years of research. *Psychological Bulletin, 132*, 959–92.

Toossi, M. (2006). A new look at long-term labor force projections to 2050. *Monthly Labor Review, 129*, 19–39.

Treynor, W., Gonzalez, R., & Nolen-Hoeksema, S. (2003). Rumination reconsidered: A psychometric analysis. *Cognitive Therapy and Research, 27*, 247–59.

Tuinstra, J., Hagedoorn, M., Van Sonderen, E., Ranchor, A., Van den Bos, G., Nijboer, C., et al. (2004). Psychological distress in couples dealing with colorectal cancer: Gender and role difference and intracouple correspondence. *British Journal of Health Psychology, 9*, 465–78.

Turner, J. B., Turse, N. A., & Dohrenwend, B. P. (2007). Circumstances of service and gender differences in war-related PTSD: Findings from the National Vietnam Veteran Readjustment Study. *Journal of Traumatic Stress, 20*, 643–9.

Turner, R. J., & Avison, W. R. (1989). Gender and depression: Assessing exposure and vulnerability to life events in a chronically strained population. *Journal of Nervous and Mental Disease, 177*, 443–55.

U.S. Coast Guard and Departments of Defense and Veterans Affairs (2008). Statistics on women in the military, from http://www.womensmemorial.org/PDFs/StatsonWIM.pdf

U.S. Department of Justice (2008). Expanded homicide data table 1, from http://www.fbi.gov/ucr/cius2007/offenses/expanded_information/data/shrtable_01.html

van Doornen, L. J. P. (1986). Sex differences in physiological reactions to real life stress and their relation to psychological variables. *Psychophysiology, 23*, 657–62.

Van Well, S., Kolk, A. M., & Klugkist, I. G. (2008). Effects of sex, gender role identification, and gender relevance of two types of stressors on cardiovascular and subjective responses. *Behavior Modification, 32*, 427–49.

Vitaliano, P. P., Maiuro, R. D., Russu, J., & Becker, J. (1987). Raw versus relative scores in the assessment of coping strategies. *Journal of Behavioral Medicine, 10*, 1–18.

Vitaliano, P. P., Zhang, J., & Scanlan, J. M. (2003). Is caregiving hazardous to one's physical health? A meta-analysis. *Psychological Bulletin, 129*, 946–72.

Vogt, D. S., Pless, A. P., King, L. A., & King, D. W. (2005). Deployment stressors, gender, and mental health outcomes among Gulf War I veterans. *Journal of Traumatic Stress, 18*, 115–27.

Wadsworth, M. E. J., Montgomery, S. M., & Bartley, M. J. (1999). The persisting effect of unemployment on health and social well-being in men early in working life. *Social Science & Medicine, 48*, 1491–9.

Weich, S., Sloggett, A., & Lewis, G. (1998). Social roles and gender difference in the prevalence of common mental disorders. *British Journal of Psychiatry, 173*, 489–93.

Whiffen, V. E., & Gotlib, I. H. (1989). Stress and coping in maritally distressed and nondistressed couples. *Journal of Personality and Social Psychology, 6*, 327–44.

Williams, S. L., & Frieze, I. H. (2005). Patterns of violent relationships, psychological distress, and marital satisfaction in a national sample of men and women. *Sex Roles, 52*, 771–84.

World Factbook (2007). Field listing: Life expectancy at birth Retrieved February 26, 2007, from www.cia.gov/cia/publications/factbook/fields/2102.html

Wupperman, P., & Neumann, C. S. (2006). Depressive symptoms as a function of sex-role, rumination and neuroticism. *Personality and Individual Differences, 40*, 189–201.

Yee, J. L., & Schulz, R. (2000). Gender differences in psychiatric morbidity among family caregivers: A review and analysis. *Gerontologist, 40*, 147–64.

Zhang, J., Vitaliano, P. P., & Lin, H.-H. (2006). Relations of caregiving stress and health depend on the health indicators used and gender. *International Journal of Behavioral Medicine, 13*, 173–81.

Affiliation and Stress

Shelley E. Taylor

Abstract

Affiliation with others is a basic human coping response for managing a broad array of stressful circumstances. Affiliating with others is both psychologically and biologically comforting, and biologically may depend upon oxytocin and brain opioid pathways. The origins of affiliative responses to stress include early life experiences, genetic factors, and epigenetic processes that interact with the availability of supportive others during times of stress. The beneficial consequences of affiliation for mental and physical health are strong and robust. Future research will continue to clarify the underlying biopsychosocial pathways that explicate why this is the case.

Keywords: affiliation, coping, fight-or-flight, social support, stress, tend-and-befriend

Affiliation with others is one of human beings' most basic coping responses to threat. Whereas other animals have weapons, such as sharp teeth or claws, and defensive resources, such as speed or thick skin, primates, including human beings, depend critically on one another for survival. Correspondingly, social isolation and rejection from a social group are among the most distressing experiences people report (Eisenberger, Lieberman, & Williams, 2003), and social isolation is associated not only with risks to safety, but with long-term mental and physical health risks as well (Cacioppo & Hawkley, 2003). This chapter explores the conceptual basis for understanding the relation of affiliation to stress, the origins of affiliative responses to stress, psychological and biological mechanisms underlying these responses, and consequences of these responses for physical and mental health.

Affiliative Responses to Threat

Social relationships have long been known to sustain human beings in non-threatening as well as

threatening times. In recent decades, convincing evidence that affiliation and its consequences also affect biological responses to stress and ultimately physical health has emerged. Thus, social relationships, especially in times of stress, have benefits at both the psychological and biological levels across the lifespan (Taylor, 2009).

Fight or flight/tend and befriend

In the past, when scientists have characterized stress responses, they usually have done so in terms of fight or flight, a response pattern first characterized by Walter Cannon (1932). Fight or flight refers to the fact that in response to threat, an animal or person can become aggressive and mount an antagonistic response to the threatening circumstances, or it can flee, either literally or metaphorically, from the stressor. Among the responses that stress researchers interpret as flight behavior are social withdrawal and substance use, especially drug and alcohol abuse. Fight and flight represent valuable individual responses for coping with stress, in that either fighting or fleeing has the potential to protect oneself from threats. However, humans are profoundly social and never more so than when the environment is threatening. Accordingly, it is important to characterize these affiliative responses to stress as well. To address the human tendency to affiliate under stress, we developed the term "tend and befriend" (Taylor, 2002; Taylor, Klein, Lewis, Gruenewald, Gurung, & Updegraff, 2000). In contrast to fight or flight, tending to offspring and affiliating with others represent social responses to stress.

The theory, tend and befriend, maintains that there is a biological signaling system that comes into play if one's affiliations fall below an adequate level, a condition that may occur in response to stress. The affiliative neurocircuitry then prompts affiliation in many animal species and in humans. As such, this system regulates social approach behavior and does so in much the same way as occurs for other appetitive needs. Once signaled, this appetitive need is met through purposeful social behaviors, such as affiliation and protecting offspring. As will be noted, oxytocin and endogenous opioid peptides appear to play a role in this system. As we will note later, the biological impetus to affiliate under stress, coupled with the psychological need for contact with others under stress, may represent redundant biobehavioral protective mechanisms that ensure affiliation and corresponding safety when the environment is threatening.

Tend and befriend has its origins in evolutionary theory, and as such tending and befriending may be somewhat more characteristic of women than men as responses to stress (Taylor et al., 2000). During the time that human stress responses evolved, men and women faced somewhat different adaptive challenges due to the division of labor they assumed. Whereas men were primarily responsible for hunting and for group protection, women were typically responsible for childcare and foraging. Consequently, women's responses to stress are likely to have evolved so as to protect not only self but also offspring during times of stress. Consistent with this position, women are more likely than men to respond to stress by turning to others (Luckow, Reifman, McIntosh, 1998; Tamres, Janicki, & Helgeson, 2002). However, men, too, show social responses to stress, and the gender difference in affiliation in response to stress, although robust, is relatively modest in magnitude. Thus, affiliation in response to stress occurs among both men and women.

Functions of affiliation

Affiliation serves several vital functions with respect to stress or threat. First, affiliating with others serves to calibrate or shape the biological stress systems that regulate responses to stress across the lifespan. As will be addressed, caregiving relationships, especially those early in life, help to serve this function. Beginning in the early environment, the quality of caregiving an infant receives can permanently affect that infant's biological, emotional, and social responses to stressful conditions. These effects can occur in the form of how genes are manifested in phenotypes and can exert permanent organizational effects on the regulatory systems that shape responses to stress, an issue addressed in more detail later in this chapter. Ultimately, these responses to stress also predict a broad array of chronic health disorders as well as longevity.

Social affiliation also affects the regulation of stress responses on an acute basis. During daily interactions, as a person copes with more or less stressful circumstances, affiliation influences the magnitude of stress responses. Contacts with others can increase tension and exaggerate responses to stress, but more commonly, affiliation buffers an individual against the deleterious biological effects of stress. These proximal functions of affiliation in response to stress interact with the more distal calibration of stress systems just described, such that people's responses to stress depend both on the early development of their biological stress regulatory systems as shaped by early relationships, and also on current circumstances that moderate these biological responses to stress.

Affiliation serves practical functions with respect to stress. For example, other people transmit important knowledge about the environment in which stress occurs. This informational function may be direct, as when one person warns another about an impending stressor, or it may be indirect, such that how others respond to a threat provides useful information for the self. Other people can provide tangible aid and assistance that better enables the recipient to cope with stressful events. For example, in harsh economic times, a loan of money from relatives or the opportunity to share living spaces may provide badly needed resources. Thus, social relationships can act as a barometer of how stressful an environment is and provide assistance for managing a stressful environment (Taylor & Gonzaga, 2006). Finally, affiliation in response to stress can reduce psychological distress. Those with whom one affiliates or from whom one seeks contact may be emotionally supportive and exert calming, soothing effects on the person seeking contact.

Origins of affiliative responses to stress

Affiliation is vital to the survival of human beings. As such, there are likely to be biobehavioral mechanisms that are sensitive to social threat or to loss of social contact, resulting in social distress and efforts to remedy the situation. A large literature on separation distress attests to such processes in young animals and human infants. When the young are separated from the mother, separation distress can result, especially during particular developmental periods. The experience of separation leads to distress vocalizations (e.g., crying in human infants) or active searching for the caregiver that may prompt the caregiver's return (Panksepp, 1998).

This system appears to depend in part on brain opioids. Evidence consistent with this pathway includes the fact that brain opioids reduce separation distress, and opioid-based drugs such as morphine reduce distress vocalizations in response to separation (Panksepp, 1998). There also appear to be genetic bases for these processes that likewise depend on opioid-based processes. For example, mice that lack the μ-opioid receptor gene emit few distress vocalizations when separated from their mothers, suggesting that endogenous opioid binding is a significant basis of infant attachment behavior (Moles, Kieffer, & D'Amato, 2004).

Oxytocin also appears to be implicated in infant bonding, separation, and reunification (Panksepp, 1998). For example, in an experimental study with rats, Nelson and Panksepp (1996) found that attraction to the mother was blocked in animals who had received an oxytocin antagonist, suggesting that oxytocin is implicated in the neurocircuitry that underlies separation and reunification. Oxytocin is also implicated in social distress in adults. Just as infants and young children experience gaps in their social relationships, so adults may experience an analog of separation distress, which may implicate the same biological systems as in the young. Both animal (Grippo et al., 2007) and human studies support this conclusion. For example, a study from our laboratory found that women who experienced reduced contact with their mothers, with their best friends, with a pet, and with their social groups had especially high levels of oxytocin. Oxytocin levels were also elevated in response to the absence of positive relationships with a partner. Similar results have been found by Turner and colleagues (Turner, Altimus, Enos, Cooper, & McGuiness, 1999). Grippo, Carter, and colleagues (Grippo et al., 2007) isolated female prairie voles and found that social isolation led to increases in oxytocin, thus confirming

the directionality of the effect. Of note, in humans, the evidence to date suggests that oxytocin levels rise primarily in women in response to social stress.

If oxytocin and endogenous opioid peptides are related to social distress, then as part of the affiliative neurocircuitry, they may provide an impetus for social contact to ameliorate stress. Indeed, numerous studies attest to the fact that exogenously administered oxytocin can act as an impetus to affiliation. Experimental studies with several animal species have found that the administration of oxytocin causes an increase in social contact and in grooming, among other pro-social activities (Argiolas & Gessa, 1991; Carter, De Vries, & Getz, 1995; Witt, Winslow, & Insel, 1992). For example, social contact is enhanced and aggression is diminished following central administration of oxytocin in estrogen-treated prairie voles (Witt, Carter, & Walton, 1990). Although human evidence for this point is more limited, Uvnäs-Moberg (1996) found that women who were breastfeeding (and therefore very high in plasma oxytocin concentration) rated themselves as more sociable than age-matched women not breastfeeding or pregnant.

Biological Effects of Affiliation
Biological responses to stress: Overview

Researchers have focused heavily on potential physiological, neuroendocrine, and immunological pathways by which affiliation in response to stress may achieve beneficial effects on stress regulation. What are these pathways? During times of stress, the body releases the catecholamines epinephrine and norepinephrine with concomitant sympathetic nervous system arousal. Stress may also engage the HPA (hypothalamic-pituitary-adrenocortical) axis, involving the release of corticosteroids, including cortisol. These responses have short-term protective effects under stressful circumstances because they mobilize the body to meet the demands of pressing situations.

However, with chronic or recurrent activation, they can be associated with deleterious long-term implications for health (e.g., Seeman & McEwen, 1996; Uchino, Cacioppo, & Kiecolt-Glaser, 1996). For example, excessive or repeated discharge of epinephrine or norepinephrine can lead to the suppression of cellular immune function, produce hemodynamic changes such as increases in blood pressure and heart rate, provoke abnormal heart rhythms such as ventricular arrhythmias, and produce neurochemical imbalances that may relate to psychiatric disorders (McEwen & Stellar, 1993).

Intense, rapid, and/or long-lasting sympathetic responses to repeated stress or challenge have been implicated in the development of hypertension and coronary artery disease.

Stress can also suppress immune functioning in ways that leave a person vulnerable to opportunistic diseases and infections. Corticosteroids have immunosuppressive effects, and stress-related increases in cortisol have been tied to decreased lymphocyte responsivity to mitogenic stimulation and to decreased lymphocyte cytotoxicity. Such immunosuppressive changes may be associated with increased susceptibility to infectious disorders and to destruction of neurons in the hippocampus as well (McEwen & Sapolsky, 1995).

An immunosuppression model does not explain how stress might influence diseases whose central feature is excessive inflammation (Miller, Cohen, & Ritchey, 2002); such diseases include allergic, autoimmune, rheumatologic, and cardiovascular disorders, among other disorders that are known to be exacerbated by stress. Miller and colleagues (2002) hypothesized that chronic stress may diminish the immune system's sensitivity to glucocorticoid hormones that normally terminate the inflammatory cascade that occurs during stress. They found a buffering effect of social support on this process, such that among healthy individuals, glucocorticoid sensitivity bore no relation to social support; however, among parents of children with cancer (a population under extreme stress), those who reported receiving a high level of support from others had higher glucocorticoid sensitivity.

Extensive evidence suggests that these systems—the HPA axis, the immune system, and the sympathetic nervous system (SNS)—influence each other and thereby affect each other's functioning. For example, links between HPA axis activity and sympathetic nervous system activity suggest that chronic activation of the HPA axis could potentiate overactivation of sympathetic functioning (Chrousos & Gold, 1992). Proinflammatory cytokines, which are involved in the inflammatory processes just noted, can activate the HPA axis and may contribute not only to the deleterious effects that chronic activation of this system may cause, but also potentially to depressive symptoms, which have previously been tied to HPA axis activation (Capuron, Ravaud, & Dantzer, 2000; Maier & Watkins, 1998). To the extent, then, that social contact can help keep sympathetic nervous system or HPA axis responses to stress low, it may have a beneficial impact on other systems as well (Seeman &

McEwen, 1996; Uchino, Cacioppo, & Kiecolt-Glaser, 1996). In turn, these benefits may affect health in a positive direction.

The Early Social Environment

Substantial evidence from both animal and human studies indicates that nurturant affiliative contacts in early life help to determine the parameters of these stress systems, and consequently have beneficial effects not only on responses to stress but also on mental and physical health across the lifespan.

Biological consequences of affiliative contact in early life: Animal studies

An early study by Harlow and Harlow (1962) found that monkeys who were raised with an artificial terrycloth mother and who were isolated from other monkeys during the first 6 months of life showed disruptions in their adult social contacts. They were less likely to engage in normal social behavior, such as grooming, their sexual responses were inappropriate, mothering among the females was deficient, and they often showed either highly fearful or abnormally aggressive behavior toward their peers, which, not surprisingly, led to social rejection. These findings suggest that social and emotional regulation skills may be critically engendered by nurturant contact in early life. Of interest, social deficiencies that result from deficient mothering appear to involve precisely the skills that would interfere with an adult offspring's ability to enlist social contact in adulthood.

Building on this work, Meaney and colleagues (Francis, Diorio, Liu, & Meaney, 1999; Liu et al., 1997) linked nurturant maternal contact to the development of stress responses in offspring and showed that these contacts affect emotional and neuroendocrine responses to stress throughout the animals' lives. In their paradigm, infant rats are removed from the nest, stroked, and then returned to the nest. The response of the mother to this separation and reunification is licking, grooming, and arched-back nursing, especially in species with a genetic predisposition to these behaviors. These contacts provide the pup with nurturant, soothing, immediate stimulation, and in the short term reduce SNS and HPA axis responses to stress in the pup (and in the mother as well).

Over the long term, this maternal behavior results in a better-regulated HPA axis response to stress and better regulation of somatic growth and neural development, especially hippocampal synaptic development. Rat pups exposed to highly nurturant mothering show less emotionality to novel circumstances and more normative social behavior, including mothering in adulthood, compared to recipients of normal mothering. These pups show more open field exploration, suggesting lower levels of fear as well (Francis, Diorio, Liu, & Meaney, 1999; Weaver et al., 2004).

This compelling animal model indicates that nurturant stimulation by the mother early in life modulates the physiological, neuroendocrine, and behavioral responses of offspring to stress in ways that have permanent effects on behavior and on the offspring's developing HPA axis. Studies with monkeys have shown similar effects. For example, Suomi (1987) reported that highly reactive monkeys cross-fostered to nurturant mothers develop good socioemotional skills and achieve high status in the dominance hierarchy, whereas monkeys with reactive temperaments who are peer-raised develop poor socioemotional skills and end up at the bottom of the dominance hierarchy.

An early nurturant environment can also induce lasting changes in the function of genes, which is an additional mechanism by which early affiliative experience can induce long-term alterations in behavior. Specifically, the long-term behavioral effects of early-life maternal care appear to result at least in part from epigenetic structural alterations (methylation) to the glucocorticoid receptor gene that occur in the first week after birth and affect its expression throughout the lifespan (Meaney & Szyf, 2005). Mothers expressing high levels of nurturant behavior exhibited greater increases in oxytocin receptors during pregnancy, which is thought to trigger maternal responsivity (Meaney, 2001), and have higher levels of dopamine release when caring for their pups (Champagne, Chretien, Stevenson, Zhang, Gratton, & Meaney, 2004). The nurturant mothering that results triggers greater increases in serotonin turnover in the pup, which initiates a cascade leading to altered glucocorticoid receptor expression that beneficially affects adult reactivity to stress (Meaney & Szyf, 2005).

Biological consequences of affiliative contact in early life: Human studies

Similar processes and mechanisms have been identified in humans. Warm, nurturant, supportive contact with a caregiver early in life affects physiological and neuroendocrine stress responses in human infants and children (see Repetti, Taylor, & Seeman, 2002, for a review). Early research on orphans, analogous to the Harlow monkey studies, found high levels of emotional disturbance, especially depression, in infants who failed to receive nurturant, stimulating contact from a caregiver (Spitz & Wolff, 1946). More recent findings from Eastern European abandoned infants confirm that without the affectionate attention of caregivers, infants may fail to thrive and many die (Carlson & Earls, 1997).

Similarly, families characterized by unsupportive relationships have damaging outcomes for the mental, physical, and social health of their offspring, not only in the short term but across the lifespan. Overt family conflict, manifested in recurrent episodes of anger and aggression, cold non-nurturant behavior, or neglect have been associated with a broad array of adverse mental and physical health outcomes long into adulthood (Repetti, Taylor, & Seeman, 2002; Repetti, Taylor, & Saxbe, 2007). The chronic stress of unsupportive families and/or chronic stress unabated by supportive family contacts may produce repeated or chronic SNS activation in children, which in turn may lead to wear and tear on the cardiovascular system. Over time, such alterations may lead to pathogenic changes in sympathetic or parasympathetic functioning or both. These changes may contribute to adult chronic health disorders such as hypertension and coronary heart disease.

Recurrent or chronic engagement of the HPA axis in response to stress can compromise the efficient functioning of this biological stress regulatory system as well. Specifically, in response to the stress of a harsh early childhood environment, functioning of the HPA axis may be compromised in any of several ways. Daily cortisol patterns may be altered. Normally, cortisol levels are high upon waking in the morning but decrease across the day (although peaking following lunch) until they flatten out at low levels in the afternoon. People under chronic stress, however, can show elevated cortisol levels long into the afternoon or evening (Powell et al., 2002) or a general flattening of the diurnal rhythm. In response to acute stress, an elevated flat response to stress (Taylor, Lerner, Sage, Lehman, & Seeman, 2004), an exaggerated cortisol response, a protracted cortisol response, or poor recovery may be seen (McEwen, 1998). Any of these patterns is suggestive of compromises in the ability of the HPA axis to respond to and recover from stress (McEwen, 1998; Pruessner, Hellhammer, Pruessner, & Lupien, 2003).

Attachment is implicated in these processes. Specifically, securely attached infants are less likely to show elevated cortisol responses to normal stress than insecurely attached offspring (Gunnar, Brodersen,

Krueger, & Rigatuso, 1996; see also Nachmias, Gunnar, Mangelsdorf, Parritz, & Buss, 1996). The protective effects of secure attachment are especially significant for socially fearful or inhibited children, temperamental characteristics that have a genetic basis.

Early nurturant and supportive contacts are also important for the development of social and emotional regulation skills, especially those involving responses to stress or threat. A broad array of evidence supports the point that children from harsh families are less likely than those from nurturant families to develop effective emotion regulation skills and social competencies (Repetti et al., 2002).

Is the calibration and regulation of stress responses confined to early environment? Just as evidence increasingly points to the important role that maternal nurturance plays in the biological stress responses of offspring, some research is beginning to uncover the ways in which adults' affiliative contacts may influence each other's biology as well. An early study (McClintock, 1971) found that roommates' menstrual cycles become synchronized over time, probably because of olfactory cues (McClintock, 2002). Research examining physiological concordance between clients and clinical psychologists suggests that such concordance is tied to ratings of therapist empathy (Marci, Ham, Moran, & Orr, 2007). These processes may be especially significant in close relationships, and, to a degree, partners may co-regulate or synchronize their physiological and affective states (Diamond, 2001; Sbarra & Hazan, 2008; Pietromonaco, Barrett, & Powers, 2006). Substantial evidence indicates reciprocity of negative affective processes and concomitant physiological arousal in marital couples (e.g., Gottman, Coan, Carrere, & Swanson, 1998; Levenson & Gottman, 1983); that is, one partner's hostility is likely to arouse the other's. In happier marriages, arousal in conflict situations is more often not in synchrony, possibly because one partner may be attempting to calm the more agitated partner (Saxbe, 2009). Hofer (1984) suggested that cohabiting partners influence each other's regulatory symptoms and routine so much that some of the consequences of bereavement, such as disturbed sleep, reduced appetite, and social withdrawal, might result from the loss of this biological regulatory influence. Until recently, physiological underpinnings of these processes had not been addressed. There is now some evidence that couples' HPA axis activity may be coordinated (Berg & Wynne-Edwards, 2002; Schreiber et al., 2006).

Overall, however, negative emotional states may be more "contagious" than positive ones, suggesting the possibility of the exacerbation of stress within close relationships rather than its amelioration. Such effects may depend on whether both members of a couple are facing a particular stressor or whether only one person is.

Whether adults can influence each other's biology on a chronic basis in the same ways as occur in the mother–infant relationship is unknown, but the answer may be not to the same degree. Maternal influences occur at the time that biological stress regulatory systems are just developing, and so their effects may be more profound and long-lasting than is true in adult biological co-regulation. Nonetheless, the idea that chronic cohabitation exerts ongoing effects on the biological functioning of both parties, resulting, in some cases, in biological synchrony, merits additional attention.

Affiliation and genetic pathways
Socioemotional skills that underpin affiliation may have an epigenetic basis in humans as well. This research is in its infancy, and so there is much still to be discovered, but to date, genes involved in the regulation of monoamine oxidase-A (MAOA), serotonin, and dopamine appear to be implicated. MAOA is an enzyme that breaks down neurochemicals such as serotonin and dopamine (Shih, Chen, & Ridd, 1999). The MAOA gene that regulates the enzyme has been implicated in antisocial behavior (e.g., Eisenberger, Way, Taylor, Welch, & Lieberman, 2007). For example, in epidemiological studies, men with the low expressing alleles of the MAOA-uVNTR are more likely to engage in aggressive and antisocial activity than men with high expressing alleles; of interest, these effects appear to be especially likely when those with the genetic risk have also been exposed to maltreatment in childhood (Caspi et al., 2002; Kim-Cohen et al., 2006).

The harshness or nurturance of the early family environment also influences the expression of the serotonin transporter gene (5-HTTLPR). People with two copies of the 5-HTTLPR short allele (short/short) who have experienced childhood maltreatment are more likely to be diagnosed with major depressive disorder than individuals with one or two copies of the long allele who have experienced similar environments (Caspi et al., 2003; Kaufman et al., 2004), although these effects do not always replicate (Risch et al., 2009). A study from our laboratory (Taylor, Way, Welch, Hilmert, Lehman, & Eisenberger, 2006), which may help to explain these inconsistencies, indicates that the short allele may not function as a risk allele for depression in the face of an adverse environment, but as a general sensitivity allele, providing protection from symptoms of depression when the environment is nurturant. We found a significant gene-by-environment interaction, such that individuals with two copies of the short allele had greater depressive symptomatology if they had experienced early familial adversity compared to participants with the short/long or long/long genotypes, but significantly less depressive symptomatology if they reported a supportive early environment. Notably, the adverse early family environments studied were fairly mild, consisting of some conflict, moderate household chaos, and/or cold, unaffectionate, and distant behaviors, rather than explicit maltreatment in the form of physical or sexual abuse. Thus, nurturant, affiliative contacts in early life can shape the expression of genes in ways that can have lifelong effects on social behavior (such as aggression) and on susceptibility to stress in the social environment.

Certain genes in the dopamine system may show a similar pattern. Researchers have found that, when exposed to non-nurturant parenting, people with the long allele of the polymorphism DRD4 are at higher risk for externalizing behaviors than individuals with other alleles (e.g., Bakermans-Kranenburg & van IJzendoorn, 2006). However, recent evidence indicates that the long allele may increase sensitivity to positive as well as negative parental influences. In one study, when the environment was nurturant, individuals with the long DRD4 allele had low levels of externalizing behavior, but when the environment was harsh, individuals with the same allele had high levels of externalizing behavior. The behavior of individuals with the other alleles was less responsive to parenting quality (Bakermans-Kranenburg & van IJzendoorn, 2007). Bakermans-Kranenburg and colleagues (2008) also found that toddlers with the long allele of DRD4 were more responsive to a parental educational program designed to reduce externalizing behavior through increasing the attentiveness of parenting than those with other alleles. Findings such as these offer significant evidence that the social environment early in life can powerfully shape expression of genes related to social behavior across the lifespan.

Affiliative responses to acute stress

A variety of empirical studies have shown that affiliative contact can be protective against the psychological and biological effects of acute stress as well. For example, experimental studies demonstrate that the presence of a supportive person when one is going through a stressful task can reduce cardiovascular and HPA axis responses to stress; these benefits can be experienced whether the supportive person is a partner, a friend, or a stranger (e.g., Christenfeld et al., 1997; Gerin, Pieper, Levy, & Pickering, 1992; Gerin, Milner, Chawla, & Pickering, 1995; Kamark, Manuck, & Jennings, 1990; Kors, Linden, & Gerin, 1997; Lepore, Allen, & Evans, 1993; Sheffield & Carroll, 1994; see Lepore, 1998 for a review).

Oxytocin may play a role in these processes. In response to stress, animals and humans experience a cascade of hormonal responses that begins, at least under some stressful conditions, with the rapid release of oxytocin. Consistent evidence suggests that oxytocin is released in response to stress and that oxytocin is associated with reduced SNS and HPA axis responses to stress (see Taylor, Dickerson, & Klein, 2002). For example, oxytocin is associated with parasympathetic (vagal) functioning that plays a counterregulatory role in fear responses to stress (e.g., Dreifuss, Dubois-Dauphin, Widmer, & Raggenbass, 1992; McCarthy, 1995; Sawchenko & Swanson, 1982; Swanson & Sawchenko, 1980). In experimental studies, oxytocin enhances sedation and relaxation, reduces anxiety, and decreases sympathetic activity (Altemus, Deuster, Galliven, Carter, & Gold, 1995; Uvnäs-Moberg, 1997). Exogenous administration of oxytocin in rats results in decreases in blood pressure, pain sensitivity, and corticosteroid levels, among other findings indicative of a reduced stress response (Uvnäs-Moberg, 1997). Oxytocin appears to inhibit the secretion of adrenocorticotropin hormone (ACTH) and cortisol in humans as well (Chiodera & Legros, 1981; Legros, Chiodera, & Demy-Ponsart, 1982).

Oxytocin may be implicated in the clinical benefits of affiliation as well. A study by Detillion and colleagues (Detillion, Craft, Glasper, Prendergast, & DeVries, 2004) reported a role for oxytocin in wound healing. In this study, Siberian hamsters received cutaneous wounds and were then exposed to immobilization stress. The stressor increased cortisol concentrations and impaired wound healing. However, these effects occurred only in socially isolated and not in socially housed animals. Thus, social housing acted as a stress buffer. The studies went further to tie down the mechanism underpinning this effect. The researchers found that eliminating cortisol via adrenalectomy eliminated the impact of the stressor on wound healing, thereby implicating the HPA axis in the wound healing process. Of particular relevance for the role of oxytocin in the wound healing process, treating the isolated hamsters with oxytocin eliminated the stress-induced increases in cortisol and facilitated wound healing; treating socially housed hamsters with an oxytocin antagonist, however, delayed wound healing. This evidence strongly implies that affiliation can be protective against adverse effects of stress through a mechanism that implicates oxytocin-induced suppression of the HPA axis. Moreover, it confirms a role for oxytocin in a clinically significant health-related outcome (wound healing).

The potential roles of oxytocin in the down-regulation of SNS and HPA axis responses to stress, in the tendency to turn to others, and in health-related outcomes at present are hypotheses with animal evidence to support them, but less evidence from human studies. Consequently, these issues currently represent a direction for research rather than an established biological pathway by which social contact may exert protective effects on health. Moreover, there may be roles for other hormones both in promoting social support initially and in regulating its biological effects, which include vasopressin, norepinephrine, serotonin, and prolactin (Nelson & Panksepp, 1998; Taylor, Dickerson, & Klein, 2002).

Research has also focused on the neural mechanisms whereby social contact affects physiological processes that, in turn, affect health outcomes. A three-part investigation (Eisenberger, Taylor, Gable, Hilmert, & Lieberman, 2007) (1) had participants complete a daily diary that recorded the supportiveness of social interactions, (2) used fMRI to scan reactions to a social exclusion manipulation, and (3) recorded physiological and HPA axis reactivity to laboratory-induced social stressors. The results indicated that people who interacted regularly with supportive people on a day-to-day basis showed diminished cortisol reactivity to a social stressor. Moreover, both greater social support and a diminished cortisol response were associated with lower reactivity during the social exclusion task in two brain regions that have been previously tied to distress induced by social separation, namely the dorsal anterior cingulate cortex (dACC) and Brodmann area 8 (BA 8). Mediational analyses revealed that individual differences in dACC and BA 8 reactivity mediated the relationship between high daily social support and low cortisol reactivity to social stress; that is, those people experiencing greater social support showed reduced neurocognitive reactivity to social exclusion, which, in turn, was tied to reduced neuroendocrine stress responses to laboratory challenges. This study, then, helps to document the neural mechanisms underpinning the relationship between social support and health-relevant outcomes and suggests a mechanism by which social support may benefit health, namely by diminishing neural and physiological reactivity to stress.

Physical and Mental Health Consequences of Affiliation Under Stress

In response to their affiliative efforts, people commonly experience social support. Social support is defined as the perception or experience that one is loved and cared for by others, esteemed and valued, and part of a social network of mutual assistance and obligations (Wills, 1991). Social support may come from a partner, relatives, friends, coworkers, social and community ties, strangers, and even a devoted pet.

Mapping onto the functions of affiliation more generally, taxonomies of social support typically classify it into several specific forms. Informational support occurs when one person helps another to understand a stressful event better by providing information about the event. Instrumental support involves the provision of tangible assistance, such as services, financial assistance, and other specific aid or goods. Emotional support involves providing warmth and assistance to another person and reassuring that person that he or she is a valuable person for whom others care. Social support may involve the reality of using the social network for benefits such as these, but it can also involve simply the perception that such resources are available should they be needed. In other words, just knowing that one is cared for and that one could request support from others is often comforting in its own right.

The beneficial effects of affiliation and social support on mental and physical health are well established. Social support reduces psychological distress such as depression or anxiety during times of stress (e.g., Fleming, Baum, Gisriel, & Gatchel, 1982; Lin, Ye, & Ensel, 1999; Sarason, Sarason, & Gurung, 1997). It promotes psychological adjustment to chronically stressful conditions, such as coronary artery disease (Holahan, Moos, Holahan, & Brennan, 1997), diabetes, HIV (Turner-Cobb et al., 2002), cancer (Penninx, van Tilburg, Boeke, Deeg, Kriegsman, & van Eijk, 1998; Stone, Mezzacappa, Donatone, & Gonder, 1999), rheumatoid arthritis (Goodenow, Reisine, & Grady, 1990), kidney disease (Dimond, 1979), childhood leukemia (Magni, Silvestro, Tamiello, Zanesco, & Carl, 1988), and stroke (Robertson & Suinn, 1968), among other disorders.

Social support has been tied to a variety of specific health benefits among individuals sustaining health risks. These include fewer complications during pregnancy and childbirth (Collins, Dunkel-Schetter, Lobel, & Scrimshaw, 1993), less susceptibility to herpes attacks among infected individuals (VanderPlate, Aral, & Magder, 1988), lower rates of myocardial infarction among individuals with diagnosed disease, a reduced likelihood of mortality from myocardial infarction (Kulik & Mahler, 1993; Wiklund, Oden, Sanne, Ulvenstam, Wilhemsson, & Wilhemsen, 1988), faster recovery from coronary artery disease surgery (King, Reis, Porter, & Norsen, 1993; Kulik & Mahler, 1993), better diabetes control (Marteau, Bloch, & Baum, 1987), better compliance and longer survival in patients with end-stage renal disease (Cohen, Sharma, Acquaviva, Peterson, Patel, & Kimmel, 2007), and less pain among arthritis patients (Brown, Sheffield, Leary, & Robinson, 2003). Social support protects against cognitive decline in older adults (Seeman, Lusignolo, Albert, & Berkman, 2001), heart disease among the recently widowed (Sorkin, Rook, & Lu, 2002), and psychological distress in response to traumatic events, such as 9/11 (Simeon, Greenberg, Nelson, Schmeider, & Hollander, 2005).

Social support contributes to longevity (e.g., Rutledge et al., 2004). In a classic study that documented this point, epidemiologists Lisa Berkman and Leonard Syme (1979) followed nearly seven thousand California residents over a 9-year period to identify factors that contributed to their longevity or early death. They found that people who lacked social and community ties were more likely to die of all causes during the follow-up period than those who cultivated or maintained their social relationships. Having social contacts predicted an average 2.8 years increased longevity among women and 2.3 years among men, and these differences persisted after controlling for socioeconomic status, health status at the beginning of the study, and health habits (Berkman & Syme, 1979). Of particular significance is the fact that the positive impact of social ties on health is as powerful, and in some cases more powerful, a predictor of health and longevity than well-established risk factors for chronic disease and mortality, with effect sizes on par with smoking, blood pressure, lipids, obesity, and physical activity (House, Landis, & Umberson, 1988).

In prospective studies controlling for baseline health status, people with a higher quantity and quality of social relationships have consistently been shown to be at lower risk of early death (Herbst-Damm & Kulik, 2005; Seeman, 1996), and in studies of both humans and animals, social isolation has been found to be a major risk factor for early mortality (House, Landis, & Umberson, 1988).

When affiliation is not experienced as supportive

Not all research shows beneficial effects of affiliation in challenging circumstances, however. Sometimes the presence of a friend or stranger actually increases sympathetic reactivity among those undergoing stress (e.g., Allen, Blascovich, Tomaka, & Kelsey, 1991; Mullen, Bryant, & Driskell, 1997). Whereas the presence of a partner typically reduces stress-related physiological and neuroendocrine reactivity among men, the presence of a male partner often enhances reactivity among women (Kiecolt-Glaser & Newton, 2001). The presence of a friend or partner may increase evaluation apprehension over whether important others' perceptions of the self may decline, and so this apprehension may eliminate any beneficial effect of support (Lepore, 1998).

Sometimes efforts to provide social support are experienced as intrusive, or would-be support providers may give poor advice or fail to provide the right kind of social support, thereby reducing the effectiveness of the effort (Bolger, Foster, Vinokur, & Ng, 1996; Burg & Seeman, 1994; Dakof & Taylor, 1990). Social support efforts may also be perceived as controlling or directive by the recipient. For example, chronically ill patients sometimes report that a spouse's efforts to co-manage the disorder can lead to conflict in the couple (e.g., Fisher, La Greca, Greco, Arfken, & Schneiderman, 1997). Social support may reinforce symptom experiences if it becomes contingent on a person's expression of psychological or physical distress (Itkowitz, Kerns, & Otis, 2003).

When people are under threat, they are especially vulnerable to perceived or actual threats to the self. In other words, although people are often receptive to negative or threatening information when they are in a positive state of mind (see Fiske & Taylor, 2008, for a review), under threat, people typically need to shore up a sense of self. As such, having to ask for help or solace or receiving obvious forms of assistance may be perceived as threats to the self. Consistent with this argument, Bolger and colleagues have suggested that the most effective kinds of social support are those that are invisible to the recipient. In a series of studies with couples, they showed that supportive efforts identified by a partner but not perceived by the recipient had greater effects on the recipient's emotional well-being than support efforts experienced by both the supportive person and the recipient as intended (Bolger & Amarel, 2007; Bolger, Zuckerman, & Kessler, 2000). Visible acts of social support can raise a sense of obligation or indebtedness and lower self-esteem, particularly when the recipient is under stress.

Other factors may compromise the efficacy of socially supportive efforts as well. In their "matching hypothesis," Cohen and McKay (1984) suggest that to be supportive, the actions of a support provider must meet the specific needs of the recipient. For example, if a person needs emotional support but receives advice instead, the misfired effort at support may actually increase psychological distress (Thoits, 1986). Consistent with this perspective, Helgeson and Cohen (1996) examined the impact of social contact on adjustment to cancer and found that emotional support was most desired by patients and appeared to have the greatest beneficial effects on adjustment. However, when that support was provided in a peer group setting, it did not, for the most part, have benefits; rather, educational groups that provided information were perceived more positively. It may be that emotional support is best provided by people close to the patient such as family and friends (Dakof & Taylor, 1990), and that educational needs are better satisfied by educational interventions (Helgeson & Cohen, 1996).

Recent research suggests that certain adverse effects of social support may be more acutely experienced by East Asians than by European Americans. Although social support appears to be universally beneficial for mental and physical health, there are cultural influences on how it is experienced. East Asians and Asian Americans are more reluctant to explicitly ask for social support from close others than European Americans, because they are more concerned about the potential negative relational consequences of such behaviors (Taylor, Sherman, Kim, Jarcho, Takagi, & Dunagan, 2004). Instead, they are more likely to use and benefit from forms of social support that do not involve explicit disclosure of personal stressful events and disclosure of distress.

Accordingly, one may distinguish between implicit and explicit social support (Taylor, Welch, Kim, & Sherman, 2007). Explicit social support involves the specific recruitment and use of a social network in response to specific stressful events and involves the elicitation of advice, instrumental aid, or emotional comfort. Implicit social support, by contrast, involves the emotional comfort that one can obtain from social networks without necessarily disclosing or discussing one's problems vis-à-vis specific stressful events. Implicit support may take the form of reminding oneself of close others, affiliating with close others without discussing problems, or simply perceiving social support to be available without actually making use of it.

In a series of studies (Kim, Sherman, & Taylor, 2008; Taylor, Sherman, et al., 2004; Taylor et al., 2007), we found that Asians and Asian Americans sought less social support than European Americans, and when they were put in a position of needing to ask for social support, experienced more psychological distress and stronger arousal. They were, however, psychologically and biologically buffered by the process of merely thinking about their close relationships. European Americans, in contrast, were more comfortable with seeking explicit social support, namely asking others for help, but were not benefitted by merely thinking about their social relationships. On the surface, these findings regarding European Americans would appear to contradict the findings on invisible support by Bolger's research group; however, it may be that European Americans are comfortable with asking for social support on their own terms, but that unsolicited social support from close others in times of threat creates a sense of indebtedness or a threat to self-esteem.

As the research on unintended negative effects of social support efforts suggests, there is a disjunction between findings concerning the benefits of affiliation and those attesting to the risks of socially supportive efforts. Research consistently finds that strong social networks have a positive effect on mental and physical health in both stressful and non-stressful times (Thoits, 1995). Research on actual support transactions, however, suggests that under many conditions, efforts at support misfire for a host of reasons. Although the difference between the two types of studies may depend on the particular type of evidence gathered and paradigms used, to the extent that it reflects a reality about social contact, it implies that mere social contact and the ability to affiliate with others under stress may be more beneficial than extracting social support from others. If you think back to an occasion when you were ill, you may remember that it was comforting just to leave the bedroom door open so you could hear other people moving about in the house. Similarly, spouses may experience much of the benefit of their contact with each other simply by knowing that the other is around and available and not through the specific social interactions that occur. Carrying this argument one step further, what scientists construe as social support may be a basic biopsychosocial process that depends heavily on proximity and/or awareness of others' availability more than on the explicit social support transactions that have been so widely studied.

Future directions

Substantial empirical progress has been made in understanding the biopsychosocial underpinnings of affiliation in response to stress. In the near future, we can expect to see additional insights regarding the roles of oxytocin, vasopressin, and the opioid system in eliciting and responding to affiliative contact. We may also see additional clarity regarding genetic bases of social support needs and perceptions. On the social psychological side, the benefits of giving as well as receiving social support will become increasingly understood (e.g., Brown, Nesse, Vinokur, & Smith, 2003).

Our current conceptualization of the role of affiliation in protection against stress may require some rethinking. Human biological systems are marked by substantial redundancy. In other words, activities that are vital to survival are often maintained by more than one biological process. There are, for example, five different ways by which the stomach can produce hydrochloric acid for the digestion of food. Other more obvious examples of redundancy include the fact that people have two eyes, two hands, two lungs, two kidneys, and so on. This is not to say that all vital biological systems are backed up through redundancy, the heart being an obvious counterexample. Nonetheless, it may be useful to think about psychological processes as implicated in this redundancy. That is, vital processes may be backed up not only through multiple biological mechanisms, but through a combination of psychological and biological mechanisms as well. In this viewpoint, the human impetus toward group living as well as human beings' tendencies to affiliate with others in stressful times may have multiple psychological and biological origins. Affiliation is psychologically satisfying, and during times of stress, human beings experience a psychological need, as well as a biological impetus, toward affiliating with others. It is possible that the psychological architecture that leads people toward comforting social relationships represents redundancy within the biopsychosocial system, whereby either the psychological impetus toward others or the biological impetus or both ensure that affiliative efforts are undertaken in times of threat. Future research will clarify whether this conceptualization is theoretically and empirically useful.

Conclusions

The tendency to affiliate with others under stressful conditions is one of the most basic responses that human beings have for coping with a broad array of stressful and threatening circumstances. Unlike the fight-or-flight response that has typically guided research, tend and befriend characterizes the fact that humans come together for mutual protection and solace and to protect offspring. These affiliative responses to stress have both biological and psychological origins and effects. Affiliating with others is inherently comforting under most conditions, and so people often choose to affiliate with others when times are stressful so as to gain emotional comfort, information about a stressor, tangible assistance, and reduced physiological reactivity. Biologically, these effects may depend upon oxytocin and brain opioid pathways that provide a signal to the organism that the social environment is lacking and that provide an impetus to seeking social contact. Part and parcel of this response is the fact that social isolation is experienced as aversive, and rising endogenous oxytocin levels in response to isolation may prompt affiliative behavior.

The biological benefits of affiliation are clear. Studies of early life experience provide unequivocal evidence that nurturant mothering helps to shape biological stress regulatory systems as well as craft socioemotional skills that aid in the creation of social networks and the seeking of social support across the lifespan. Genetic factors and epigenetic processes are also implicated in these pathways. The interplay of these early influences with the availability of supportive others during times of acute stress leads reliably to ameliorative effects on both psychological distress and biological responses to acute stressors.

The consequences of affiliation under stress for mental and physical health are very well established. Although there are circumstances under which efforts at social support backfire and may actually worsen the situation, social support nonetheless has effects on health on par with smoking, lipids, and other well-established biological risk factors. On the whole, the perception that one has social support available appears to have as many mental and physical health benefits as the reality, and under some circumstances, may suffice for protecting against the ravages of stress.

Author Note

Preparation of this manuscript was supported by grants from NIA (AG-030309) and NSF (SES-0525713 and BCS-0729532).

References

Allen, K. M., Blascovich, J., Tomaka, J., & Kelsey, R. M. (1991). Presence of human friends and pet dogs as moderators of autonomic responses to stress in women. *Journal of Personality and Social Psychology, 61*, 582–9.

Altemus, M. P., Deuster, A., Galliven, E., Carter, C. S., & Gold, P. W. (1995). Suppression of hypothalamic-pituitary-adrenal axis response to stress in lactating women. *Journal of Clinical Endocrinology and Metabolism, 80*, 2954–9.

Argiolas, A., & Gessa, G. L. (1991). Central functions of oxytocin. *Neuroscience and Biobehavioral Reviews, 15*, 217–31.

Bakermans-Kranenburg, M. J., & van IJzendoorn, M. H. (2006). Gene-environment interaction of the dopamine D4 receptor (DRD4) and observed maternal insensitivity predicting externalizing behavior in preschoolers. *Developmental Psychobiology, 48*, 406–9.

Bakermans-Kranenburg, M. J., & van IJzendoorn, M. H. (2007). Research review: genetic vulnerability or differential susceptibility in child development: the case of attachment. *Journal of Child Psychology and Psychiatry, 48*, 1160–73.

Bakermans-Kranenburg, M. J., van IJzendoorn, M. H., Pijlman, F. T., Mesman, J., & Juffer, F. (2008). Experimental evidence for differential susceptibility: dopamine D4 receptor polymorphism (DRD4 VNTR) moderates intervention effects on toddlers' externalizing behavior in a randomized controlled trial. *Developmental Psychobiology, 44*, 293–300.

Berg, S. J., & Wynne-Edwards, K. E. (2002). Salivary hormone concentrations in mothers and fathers becoming parents are not correlated. *Hormones and Behavior, 42*, 424–36.

Berkman, L. F., & Syme, S. L. (1979). Social networks, host resistance, and mortality: A nine-year followup study of Alameda County residents. *American Journal of Epidemiology, 109*, 186–204.

Bolger, N., & Amarel, D. (2007). Effects of support visibility on adjustment to stress: Experimental evidence. *Journal of Personality and Social Psychology, 92*, 458–75.

Bolger, N., Foster, M., Vinokur, A. D., & Ng, R. (1996). Close relationships and adjustments to a life crisis: The case of breast cancer. *Journal of Personality and Social Psychology, 70*, 283–94.

Bolger, N., Zuckerman, A., & Kessler, R. C. (2000). Invisible support and adjustment to stress. *Journal of Personality and Social Psychology, 79*, 953–61.

Brown, S. L., Nesse, R. M., Vinokur, A. D., & Smith, D. M. (2003). Providing social support may be more beneficial than receiving it: Results from a prospective study of mortality. *Psychological Science, 14*, 320–7.

Brown, J. L., Sheffield, D., Leary, M. R., & Robinson, M. E. (2003). Social support and experimental pain. *Psychosomatic Medicine, 65*, 276–83.

Burg, M. M., & Seeman, T. E. (1994). Families and health: The negative side of social ties. *Annals of Behavioral Medicine, 16*, 109–15.

Cacioppo, J. T., & Hawkley, L. C. (2003). The anatomy of loneliness. *Current Directions in Psychological Science, 12*, 71–4.

Cannon, W. B. (1932). *The wisdom of the body.* New York: Norton.

Caputon, L., Ravaud, A., & Dantzer, R. (2000). Early depressive symptoms in cancer patients receiving interleukin-2 and/or interferon alpha-2b therapy. *Journal of Clinical Oncology, 18*, 2143–51.

Carlson, M., & Earls, F. (1997). Psychological and neuroendocrinological sequelae of early social deprivation in institutionalized children in Romania. *Annals of the New York Academy of Sciences, 807*, 419–28.

Carter, C. S., DeVries, A. C., & Getz, L. L. (1995). Physiological substrates of mammalian monogamy: The prairie vole model. *Neuroscience and Biobehavioral Reviews, 19*, 303–14.

Caspi, A., McClay, J., Moffitt, T. E., Mill, J., Martin, J., Craig, I. W., et al. (2002). Role of genotype in the cycle of violence in maltreated children. *Science, 297*, 851–4.

Caspi, A., Sugden, K., Moffitt, T. E., Taylor, A., Craig, I. W., Harrington, H., et al. (2003). Influence of life stress on depression: moderation by a polymorphism in the 5-HTT gene. *Science, 301*, 386–9.

Champagne, F. A., Chretien, P., Stevenson, C. W., Zhang, T. Y., Gratton, A., & Meaney, M. J. (2004). Variations in nucleus accumbens dopamine associated with individual differences in maternal behavior in the rat. *Journal of Neuroscience, 24*, 4113–23.

Chiodera, P., & Legros, J. J. (1981). L'injection intraveineuse d'ocytocine entraîne une diminution de la concentration plasmatique de cortisol chez l'homme normal. *Comptes Rendus des Séances de la Société de Biologie et de Ses Filiales (Paris), 175*, 546–9.

Christenfeld, N., Gerin, W., Linden, W., Sanders, M., Mathur, J., Deich, J. D., & Pickering, T. G. (1997). Social support effects on cardiovascular reactivity: Is a stranger as effective as a friend? *Psychosomatic Medicine, 59*, 388–98.

Chrousos, G. P., & Gold, P. W. (1992). The concepts of stress and stress system disorders: Overview of physical and behavioral homeostasis. *Journal of the American Medical Association, 267*, 1244–52.

Cohen, S., & McKay, G. (1984). Social support, stress, and the buffering hypothesis: A theoretical analysis. In A. Baum, S. E. Taylor, and J. Singer (Eds.), *Handbook of psychology and health* (Vol. 4, pp. 253–268). Hillsdale, NJ: Erlbaum.

Cohen, S. D., Sharma, T., Acquaviva, K., Peterson, R. A., Patel, S. S., & Kimmel, P. L. (2007). Social support and chronic kidney disease: An update. *Advances in Chronic Kidney Disease, 14*, 335–44.

Collins, N. L., Dunkel-Schetter, C., Lobel, M., & Scrimshaw, S. C. M. (1993). Social support in pregnancy: Psychosocial correlates of birth outcomes and post-partum depression. *Journal of Personality and Social Psychology, 65*, 1243–58.

Dakof, G. A., & Taylor, S. E. (1990). Victims' perceptions of social support: What is helpful from whom? *Journal of Personality and Social Psychology, 58*, 80–9.

Detillion, C. E., Craft, T. K. S., Glasper, E. R., Prendergast, B. J., & DeVries, A. C. (2004). Social facilitation of wound healing. *Psychoneuroendocrinology, 29*, 1004–11.

Diamond, L. M. (2001). Contributions of psychophysiology to research on adult attachment: Review and recommendations. *Personality and Social Psychology Review, 5*, 276–95.

Dimond, M. (1979). Social support and adaptation to chronic illness: The case of maintenance hemodialysis. *Research in Nursing and Health, 2*, 101–8.

Dreifuss, J. J., Dubois-Dauphin, M., Widmer, H., & Raggenbass, M. (1992). Electrophysiology of oxytocin actions on central neurons. *Annals of the New York Academy of Science, 652*, 46–57.

Eisenberger, N. I., Lieberman, M. D., & Williams, K. D. (2003). Does rejection hurt? An fMRI study of social exclusion. *Science, 302*, 290–2.

Eisenberger, N. I., Taylor, S. E., Gable, S. L., Hilmert, C. J., & Lieberman, M. D. (2007). Neural pathways link social support to attenuated neuroendocrine stress responses. *Neuroimage, 35*, 1601–12.

Eisenberger, N. I., Way, B. M., Taylor, S. E., Welch, W. T., & Lieberman, M. D. (2007). Understanding genetic risk for aggression: Clues from the brain's response to social exclusion. *Biological Psychiatry, 61*, 1100–8.

Fisher, E. B., La Greca, A. M., Greco, P., Arfken, C., & Schneiderman, N. (1997). Directive and nondirective social support in diabetes management. *International Journal of Behavioral Medicine, 4*, 131–44.

Fiske, S. T., & Taylor, S. E. (2008). *Social cognition: From brains to culture* (1st ed.). New York: McGraw-Hill.

Fleming, R., Baum, A., Gisriel, M. M., & Gatchel, R. J. (1982). Mediating influences of social support on stress at Three Mile Island. *Journal of Human Stress, 8*, 14–22.

Francis, D., Diorio, J., Liu, D., & Meaney, M. J. (1999). Nongenomic transmission across generations of maternal behavior and stress responses in the rat. *Science, 286*, 1155–8.

Gerin, W., Pieper, C., Levy, R., & Pickering, T. G. (1992). Social support in social interaction: a moderator of cardiovascular reactivity. *Psychosomatic Medicine, 54*, 324–36.

Gerin, W., Milner, D., Chawla, S., & Pickering, T. G. (1995). Social support as a moderator of cardiovascular reactivity: A test of the direct effects and buffering hypothesis. *Psychosomatic Medicine, 57*, 16–22.

Goodenow, C., Reisine, S. T., & Grady, K. E. (1990). Quality of social support and associated social and psychological functioning in women with rheumatoid arthritis. *Health Psychology, 9*, 266–84.

Gottman, J. M., Coan, J., Carrere, S., & Swanson, C. (1998). Predicting marital happiness and stability from newly-wed interactions. *Journal of Marriage and the Family, 60*, 5–22.

Gunnar, M. R., Brodersen, L., Krueger, K., & Rigatuso, J. (1996). Dampening of adrenocortical responses during infancy: Normative changes and individual differences. *Child Development, 67*, 877–89.

Grippo, A. J., Gerena, D., Huang, J., Kumar, N., Shah, M., Ughreja, R., & Carter, C. S. (2007). Social isolation induces behavioral and neuroendocrine disturbances relevant to depression in female and male prairie voles. *Psychoneuroendocrinology, 32*, 966–80.

Harlow, H. F., & Harlow, M. K. (1962). Social deprivation in monkeys. *Scientific American, 207*, 136–46.

Helgeson, V. S., & Cohen, S. (1996). Social support and adjustment to cancer: Reconciling descriptive, correlational, and intervention research. *Health Psychology, 15*, 135–48.

Herbst-Damm, K. L., & Kulik, J. A. (2005). Volunteer support, marital status, and the survival times of terminally ill patients. *Health Psychology, 24*, 225–9.

Hofer, M. (1984). Relationships as regulators. *Psychosomatic Medicine, 46*, 183–97.

Holahan, C. J., Moos, R. H., Holahan, C. K., & Brennan, P. L. (1997). Social context, coping strategies, and depressive symptoms: An expanded model with cardiac patients. *Journal of Personality and Social Psychology, 72*, 918–28.

House, J. S., Landis, K. R., & Umberson, D. (1988). Social relationships and health. *Science, 241*, 540–5.

Itkowitz, N. I., Kerns, R. D., & Otis, J. D. (2003). Support and coronary heart disease: The importance of significant other responses. *Journal of Behavioral Medicine, 26*, 19–30.

Kamarck, T. W., Manuck, S. B., & Jennings, J. R. (1990). Social support reduces cardiovascular reactivity to psychological challenge: A laboratory model. *Psychosomatic Medicine, 52*, 42–58.

Kaufman, J., Yang, B. Z., Douglas-Palumberi, H., Houshyar, S., Lipschitz, D., Krystal, J. H., & Gelernter, J. (2004). Social supports and serotonin transporter gene moderate depression in maltreated children. *Proceedings of the National Academy of Sciences U S A, 101*, 17316–21.

Kiecolt-Glaser, J. K., & Newton, T. L. (2001). Marriage and health: His and hers. *Psychological Bulletin, 127*, 472–503.

Kim, H. S., Sherman, D. K., & Taylor, S. E. (2008). Culture and social support. *American Psychologist, 63*, 518–26.

King, K. B., Reis, H. T., Porter, L. A., & Norsen, L. H. (1993). Social support and long-term recovery from coronary artery surgery: Effects on patients and spouses. *Health Psychology, 12*, 56–63.

Kim-Cohen, J., Caspi, A., Taylor, A., Williams, B., Newcombe, R., Craig, I. W., & Moffitt, T. E. (2006). MAOA, maltreatment, and gene-environment interaction predicting children's mental health: new evidence and a meta-analysis. *Molecular Psychiatry, 11*, 903–13.

Kors, D., Linden, W., & Gerin, W. (1997). Evaluation interferes with social support: Effects on cardiovascular stress reactivity. *Journal of Social and Clinical Psychology, 16*, 1–23.

Kulik, J. A., & Mahler, H. I. M. (1993). Emotional support as a moderator of adjustment and compliance after coronary artery bypass surgery: A longitudinal study. *Journal of Behavioral Medicine, 16*, 45–64.

Legros, J. J., Chiodera, P., & Demy-Ponsart, E. (1982). Inhibitory influence of exogenous oxytocin on adrenocorticotropin secretion in normal human subjects. *Journal of Clinical Endocrinology and Metabolism, 55*, 1035–9.

Lepore, S. J. (1998). Problems and prospects for the social support-reactivity hypothesis. *Annals of Behavioral Medicine, 20*, 257–69.

Lepore, S. J., Allen, K. A. M., & Evans, G. W. (1993). Social support lowers cardiovascular reactivity to an acute stress. *Psychosomatic Medicine, 55*, 518–24.

Levenson, R. W., & Gottman, J. M. (1983). Marital interaction: Physiological linkage and affective exchange. *Journal of Personality and Social Psychology, 45*, 587–97.

Lin, N., Ye, X., & Ensel, W. (1999). Social support and depressed mood: A structural analysis. *Journal of Health and Social Behavior, 40*, 344–59.

Liu, D., Diorio, J., Tannenbaum, B., Caldji, C., Francis, D., Freedman, A., et al. (1997). Maternal care, hippocampal glucocorticoid receptors, and hypothalamic-pituitary-adrenal responses to stress. *Science, 277*, 1659–62.

Luckow, A., Reifman, A., & McIntosh, D. N. (1998, August). *Gender differences in coping: A meta-analysis.* Poster presented to the annual meetings of the American Psychological Association, San Francisco, CA.

Magni, G., Silvestro, A., Tamiello, M., Zanesco, L., & Carl, M. (1988). An integrated approach to the assessment of family adjustment to acute lymphocytic leukemia in children. *Acta Psychiatrica Scandinavia, 78,* 639–42.

Maier, S. F., & Watkins, L. R. (1998). Cytokines for psychologists: Implications of bidirectional immune-to-brain communication for understanding behavior, mood, and cognition. *Psychological Review, 105,* 83–107.

Marci, C. D., Ham, J., Moran, E., & Orr, S. P. (2007). Physiologic correlates of perceived therapist empathy and social-emotional process during psychotherapy. *Journal of Nervous and Mental Disease, 195,* 103–11.

Marteau, T. M., Bloch, S., & Baum, J. D. (1987). Family life and diabetic control. *Journal of Child Psychology and Psychiatry, 28,* 823–33.

McCarthy, M. M. (1995). Estrogen modulation of oxytocin and its relation to behavior. In R. Ivell and J. Russell (Eds.), *Oxytocin: Cellular and molecular approaches in medicine and research* (pp. 235–242). New York: Plenum Press.

McClintock, M. (1971). Menstrual synchrony and suppression. *Nature, 229,* 244–5.

McClintock, M. (2002). The neuroendocrinology of social chemosignals in humans and animals: Odors, pheromones and vasanas. *Hormones, Brain, and Behavior, 1,* 797–870.

McEwen, B. S. (1998). Protective and damaging effects of stress mediators. *New England Journal of Medicine, 338,* 171–9.

McEwen, B. S., & Sapolsky, R. M. (1995). Stress and cognitive function. *Current Opinion in Neurobiology, 5,* 205–16.

McEwen, B. S., & Stellar, E. (1993). Stress and the individual: Mechanisms leading to disease. *Archives of Internal Medicine, 153,* 2093–101.

Meaney, M. J. (2001). Maternal care, gene expression, and the transmission of individual differences in stress reactivity across generations. *Annual Review of Neuroscience, 24,* 1161–92.

Meaney, M. J., & Szyf, M. (2005). Environmental programming of stress responses through DNA methylation: life at the interface between a dynamic environment and a fixed genome. *Dialogues in Clinical Neuroscience, 7,* 103–23.

Miller, G. E., Cohen, S., & Ritchey, A. K. (2002). Chronic psychological stress and the regulation of pro-inflammatory cytokines: A glucocorticoid-resistance model. *Health Psychology, 21,* 531–41.

Moles, A., Kieffer, B. L., & D'Amato, F. R. (2004). Deficit in attachment behavior in mice lacking the μ-opioid receptor gene. *Science, 304,* 1983–5.

Mullen, B., Bryant, B., & Driskell, J. E. (1997). Presence of others and arousal: An integration. *Group Dynamics: Theory, Research, and Practice, 1,* 52–64.

Nachmias, M., Gunnar, M. R., Mangelsdorf, S., Parritz, R. H., & Buss, K. (1996). Behavioral inhibition and stress reactivity: The moderating role of attachment security. *Child Development, 67,* 508–22.

Nelson, E., & Panksepp, J. (1996). Oxytocin mediates acquisition of maternally associated odor preferences in preweanling rat pups. *Behavioral Neuroscience, 110,* 583–92.

Nelson, E., & Panksepp, J. (1998). Brain substrates of infant-mother attachment: contributions of opioids, oxytocin, and norepinephrine. *Neuroscience and Biobehavioral Reviews, 22,* 437–52.

Panksepp, J. (1998). *Affective neuroscience.* New York: Oxford University Press.

Penninx, B. W. J. H., van Tilburg, T., Boeke, A. J. P., Deeg, D. J. H., Kriegsman, D. M. W., & van Eijk, J. T. M. (1998). Effects of social support and personal coping resources on depressive symptoms: Different for various chronic diseases? *Health Psychology, 17,* 551–8.

Pietromonaco, P. R., Barrett, L. F., & Powers, S. I. (2006). Adult attachment theory and affective reactivity and regulation. In D. K. Snyder, J. A. Simpson, and J. N. Hughes (Eds.), *Emotion regulation in couples and families: Pathways to dysfunction and health* (pp. 57–74). Washington, DC: American Psychological Association.

Powell, L. H., William, R. L., Matthews, K. A., Meyer, P., Midgley, A. R., Baum, A., et al. (2002). Physiologic markers of chronic stress in premenopausal, middle-aged women. *Psychosomatic Medicine, 64,* 502–9.

Pruessner, M., Hellhammer, D. H., Pruessner, J. C., & Lupien, S. J. (2003). Self-reported depressive symptoms and stress levels in healthy young men: Associations with the cortisol response to awakening. *Psychosomatic Medicine, 65,* 92–9.

Repetti, R. L., Taylor, S. E., & Saxbe, D. (2007). The influence of early socialization experiences on the development of biological systems. In J. Grusec and P. Hastings (Eds.), *Handbook of socialization* (pp. 124–52). New York: Guilford.

Repetti, R. L., Taylor, S. E., & Seeman, T. E. (2002). Risky families: Family social environments and the mental and physical health of offspring. *Psychological Bulletin, 128,* 330–66.

Risch, N., Herrell, R., Lehner, T., Liang, K., Eaves, L., Hoh, J., et al. (2009). Interaction between the serotonin transporter gene (5-HTTLPR), stressful life events, and risk of depression: A meta-analysis. *Journal of the American Medical Association, 301,* 2462–71.

Robertson, E. K., & Suinn, R. M. (1968). The determination of rate of progress of stroke patients through empathy measures of patient and family. *Journal of Psychosomatic Research, 12,* 189–91.

Rutledge, T., Reis, S. E., Olson, M., Owens, J., Kelsey, S. F., Pepine, C. J., et al. (2004). Social networks are associated with lower mortality rates among women with suspected coronary disease: The National Heart, Lung, and Blood Institute-sponsored women's ischemia syndrome evaluation study. *Psychosomatic Medicine, 66,* 882–8.

Sarason, B. R., Sarason, I. G., & Gurung, R. A. R. (1997). Close personal relationships and health outcomes: A key to the role of social support. In S. Duck (Ed.), *Handbook of personal relationships* (pp. 547–73). New York: Wiley.

Sawchenko, P. E., & Swanson, L. W. (1982). Immunohistochemical identification of neurons in the paraventricular nucleus of the hypothalamus that project to the medulla or to the spinal cord in the rat. *Journal of Comparative Neurology, 205,* 260–72.

Saxbe, D. (2009). For better or worse? Coregulation of couples' cortisol levels and mood states. Manuscript under review.

Schreiber, J. E., Shirtcliff, E., Van Hulle, C., Lemery-Chalfant, K., Klein, M. H., Kalin, N. H., et al. (2006). Environmental influences on family similarity in afternoon cortisol levels: Twin and parent-offspring designs. *Psychoneuroendocrinology, 31,* 1131–7.

Sbarra, D. A., & Hazan, C. (2008). Coregulation, dysregulation, self-regulation: An integrative analysis and empirical agenda for understanding adult attachment, separation, loss, and recovery. *Personality and Social Psychology Review, 12,* 141–67.

Seeman, T. E. (1996). Social ties and health: The benefits of social integration. *Annals of Epidemiology, 6,* 442–51.

Seeman, T. E., Lusignolo, T. M., Albert, M., & Berkman, L. (2001). Social relationships, social support, and patterns of cognitive aging in healthy, high-functioning older adults: MacArthur Studies of Successful Aging. *Health Psychology, 20,* 243–55.

Seeman, T. E., & McEwen, B. (1996). Impact of social environment characteristics on neuroendocrine regulation. *Psychosomatic Medicine, 58,* 459–71.

Shih, J. C., Chen, K., & Ridd, M. J. (1999). Monoamine oxidase: From genes to behavior. *Annual Review of Neuroscience, 22,* 197–217.

Sheffield, D., & Carroll, D. (1994). Social support and cardiovascular reactions to active laboratory stressors. *Psychology and Health, 9,* 305–16.

Simeon, D., Greenberg, J., Nelson, D., Schmeider, J., & Hollander, E. (2005). Dissociation and posttraumatic stress 1 year after the World Trade Center disaster: Follow-up of a longitudinal study. *Journal of Clinical Psychiatry, 66,* 231–7.

Sorkin, D., Rook, K. S., & Lu, J. L. (2002). Loneliness, lack of emotional support, lack of companionship, and the likelihood of having a heart condition in an elderly sample. *Annals of Behavioral Medicine, 24,* 290–8.

Spitz, R. A., & Wolff, K. M. (1946). Anaclitic depression: An inquiry into the genesis of psychiatric conditions in early childhood, II. In A. Freud et al. (Eds.), *The psychoanalytic study of the child* (Vol. 2, pp. 313–42). New York: International Universities Press.

Stone, A.A., Mezzacappa, E.S., Donatone, B.A., & Gonder, M. (1999). Psychosocial stress and social support are associated with prostate-specific antigen levels in men: Results from a community screening program. *Health Psychology, 18,* 482–6.

Suomi, S. J. (1987). Genetic and maternal contributions to individual differences in rhesus monkey biobehavioral development. In N. A. Krasnagor, E. M. Blass, M. A. Hofer, and W. P. Smotherman (Eds.), *Perinatal development: A psychobiological perspective* (pp. 397–420). New York: Academic Press.

Swanson, L. W., & Sawchenko, P. E. (1980). Paraventricular nucleus: A site for the integration of neuroendocrine and autonomic mechanisms. *Neuroendocrinology, 31,* 410–7.

Tamres, L., Janicki, D., & Helgeson, V. S. (2002). Sex differences in coping behavior: A meta-analytic review. *Personality and Social Psychology Review, 6,* 2–30.

Taylor, S. E. (2002). *The tending instinct: How nurturing is essential to who we are and how we live.* New York: Holt.

Taylor, S. E. (2009). Social support: A review. In H. S. Friedman (Ed.), *Oxford handbook of health psychology.* New York: Oxford University Press.

Taylor, S. E., Dickerson, S. S., & Klein, L. C. (2002). Toward a biology of social support. In C.R. Snyder and S.J. Lopez (Eds.), *Handbook of positive psychology.* London: Oxford University Press.

Taylor, S. E., & Gonzaga, G. (2006). Evolution, relationships, and health: The social shaping hypothesis. In M. Schaller, J. Simpson, and D. Kenrick (Eds.), *Evolution and social psychology* (pp. 211–36). New York: Psychology Press.

Taylor, S. E., Klein, L. C., Lewis, B. P., Gruenewald, T. L., Gurung, R. A. R., & Updegraff, J. A. (2000). Biobehavioral responses to stress in females: Tend-and-befriend, not fight-or-flight. *Psychological Review, 107,* 411–29.

Taylor, S. E., Lerner, J. S., Sage, R. M., Lehman, B. J., & Seeman, T. E. (2004). Early environment, emotions, responses to stress, and health. Special Issue on Personality and Health. *Journal of Personality, 72,* 1365–93.

Taylor, S. E., Sherman, D. K., Kim, H. S., Jarcho, J., Takagi, K., & Dunagan, M. S. (2004). Culture and social support: Who seeks it and why? *Journal of Personality and Social Psychology, 87,* 354–62.

Taylor, S. E., Way, B. M., Welch, W. T., Hilmert, C. J., Lehman, B. J., & Eisenberger, N. I. (2006). Early family environment, current adversity, the serotonin transporter polymorphism, and depressive symptomatology. *Biological Psychiatry, 60,* 671–6.

Taylor, S. E., Welch, W. T., Kim, H. S., & Sherman, D. K. (2007). Cultural differences in the impact of social support on psychological and biological stress responses. *Psychological Science, 18,* 831–7.

Thoits, P. A. (1986). Social support as coping assistance. *Journal of Consulting and Clinical Psychology, 54,* 416–23.

Thoits, P. A. (1995). Stress, coping and social support processes: Where are we? What next? *Journal of Health and Social Behavior, (Extra Issue),* 53–79.

Turner, R. A., Altemus, M., Enos, T., Cooper, B., & McGuinness, T. (1999). Preliminary research on plasma oxytocin in normal cycling women: investigating emotion and interpersonal distress. *Psychiatry, 62,* 97–113.

Turner-Cobb, J. M., Gore-Felton, C., Marouf, F., Koopman, C, Kim, P., Israelski, D., & Spiegel, D. (2002). Coping, social support, and attachment style as psychosocial correlates of adjustment in men and women with HIV/AIDS. *Journal of Behavioral Medicine, 25,* 337–53.

Uchino, B., Cacioppo, J., & Kiecolt-Glaser, J. (1996). The relationship between social support and physiological processes: A review with emphasis on underlying mechanisms and implications for health. *Psychological Bulletin, 119,* 488–531.

Uvnäs-Moberg, K. (1996). Neuroendocrinology of the mother-child interaction. *Trends in Endocrinology and Metabolism, 7,* 126–31.

Uvnäs-Moberg, K. (1997). Oxytocin linked antistress effects: the relaxation and growth response. *Acta Psychologica Scandinavica, 640* (Suppl), 38–42.

VanderPlate, C., Aral, S. O., & Magder, L. (1988). The relationship among genital herpes simplex virus, stress, and social support. *Health Psychology, 7,* 159–68.

Weaver, I. C., Cervoni, N., Champagne, F. A., D'Alessio, A. C., Sharma, S., Seckl, J. R., et al. (2004). Epigenetic programming by maternal behavior. *Nature Neuroscience, 7,* 847–54.

Wiklund, I., Oden, A., Sanne, H., Ulvenstam, G., Wilhemsson, C., & Wilhemsen, L. (1988). Prognostic importance of somatic and psychosocial variables after a first myocardial infarction. *American Journal of Epidemiology, 128,* 786–95.

Wills, T. A. (1991). Social support and interpersonal relationships. In M. S. Clark (Ed.), *Prosocial behavior* (pp. 265–89). Newbury Park, CA: Sage.

Witt, D. M., Carter, C. S., & Walton, D. (1990). Central and peripheral effects of oxytocin administration in prairie voles (*Microtus ochrogaster*). *Pharmacology, Biochemistry, and Behavior, 37,* 63–9.

Witt, D. M., Winslow, J. T., & Insel, T. R. (1992). Enhanced social interactions in rats following chronic, centrally infused oxytocin. *Pharmacology, Biochemistry, and Behavior, 43,* 855–86.

Tracey A. Revenson *and* Anita DeLongis

Abstract

This chapter reviews current theoretical frameworks on dyadic coping processes among couples coping with the stresses of chronic illness. These frameworks are set in their historical context to illustrate how they emerged from individual stress and coping models. The empirical literature on couples coping with chronic illness, in particular cancer and rheumatoid arthritis, is reviewed to examine which models have been supported and to identify gaps for future research. Using a social contextual framework, the chapter examines how partners experience unique stresses as a result of living with a chronically ill person, how psychosocial adaptation is shaped by the complex interplay of personality and relationship characteristics, and how sociocultural characteristics, such as gender, affect dyadic coping processes. The chapter addresses current methods in dyadic coping and the translation of research into clinical practice.

Keywords: coping, dyadic coping, couples, illness, marriage, social support, cancer, arthritis, relationship-focused coping, protective buffering

Introduction

When one member of a family is experiencing ongoing, complex stressors or life strains, other members of the family are affected as well: by the stressor itself, by its psychological impact on the affected individual, and by its cumulative effect on family functioning. Stress significantly influences marital communication, marital satisfaction, and the development of close relationships (Bodenmann, 2000; Neff & Karney, 2004; Repetti, Wang, & Saxbe, 2009; Story & Bradbury, 2004). Marriages subjected to chronic stress have a higher probability of ending in divorce (Bodenmann, 2000; Karney, Story, & Bradbury, 2005), and marital distress exerts significant and deleterious effects on immune functions and health outcomes (Burman & Margolin,

1992; Kiecolt-Glaser & Newton, 2001; Robles & Kiecolt-Glaser, 2003).

At the same time, many studies have demonstrated the beneficial effects of social support from family members when one is facing a major life stressor (e.g., Cutrona, 1996; Lyons, Sullivan, Ritvo, & Coyne, 1996). Individuals reporting better marital adjustment are less emotionally reactive to family stressors and may be more adept at managing or resolving tension when it occurs (O'Brien, DeLongis, Pomaki, Puterman, & Zwicker, 2009). In one study (DeLongis, Capreol, Holtzman, O'Brien, & Campbell, 2004) couples higher in marital adjustment recovered from the previous day's tension more quickly than those with worse marriages. Having a satisfying marriage may serve a protective function during times of stress, particularly for women. Thus, it is critical to investigate how couples cope with chronic life stressors in order to identify which coping strategies are effective in managing stress and which will prove to have a negative impact on close relationships.

This focus on couples is fairly new in the stress and coping literature. Relatively few researchers have investigated how family members cope with the stressors they face as a couple or as a family, or how the coping efforts of family members mutually influence each other, for better or for worse. A number of conceptual frameworks appeared in the 1990s, for the most part expanding on Lazarus and colleagues' stress and coping paradigm (Lazarus & DeLongis, 1983; Lazarus & Folkman, 1984). These frameworks identified a missing piece of the original paradigm, interpersonal processes, which has been described subsequently in terms of relationship-focused coping (Coyne & Fiske, 1992; DeLongis & O'Brien, 1990), coping congruence (Revenson, 1994), and dyadic coping (Bodenmann, 1997).

Chronic illness provides a good opportunity for exploring how coping occurs in the interpersonal context. In this chapter, we focus on how couples cope with the chronic physical illness of one partner in order to understand couples coping processes more generally. We begin by reviewing current theories and frameworks of dyadic coping, setting them in their historical context within individual stress and coping models. To illustrate these theoretical frameworks, we turn to the empirical literature on couples coping with illness, examining which models have received empirical support and identifying gaps. Central to all frameworks is the way in which both gender and social role (i.e., whether one is the patient or the spouse) influences couples coping. We then address the current state of methodology for studying couples coping and end with challenges for the next generation of work.

Two caveats are in order. First, dyadic or couples coping involves two people in a marital or committed relationship, of the same or opposite sex. However, most of the literature on couples coping with illness involves heterosexuals and legally married couples, with the exception of a small number of studies of couples with HIV. Second, although we want to make conclusions about illness, writ large, most of the studies focus on a specific disease and often patients of one gender (e.g., men with heart disease and their wives, women with breast cancer and their husbands). Sometimes this is because of the prevalence of the illness and sometimes because

of sampling decisions, but it is important when making broad conclusions about the literature. We emphasize two illnesses—cancer and arthritis—in this chapter. These illnesses have received the lion's share of research attention; moreover, the diversity of coping tasks they present brings out both commonalities of coping across illnesses and the uniqueness of each illness. At the same time, we expect that our conclusions will be applicable to couples with many different chronic illnesses.

Chronic Illness as a Dyadic Stressor

Evidence is accumulating to suggest that one needs to consider a couples perspective to understand the phenomenon of adjustment to illness. Translating Moos' seminal work on the adaptive tasks of illness (Moos & Tsu, 1977) from the individual to the marital level, each adaptive (or coping) task that patients confront has a counterpart in marital functioning. Medical uncertainty about prognosis and disease progression is mirrored in uncertainty about the future functioning of the marriage and the family. What will happen to daily schedules if the ill spouse is in severe pain? Which family activities may be sacrificed in order to accommodate a demanding treatment regimen or its effects? Even small chores or events, such as doing laundry or going to a child's soccer game, may become transformed into chronic strains that overshadow other aspects of family life. "Disruptive events acquire much of their stressful character not by their own *direct* impact but by disrupting and dislocating the more structured elements of peoples' lives" (Pearlin & Turner, 1987, p. 148; see also Repetti et al., 2009).

A diagnosis of chronic illness unleashes multiple stressors or adaptive tasks for the couple, which is why illness needs to be understood as an interpersonal experience. Some stressors emanate directly from caregiving, for example making treatment decisions, managing treatment, and providing hands-on care if the patient is frail or disabled (Martire & Schulz, in press). Other stressors emerge from the need to restructure family roles and responsibilities as the disease progresses or presents new challenges. Chronic illness often affects sexual desire and beliefs about the relationship (Samelson & Hannon, 1999). These stressors are both continuous and shape-shifting, as patients go through different stages of the illness trajectory, from diagnosis to initial treatment to reentry into their pre-illness lives (Stanton, Revenson & Tennen, 2007). Still other stressors are filtered through the lens of the patient's or partner's experience, as in the case of one partner feeling unable to help the other cope with pain or an altered body image (Revenson & Majerovitz, 1990). There are societal expectations that spouses care for each other "in sickness and in health," but few prescriptions for how to cope with one's own feelings of anger, resentment, imminent loss, or exhaustion.

Spouses often take on new or additional responsibilities when the patient becomes physically disabled (Martire & Schulz, in press). Sometimes these changes in role responsibilities may lie outside traditional gender roles (e.g., Rose, Suls, Green, Lounsbury, & Gordon, 1996). For example, when married women are afflicted with a disabling illness, such as rheumatoid arthritis, husbands often need to take on a greater share of household chores and childcare (Abraído-Lanza & Revenson, 2006). Similarly, some wives of men whose employment is terminated by disability find that they need to work outside the home for the first time. And, at times, partners need to take on new roles in the treatment process. In a qualitative study of men with prostate cancer and their wives, Gray, Fitch, Phillips, Labreque, and Fergus (2000) found it was rare for men to disclose information about the illness to anyone but their wives, so that the wives had to become the information conduit between spouse and doctor.

Thus, people in intimate, committed relationships, including both legal marriage and domestic partnerships, are faced with dual challenges in the process of coping with illness. They are expected to provide support to their partners while coping with their own emotional distress. Many couples report that the illness brought them closer together, but at the same time report many illness-related changes in their relationship and daily lives (e.g., Dorval, Guay, Mondor, Mâsse, Falardeau, Robidoux, Deschênes, & Maunsell, 2005).

Theoretical Approaches
The stress and coping paradigm

Since its inception, research on stress and coping has focused almost exclusively on the coping efforts of individuals. Whether described as an ego defense mechanism (Haan, 1978), a personality disposition (Ouellette, 1993), or a process that changes in response to situational cues (Folkman, Lazarus, Dunkel-Schetter, DeLongis, & Gruen, 1986), coping has been conceptualized as something an *individual* thinks or does. The process model of psychologist Richard Lazarus, along with colleagues on the Berkeley Stress and Coping Project in the

1980s, led to a transactional paradigm of stress and coping that has served as the guiding framework for many researchers in the following three decades. This paradigm (Lazarus, 1966; Lazarus, Averill, & Opton, 1974; Lazarus & DeLongis, 1983; Lazarus & Folkman, 1984; Lazarus & Launier, 1978; Lazarus, 1981) brought together two ideas: first, that individuals' experience of stress is dependent on their cognitive and affective appraisals of an event and second, that coping is shaped by both personal resources and situational determinants.

Within this stress and coping paradigm, coping strategies were described as serving problem- and emotion-focused functions. In the former, coping efforts are aimed at managing or eliminating the source of stress; in the latter, coping is directed toward managing the emotional distress that arises from stress appraisals. In this work, supportive relationships were conceptualized primarily as available resources that could aid the individual's coping in a number of ways—by providing information about coping options, feedback validating or criticizing the individual's coping choices, instrumental assistance in carrying out the coping actions, or emotional sustenance to help sustain coping efforts. As such, social support was conceptualized as coping assistance (Thoits, 1986).

Much of the literature on social support has adopted Lazarus' paradigm. These earlier studies focused largely on the exchange of social support as a factor in adjustment to chronic illness. A supportive relationship was shown to both enhance patients' mental health and strengthen the relationship over the illness trajectory (e.g., Manne, 1998). Across a number of illnesses, patients identified emotional support as the most helpful type of support from partners (e.g., Dakof & Taylor, 1990; Kayser, 2005; Lanza, Cameron, & Revenson, 1995). Following this, patients report better emotional adjustment if their partners are highly supportive (e.g., Kayser, 2005; Northouse, Templin, & Mood, 2001).

A number of studies examined the effects of chronic illness on the spouse (see reviews by Manne & Badr, 2008; Manne & Zautra, 1990; see also Stephens, Martire, Cremeans-Smith, Druly, & Wojno, 2006; Strating, Van Duihn, can Schuur, & Surrmeijer, 2007). These studies, although not involving both members of the couple directly, were important because they laid the groundwork for researchers to argue that both patients and partners experienced psychological distress when illness struck. Many studies, though not all, found that spouses experienced even greater psychological distress than patients did. A recent meta-analysis attributed this difference not to role (patient vs. partner) but to gender (Hagedoorn, Sanderman, Bolks, Tuinistra, & Coyne, 2008). Even in some studies that ostensibly studied couples coping, the only goal of coping considered was the patient's adjustment to the illness. One group of researchers (Maliski, Heilemann, & McCorkle, 2001) categorized couples coping strategies as his work, her work, and their work, but his work was regaining mastery and her work was labeled "supportive presence." The wife's coping strategies were all about helping him cope, making dealing with her own distress secondary.

Thus, until recently, research in health psychology largely focused on the psychosocial effects of illness on patients, with much less attention to partners. Even less research examined the impact of illness on the marital relationship or functioning of the family. An edited volume by Schmaling and Sher (2000) provided the state of the science of the impact of illness on couples, but lacked a dyadic perspective.

Dyadic coping

Broadly cast, dyadic coping recognizes mutuality and interdependence in coping responses to a specific shared stressor, indicating that couples respond to stressors as interpersonal units rather than as individuals in isolation. The construct of dyadic coping goes beyond the exchange of social support, although that is a central component in most definitions (Berg & Upchurch, 2007; Bodenmann, 1997; Manne & Badr, 2008). In dyadic coping, the members of the couple negotiate the emotional aspects of their shared experience (e.g., Coyne & Smith, 1991) or engage in collaborative coping efforts, such as joint problem-solving (Berg & Upchurch, 2007). Ideally, couples coping involves taking a "we" approach whereby both persons maintain a couples identity and work together to maintain the quality of their relationship while they jointly manage their shared stress (Acitelli & Badr, 2005; Badr, Acitelli, & Carmack Taylor, 2007; Kayser, Watson & Andrade, 2007).

Any relationship that endures long enough to allow both partners to form attitudes and beliefs about each other and about the relationship (as most marriages do) can be viewed as exhibiting psychological interdependence (Huston & Robins, 1982). Thus, dyadic models must consider how each partner implicitly or explicitly influences the other partner's cognitions, emotions, and actions. For

example, it is not enough to know that one partner was trying to be supportive; it is also critical to know whether that support was perceived as helpful by the recipient (Lanza et al., 1995).

When spouses report receiving helpful support they tend to engage in more adaptive ways of coping with chronic stress. Holtzman, Newth, and DeLongis (2004) examined the role of support in coping and pain severity among patients with rheumatoid arthritis and found that such support influences pain severity indirectly, both through encouraging the use of specific coping strategies, such as positive reappraisal, as well as by affecting the effectiveness with which these coping strategies were employed. Moreover, support from the spouse attenuated the impact of maladaptive responses to pain, disrupting the vicious cycle of catastrophizing and pain (Holtzman & DeLongis, 2007).

The coping literature has been plagued by inconsistencies regarding which strategies should be considered adaptive versus maladaptive (Coyne & Gottlieb, 1996). One reason for these inconsistencies may be that the effectiveness of any given coping strategy depends at least in part upon the response of the spouse to the use of that strategy. For example, in a study of parents coping with their child's chronic illness, Marin, Holtzman, DeLongis, & Robinson (2007) found that the use of cognitive restructuring was effective in reducing levels of psychological distress only in the presence of a positive response from the spouse. Among parents who reported *negative* responses from the spouse, the use of cognitive restructuring was associated with *higher* levels of distress. This pattern of findings is consistent with research on couples suggesting that the benefits of accommodation (i.e., one's willingness to respond in a constructive manner when a partner has behaved negatively) may depend on the extent to which these responses are met with accommodating responses by one's partner (O'Brien & DeLongis, 1997; Rusbult, Verette, Whitney, Slovik, & Lipkus, 1991). If one spouse engages in efforts to compromise and provide empathy during stressful situations, and his or her spouse does not reciprocate, these coping efforts, although generally expected to have positive effects, may actually result in heightened levels of distress.

Relationship-focused coping

In a reformulation of the stress and coping paradigm, Coyne (Coyne & Smith, 1991; Coyne & Fiske, 1992) and DeLongis (DeLongis & O'Brien, 1990;

O'Brien & DeLongis, 1997) added a third and possibly superordinate coping function: *relationship-focused or relational coping*. We use the term "relationship-focused" coping to refer to cognitive and behavioral efforts to manage and sustain social relationships during stressful episodes. Relationship-focused coping involves efforts to attend to the other partner's emotional needs while maintaining the integrity of the relationship, and efforts to manage one's own stress without creating upset or problems for others. It involves trying to maintain a balance between self and other, with the goal of maintaining the integrity of the relationship above either partner's needs. Relationship-focused coping modes include negotiating or compromising with others, considering the other person's situation, and being empathic (DeLongis & O'Brien, 1990; Manne & Badr, 2009; O'Brien et al., 2009).

This conceptualization of relationship-focused coping rests on the assumption that maintaining relatedness with others is a fundamental human need, as fundamental to coping as emotional regulation or problem-solving. Successful coping involves not only solving the problem and managing negative emotions generated by stress, but also involves maintaining relationships during stressful periods, particularly when those stressors affect the family. Interpersonal stressors have a particularly deleterious effect on physical and psychological well-being (Baumeister & Leary, 1995; Bolger, DeLongis, Kessler, & Schilling, 1989). Maintaining close relationships in the face of stress protects individuals from the negative effects of those stressful episodes (e.g., Badr et al, 2007), making it important to focus on relationship maintenance during times of stress.

One critical determinant of maintaining satisfying relationships during times of stress may be the extent to which persons can respond with an empathic orientation. Empathy has long been considered a quintessential footing of emotional attunement, promoting pro-social and caring actions between people (Eisenberg, 2000). Though few coping measures tap empathy as a mode of coping, the notion that people use empathy as a means of managing stress within the social context is not new. Haan (1977) identified empathy as a mode of coping that involves attempts to formulate an understanding of another person's feelings and thoughts. In stressful marital and family contexts, *empathic responding* may serve a myriad of purposes, such as managing or preventing conflict, dealing

with the distress of loved ones, minimizing negative attributions or blaming orientations towards others, and maintaining closeness, emotional intimacy, and relationship quality and satisfaction (Davis, 1994; Gottman, 1998; O'Brien & DeLongis, 1997).

Empathic responding as a mode of relationship-focused coping differs significantly from emotion-focused modes of social support-seeking. Emotion-focused modes of support-seeking are generally construed as efforts to get support from another person. Empathic responding is construed as efforts to understand another person and efforts to respond to the other person in the stressful situation in a supportive, caring manner as a means to defuse interpersonal stress and maintain the relationship. With empathic responding, it is the coper who engages in empathic processes and who provides caring gestures to the other person in the stressful situation. With social support seeking, it is the coper who tries to elicit support from others.

Research conducted in laboratory settings indicates that marital tension or conflict is diminished when partners convey empathy during interactions (Gottman, 1998). Couples in higher-quality marriages tend to communicate in a more relationship-maintaining manner during conflict (e.g., less negative affect reciprocity, less cross-complaining, and more expressions of empathy, understanding, and validation). These communication patterns may allow couples with better marital quality to manage conflict more effectively (Fincham & Beach, 1999).

Using a measure of relationship-focused coping that incorporates empathic responding, Bodenmann and colleagues (Bodenmann & Cina, 2005; Bodenmann, Pihet, & Kayser, 2006) found that it predicted marital quality and stability among community-residing couples 2 to 5 years later. In an intervention study, improving these coping skills resulted in higher marital satisfaction in the intervention group relative to the control group (Bodenmann & Shantinath, 2004). Observational studies also suggest that using empathic responding leads to higher interaction satisfaction in both members of the couple (Cutrona & Suhr, 1992).

Two relationship-focused coping strategies that have dominated the literature are active engagement and protective buffering (Coyne & Smith, 1991). *Active engagement* strategies involve the partner in discussions, asking how she or he feels, and are characterized by instrumental or problem-focused coping efforts. *Protective buffering* involves hiding concerns from the partner and not disclosing personal worries and concerns in order to protect the patient from upset and conflict. (Although we are classifying these as coping efforts, they also can be conceptualized as ways that partners attempt to provide support to each other.)

But are these relationship-focused strategies effective in managing stress and maintaining the quality of the relationship? Active engagement has been found to be related to the patient's well-being in couples coping with a myocardial infarction (Buunk, Berkhuysen, Sanderman, Nieuwland, & Ranchor, 1996) and to marital satisfaction among persons with cancer (Buunk et al., 1996; Hagedoorn, Kuijer, Buunk, DeJong, Wobbes, & Sanderman, 2000; Kuijer, Ybema, Buunk, DeJong, Thijs-Boer, & Sanderman, 2000) and their partners (Ybema, Kujer, Buunk, DeJong, & Sanderman, 2001). Patients with the greatest physical impairment or psychological distress seem to benefit the most (Hagedoorn et al., 2000).

Active engagement may allow patients to regain control over their lives (Hagedoorn et al., 2000); at the same time, it may signify that the partner sees the illness as a stressor that he or she shares. Active engagement by partners appears to be a response to the patient's coping with the illness; those who were perceived as coping better were provided more active engagement coping (Kuijer et al., 2000) Similarly, in a German study of couples facing cancer, partners provided the most support to patients who used a good deal of instrumental coping and actively mobilized support and the least support to patients who had accepted the illness but weren't coping actively (Luszczynska, Gerstorf, Boehmer, Knoll, & Schwarzer, 2007). Ironically, those who were in most need of support may not have received the "best," most active type of support from partners.

Protective buffering is ostensibly used to avoid disagreements and "protect" the relationship, but across many studies of different illnesses, it appears to exact psychological costs for the person using it. In studies of couples coping with a husband's myocardial infarction (Coyne & Smith, 1991; Suls, Green, Rose, Lounsbury, & Gordon, 1997), wives' coping efforts to shield husbands from stress in the post-MI period may have contributed to their own distress, as did husbands' efforts to protect their wives. In a study of spouses of rheumatoid arthritis patients, the wives of ill men confided that they had lessened their own requests for emotional support, for fear of increasing their ill husbands' distress (Revenson & Majerovitz, 1990, 1991). The evidence

for studies of cancer is mixed; in one study of patients with various cancers (Kuijer et al., 2000), protective buffering had no effect on patients' distress. In a study of women with breast cancer and their partners (Manne, Dougherty, Veach, & Kless, 1999), greater use of protective buffering (by patient or partner) was associated with greater distress experienced by the person engaging in that coping strategy. This association was even stronger for patients who rated their relationships as more (vs. less) satisfactory (Manne, Norton, Ostroff, Winkel, Fox, & Grana, 2007).

Perhaps this happens because the partner using protective buffering feels constrained to express negative emotions or worries to the other person. However, protective buffering does not appear to harm the spouse (i.e., the person being "protected"). Thus, this form of relationship-focused coping may require a tradeoff between protecting one's own well-being and that of one's partner.

Mutual influence models

Communication processes and relationship maintenance strategies have been studied under the aegis of relationship-focused coping as well. In a separate analysis of communication styles among the breast cancer patients and husbands described above (Manne, Ostroff, Norton, Fox, Goldstein, & Grana, 2006), patients' ratings of three relationship communication styles—mutual constructive communication, demand–withdraw communication, and mutual avoidance—were related in the expected directions to the partner's psychological distress 9 months later; moreover, both mutual constructive communication and demand–withdraw communication were associated with relationship satisfaction as well (but mutual avoidance was not). Similarly, in a study of recently diagnosed lung cancer patients and their partners, engaging in relationship maintenance early on was associated with the psychological and marital adjustment of both patients and partners both concurrently and over the next 6 months (Badr, Acitelli, & Taylor, 2008; Badr & Taylor, 2008).

In essence, this type of research could be categorized as using a theoretical model of "mutual influence" (Revenson, 2003). Mutual influence models focus on the effects of one partner's coping on the other partner's coping and adjustment (e.g., Manne & Zautra, 1990). A study by Berghuis and Stanton (2002) of adjustment to infertility provides a nice illustration of the mutual influence model, in that it untangles three possible mechanisms through which each partner's coping influences her or his adjustment as well as the other partner's adjustment. The first mechanism is essentially an additive, or separate influence model: each person's adjustment is independently affected by her or his coping and her or his partner's coping. The two other mechanisms are interaction models in which the relation between one partner's coping and her or his adjustment is tempered by what the other person is (or is not) doing.

In Berghuis and Stanton's study, husbands and wives completed measures of coping, depression, and marital satisfaction prior to participating in a medical procedure (artificial insemination by the husband) and after receiving a negative pregnancy test result. The relationship between women's use of emotional approach coping and depression was a function of their husbands' use of emotional-approach coping. If women used primarily emotional-approach coping, their husbands' use of that strategy was less influential on her depression. If women used very little emotional-approach coping, her husband's use of emotional-approach coping was more strongly related to her depression level. Conversely, if husbands engaged in emotional-approach coping while the wives did *not*, the women had relatively low depression scores. But if husbands also did not use this strategy—that is, both members of the couple used little emotional-approach coping—women were more depressed after the failed insemination attempt. This pattern of findings suggests a compensatory coping model, in which one person in the family has to use an effective coping strategy (effective, that is, relative to the target stressor).

Although reciprocal influences could be tested, many studies using the mutual influence model test only the influence of one partner on the other and do not analyze the couple as a unit. As a result, researchers in clinical psychology, health psychology, and interpersonal relationships began to develop theoretical frameworks for studying how couples cope together with life stress.

The systemic-transactional model of dyadic coping

The systematic-transactional model of Swiss psychologist Guy Bodenmann conceptualizes and measures dyadic coping as a dynamic and transactional stress management process (Bodenmann, 1997, 2005). Dyadic coping goes beyond individual coping efforts within the context of a relationship and beyond the effects of one person's coping on the other

(mutual influence model). It emphasizes the importance of partners relating to each other as people, rather than simply assuming the roles of "patient" and "partner" (Manne & Badr, 2008).

Each partner's well-being depends upon the other partner's well-being, as well as the couple's ability to draw on other social resources. When faced with a shared stressor, partners cope both individually and collectively as a unit. At the individual level, a stress communication process is triggered whereby each partner communicates his or her own stress to the other in hopes of receiving support and coping feedback. The other partner can respond in either a supportive or unsupportive fashion. Supportive responses include providing advice and practical help with daily tasks, showing empathy and concern, expressing solidarity, and helping one's partner to relax and engage in positive reframing. Unsupportive responses include showing disinterest, providing support that is accompanied by criticism, distancing, or sarcasm, and minimizing the severity of the stressor. At the couple level, relational well-being is affected by the couple's ability to work as a team to manage aspects of the dyadic stressor that affect both of them. This coordinated effort also has both positive and negative forms. Common positive dyadic coping involves joint problem-solving, coordinating everyday demands, relaxing together, as well as mutual calming, sharing, and expressions of solidarity. Common negative dyadic coping involves strategies such as mutual avoidance and withdrawal.

In a number of studies of community-living couples, couples in marital therapy, or couples coping with a specific stressor, dyadic coping has been associated with higher marital quality, lower stress experience, and better psychological and physical well-being in studies with self-report (e.g., Badr, 2004; Bodenmann, 2000; Bodenmann et al., 2006; Dehle, Larsen, & Landers, 2001; Walen & Lachman, 2000) and observational data (e.g., Bodenmann, 2000; Cutrona & Suhr, 1992; Pasch & Bradbury, 1998). A study of community-dwelling adults found that couples who reported low levels of common positive dyadic coping at study entry were more likely to divorce or separate 5 years later (Bodenmann & Cina, 2005). Dyadic coping has been shown to be positively associated with marital quality through two mechanisms: first by alleviating the negative impact of stress on marriage and second by strengthening feelings of mutual trust and intimacy, and the cognitive representation of the relationship as helpful and supportive (Bodenmann, 2005).

Dyadic Coping with Chronic Illness

Dyadic coping has been explored only recently within the context of chronic illness. Consistent with the findings from community samples, studies show that dyadic coping is significantly associated with a higher level of marital and psychosocial adjustment among patients with breast, colon, and lung cancer, heart disease, rheumatoid arthritis, and psychiatric illness (Revenson, Kayser, & Bodenmann, 2005). For example, Berg, Wiebe, Butner, Bloor, Bradstreet, Upchurch, and Patton (2008) examined whether collaborative coping (a construct similar to positive dyadic coping) was related to positive and negative mood among men with prostate cancer and their wives, using a diary methodology. Perceptions of collaborative coping were associated with more same-day positive emotions for both the male patients and their female partners and less same-day negative emotion for the wives only. Thus, both partners benefited.

In a recent longitudinal study of couples facing metastatic breast cancer (Badr, Carmack Taylor, Kashy, Cristofanilli, & Revenson, 2010) positive dyadic coping was shown to decrease cancer-related distress and increase marital adjustment after controlling for the effects of positive and negative support exchange. Common negative dyadic coping was associated with greater cancer-related distress and poorer marital adjustment, even after controlling for the length of the relationship and support exchange. Thus, this study demonstrated that dyadic coping involves support exchange, but also is more than social support.

Recently, Berg and Upchurch (2007) proposed a model of coping that draws together all of these approaches. In their developmental-contextual model, they conceptualize dyadic coping as having four different types: collaborative coping (joint problem-solving, involving the active engagement of spouses in pooling resources); uninvolved coping (strategies in which an individual acts on her or his own, most similar to the Lazarus and Folkman [1984] paradigm's notions of individual coping); supportive strategies (one spouse providing support to the other); and social control strategies. At this point, these four modes have not been tested together or compared.

Coping congruence

Strongly influenced by person-environment fit theory (French, Rodgers, & Cobb, 1974), family systems theories (e.g., Patterson & Garwick, 1994), and the earlier work on relational coping (Coyne & Fiske, 1992; DeLongis & O'Brien, 1990),

Revenson (1994, 2003) proposed the idea of coping congruence to examine dyadic processes. This construct emphasizes the congruence between partners' coping responses as a predictor of both individual- and couple-level adaptation. Most simply, couples coping involves efforts to maximize the congruence or "fit" between the partners' coping styles, in order to cope most effectively as a couple.

Congruence, however, can involve either similarity or complementarity of partners' coping styles, and this may depend on the function of coping. Partners who use similar coping strategies mutually reinforce each other's efforts, perhaps paving the way for better adjustment. Complementary coping styles can be congruent when they work in concert to reach a desired goal, either enhancing the other person's strategy or filling a coping "gap," or when they prevent one partner's coping from damaging the situation. Alternately, complementary strategies may be more effective than when partners use identical strategies because the couple, as a unit, would have a broader coping repertoire. However, strategies that work in direct opposition or cancel each other out would be considered incongruent and lead to worse psychosocial outcomes.

Further, there is some evidence that whether similarity or complementarity indicates congruence (and better adjustment) may depend on the function of coping. Similarity in coping may be more adaptive with strategies that focus on solving or minimizing the problem, or ones characterized as "approach" coping (Suls & Fletcher, 1985) or a "team" perspective (Haggan, 2002; Sterba, DeVellis, Lewis, Baucom, Jordan, & DeVellis, 2007). Not only may they get the couple "to the goal" (to overuse the sports metaphor), but they prevent one partner from blocking the other partner's coping efforts. Complementarity might be more effective for strategies characterized by avoidance or emotional expression (for example, in the Berghuis & Stanton, 2002, study described earlier). If both partners avoid making a treatment decision or engage in negative emotional expression, distress may be exacerbated.

Empirical evidence for coping congruence

There has been little research testing the congruence hypothesis, and the findings are mixed. Revenson first tested the coping congruence approach in a cross-sectional study of 113 heterosexual married couples with rheumatic disease (Revenson, 2003; Revenson, Abraido-Lanza, Majerovitz, & Jordan, 2005) using cluster analysis techniques that joined both partners' coping strategies so that the couple was the unit of analysis. The largest cluster of couples, dubbed Effortful Partnerships, was largely congruent in their coping, and their coping was characterized primarily by the instrumental strategies of Positive Problem-Solving and Rational Thinking. These couples stood apart from the others in several ways: Patients had greater levels of depressive symptoms (with half having scores indicative of clinical depression) and the healthy spouses perceived a much greater degree of interpersonal stress with family and friends, greater illness intrusion, and a higher degree of caregiver burden. At the same time, both patients and partners in the Effortful Partnership cluster had *higher* scores on an early measure of personal growth developed to assess the positive outcomes of illness (Felton & Revenson, 1984). Thus, despite their distress, these actively coping couples were able to reappraise their illness in a more positive light and could see benefits from their struggle.

This study lends support to the notion that similarity in coping congruence is adaptive when applied to instrumental, problem-focused strategies. In a small sample of couples with which one partner had multiple sclerosis, Pakenham (1998) found that less discrepancy (indicating more congruence) in problem-focused coping was related to lower levels of collective depression and better individual adjustment of both patients and partners. More recently, in a study of mixed illnesses, Badr (2004) found that couples who were more congruent in their use of active engagement as a coping strategy reported greater marital adjustment.

The story is somewhat different for emotion-focused coping. In Revenson's (2003) study, couples who were more complementary in their use of protective buffering and avoidance coping—both emotion-focused strategies—showed better adjustment. Thus, for the more emotion-focused strategies, better adjustment was signaled by a "seesaw" on which one partner sat high (i.e., used that strategy a lot) and the other low. Pakenham (1998) found no effects of congruence in emotion-focused coping on either individual adjustment or collective depression among his sample of multiple sclerosis couples, although the raw difference scores were related in the predicted direction to adjustment outcomes in bivariate analyses. In a study of breast cancer patients and their partners, Ben-Zur, Gilbar, and Lev (2001) found that when both partners coped by using emotion-focused strategies, the patients reported greater psychological distress and poorer functioning, but this was also true even when only one partner used a high level of emotion-focused coping, blurring whether it is congruence or the type of coping that matters.

Several studies of couples coping with prostate cancer have tested the congruence model, also producing mixed results. A small qualitative study of men with prostate cancer and their wives (Lavery & Clarke, 1999) suggested much incongruence in spouses' coping styles of emotional disclosure. Relatively few wives reacted with stoic acceptance, but this strategy was used a great deal by their husbands. Wives tended to engage in more instrumental coping than did their husbands. In contrast, Yoshimoto, Ghorbani, Baer, Cheng, Banthhia, Malcarne, Sadler, Greenbergs, and Varni (2006) found that when both men with prostate cancer and their wives used religious coping, they showed decreases over time in the coping strategy of skillful problem-solving. Whether it was the type of coping or whether this shared coping reflects better communication about coping is unknown. In another study of prostate cancer, Berg et al. (2008) found that partners' perceptions of collaborative coping were related to more same-day positive emotion for both husbands and wives and to less same-day negative emotion for wives but not husbands (who were the patients), except when husbands perceived that mode of coping to be effective.

Other studies have examined congruence in illness perceptions. It should be pointed out, however, that these studies examined individual beliefs and their impact on one partner's functioning, so they are not truly dyadic. Sterba, DeVellis, Lewis, DeVellis, Jordan, and Baucom (2008) studied married women with rheumatoid arthritis and their husbands and found that congruence in perceptions about the cyclic nature of the disease and personal control was related to better patient adjustment; however, congruence on other illness dimensions was not. They also developed a measure of each partners' beliefs in the dyad's coping efficacy as a unit concerning general coping and symptom management, which was related to better marital quality. However, because the data were cross-sectional, it is equally possible that marital quality predicted greater beliefs in dyadic efficacy.

In a small study of patients with Huntington's disease and their partners (Kaptein, Scharloo, Helder, Snoei, van Kempen, Weinman, van Houwelingen, & Roos, 2007), one partner's illness perceptions had minimal effect on the other partner's quality of life (whether they were the patient or the healthy spouse), but this may have been due to the fact that partners' illness perceptions were highly congruent. Barnoy, Bar-Tal, and Zisser (2006) examined how similar it was for patients with various types of cancer and their spouses to have similar approaches to seeking medical information. While similar styles affected psychological distress, this finding occurred only for patients, not partners, and was dependent on gender: It was important for female patients to be congruent with their spouses on monitoring (high information-seeking) but better for male patients to be congruent on blunting. The interpretation made was individualistic and gender-stereotyped: Information gives women a sense of control and men gain control by avoiding threatening information. Congruence was deemed important so that patients could feel supported in their preferred informational coping styles.

In sum, the jury is still out on whether congruent coping is better, and what congruent coping is. Dissimilar coping styles within a couple do not always signal a greater level of psychological or marital problems (Revenson, 2003). What is important may be that the partners' different modes of coping did not cancel each other out, but complement each other, producing a wider repertoire of coping options.

What Makes a Theory of Dyadic Coping Dyadic?

This is the most important and trickiest question, and to answer it theory cannot be disentangled from method. We will answer this question first on conceptual grounds and then move to methodological considerations.

First, and most importantly, the dyad or couple should be the unit of analysis at all stages of the research process, from conceptualizing the research question through measurement of coping processes (including outcomes) to data analysis and interpretation. Conceptualization and measurement of the coping process within the dyad—in Lazarus' terms, the person-environment transaction (where the environment is the other person)—is the essential starting point for all dyadic coping research. This requires obtaining data from both members of the couple, acknowledging its interdependence, and using it in analyses. One person's view of her own coping and her partner's does not make for dyadic coping. For example, it is not enough to know that the one partner was trying to be supportive; it is also critical to know whether that support was perceived as helpful by the recipient (Lanza et al., 1995).

Neither do correlations between a group of husbands and a group of wives make a study "dyadic." Often, the information about spouses is obtained from the patients, so that the spouses' own perspectives and experiences are not captured. In a later section of this chapter, we review current methods and measures for studying dyadic coping among couples facing chronic illness.

Second, echoing a basic tenet of Lazarus' stress and coping paradigm, dyadic coping is a dynamic, unfolding process. Applying this to a social contextual framework (DeLongis & Holtzman, 2005), we can posit that one partner's stress appraisals and coping responses influence the other, which in turn influence the "stressed" partner. Thus, theoretically, we need to allow for immediate, short-term, and longer-term influences between partners' coping efforts. And, because these reciprocal influences may be split-second in time, self-report methods cannot capture this.

Third, dyadic coping unfolds on multiple levels of analysis. While most frameworks emphasize coping as a team or a unit, there is an implicit recognition that each partner brings something unique to the situation and that individuals' coping is directed toward their own well-being, as well as the well-being of the partner and of the relationship. These goals may have differential preference. For example, in protective buffering (Coyne & Smith, 1991) wives shield their husbands from the stresses of their illness, often at the expense of their own well-being. In this way, the well-being of the partner takes priority. In other instances, one partner needs to emphasize her own well-being—for example, a breast cancer patient struggling though the physical effects of chemotherapy. In other circumstances, the couple focuses on the well-being of the relationship—for example, the relationship enhancement model of social support (Cutrona, Russell, & Gardner, 2005).

Fourth, couples coping must be studied within its political, cultural, and temporal context to be understood (Revenson, 1990, 2003). Contextual variables have direct influences on coping processes but also may serve as moderators of these processes and reflect the coping resources available to the couple. Revenson (1990, 2003) proposed a contextual model for studying stress and coping processes within illness. This model serves more as deep structure for research than an empirically testable model. The *sociocultural context* includes molar variables such as age, gender, socioeconomic status, and culture and may set boundaries for coping responses.

For example, the gendered traits of agency, communion, and unmitigated communion affect couples' adaptive processes (Helgeson, 1993). The *situational context* encompasses those aspects of the proximal environment that create or alleviate stress, including pain, disability, or life threat. The situational context also includes other major and minor stressors that people confront as they live with the illness, such as unemployment and daily childcare. The *temporal context* encompasses both the timing of the stressor within the individual's life and the lifespan of the stressor, thus taking a developmental perspective. Disease stage or current treatment provides clues as to what coping tasks are most salient at a given time. At the same time, the time of occurrence in the person's life is critical. Life transitions or unexpected events that occur "off-time" in the normative life cycle are likely to be perceived as more stressful than those that are experienced "on-time," particularly if they occur suddenly, leaving the couple no time for anticipatory coping or planning. The temporal context is also reflected in questions of "when" and "for how long" partners' coping efforts affect each other. The *interpersonal context* encompasses the full spectrum of an individual's social relations, including family, friends, group affiliations, social networks, and formal and informal helping systems. The social context connects individuals with others in their world. A couple constitutes a social system in itself, but it also exists within a number of interdependent social systems.

Given the primacy of social processes when examining dyadic coping, we now turn to several processes that have been studied within the couples coping literature and show promise for future work.

Social Support and Communication

Although we have focused on dyadic models of couples coping, a central aspect of couples coping involves the transaction of social support (Bodenmann, 2005; Cutrona, 1996).

A decade of research has shown that social support from spouses is an important predictor of patients' adaptation to serious illnesses such as arthritis (e.g., Holtzman & DeLongis, 2007), cancer (e.g., Manne, Sherman, Ross, Ostroff, Heyman, & Fox, 2004). and heart disease (Case, Moss, Case, McDermott, & Eberly, 1992). Partners provide love and affection, especially the assurance that the patient is loved despite the changes in his or her body, functional abilities, or personality. They provide tangible assistance with day-to-day responsibilities and special needs created by treatment, validate their partners'

emotions or coping choices, and help reappraise the meaning of the illness. Partners share the existential and practical concerns about how the illness may affect the marriage and family in the future. They provide continuity and security in a life disrupted by the physical indications and emotional meanings of illness.

However, not all studies show that spousal support minimizes patients' distress (Bolger, Foster, Vinokur, & Ng, 1996; Revenson, Schiaffino, Majerovitz, & Gibofsky, 1991). For example, in a study of women with rheumatoid arthritis, Revenson et al. (1991) showed that spouses could provide both positive and problematic support, and that the problematic support could cancel out the positive effects. In a study of breast cancer patients, significant others (combining spouses and other close family members and friends) provided support when the person was more physically disabled but withdrew it in response to emotional distress (Bolger et al., 1996). Different social resources from different people make different, potentially complementary, contributions to patients' and partners' well-being (Dakof & Taylor, 1990; Lanza et al., 1995). Particularly when the disease is severe, or the spouse emotionally exhausted from providing support, support from other social network members may play a compensatory role (Cutrona, 1996; Schiaffino, Revenson, & Gibofsky, 1991).

Most marriages evidence both support and conflict, with spouses enjoying the benefits of each other's support while also suffering the consequences of marital tension and conflict. Day-to-day supportive and negative interactions with the spouse each make significant, independent contributions to the well-being of each member of the couple (DeLongis, et al., 2004). However, the impact of marital conflict on well-being appears to be greater than the beneficial effects of marital support, with the negative effects of marital tension and conflict amplified for those with poor marital adjustment. Further, those with low marital satisfaction are particularly vulnerable to mood disturbance on days when there is an absence of positive interactions with the spouse. Those high in marital satisfaction are better able to weather the natural vicissitudes of married life (DeLongis et al., 2004). Negative responses from significant others can decrease the desire to cope and can lead to greater use of maladaptive coping and to increased negative affect and pain and poorer disease status in the long term (Griffin, Friend, Kaell, & Bennett, 2001; Holtzman & DeLongis, 2007; Lepore, Silver, Wortman, &

Wayment, 1996; Manne & Zautra, 1989). In a study of parents with a child with disability, positive spouse response attenuated the effect of maladaptive coping responses (such as interpersonal withdrawal, escape avoidance, and confrontive coping) on psychological distress (Marin et al., 2007).

Support that is not offered at the right time, is not of the right type, or is not offered by the right person may hinder adaptation more than it helps among both arthritis (Lanza et al., 1995; Manne & Zautra, 1989) and cancer patients (Hagedoorn et al., 2000). What has been called negative or problematic support includes not only these miscarried efforts at helping (Coyne, Wortman, & Lehman, 1988) but also outright negative behaviors, including partner avoidance and criticism (Manne, 1999; Manne & Zautra, 1989). In a study of cancer patients and spouses, Manne et al. (2006) described three communication styles: mutual constructive communication, mutual avoidance, and demand–withdraw communication. All three styles were related to distress 9 months later, with demand–withdraw communication associated with the highest distress and lowest relationship satisfaction for both patients and partners.

Healthy spousal communication is important for couples facing chronic illness and has been associated with lower psychological distress and better relationship quality for both adults with illness and their partners (Carmack Taylor, Badr, Lee, Fossella, Pisters, Gritz, & Schover, 2008; Manne et al., 2006). Open communication about cancer-related concerns has been associated with less distress and more relationship satisfaction (Manne et al., 2006). Yet research with many illnesses suggests that patients and partners often avoid discussing how the diagnosis and its treatment affect their emotions, marital relationship, and sexual relationship. Avoidance of critical issues and withdrawing from communication has been related to higher distress for both patients and their partners (Badr & Carmack Taylor, 2008), especially in the context of a poor marital relationship (Ey, Compas, Epping-Jordan, & Worsham, 1998).

Emotional Disclosure and Social Constraints

People with chronic illness need to disclose thoughts and feelings to others in order to make sense of their illness; feeling that one cannot disclose to others can lead to rumination and prolonged intrusive thoughts, which can be distressing (Lepore, 2001).

Social constraints are objective social conditions and individuals' construal of those conditions that lead them to refrain from or modify their disclosure of stress- and trauma-related thoughts, feelings, or concerns (Lepore & Revenson, 2007). Social constraints are likely to emerge when responses from intimate relationships lead individuals to feel unsupported or misunderstood when they are seeking social support or attempting to express their thoughts, feelings, or concerns. Social constraints on disclosure may arise because of disadvantageous conditions (for example, the spouse is also ill and is less able to provide support) but are not dependent on objective circumstances. For example, although a spouse may not know how to respond effectively to a patient's expression of fear of recurrence of their cancer, the patient may be able to shape the conversation to improve interpersonal communication and, consequently, not feel socially constrained. Alternately, a patient may not interpret a partner's inability to respond in a desired manner as a social constraint, but as a lifelong "personality trait" or an understandable short-term reaction to an acute stressor.

Social constraints are envisioned as a dynamic variable that changes over time and emerges through dyadic transactions. Interpersonal exchanges may be perceived as more or less constraining at various times in the coping process, and this perception may change as a result of changes within the illness context, network members' responses, or the relationship itself.

The best illustrations of the transactional and dynamic qualities of social constraints on disclosure come from qualitative research studies (e.g., Badr and Carmack Taylor, 2006; Pistrang & Barker, 2005) For example, Badr and Carmack Taylor (2006) examined social constraints in communication between recently diagnosed lung cancer patients and their spouse. Slightly over a third of the sample reported avoiding or having difficulties talking about the cancer in general, and two thirds of the spouses had difficulties or avoided discussing prognosis, death, or funeral arrangements, ostensibly for fear of upsetting the patient. Some patients reported that their partner's denial and avoidance was distressing, made them change how they interacted with the partner, and strained the marital relationship.

Research has shown that social constraints on disclosure are associated with heightened psychological distress and lower psychological adjustment across a number of illnesses, primarily cancer (Cordova, Cunningham, Carlson, & Andrykowski 2001; Eton, Lepore, & Helgeson, 2001; Lepore, 2001; Lepore & Helgeson, 1998; Lepore & Ituarte, 1999; Manne, DuHamel, & Redd 2000; Manne, Ostroff, Winkel, Grana, & Fox, 2005; Schmidt & Andrykowski, 2004; Widows, Jacobsen, & Fields 2000; Zakowski, Ramati, Morton, Johnson, & Flanigan 2003; Zakowski, 2004) but also rheumatoid arthritis (Danoff-Burg, Revenson, Trudeau, & Paget 2004), HIV infection (Ullrich, Lutgendorf, & Stapleton, 2002), traumatic injuries (Cordova Walser, Neff, Ruzek 2005), and chronic pain (Herbette & Rime, 2004; Hoffman, Meier, & Council, 2002). In the cancer literature, studies have shown both a direct positive association between level of social constraints and level of intrusive thoughts (e.g., Lepore & Helgeson, 1998; Manne, Ostroff, Winkel, Grana, & Fox 2005; Schmidt & Andrykowski, 2004; Zakowski et al., 2004) and moderational effects of social constraints on the relation between intrusive thoughts and distress (Lepore, 2001; Lepore & Helgeson, 1998; Manne, 1999).

Several studies of cancer patients suggest important gender differences in the psychological impact of social constraints, particularly from a spouse. In a study of prostate cancer patients, Lepore and Helgeson (1998) found that spousal constraints were more strongly related to psychological distress than constraints from friends and family. Zakowski et al. (2003) found that the association between perceived spousal constraints on mood disturbances was stronger among men (with prostate cancer) than among women (with gynecological cancer). Men's reliance on their spouse as a primary outlet for disclosing their concerns and feelings related to cancer may make them more vulnerable when they perceive spouse constraints on disclosure; fortunately for married men, women appear to be more receptive and less constraining than men when others disclose to them. Quartana, Schmaus, and Zakowski (2005) suggest that men may have difficulty in responding to expressions of negative emotions because it communicates neediness and interdependence, which challenges their sense of autonomy.

Because women tend to rely on a broader support network than men (Harrison, Maguire, & Pitcealthy, 1995), they may be more likely than men to find extramarital, non-constraining social outlets for disclosure. Alternately, emotional-approach coping, involving both the processing and expression of emotions, may be more advantageous for women than for men (Stanton et al., 2000).

Partner's Mood as a Factor in Dyadic Coping

Spouse depression may play a critical role in the ability to deal effectively with stress (DeLongis, Holtzman, Puterman, & Lam, 2010). The depressive symptoms of one partner may "infect" the other partner in what has been called "mood contagion." Consistent with cognitive models that consider attributions to play a key role in depression, Joiner and Katz (1999) argue that mood contagion can occur when one spouse makes negative attributions about his or her partner's distress or depression. In addition, depressive symptoms may be transmitted to the spouse because of the depressed partner's inability to provide response-contingent positive reinforcement, leading to a depleted interpersonal environment lacking in support.

Similarly, Coyne and Benazon (2001) have argued that when spouses are depressed they may be less likely to provide satisfactory support to their partners. Depressed persons have a tendency to be critical and hostile towards their spouses, which can magnify or lead to depressive symptoms. In a study of couples in which one partner was diagnosed with rheumatoid arthritis, Manne and Zautra (1989) found that patients with highly critical spouses were more likely to display maladaptive coping strategies and to exhibit poorer psychological adjustment than those with less critical spouses. Taken together with other studies on adjustment to rheumatoid arthritis showing a link between coping and well-being (e.g., Holtzman & DeLongis, 2007; Newth & DeLongis, 2004), it seems reasonable to posit a cascade of events in which depressed spouses criticize their chronically ill partners, who in turn cope poorly with their disease. This results in more negative outcomes, including poor mood for the (previously) non-depressed partner. Consistent with this, in a recent study investigating psychosocial factors affecting the disease course of rheumatoid arthritis, spouse depression was found to play a key role (Lam, Lehman, Puterman & DeLongis, 2009). Higher levels of spouse depression predicted worse disease course over a 1-year period for rheumatoid arthritis patients, as indicated by higher reports of subsequent disability and disease activity. These findings held even after controlling for initial levels of depression, disability, disease activity, age, number of years married, education, disease duration, and employment.

Methodological Considerations in Studying Couples Coping with Illness

The study of dyadic coping is fraught with complexities that present methodological challenges for researchers. Findings from research on couples coping is often difficult to interpret, as many studies have focused on only one member of the couple, not specified the coping task, or collapsed across different types of stressors, failing to control for a number of variables related to outcomes. Given the difficulty in obtaining data from sufficient numbers of couples in which one member has been diagnosed with a chronic illness, it is often the case that contextual variables, such as disease type or stage, socioeconomic status, age, relationship history, or presence of children in the family home, are left unexamined. Further, the role of gender and social role (i.e., patient vs. partner) are often confounded, as discussed below.

As we noted earlier, despite decades of research, the study of coping is plagued by contradictory and often inconsistent results (Somerfield & McCrae, 2000), and although the study of dyadic coping is relatively new, it faces many of the same methodological challenges, as well as some additional ones. Some critics contend that the discrepancies in the coping literature are due to an over-reliance on cross-sectional, between-person (and between-couple), retrospective research designs (e.g., Tennen, Affleck, Armeli, & Carney, 2000). Coping is often assessed with self-report questionnaires asking one or both member of the couple to recall a single stressful event in the past week, month, year or more and then to indicate if, and to what extent, they used a variety of coping strategies.

This methodology is problematic for a number of reasons. First, the cross-sectional methodology fails to capture the dynamic nature of the coping process (Bolger & Zuckerman, 1995; Coyne & Gottlieb, 1996; Tennen et al., 2000). Coping involves the concept of changing cognitive and behavioral efforts to manage psychological stress; it is by definition a process (Folkman et al., 1986). A single assessment cannot reveal such a pattern or process. Similarly, a between-person or between-couple design may indicate group-level patterns that are not reflective of the pattern for a single individual or couple. For example, a between-person positive association can emerge without a single individual demonstrating that positive association at the within-person level of analysis (Kenny, Kashy, & Bolger, 1998; Tennen & Affleck, 1996). Using single assessments to examine coping between individuals or couples has inherently missed the within-person, idiographic process of coping over time.

Second, reports of long-past coping responses tend to be plagued by memory biases and distortions (Bolger, Stadler, Paprocki, & DeLongis, 2010; DeLongis, Hemphill, & Lehman, 1992; Schwarz, 1999). Ptacek, Smith, and colleagues (Ptacek, Smith, Espe, & Raffety, 1994; Smith, Leffingwell, & Ptacek, 1999) examined the relationship between daily and retrospective measures of coping in two studies. They found that retrospective measures were poor reflections of daily reports, with only 26% and 37% of shared variance. Moreover, the correspondence between daily record and retrospective measures of coping was lower when the participant was experiencing greater stress. These authors suggest that the insidious use of retrospective studies, which have dominated the field, may have contributed to the inconclusive and contradictory findings that have frequently occurred in the coping literature. Given the plentiful evidence of inaccuracy and bias in retrospective accounts in other fields (e.g., Henry, Moffitt, Caspi, Langley, & Silva, 1994; Hyman & Loftus, 1998) it is hardly surprising that the same problems are present in dyadic coping research.

A related methodology frequently relied upon in research on couples coping with illness is to ask each member of the couple how he or she "typically" responds to some aspect of the disease, or the disease more generally. This methodology is problematic because research has demonstrated that coping often varies by situation (e.g., Folkman et al., 1986; Lee-Baggley, Preece, & DeLongis, 2005; O'Brien & DeLongis, 1996). Glossing over the stressor ignores the important contribution that situation can make to the coping response. In addition, when participants are asked how they *usually* cope, we may be asking them to tell us more than they can know. How does a participant go about aggregating in his or her head across multiple episodes with different stressors to report "typical" coping? Do participants report coping with a salient stressor? Or do they report coping with a recent stressor? Members of the couple likely vary in how they aggregate their coping episodes in their own heads, and likely this variability is systematically related to participant personality and to their history of stressful experiences. The gender differences or patient versus partner differences that are found in coping may be due to response biases rather than to actual differences in coping.

Further, the answer to the question of "What is effective dyadic coping?" may depend upon the time frame in which we look. The effects of coping can vary from one day to the next, with some strategies having effects that are limited to the same day and others persisting across days or even shifting direction from one day to the next. For example, on days when husbands reported family stress, their empathic responding was surprisingly associated with increases in same-day marital tension (O'Brien et al., 2009). However, lagged analyses revealed that empathic responding in husbands was associated with lower marital tension by the following day. In this case, the apparently adverse short-term effects of this strategy were compensated for by later positive effects.

Daily process methodology

Daily process methodology has been offered as a way to address many of these concerns (Bolger et al., 2010; DeLongis et al., 1992). It involves multiple assessments over time: each member of the couple is asked to report on his or her coping on a daily basis or multiple times per day. Couples typically report their experiences for a week, month, or more. For example, in a study of couples coping with rheumatoid arthritis, each member of the couple reported coping twice daily for a period of one week (DeLongis et al., 2010). Bolger and Kelleher (1993) recommended that researchers use this type of information in characterizing the quality of interpersonal relationships.

Daily process methodology permits a more accurate assessment of coping because it can examine antecedents, behaviors, and outcomes closer to their real-time occurrence. Diary measures can capture important details such as timing, frequency, and emotional reactivity that cannot be assessed using conventional self-report measures (Bolger et al., 2010). This proximity to events is important in examining changes in rapidly fluctuating processes, such as dyadic coping and well-being. Having obtained multiple assessments from both members of the couple, the researcher can examine patterns of dyadic coping as they unfold across time, instead of just a "snapshot" of the couple from a single assessment. Daily process methodology reduces the retrospective nature of reporting and therefore minimizes the inaccuracy of memory (Pearson, Ross, & Dawes, 1992; Ross & Conway, 1986).

Although daily process studies are labor-intensive research designs and debate continues regarding ways to improve the methodology

(Tennen, Affleck, Coyne, Larsen & DeLongis 2006), they offer a promise for allowing insights into dyadic coping (Bolger et al., in press). Potentially, such a method may help clarify the contradictory results in the field and lead to a better understanding of the role of dyadic coping in health and well-being. However, researchers need to be particularly sensitive to the problem of burdening couples with overly demanding methods of data collection, especially when participants are also struggling with health problems or other stressors. Compliance with a complex research protocol is likely to be reduced as burden increases. Thus, researchers must consider carefully the minimum number of time points necessary to address the research question under investigation. The use of even as few as three time points per day may result in excessive burden for many study participants, particularly those coping with chronic pain or other severe stressors. Further, researchers should carefully consider the length of time over which they are going to ask couples to keep records.

When putting extensive research demands on couples, development of rapport is essential to a successful and accurate data collection process. Many researchers achieve this by conducting initial one-on-one interviews with each member of the couple prior to the daily reporting (e.g., Holtzman & DeLongis, 2007). These initial interviews allow the researcher to (1) engage the couple fully in the research process, (2) introduce the diary method of data collection, and (3) discuss the potential challenges. When diary completion times are linked to daily activities, such as mealtimes and bedtime, adherence rates are likely to improve. Just as patient adherence to taking medication is increased when it is tied to routine daily events (Dunbar-Jacob & Schlenk, 2000), rates of adherence for couples in diary studies are likely to improve when tied to other daily activities. When entries match natural events in the couple's day, such as lunchtime and bedtime, then even participants who are ill, have children to care for, or have other daily commitments, can participate fully in the research. The use of electronic time-stamps, iPhones, or PDAs is ideal for obtaining the exact timing of diary entries. With couples in which one member has a disabling condition such as arthritis, or a fatiguing one, such as intensive chemotherapy, daily or twice-daily telephone interviews may be more appropriate. Particularly when studying elderly couples who might not be comfortable with technology, or when we wish to ask open-ended questions that are not easily answered in an electronic format, telephone "diaries" may be preferred (Green, Rafaeli, Bolger, Shrout, & Reis, 2006).

Multi-level modeling of dyadic data

The development of multi-level statistical models has permitted a more meaningful examination of couples data, particularly longitudinal data. Multi-level modeling takes into account the dependency in the data caused by both multiple data points and couples that standard regression analysis is unable to account for (Bryk & Raudenbush, 1992; Kashy & Kenny, 2000, Kenny, Kashy, & Cook, 2006). Multi-level modeling allows for the simultaneous analysis of within-person and between-person variation, within and between dyads, and in the case of longitudinal data, same-day and cross-day effects (Bryk & Raudenbush, 1992; Kenny et al., 1998, 2006). Thus, the coping of each member of the dyad can be examined within the context of his or her own coping across time, as well as within the context of the spouse's coping and the coping of other couples. Days can be nested within individuals (patients and partners). In turn, these individuals are nested within couples. In the case of families, children can be nested within the parental structure (Snijders & Bosker, 1999). We urge couples researchers to take advantage of these newer methodologies and statistics in order to understand the dynamic and intricate nature of couples coping. For more detail on ways to conceptualize and analyze dyadic data, see Bolger et al. (2010), Kashy and Kenny (2000), and Kenny et al. (2006).

A Note on Gender

We have made mention of the influence of gender on couples coping at several points in the chapter, but want to emphasize a few "take-home" points. In part because of funding priorities and practical constraints, most studies of couples coping with illness focus on a specific disease. And, because many diseases vary in their prevalence among men and women, most studies of coping with illness include respondents of only one sex. Thus, it is difficult, if not impossible, to disentangle the influences of the illness context and of gender, or conclude whether the experience of coping with the "same" illness differs for men and women.

Wives face a greater burden than husbands, whether they are the partner with the illness or the spouse-caregiver (Schmaling & Sher, 2000). Michela (1987) found such substantial differences in husbands' and wives' experience of men's recovery from a myocardial infarction that he wrote, "*His* experience is filtered through concerns about surviving and recovering from the MI with a minimum of danger or discomfort, while *her* experience is filtered through the meaning of the marital relationship to her—what the marriage has provided and, hence, what is threatened by the husband's potential death or what is lost by his disability" (p. 272). A prominent question in the literature is whether effects of social role—whether the individual is the person with the illness or the (presumably) healthy spouse—are truly about role or really about gender. Across the literature, comparisons are made between female patients and their husbands, male patient and their wives, male and female patients, male and female partners. In general, wives of male patients show higher distress than do their partners (e.g., Baider, Koch, Eascson, & Kaplan De-Nour, 1998; Kornblith, Herr, Ofman, Scher, & Holland, 1994; Morse & Fife, 1998) and experience different stressors. For example, in a study of prostate cancer patients and their wives, Harden, Schafenacker, Northouse, Mood, Smith, Pienta, Hussaind, Baranowri (2002) found that wives were more concerned with the possibility of their partners' death, while the men were more concerned with their sexual dysfunction. Mirroring this, men often report higher levels of social support and marital satisfaction than do women, whether they are the patient or the spouse (e.g., Goldzweig, Hubert, Walach, Brenner, Perry, Andritsch, Elisabeth, & Baider, 2009; Revenson et al., 2005).

A recent meta-analysis (Hagedoorn et al., 2008) examined the relative importance of social role (patient vs. partner) and gender in understanding the effects of cancer on couples. Combining the findings of 38 studies, Hagedoorn and colleagues found patient–partner differences in distress were dependent on gender: Cancer patients reported more distress when the patient was female and partners report more distress when the patient was male—that is, women report greater distress than men, regardless of whether they are the patient or the partner.

Why? Women typically report larger social networks than men, and men tend to rely primarily on their partner for support (Antonucci & Akiyama 1987; Harrison et al., 1995; see review by Helgeson and Cohen, 1996). Potentially because of this, men tend to be more satisfied with the support they receive from their partners and report greater marital satisfaction (e.g., Goldzweig, 2009). We urge all couples researchers to be cognizant of how gender may play a role in their study design and findings, and take care not to confound it with the patient versus partner role.

Applications to Clinical Practice

If indeed couples cope with chronic illness as a unit, it would follow that psychosocial interventions to enhance adjustment would be couples-based. These interventions can bring the partner into the patient's treatment (Martire, Lustig, Schulz, Miller, & Helgeson, 2004) or be directed wholly at the couple. They can enhance disclosure and communication processes among partners (e.g., Martire, Schulz, Keefe, Rudy, & Starz, 2007; Porter, Keefe, Baucom, Hurwitz, Moser, Patterson, & Kim, 2009), teach coping skills (Keefe, Blumenthal, Baucom, Affleck, Waugh, Caldwell, Beaupre, Kashikar-Zuck, Wright, Egert, & Lefebvre, 2004), or combine several strategies (Northouse, Mood, Schafenacker, Montie, Sandler, Forman, Hussain, Pienta, Smith, & Kershaw, 2007; Scott, Halford, & Ward, 2004). A review of intervention studies or current intervention techniques is beyond the scope of this chapter; for this, the reader is referred to work that focuses on the translation of dyadic research into clinical practice (Kayser & Scott, 2008; Widmer, Cina, Charvoz, Shantinath, & Bodenmann, Kayser, 2005). At this time, there are few well-designed studies of interventions for couples facing chronic illnesses, and most of these involve couples living with cancer. Moreover, the evidence for strong or consistent treatment effects for family-based interventions is thin (Martire & Schulz, 2007). To provide the evidence base for such interventions, we need randomized clinical trials that assess theoretically grounded couples-based interventions with outcomes measured for both partners and for the relationship, and that consider contextual variables, such as marital quality, as moderators.

Conclusion

Living with a serious, chronic illness involves adaptive tasks in many domains: illness management, daily tasks of medical care, family and social relationships, maintaining self-esteem, and existential questions related to life threat and bodily integrity (Moos, 1977; Stanton & Revenson, 2010; Stanton, et al., 2007). Patients and spouses typically face the challenges presented by an illness diagnosis together. The study of coping on a dyadic level represents a next step in understanding process as well as outcome, particularly when individuals are coping with a chronic stressor that affects both spouses.

Future Directions

The study of couples coping is still in its childhood. In the past decade there have been many advances, including a wide range of research designs and methods across studies, new concepts added to the study of dyadic coping, such as social constraints, and new methods to assess dyadic coping. At the same time, however, there is opportunity for growth and development, solidifying the identity of the field, and taking intellectual risks. We identify four broad areas for future work:

1. **Move toward including the larger social context in the study of dyadic coping**. How do gender roles affect dyadic coping? How do family environments and cultural mores affect dyadic coping? Does dyadic coping differ in same-sex and opposite-sex couples? How do we merge paradigms from different disciplines to create a more complete and integrated picture of dyadic coping processes?

2. **Identify the developmental trajectory or trajectories of couples coping with a stressful episode or chronic stressor**. Is there consistency in dyadic coping over time and situations? What is the developmental trajectory of dyadic coping over the lifespan? Is there a move toward greater consistency over time? How does the preexisting relationship affect dyadic coping?

3. **Conduct research at multiple levels of analysis with multiple methods**. How do we link individual-level coping processes to dyadic coping? How do we focus on microanalytic processes without losing the larger relationship context? How do we measure the relationship and family context?

4. **Translate the research findings into interventions and test the efficacy and effectiveness of those interventions**. Why do some interventions for couples fail? What aspects of the intervention affect couple-level outcomes? Where, when, for whom and how should we intervene to change dyadic coping processes?

References

Abraído-Lanza, A. F., & Revenson, T. A. (2006). Illness intrusion and psychological adjustment to rheumatic diseases: A social identity framework. *Arthritis and Rheumatism: Arthritis Care & Research, 55,* 224–32.

Acitelli, L. K., & Badr, H. J. (2005). My illness or our illness? Attending to the relationship when one partner is ill. In T. A. Revenson, K. Kayser, & G. Bodenmann (Eds.), *Couples coping with stress: Emerging perspectives on dyadic coping* (pp. 121–36). Washington, DC: American Psychological Association.

Antonucci, T. C., & Akiyama, H. (1987). Social networks in adult life and a preliminary examination of the convoy world. *Journal of Gerontology, 42*, 519–27.

Badr, H. (2004). Coping in marital dyads: A contextual perspective on the role of gender and health. *Personal Relationships, 11*, 197–211.

Badr, H., Acitelli, L. K., & Carmack Taylor, C. L. (2007). Does couple identity mediate the stress experienced by caregiving spouses. *Psychology and Health, 22*, 211–29.

Badr, H., Acitelli, L. K., & Carmack Taylor, C. L. (2008). Does talking about their relationship affect couples' marital and psychological adjustment to lung cancer? *Journal of Cancer Survivorship, 2*(1), 53–64.

Badr, H., & Carmack Taylor, C. L. (2006). Social constraints and spousal communication in lung cancer. *Psycho-Oncology, 15*, 673–83.

Badr, H. & Carmack Taylor, C. L. (2008). Effects of relationship maintenance on psychological distress and dyadic adjustment among couples coping with lung cancer. *Health Psychology, 27*(5) 616–27.

Badr, H., Carmack, C. L., Kashy, D. A., Cristofanilli, M., & Revenson, T. A. (2010). Dyadic coping in metastatic breast cancer. *Health Psychology, 29*, 169–80.

Baider, L., Koch, U., Eascson, R. & Kaplan De-Nour, A. (1998). Prospective study of cancer patients and their spouses: The weakness of marital strength. *Psycho-Oncology, 7*, 49–56.

Barnoy, S., Bar-Tal, Y., & Zisser, B., (2006). Correspondence in informational coping styles: How important is it for cancer patients and their spouses? *Personality and Individual Differences, 41*(1), 105–15.

Baumeister, R. F., & Leary, M. R. (1995). The need to belong: Desire for interpersonal attachments as fundamental human motivation. *Psychological Bulletin, 117*(3), 497–529.

Ben-Zur, H., Gilbar, O., & Lev, S. (2001). Coping with breast cancer: Patient, spouse, and dyad models. *Psychosomatic Medicine, 63*(1), 32–9.

Berg, C. A., & Upchurch, R. (2007). A developmental-contextual model of couples coping with chronic illness across the adult life span. *Psychological Bulletin, 133*(6), 920–54.

Berg, C. A., Wiebe, D. J., Butner, J., Bloor, L., Bradstreet, C., Upchurch, R., & Patton, G. (2008). Collaborative coping and daily mood in couples dealing with prostate cancer. *Psychology and Aging, 23*(3), 505–16.

Berghuis, J. P., & Stanton, A. L. (2002). Adjustment to a dyadic stressor: A longitudinal study of coping and depressive symptoms in infertile couples over an insemination attempt. *Journal of Consulting and Clinical Psychology, 70*, 433–8.

Bodenmann, G. (1997). Dyadic coping: A systemic-transactional view of stress and coping among couples: Theory and empirical findings. *European Review of Applied Psychology, 47*, 137–40.

Bodenmann, G. (2000). *Stress and Coping bei Paaren* [Stress and coping in couples]. Göttingen, Germany: Hogrefe.

Bodenmann, G. (2005). Dyadic coping and its significance for marital functioning. In T. A. Revenson, K. Kayser, & G. Bodenmann (Eds.), *Couples coping with stress: Emerging perspectives on dyadic coping* (pp. 33–50). Washington, DC: American Psychological Association.

Bodenmann, G., & Cina, A. (2005). Stress and coping among stable-satisfied, stable-distressed and separated/divorced Swiss couples: A 5-year prospective longitudinal study. *Journal of Divorce & Remarriage, 44*, 71–89.

Bodenmann, G., Pihet, S., & Kayser, K. (2006). The relationship between dyadic coping and marital quality: A 2-year longitudinal study. *Journal of Family Psychology, 20*(3), 485–93.

Bodenmann, G., & Shantinath, S. D. (2004). The couples coping enhancement training (CCET): A new approach to prevention of marital distress based upon stress and coping. *Family Relations, 53*, 477–84.

Bolger, N., DeLongis, A., Kessler, R. C., & Schilling, E. A. (1989). Effects of daily stress on negative mood. *Journal of Personality and Social Psychology, 57*(5), 808–18.

Bolger, N., Foster, M., Vinokur, A. D., & Ng, R. (1996). Close relationships and adjustments to a life crisis: The case of breast cancer. *Journal of Personality and Social Psychology, 70*(2), 283–94.

Bolger, N., & Kelleher, S. (1993). Daily life in relationships. In S. W. Duck (Ed.), *Social context and relationships* (pp. 100–9). Newbury Park, CA: Sage.

Bolger, N., Stadler, G., Paprocki, C., & DeLongis, A. (2010). Grounding social psychology in behavior in daily life: The case of conflict and distress in couples. In C. Agnew, D. E. Carlston, W. G. Graziano, & J. R. Kelly (Eds.), *Then a miracle occurs: Focusing on behavior in social psychological theory and research.* (pp. 368–390). NY: Oxford University Press.

Bolger, N., & Zuckerman, A. (1995). A framework for studying personality in the stress process. *Journal of Personality and Social Psychology, 69*(5), 890–902.

Bryk, A. S., & Raudenbush, S. W. (1992). *Hierarchical linear models: Applications and data analysis methods.* Newbury Park, CA: Sage.

Burman, B. U., & Margolin, G. (1992). Analysis of the association between marital relationships and health problems: An interactional perspective. *Psychological Bulletin, 112*(1), 39–63.

Buunk, B. P., Berkhuysen, M. A., Sanderman, R., Nieuwland, W., & Ranchor, A. V. (1996). Actieve bektrokkenheid, beschermend bufferen en overbescherming: Meetinstrumenten voor de rol van de partner bij hartrevalidate [The role of the partner in heart disease: Active engagement, protective buffering, and overprotection]. *Gedrag & Gezondheid, 24*, 304–13.

Carmack Taylor, C. L., Badr, H., Lee, L., Pisters, K., Fossella, F., Gritz, E. R., & Schover, L. (2008). Lung cancer patients and their spouses: Psychological and relationship functioning within one month of treatment initiation. *Annals of Behavioral Medicine, 36*(2), 129–40.

Case, R. B., Moss, A. J., Case, N., McDermott, M., & Eberly, S. (1992). Living alone after myocardial infarction: Impact on prognosis. *Journal of the American Medical Association, 267*, 515–9.

Cordova, M. J., Cunningham, L. L., Carlson, C. R., & Andrykowski, M. A. (2001). Social constraints, cognitive processing, and adjustment to breast cancer. *Journal of Consulting and Clinical Psychology, 69*(4), 706–11.

Cordova, M. J., Walser, R., Neff, J., & Ruzek, J. I. (2005). Predictors of emotional adjustment following traumatic injury: personal, social, and material resources. *Prehospital & Disaster Medicine, 20*(1), 7–13.

Coyne, J. C., & Benazon, N. R. (2001). Not agent blue: Effects of marital functioning on depression and implication for treatment. In S. R. H. Beach (Ed.), *Marital and family processes in depression: A scientific foundation for clinical practice* (pp. 25–43). Washington, DC: American Psychological Association.

Coyne, J.C., & Fiske, V. (1992). Couples coping with chronic and catastrophic illness. In M. A. P. Stephens, S. E. Hobfoll, & J. Crowther (Eds.), *Family health psychology* (pp. 129–49). Washington DC: Hemisphere.

Coyne, J. C., & Gottlieb, B. H. (1996). The mismeasure of coping by checklist. *Journal of Personality, 64*(4), 959–91.

Coyne, J. C., & Smith, D. A. F. (1991). Couples coping with a myocardial infarction: A contextual perspective on wives distress. *Journal of Personality and Social Psychology, 61*(3), 404–12.

Coyne, J. C., Wortman, C. B., & Lehman, D. R. (1988). The other side of support: Emotional overinvolvement and miscarried helping. In B. Gottlieb (Ed.), *Marshaling social support: Formats, processes, and effects.* (pp. 305–30). New York: Sage Publications, Inc.

Cutrona, C.E. (1996). *Social support in couples.* Thousand Oaks, CA: Sage.

Cutrona, C. E., Russell, D. W., & Gardner, K. A. (2005). The relationship enhancement model of social support. In T.A. Revenson, K. Kayser, & G. Bodenmann (Eds.), *Couples coping with stress: Emerging perspectives on dyadic coping* (pp. 73–95). Washington, DC: American Psychological Association.

Cutrona, C. E., & Suhr, J. A. (1992). Controllability of stressful events and satisfaction with spouse support behaviours. *Communication Research, 19*(2), 154–74.

Dakof, G. A., & Taylor, S. E. (1990). Victims' perceptions of social support: what is helpful from whom? *Journal of Personality and Social Psychology, 58*(1), 80–9.

Danoff-Burg, S., Revenson, T. A., Trudeau, K. J., & Paget, S. A. (2004). Unmitigated communion, social constraints, and psychological distress among women with rheumatoid arthritis. *Journal of Personality, 72,* 29–46.

Davis, M. H. (1994). *Empathy: A social psychological approach.* Madison, WI: Brown & Benchmark.

Dehle, C., Larsen, D., & Landers, J. E. (2001). Social support in marriage. *American Journal of Family Therapy, 29*(4), 307–24.

DeLongis, A., Capreol, M. J., Holtzman, S., O'Brien, T. B., & Campbell, J. (2004). Social support and social strain among husbands and wives: A multilevel analysis. *Journal of Family Psychology, 18,* 470–9.

DeLongis, A., Hemphill, K. J., & Lehman, D. R. (1992). A structured diary methodology for the study of daily events. In F. B. Bryant, J. Edwards, R. S. Tindale, E. J. Posavac, L. Heath, E. Henderson, & Y. Suarez-Balcazar (Eds.), *Methodological issues in applied social psychology* (pp. 83–109). New York: Plenum Press.

DeLongis, A., & Holtzman, S. (2005). Coping in context: The role of stress, social support, and personality in coping. *Journal of Personality, 73,* 1633–56.

DeLongis, A., Holtzman, S, Puterman, E., & Lam, M. (2010). Dyadic coping: Support from the spouse in times of stress. In K. Sullivan & J. Davila (Eds.), *Support Processes in Intimate Relationships.* (pp. 153–174). New York: Oxford UniversityPress.

DeLongis, A., & O'Brien, T. B. (1990). An interpersonal framework for stress and coping: An application to the families of Alzheimer's patients. In M. A. P. Stephens, J. H. Crowther, S. E. Hobfoll, & D. L. Tennenbaum (Eds.), *Stress and coping in later-life families* (pp. 221–39). Washington, DC: Hemisphere Publishing Corp.

Dorval, M., Guay, S., Mondor, M., Mâsse, B., Falardeau, M., Robidoux, A., Deschênes, L., & Maunsell, E. (2005). Couples who get closer after breast cancer: Frequency and predictors in a prospective investigation. *Journal of Clinical Oncology, 23,* 3588–96.

Dunbar-Jacob, J., & Schlenk, E. (2000). Patient adherence to treatment regimen. In A. Baum, T. A. Revenson, & J. E. Singer (Eds.), *Handbook of health psychology* (pp. 571–80). Hillsdale, NJ: Lawrence Erlbaum Associates.

Eisenberg, N. (2000). Emotion, regulation, and moral development. *Annual Review of Psychology, 51,* 665–97.

Eton, D. T., Lepore, S. J., & Helgeson, V. S. (2001). Early quality of life in patients with localized prostate carcinoma: An examination of treatment-related, demographic, and psychosocial factors. *Cancer, 92,* 1451–9.

Ey, S., Compas, B. E., Epping-Jordan, J. E., & Worsham, N. (1998) Stress responses and psychological adjustment in patients with cancer and their spouses. *Journal of Psychosocial Oncology, 16,* 59–77.

Felton, B. J., & Revenson, T. A. (1984). Coping with chronic illness: A study of illness controllability and the influence of coping strategies on psychological adjustment. *Journal of Consulting and Clinical Psychology, 52,* 343–53.

Fincham, F. D., & Beach, S. R. H. (1999). Conflict in marriage: Implications for working with couples. *Annual Review of Psychology, 50,* 47–77.

Folkman, S., Lazarus, R. S., Dunkel-Schetter, C., DeLongis, A., & Gruen, R. J. (1986). Dynamics of a stressful encounter: Cognitive appraisal, coping, and encounter outcomes. *Journal of Personality and Social Psychology, 50,* 992–1003.

French, J. R. P., Jr., Rodgers, W., & Cobb, S. (1974). Adjustment as person-environment fit. In G. V. Coelho, D. A. Hamburg, & J. E. Adams (Eds.), *Coping and adjustment* (pp. 316–33). New York: Basic Books.

Goldzweig, G., Hubert, A., Walach, N., Brenner, B., Perry, S., Andritsch, Elisabeth, & Baider, L. (2009). Gender and psychological distress among middle- and older-aged colorectal cancer patients and their spouses: An unexpected outcome. *Critical Reviews in Oncology/Hematology, 70,* 71–82.

Gottman, J. M. (1998). Psychology and the study of marital processes. *Annual Review of Psychology, 49,* 169–97.

Gray, R. E., Fitch, M., Phillips, C., Labrecque, M., & Fergus, K. (2000). Managing the impact of illness: The experiences of men with prostate cancer and their spouses. *Journal of Health Psychology, 5,* 531–48.

Green, A. S., Rafaeli, E., Bolger, N., Shrout, P. E., & Reis, H. T. (2006). Paper or plastic? Data equivalence in paper and electronic diaries. *Psychological Methods, 11*(1), 87–105.

Griffin, K. W., Friend, R., Kaell, A. T., & Bennett, R. S. (2001). Distress and disease status among patients with rheumatoid arthritis: Roles of coping styles and perceived responses from support providers. *Annals of Behavioral Medicine, 23*(2), 133–8.

Haan, N. (1977). *Coping and defending: Processes of self-environment organization.* New York: Academic Press.

Haan, N. (1978). Two moralities in action contexts: Relationships to thought, ego regulations, and development. *Journal of Personality and Social Psychology, 36*(3), 286–305.

Hagedoorn, M., Kuijer, R. G., Buunk, B. P., DeJong, G. M., Wobbes, T., & Sanderman, R. (2000). Marital satisfaction in patients with cancer: Does support from intimate partners benefit those who need it most? *Health Psychology, 19,* 274–82.

Hagedoorn, M., Sanderman, R., Bolks, H., Tuinstra, J., & Coyne, J. C. (2008). Distress in couples coping with cancer: A meta-analysis and critical review of role and gender effects. *Psychological Bulletin, 134,* 1–30.

Haggan, P. (2002) Family resilience through sports: The family as a team. *Journal of Individual Psychology, 58,* 279–89.

Harden, J., Schafenacker, A., Northouse, L., Mood, D., Smith, D., Pienta, K., Hussain, M., & Baranowski, K. (2002). Couples' experiences with prostate cancer: focus group research. *Oncology Nursing Forum, 29*(4), 701–9.

Harrison, J., Maguire, P., & Pitceathly, C. (1995). Confiding in crisis: gender differences in pattern of confiding among cancer patients. *Social Science & Medicine, 41,* 1255–60.

Helgeson, V.S. (1993). Implications of agency and communion for patient and spouse adjustment to a first coronary event. *Journal of Personality and Social Psychology, 64,* 807–16.

Helgeson, V. S., & Cohen, S. (1996). Social support and adjustment to cancer: reconciling descriptive, correlational, and intervention research. *Health Psychology, 15,* 135–48.

Henry, B., Moffitt, T. E., Caspi, A., Langley, J., & Silva, P. A. (1994). On the 'remembrance of things past': A longitudinal evaluation of the retrospective method. *Psychological Assessment, 6*(2), 92–101.

Herbette, G., & Rime, B. (2004). Verbalization of emotion in chronic pain patients and their psychological adjustment. *Journal of Health Psychology, 9,* 661–76.

Hoffman, P. K., Meier, B. P., & Council, J. R. (2002). A comparison of chronic pain between an urban and rural population. *Journal of Community Health Nursing, 19,* 213–24.

Holtzman, S., & DeLongis, A. (2007). One day at a time: The impact of daily satisfaction with spouse responses on pain, negative affect and catastrophizing among individuals with rheumatoid arthritis. *Pain, 131,* 202–13.

Holtzman, S., Newth, S., & DeLongis, A. (2004). The role of social support in coping with daily pain among patients with rheumatoid arthritis. *Journal of Health Psychology, 9,* 677–95.

Huston, T. L., & Robins, E. (1982). Conceptual and methodological issues in studying close relationships. *Journal of Marriage and the Family, 44,* 901–25.

Hyman, I. E., & Loftus, E. F. (1998). Errors in autobiographical memory. *Clinical Psychology Review, 18*(8), 933–47.

Joiner, T. E., & Katz, J. (1999). Contagion of depressive symptoms and mood: Meta-analytic review and explanations from cognitive, behavioral, and interpersonal viewpoints. *Clinical Psychology: Science and Practice, 6*(2), 149–64.

Kaptein, A. A., Scharloo, M., Helder, D. I., Snoei, L., van Kempen, G. M. J., Weinman, J., van Houwelingen, J. C., & Roos, R. A. C. (2007). Quality of life in couples living with Huntington's disease: The role of patients' and partners' illness perceptions. *Quality of Life Research: An International Journal of Quality of Life Aspects of Treatment, Care & Rehabilitation, 16*(5), 793–801.

Karney, B. R., Story, L. B., & Bradbury, T. N. (2005). Marriages in context: Interactions between chronic and acute stress among newlyweds. In T. A. Revenson, K. Kayser, & G. Bodenmann (Eds.), *Emerging perspectives on couples' coping with stress* (pp. 13–32). Washington, DC: American Psychological Association.

Kashy, D. A., & Kenny, D. A. (2000). The analysis of data from dyads and groups. In H. Reis & C. M. Judd (Eds.), *Handbook of research methods in social psychology* (pp. 451–77). New York: Cambridge University Press.

Kayser, K. (2005). Enhancing dyadic coping during a time of crisis: A theory-based intervention with breast cancer patients and their partners. In T. A. Revenson, K. Kayser, & G. Bodenmann (Eds.), *Couples coping with stress: Emerging perspectives on dyadic coping* (pp. 175–94). Washington, DC: American Psychological Association.

Kayser, K., & Scott, J. (2008). *Helping couples cope with women's cancers: An evidence-based approach for practitioners.* New York: Springer.

Kayser, K., Watson, L. E., & Andrade, J. T. (2007). Cancer as a 'we-disease': Examining the process of coping from a relational perspective. *Families, Systems & Health, 25,* 404–18.

Keefe, F. J., Blumenthal, J., Baucom, D., Affleck, G., Waugh, R., Caldwell, D. S., & Lefebvre, J. (2004). Effects of spouse-assisted coping skills training and exercise training in patients with osteoarthritic knee pain: A randomized controlled study. *Pain, 110,* 539–49.

Kenny, D. A., Kashy, D. A., & Bolger, N., (1998). Data analysis in social psychology. In D. T. Gilbert, S. T. Fiske, & G. Lindzey (Eds.), *The handbook of social psychology, Vols. 1 and 2 (4th ed.)* (pp. 233–65). New York: McGraw-Hill.

Kenny D. A., Kashy, D. A., & Cook, W. L. (2006). *Dyadic data analysis.* New York: Guilford.

Kiecolt-Glaser, J. K., & Newton, T. L. (2001). Marriage and health: His and hers. *Psychological Bulletin, 127,* 472–503.

Kornblith, A. B., Herr, H. W., Ofman, U. S., Scher, H. I., & Holland, J. C. (1994). Quality of life of patients with prostate cancer and their spouses. The value of a data base in clinical care. *Cancer, 73,* 2791–802.

Kuijer, R. G., Ybema, J. F., Buunk, B. P., De Jong, G. M., Thijs-Boer, F., & Sanderman, R. (2000). Active engagement, protective buffering, and overprotection: Three ways of giving support by intimate partners of patients with cancer. *Journal of Social & Clinical Psychology, 19,* 256–75.

Lam, M., Lehman, A. J., Puterman, E., & DeLongis, A. (2009). Spouse depression and disease course among persons with rheumatoid arthritis. *Arthritis & Rheumatism, 61,* 1011–7.

Lanza, A. F., Cameron, A. E., & Revenson, T. A. (1995). Perceptions of helpful and unhelpful support among married individuals with rheumatic diseases. *Psychology and Health, 10,* 449–62.

Lavery, J. F., & Clarke, V. A. (1999). Prostate cancer: Patients' and spouses' coping and marital adjustment. *Psychology, Health & Medicine, 4,* 289–302.

Lazarus, R. S. (1966). *Psychological stress and the coping process.* New York: McGraw-Hill.

Lazarus, R. S. (1981). The stress and coping paradigm. In C. Edisdorfer, D. Cohen, A Kleinman, & P. Maxim (Eds.), *Models for clinical psychopathology* (pp. 177–214). New York: Spectrum Medical and Scientific Books.

Lazarus, R. S., Averill, J. R., & Opton, E. M., Jr. (1974). The psychology of coping: Issues of research and assessment. In G. V. Coelho, D. A. Hamburg, & J. E. Adams (Eds.), *Coping and adaptation* (pp. 249–315). New York: Basic Books.

Lazarus, R. S., & DeLongis, A. (1983). Psychological stress and coping in aging. *American Psychologist, 38,* 245–54.

Lazarus, R. S., & Folkman, S. (1984). *Stress, appraisal, and coping.* New York: Springer.

Lazarus, R. S., & Launier, R. (1978). Stress-related transactions between person and environment. In L. A. Pervin & M. Lewis (Eds.), *Perspectives in interactional psychology* (pp. 287–327). New York: Plenum.

Lee-Baggley, D. L., Preece, M., & DeLongis, A. (2005). Coping with interpersonal stress: Role of big five traits. *Journal of Personality, 73*(5), 1141–80.

Lepore, S. J. (2001). A social-cognitive processing model of emotional adjustment to cancer. In A. Baum & B. L. Andersen (Eds.), *Psychosocial interventions for cancer* (pp. 99–116). Washington, DC: American Psychological Association.

Lepore, S. J., & Helgeson, V. S. (1998). Social constraints, intrusive thoughts, and mental health after prostate cancer. *Journal of Social and Clinical Psychology, 17*, 89–106.

Lepore, S. J., & Ituarte, P. H. G. (1999). Optimism about cancer enhances mood by reducing negative social interactions. *Cancer Research, Therapy and Control, 8*, 165–74.

Lepore. S. J., & Revenson, T. A. (2007). Social constraints on disclosure and adjustment to cancer. *Social and Personality Psychology Compass, 1*, 313–33.

Lepore, S. J., Silver, R. C., Wortman, C. B., & Wayment, H. A., (1996). Social constraints, intrusive thoughts, and depressive symptoms among bereaved mothers. *Journal of Personality and Social Psychology, 70*(2), 271–82.

Luszczynska, A., Gerstorf, D., Boehmer, S., Knoll, N., & Schwarzer, R. (2007). Patients' coping profiles and partners' support provision. *Psychology & Health, 22*, 749–64.

Lyons, R. F., Sullivan, M. J. L., Ritvo, P. G., & Coyne, J. C., (1996). *Relationships in chronic illness and disability.* Thousand Oaks, CA: Sage.

Maliski, S. L., Heilemann, M. V., & McCorkle, R. (2001). Mastery of post-prostatectomy incontinence and impotence: His work, her work, our work. *Oncology Nursing Forum, 28*, 985–92.

Manne, S. L. (1998). Cancer in the marital context: A review. *Cancer Investigations, 16*, 188–202.

Manne, S. L. (1999). Intrusive thoughts and psychological distress among cancer patients: The role of spouse avoidance and criticism. *Journal of Consulting and Clinical Psychology, 67*, 539–46.

Manne, S. L., & Badr, H. (2008). Intimacy and relationship processes in couples' psychosocial adaptation to cancer. *Cancer, 112*, 2541–55.

Manne, S. L., & Badr, H. (2009). Intimacy processes and psychological distress among couples coping with head and neck or lung cancers. *Psycho-Oncology,* DOI: 10.1002/pon.1645.

Manne, S. L., Dougherty, J., Veach, S., & Kless, R. (1999). Hiding worries from one's spouse: Protective buffering among cancer patients and their spouses. *Cancer Research Therapy and Control, 8*, 175–88.

Manne, S. L., DuHamel, K., & Redd, W. H. (2000). Association of psychological vulnerability factors to post-traumatic stress symptomatology in mothers of pediatric cancer survivors. *Psycho-Oncology, 9*, 372–84.

Manne, S., Norton, T., Ostroff, J., Winkel, G., Fox, K., & Grana, G. (2007). Protective buffering and psychological distress among couples coping with breast cancer: The moderating role of relationship satisfaction. *Journal of Family Psychology, 21*, 380–8.

Manne, S., Ostroff, J., Norton, T., Fox, K., Goldstein, L., & Grana, G. (2006). Cancer-related relationship communication in couples coping with early stage breast cancer. *Psycho-Oncology, 15*, 234–47.

Manne, S. L., Ostroff, J., Winkel, G., Grana, G., & Fox, K. (2005). Partner unsupportive responses, avoidant coping, and distress among women with early stage breast cancer: Patient and partner perspectives. *Health Psychology, 24*, 635–41.

Manne, S. L., Sherman, M., Ross, S., Ostroff, J., Heyman, R. E., & Fox, K. (2004). Couples' support-related communication, psychological distress, and relationship satisfaction among women with early stage breast cancer. *Journal of Consulting and Clinical Psychology, 72*, 660–70.

Manne, S. L., & Zautra, A. J. (1989). Spouse criticism and support: Their association with coping and psychological adjustment among women with rheumatoid arthritis. *Journal of Personality and Social Psychology, 56*, 608–17.

Manne, S. L., & Zautra, A. J. (1990). Couples coping with chronic illness: Women with rheumatoid arthritis and their healthy husbands. *Journal of Behavioral Medicine, 13*, 327–42.

Marin, T., Holtzman, S., DeLongis, A., & Robinson, L. (2007). Coping and the response of others. *Journal of Social and Personal Relationships, 24*, 951–69.

Martire, L. M., Lustig, A. P., Schulz, R., Miller, G. E., & Helgeson, V. S. (2004). Is it beneficial to involve a family member? A meta-analysis of psychosocial interventions for chronic illness. *Health Psychology, 23*, 599–611.

Martire, L. M., & Schulz, R. (2007). Involving family in psychosocial interventions for chronic illness. *Current Directions in Psychological Science, 16*, 90–4.

Martire, L.M., & Schulz, R. (in press). Caregiving and care-receiving in later life: Recent evidence for health effects and promising intervention approaches. In A. Baum, T. A. Revenson, & J. E. Singer (Eds.), *Handbook of health psychology (2nd ed.).* New York: Taylor & Francis.

Martire, L. M., Schulz, R., Keefe, F. J., Rudy, T. E., & Starz, T. W. (2007). Couple-oriented education and support intervention: Effects on individuals with osteoarthritis and their spouses. *Rehabilitation Psychology, 52*, 121–32.

Michela, J. L. (1987). Interpersonal and individual impacts of a husband's heart attack. In A. Baum & J. E. Singer (Eds.), *Handbook of psychology and health*, volume 5 (pp. 255–301). Hillsdale, NJ: Erlbaum.

Moos, R. H. (1977). *Coping with physical illness.* Oxford, England: Plenum.

Moos, R. H., & Tsu, V. D. (1977). The crisis of illness. In R. H. Moos (Ed.), *Coping with physical illness* (pp. 3–21). New York: Plenum Medical.

Morse, S. R., & Fife, B. (1998). Coping with a partner's cancer: adjustment at four stages of the illness trajectory. *Oncology Nursing Forum, 25*, 751–60.

Neff, L. A., & Karney, B. R. (2004). How does context affect relationships? Linking external stress and cognitive processes within marriage. *Personality and Social Psychology Bulletin, 30*, 134–48.

Newth, S., & DeLongis, A. (2004). Individual differences, mood, and coping with chronic pain in rheumatoid arthritis: A daily process analysis. *Psychology & Health, 19*(3), 283–305.

Northouse, L. L., Mood, D. W., Schafenacker, A., Montie, J. E., Sandler, H. M., Forman, J. D., & Kershaw, T. (2007). Randomized clinical trial of a family intervention for prostate cancer patients and their spouses. *Cancer, 110*, 2809–18.

Northouse, L., Templin, T., & Mood, D. (2001). Couples' adjustment to breast disease during the first year following diagnosis. *Journal of Behavioral Medicine, 24*, 115–36.

O'Brien, T. B., & DeLongis, A. (1996). The interactional context of problem-, emotion-, and relationship-focused coping: The role of the Big Five personality factors. *Journal of Personality, 64*, 775–813.

O'Brien, T. B., & DeLongis, A. (1997). Coping with chronic stress: An interpersonal perspective. In B. Gottlieb (Ed)., *Coping with chronic stress* (pp. 161–90). New York: Plenum Press.

O'Brien, T. B., DeLongis, A., Pomaki, G., Puterman, E., & Zwicker, A. (2009). Couples coping with stress: The role of empathic responding. *European Psychologist, 14,* 18–28.

Ouellette, S. C. (1993). Inquiries into hardiness. In L. Goldberger & S. Breznitz (Eds.), *Handbook of stress: Theoretical and clinical aspects* (2nd ed., pp. 77–100). New York: Free Press.

Pakenham, K. I. (1998). Couple coping and adjustment to multiple sclerosis in care receiver-carer dyads. *Family Relations, 47*(3), 269–77.

Pasch, L. A., & Bradbury, T. N. (1998). Social support, conflict, and the development of marital dysfunction. *Journal of Consulting and Clinical Psychology, 66*(2), 219–30.

Patterson, J. M., & Garwick, A. W. (1994). The impact of chronic illness on families: A family systems perspective. *Annals of Behavioral Medicine, 16,* 131–42.

Pearlin, L. I., & Turner, H. A. (1987). The family as a context of the stress process. In S. V. Kasl & C. L. Cooper (Eds.), *Stress and health: Issues in research methodology* (pp. 143–65). New York: John Wiley & Sons.

Pearson, R. W., Ross, M. A., & Dawes, R. M. (1992). Personal recall and the limits of retrospective questions in surveys. In J. M. Tanur (Ed.), *Questions about questions: Inquiries into the cognitive bases of surveys* (pp. 65–94). New York: Sage Foundation.

Pistrang, N., & Barker, C. (2005). How partners talk in times of stress: A process analysis approach. In T. A. Revenson, K. Kayser, & G. Bodenmann (Eds.), *Couples coping with stress: Emerging perspectives on dyadic coping* (pp. 97–119). Washington, DC: American Psychological Association.

Porter, L. S., Keefe, F. J., Baucom, D. H., Hurwitz, H., Moser, B., Patterson, E., & Kim, H. J. (2009). Partner-assisted emotional disclosure for patients with gastrointestinal cancer. *Cancer, 115 (18 suppl),* 4326–38.

Ptacek, J. T., Smith, R. E., Espe, K., & Raffety, B. (1994). Limited correspondence between daily coping reports and restrospective coping recall. *Psychological Assessment, 6*(1), 41–9.

Quartana, P. J., Schmaus, B. J., & Zakowski, S. G., (2005), Gender, neuroticism, and emotional expressivity: Effects on spousal constraints among individuals with cancer. *Journal of Consulting and Clinical Psychology, 73*(4), 769–76.

Repetti, R., Wang, S., & Saxbe, D. (2009). Bringing it all back home: How outside stressors shape families' everyday lives. *Current Directions in Psychological Science, 18,* 106–11.

Revenson, T. A. (1990). All other things are not equal: An ecological perspective on the relation between personality and disease. In H. S. Friedman (Ed.), *Personality and disease,* (pp. 65–94) New York: John Wiley.

Revenson, T. A. (1994). Social support and marital coping with chronic illness. *Annals of Behavioral Medicine, 16,* 122–30.

Revenson, T. A. (2003). Scenes from a marriage: Examining support, coping, and gender within the context of chronic illness. In J. Suls & K. Wallston (Eds.), *Social psychological foundations of health and illness* (pp. 530–59). Oxford, England: Blackwell Publishing.

Revenson, T. A., Abraído-Lanza, A. F., Majerovitz, S. D., & Jordan, C. (2005). Couples coping with chronic illness: What's gender got to do with it?. In T. A. Revenson K. Kayser & G. Bodenmann (Eds.), *Couples coping with stress: Emerging perspectives on dyadic coping* (pp. 137–156). Washington DC: American Psychological Association.

Revenson, T. A., Kayser, K., & Bodenmann, G. (Eds.). (2005). *Couples coping with stress: Emerging perspectives on dyadic coping.* Washington, DC: American Psychological Association.

Revenson, T. A., & Majerovitz, S. D. (1990). Spouses' support provision to chronically ill patients. *Journal of Social and Personal Relationships, 7,* 575–86.

Revenson, T. A., & Majerovitz, D. M. (1991). The effects of chronic illness on the spouse: Social resources as stress buffers. *Arthritis Care and Research, 4,* 63–72.

Revenson, T. A., Schiaffino, K. M., Majerovitz, D. S., & Gibofsky, A. (1991). Social support as a double-edged sword: The relation of positive and problematic support to depression among rheumatoid arthritis patients. *Social Science & Medicine, 33,* 807–13.

Robles, T. F., & Kiecolt-Glaser, J. K. (2003). The physiology of marriage: pathways to health. *Physiology & Behavior, 79,* 409–16.

Rose, G., Suls, J., Green, P. J., Lounsbury, P., & Gordon, E. (1996). Comparison of adjustment, activity, and tangible social support in men and women patients and their spouses during the six months post-myocardial infarction. *Annals of Behavioral Medicine, 18,* 264–72.

Ross, M., & Conway, M. (1986). Remembering one's own past: The construction of personal histories. In R. M. Sorrentino & E. T. Higgins (Eds.), *Handbook of motivation and cognition: Foundations of social behavior* (pp. 122–44). New York: Guilford Press.

Rusbult, C. E., Verette, J., Whitney, G. A., Slovik, L. F., & Lipkus, I. (1991). Accommodation processes in close relationships: Theory and preliminary empirical evidence. *Journal of Personality and Social Psychology, 60*(1), 53–78.

Samelson, D. A., & Hannon, R. (1999). Sexual desire in couples living with chronic medical conditions. *The Family Journal: Counseling and Therapy for Couples and Families, 7,* 29–38.

Schiaffino, K. M., Revenson, T. A., & Gibofsky, A. (1991). Assessing the role of self-efficacy beliefs in adaptation to rheumatoid arthritis. *Arthritis Care and Research, 4* (4), 150–7.

Schmaling, K. B., & Sher, T.G. (2000). *The psychology of couples and illness.* Washington DC: American Psychological Association.

Schmidt, J. E., & Andrykowski, M. A. (2004). The role of social and dispositional variables associated with emotional processing in adjustment to breast cancer: an Internet-based study. *Health Psychology, 23*(3), 259–66.

Schwarz, N. (1999). Self-reports: How the questions shape the answers. *American Psychologist, 54*(2), 93–105.

Scott, J. L., Halford, W. K., & Ward, B. G. (2004). United we stand? The effects of a couple-coping intervention on adjustment to early stage breast or gynecologic cancer. *Journal of Consulting and Clinical Psychology, 72*(6), 1122–35.

Smith, R. E., Leffingwell, T. R., & Ptacek, J. T. (1999). Can people remember how they coped? Factors associated with discordance between same-day and retrospective reports. *Journal of Personality and Social Psychology, 76*(6), 1050–61.

Snijders, T., & Bosker, R. (1999). *Multilevel analysis.* London: Sage Publications.

Somerfield, M. R., & McCrae, R. (2000). Stress and coping research: Methodological challenges, theoretical advances, and clinical applications. *American Psychologist, 55*(6), 620–5.

Stanton, A. L., Danoff-Burg, S., Cameron, C. L., Bishop, M., Collins, C. A., Kirk, S. B., et al. (2000). Emotionally expressive coping predicts psychological and physical adjustment to breast cancer. *Journal of Consulting and Clinical Psychology, 68*(5), 875–82.

Stanton, A., & Revenson, T. A. (2010). Adjustment to chronic disease: Progress and promise in research. In H. Friedman

(Ed.), *Oxford handbook of health psychology*. New York: Oxford University Press.

Stanton, A., Revenson, T. A., & Tennen, H. (2007). Health psychology: Psychological adjustment to chronic disease. *Annual Review of Psychology, 58,* 13.1–13.28.

Stephens, M. A. P., Martire, L. M., Cremeans-Smith, J. K., Druley, J. A., & Wojno, W. C. (2006). Older women with osteoarthritis and their caregiving husbands: Effects of pain and pain expression on husbands' well-being and support. *Rehabilitation Psychology, 51*(1), 3–12.

Sterba, K. R., DeVellis, R. F., Lewis, M. A., Baucom, D. H., Jordan, J. M., & DeVellis, B. (2007). Developing and testing a measure of dyadic efficacy for married women with rheumatoid arthritis and their spouses. *Arthritis & Rheumatism, 57*(2), 294–302.

Sterba, K. R., DeVellis, R. F., Lewis, M. A., DeVellis, B., Jordan, J., & Baucom, D. H. (2008). Effect of couple illness perception congruence on psychological adjustment in women with rheumatoid arthritis. *Health Psychology, 27* (2), 221–9.

Story, L. B., & Bradbury, T. N. (2004) Understanding marriage and stress: Essential questions and challenges. *Clinical Psychology Review, 23*(8), 1139–62.

Strating, M. M. H, Van Duijin, M. A. J., Van Schuur, W. H., & Suurmeijer, T. P. B. M. (2007). The differential effects of rheumatoid arthritis on distress among patients and partners. *Psychology & Health, 22*(3), 361–79.

Suls, J., & Fletcher, B. (1985). The relative efficacy of avoidant and nonavoidant coping strategies: A meta-analysis. *Health Psychology, 4,* 249–88.

Suls, J., Green, P., Rose, G., Lounsbury, P., & Gordon, E. (1997). Hiding worries from one's spouse: Associations between coping via protective buffering and distress in male postmyocardial infarction patients and their wives. *Journal of Behavioral Medicine, 20,* 333–49.

Tennen, H., & Affleck, G. (1996). Daily processes in coping with chronic pain: Methods and analytic strategies. In M. Zeidner & N. S. Endler (Eds.), *Handbook of coping: Theory, research, applications* (pp. 151–71). New York: Wiley.

Tennen, H., Affleck, G., Armeli, S., & Carney, M. A. (2000). A daily process approach to coping: Linking theory, research, and practice. *American Psychologist, 55*(6), 626–36.

Tennen, H., Affleck, G., Coyne, J. C., Larsen, R. J., & DeLongis, A. (2006). Paper and plastic in daily diary research. *Psychological Methods, 11,* 112–8.

Thoits, P. A. (1986). Social support as coping assistance. *Journal of Consulting & Clinical Psychology, 54,* 416–23.

Ullrich, P. M., Lutgendorf, S. K., & Stapleton, J. T. (2002). Social constraints and depression in HIV infection: Effects of sexual orientation and area of residence. *Journal of Social and Clinical Psychology, 21*(1), 46–66.

Walen, H. R., & Lachman, M. E. (2000) Social support and strain from partner, family, and friends: Costs and benefits for men and women in adulthood. *Journal of Social and Personal Relationships, 17*(1), 5–30.

Widmer, K., Cina, A., Charvoz, L., Shantinath, S., & Bodenmann, G. (2005). A model dyadic-coping intervention. In T. A. Revenson, K. Kayser, & G. Bodenmann (Eds.), *Couples coping with stress: Emerging perspectives on dyadic coping* (pp. 159–74). Washington, DC: American Psychological Association.

Widows, M. R., Jacobsen, P. B., & Fields, K. K. (2000). Relation of psychological vulnerability factors to posttraumatic stress disorder symptomatology in bone marrow transplant recipients. *Psychosomatic Medicine, 62*(6), 873–82.

Ybema, J. F., Kuijer, R. G., Buunk, B. P., DeJong, G. M., & Sanderman, R. (2001). Depression and perceptions of inequity among couples facing cancer. *Personality and Social Psychology Bulletin, 27* (1), 3–13.

Yoshimoto, S. M., Ghorbani, S., Baer, J. M., Cheng, K. W., Banthia, R., Malcarne, V. L., & Varni, J. W. (2006). Religious coping and problem-solving by couples faced with prostate cancer. *European Journal of Cancer Care, 15*(5), 481–8.

Zakowski, S. G., Harris, C., Krueger, N., Laubmeier, K. K., Garrett, S., Flanigan, R., Johnson, P. (2003). Social barriers to emotional expression and their relations to distress in male and female cancer patients. *British Journal of Health Psychology, 8* (Pt 3), 271–86.

Zakowski, S. G., Ramati, A., Morton, C., Johnson, P., & Flanigan, R. (2004). Written emotional disclosure buffers the effects of social constraints on distress among cancer patients. *Health Psychology, 23*(6), 555–63.

PART 4

Models of Stress, Coping, and Positive and Negative Outcomes

Conservation of Resources Theory: Its Implication for Stress, Health, and Resilience

Stevan E. Hobfoll

Abstract

Conservation of resources (COR) theory has become one of the two leading theories of stress and trauma in the past 20 years, along with the pioneering theory of Lazarus and Folkman (1984). COR theory emphasizes objective elements of threat and loss, and *common* appraisals held jointly by people who share a biology and culture. This places central emphasis on objective reality and greater focus on circumstances where clear stressors are occurring, rather than a focus on personal appraisal. Although originally formulated to focus on major and traumatic stress, COR theory has also become a major theory in the field of burnout and the emerging field of positive psychology. This chapter reviews the principles of COR theory and covers new ground by examining more closely aspects of resource gain cycles and how they might contribute to resilience.

Keywords: resource loss, resource gain, engagement, resilience, major and traumatic stress

Conservation of resources (COR) theory has become one of the two leading theories of stress and trauma in the past 20 years, along with the pioneering theory of Lazarus and Folkman (1984). Although COR theory acknowledges that humans are appraising animals, COR theory departs markedly from Lazarus and Folkman's personal appraisal theory. Rather than emphasizing individual, idiographic appraisals, COR theory emphasizes objective elements of threat and loss, and *common* appraisals held jointly by people who share a biology and culture. This places much greater emphasis on objective reality, and greater focus on circumstances where clear stressors are occurring. Although originally formulated to focus on major and traumatic stress (Benight et al., 1999; Freedy, Saladin, Kilpatrick, Resnick, & Saunders, 1994; Freedy, Shaw, Jarrell, & Masters, 1992; Hobfoll, Canetti-Nisim, &

Johnson, 2006; Ironson et al., 1997; Kaiser, Sattler, Bellack, & Dersin, 1996; Norris, Perilla, Riad, Kaniasty, & Lavizzo, 1999). COR theory has also become a major theory in the field of burnout (Brotheridge & Lee, 2002; Buchwald & Hobfoll, 2004; Freedy & Hobfoll, 1994; Hobfoll & Freedy, 1993; Hobfoll & Shirom, 2001; Ito & Brotheridge, 2003; Neveu, 2007) and the emerging field of positive psychology (Bakker, Hakanen, Demerouti, & Xanthopoulou, 2007; Halbesleben & Bowler, 2007; Ito & Brotheridge, 2003; Jawahar, Stone, & Kisamore, 2007; Sun & Pan, 2008; Zellars, Perrewe, Hochwarter, & Anderson, 2006) as it has been applied to challenging work circumstances.

In this chapter, I review the principles of COR theory. I cover new ground by examining more closely aspects of resource gain cycles and how they might contribute to resilience. Although the concept of resilience has been around in psychology for decades, there is perhaps for the first time an empirical focus on thriving in the face of stress rather than on "not succumbing to stress." At the same time, we must be careful not to romanticize this striving, as our research already shows that the initial optimism about how many people are resilient in the face of major stress (Bonanno, Galea, Bucciarelli, & Vlahov, 2007) is greatly exaggerated in circumstances where stressors are more massive or chronic (Hobfoll et al., 2009).

I will begin by detailing the principles of COR theory. Within this context, I will integrate these principles with our most current understanding of how people react to major stress and challenge, and potential processes of resilience. By resilience I mean two things. First, I refer to people's ability to withstand the most negative consequences of stressful challenges, even the traumatic challenges they face. Second, I refer to the extent people remain vigorous, committed, and absorbed in important life tasks, even amidst significant challenge.

In the first instance, we are interested in who remains relatively free of depression, post-traumatic stress disorder (PTSD), and health problems in the face of stress and trauma. The second, question represents to me the more interesting question of who remains involved and committed in their life tasks, even if they might also be suffering from difficult emotions and experience health problems. That significant life challenges and losses cause psychological and physical distress is not surprising. That people with more resources experience less of such difficulty is important, but again not surprising. That people may experience distress and disease and yet remain committed and absorbed in their life tasks as parents, partners, workers, citizens, and friends is fascinating and something we know little about. I think it is nothing less than the next horizon for research in stress. I intend to theorize on this issue in this chapter and provide initial results from studies our research group have conducted in Israel and the Palestinian Authority, where people have been forced to survive and strive amidst war, terrorism, economic upheaval, military occupation, and a future that is not seen with great hope for peace.

Principles of Conservation of Resources Theory and Resiliency

COR theory is a motivational stress theory that broadly predicts a key axis that determines people's behavior. It is especially relevant to stressful challenges as I believe that stressful challenges are a key part of people's lives. Basic to COR theory is the premise that even when stress is not occurring, the knowledge of the future possibility of stress and challenge results in people being primed biologically, socially, cognitively, and culturally to attend to current, past, and future challenge as central to their experience in the world, their internal experience, and the biological development of the species itself. COR theory is based on several principles and corollaries that must be delineated to understand the theory and apply it to the context of stress and trauma. Unlike other stress theories, COR theory emphasizes the centrality of both loss and gain cycles, and that an understanding of both is critical to understanding how people respond to stress and their potential for resiliency.

COR theory begins with the tenet that individuals strive to obtain, retain, foster, and protect those things they centrally value. This tenet means that people employ key resources in order to conduct the regulation of the self, their operation of social relations, and how they organize, behave, and fit into the greater context of organizations and culture itself. This tenet suggests that this striving both is the normal course of human responding and occurs within the contexts of most behavior. It is critical at this juncture to state that what is centrally valued is universal and includes health, well-being, peace, family, self-preservation, and a positive sense of self, even if the core elements of sense of self differ culturally. Said another way, although psychology might emphasize individual differences, to the greatest extent behavior will be predicted by how humans are biologically, the context in which they find themselves, and the roles that exist within a certain cultural context. By extension, humans will exist in, build, foster, and protect social and societal systems that enable these same valued ends. COR theory next states several key principles that have been supported in literally hundreds of studies of stress and trauma (Hobfoll, 1988, 1989, 1998, 2001; Hobfoll & Lilly, 1993).

Principle 1: The primacy of resource loss. The first *principle of COR theory is that resource loss is disproportionately more salient than resource gain.* Resources include object resources (e.g., car, house), condition resources (e.g., employment, marriage), personal resources (e.g., key skills and personal traits such as self-efficacy and self-esteem), and energy resources (e.g., credit, knowledge, money). The disproportionate impact of resource loss is seen in both degree and speed of impact, as losses have large impact and typically also affect people at rapid and accelerating speed. It might appear counterintuitive to emphasize resource loss when this chapter largely focuses on resiliency. However, loss is primary in human systems, especially when objective circumstances signal loss, and past attempts to romanticize self-actualization and positive psychology, without attending to loss, threat, and stressful conditions, have had little real-world value. COR theory suggests instead that resilient responding must counteract or complement the powerful, usually rapid, and often long-term impact of resource loss.

The concept of resources risks becoming mundane and vague, as everything that might be helpful might be a resource, and indeed this is how Lazarus and Folkman (1984) defined resources. "Psychological stress is a particular relationship between the person and environment that is appraised by the person as taxing or exceeding his or her resources and endangering his or her well-being." (g. 19). But then on page 167, "The extent to which a person feels threatened is in part a function of his or her evaluation [i.e., appraisal] of coping resources " Hence, according to Lazarus and Folkman, stress occurs when resources cannot meet challenge and resources are those things we use to meet challenge, which I have argued is fully circular (Hobfoll, 1988, 1998). In order to move from individual appraisal to identify a general set of resources, we had numerous groups of people from many walks of life develop a list of resources that they found to be critical. Groups added, subtracted, and refined the list until future groups no longer added or subtracted resources that multiple prior groups had not already resolved (Hobfoll & Lilly, 1993). This became known as the COR-Evaluation (COR-E) and is included in Appendix 7.1. The list of 74 resources is seen as comprehensive but not all-inclusive. Clearly, if we use the scale to ask individuals about their experience of resource loss and gain, we are still relying on their appraisal, but even where the COR-E has been used for its most objective items on material loss following a hurricane, it was the single best predictor of psychological distress and immune compromise (Ironson et al., 1997).

Principle 2: Resource investment. The second principle of COR theory is that people must invest resources in order to protect against resource loss, recover from losses, and gain resources. A related corollary of this (*Corollary 1*) is that *those with greater resources are less vulnerable to resource loss and more capable of orchestrating resource gain. Conversely, those with fewer resources are more vulnerable to resource loss and less capable of resource gain.*

There are several sub-principles that emerge with Principle 2 of COR theory. The first and foremost of these is that the process of resource investment requires that people must build a pool of resources or have resources at their disposal. This has led to the concept within COR theory of resource caravans (Hobfoll, 1988, 1998). As people develop, they are ideally offered circumstances that share resources with them, imbue them with resources, and teach them how to foster and maintain resources. Nurturance, family stability, family safety, neighborhood and community safety, and what became popularized as "it takes a village to raise a child" exemplify this. But many families are in dire circumstances—where safety cannot be assumed, where resources are scarce, where schools are poor or non-existent, and where survival is more the order of the day. In several key studies Rutter (2000) showed that neighborhood factors far exceed the influence of family factors in predicting childhood psychopathology—said another way, a bad neighborhood and school is far more powerful than a good family. Psychology would have us think quite the opposite.

For those with resource-enriching environments, their caravan of resources, starting with a strong, loving family, begins to develop. Many of these resources are bestowed on children, but in time they learn skills that enable them to develop resources. They also are placed in safe passageways for their caravans. For this chapter, I will for the first time use this *caravan passageways* concept, although it is inherent in much of my past writing on COR theory.

Caravan passageways

Caravan passageways are the environmental conditions that support, foster, enrich, and protect the resources of individuals, families, and organizations, or that detract, undermine, obstruct, or impoverish people's resource reservoirs. Individuals and families are able to maintain and develop their resource caravans, or fail to develop and maintain them, mainly out of circumstances that are beyond their and their families' control. The likelihood of physical safety, good schools, wealth or relative wealth, safe leisure activities, or the cleanliness of streets, the availability of good employment, or of first-class medicine, the degree of crowdedness, the extent of pollution, clean water, the availability of playgrounds, or green spaces is not something that is so much chosen as given.

Inheritance is the principal mechanism by which caravan passageways are created and preserved. This inheritance is not only directly financial, although it is centrally related to financial wealth. The first form of inheritance of these passageways is *cultural capital*. This takes the forms of linguistic style, access to certain social circles, and aesthetic preferences that de facto become the signs and signature of status (Miller & McNamee, 1998). The second form of inheritance is through family processes and is termed *inter vivos* transfers, meaning gifts between those living. These transfers are especially important as they facilitate advancement and prevent crises at critical junctures in life that are the essence of any stressful life events list. Thus, these *inter vivos* transfers include paying for children's college, a first home, getting married, getting the right job, paying a critical bill that comes due, helping with childcare, buying a car needed for transport to work or school, paying for access to safe neighborhoods, assistance with health insurance or legal aid, or a much-needed vacation. Thus, if the best universities cost today over $200,000 for tuition and living expenses and people have two children on average, this represents a transfer of $400,000 of wealth. If a 2-year master's degree is added to this, the cost rises to over half a million dollars. Some of this is in the direct purchase of these, but it is often in trading favors and expectations of exchange for persons who belong to the same country club, social class, religion, or ethnic group, and also the exclusion of those who do not. This may take the form of the "important phone call" of a contact who is an "insider." The third kind of inheritance transfer is testamentary, occurring after a person has died, through the transfer of estates. As much as 80 percent of wealth in the United States is inherited, particularly if *in vivos* transfer is included, and much of the remaining wealth is assured through the process of cultural capital (i.e., the providing of the "right behavior, right family" for entrance to the "right club," legacy acceptances at universities, etc.) (Kalmijn & Kraaykamp, 1996).

How such passageways are inherited on broader community levels is exemplified in school and neighborhood factors. Schools in the United States are deeply affected by local family income. Thus, the *inter vivos* transfer of wealth in the form of cultural capital is instituted by financing schools locally. In an important way, this passageway of good education that is vital for producing so many resources for children and their future is insured by families; the tax for schools is largely dependent on community

wealth, and wealthy communities both highly value education and have the wealth to transfer to schools in the form of what is essentially a self-imposed tax. And of course schools also provide art education, music, team sports and quality coaching, supervised academic activities, mental health counselors, college preparation coursework, and college counselors. Hence, it is not surprising that the socioeconomic status (SES) of the school district and the typical class size are the best predictors of multiple school outcomes. Poorer neighborhoods have larger average classroom size, making the problem doubly bad for low-income schools (Fowler & Walberg, 1991).

These passageways have a clear influence on physical and mental health. SES is among the best predictors of mental health. Although the United States is the wealthiest large nation in the world, it ranks 50th in life expectancy (Central Intelligence Agency, 2009a) and 180th in infant mortality (Central Intelligence Agency, 2009b). This seeming contradiction is possible because, although the wealthy and middle class have very positive health attributes, the passageways related to poverty are so strong as to place the United States alongside many of the poorer nations in the world. The inheritance of these health passageways is a central explanatory factor in such outcomes (Dubner, 2008). As Gallo and Matthews (2003) note in their comprehensive review, low-SES environments not only are stressful, but they also reduce individuals' reserve capacity to manage stress, and increase vulnerability to negative emotions and cognitions. As such, lower SES results in fewer resources and at the same time is linked to greater stressful experiences and fewer positive experiences in everyday life (Gallo, Bogart, Vranceanu, & Matthews, 2005). This pattern can be observed in disasters. For example, those who were poorer were less likely to be resilient in the face of Hurricane Katrina, and also less likely to be insured, which in turn was almost as highly related to psychological distress as was loss of loved ones (Lee, Shen, & Tran, 2009). This process can also be seen in dealing with everyday stress in adolescents. Specifically, adolescents whose parents have more education tend to be more optimistic and use more engagement coping than children whose parents have less education, and these factors combine to lower perceived distress in the adolescents whose parents have more education (Finkelstein, Kubzansky, Capitman, & Goodman, 2007).

Psychology has considered families the foremost purveyor of passageways for resource development. Although families are important in this regard, neighborhood factors greatly supersede the impact of family factors (Rutter, 2000). This is why safe neighborhoods, good schools, and activities for youth are so important. Most families now have both parents working, and single-parent families are largely working, which results in even less supervision of children. Strong schools educate well and provide nutritious meals, physical warmth, activities that build character, and safety from gangs, violence, and rape. Studies show that a positive mentor such as a team coach can have an enormous impact on a child (Holt, Bry, & Johnson, 2008), and of course a good school might afford several such mentors. To understand the concept of passageways in which resource caravans are developed and nurtured, it would be a mistake to think that only the most disenfranchised or the wealthiest are affected. Those who are middle class are also most likely to stay within a similar middle-class passageway for resource caravans. They will attend fair to good schools, have reasonable neighborhood safety, have fair to good health insurance and services, and have access to fair to good colleges and jobs. But statistics also show that they will largely neither slide into poverty, nor obtain wealth and advantage (Pew Center, 2009). If individual differences such as drive, intelligence, self-efficacy, self-esteem, depression, anxiety, optimism, and other key individual factors were actually key in these processes, then there would be much greater mobility across social classes and the passageways that resources travel within. Indeed, the percent of low- and middle-income children who are able to enter Ivy League universities is declining, not increasing (Austin, 2006; Bowen, Kurzweil, & Tobin, 2005; Lewis, 1990). A new graduate with a master's of business administration (MBA) degree from the top 10 programs in the United States earn between $109,000 and $145,000 per year median pay (U.S. News and World Report, 2008). However, for the middle-class majority with MBAs, new jobs typically pay around $50,000 per year (Payscale, 2009). If one were to be ambitious, motivated, optimistic, and self-efficacious and have good social support, an evening or long-distance MBA program might be more common for the middle-class individual, and these of course pay less. So, even if achieving an MBA is one indication of white-collar, middle-class status, the passageways principle is seen as establishing rather robust, if not rigid, pathways for resource accumulation.

If the passageway to money is seen as too material an argument, one divorced from psychological or health outcomes (as might be assumed, as psychological studies more typically control for than examine SES), this argument is quickly countered with the findings for coronary heart disease—specifically, the worse off the neighborhood, the higher the incidence of heart disease (Diez Roux et al., 2001). Among Blacks who encounter many obstacles to resource passageways, the best Black neighborhoods have worse coronary heart statistics than the worst white neighborhoods (Diez Roux et al., 2001). In the well-known Whitehall studies of British civil servants, among white-collar, middle-class workers, none of whom were poor, mortality and morbidity rates ascended as social hierarchy levels descended (Marmot, Bosma, Hemingway, Brunner, & Stansfeld, 1997; Marmot, Shipley, & Rose, 1984). Of course, this still means that for Harlem in 1990, only 37 percent of Black men survived to age 65 if they reached the age of 15, compared to 77 percent for white men nationally (Geronimus, Bound, Waidmann, Hillemeier, & Burns, 1996). These statistics show that although the extremes of the effects of resource caravan passageways reveal shocking differences, at all levels of SES the passageways in which resources travel are key.

Caravan passageways and psychosocial resources

The impact of social support is one of the most robust single markers of resiliency resources, after SES and race are accounted for (Schumm, Briggs-Phillips, & Hobfoll, 2006). Indeed, in our own work in Israel and in the Palestinian Authority, we found that when stress is extreme and chronic, personal resources such as self-efficacy are outstripped (Hobfoll et al., in preparation; Palmieri, Galea, Canetti-Nisim, Johnson, & Hobfoll, 2008) but that the beneficial impact of social support remains robust. Social support contributes to the structure of resource passageways for children (Elias & Haynes, 2008; Warren, Jackson, & Sifers, 2009), adult members of the family (Schwarzer & Knoll, 2007), and the elderly (Fiksenbaum, Greenglass, & Eaton, 2006; Tomaka, Thompson, & Palacios, 2006). It does so through material support, instrumental support, good advice, and emotional support (Haber, Cohen, Lucas, & Baltes, 2007; Uchino, Cacioppo, & Kiecolt-Glaser, 1996).

The passageways concept also helps explain the high correlation among resources and why they tend to travel in resource caravans. Although there are quite different theories, for example, for self-esteem, self-efficacy, and optimism, these three key resources are highly inter-correlated (Luszczynska, Gutierrez-Dona, & Schwarzer, 2005; Xanthopoulou, Bakker, Demerouti, & Schaufeli, 2007). Indeed, the correlation is so high as to suggest that they are intimately tied to one another developmentally. Perhaps more surprising is that they are also substantively correlated with social support (Brissette, Scheier, & Carver, 2002; Miyamoto et al., 2001; Rogers, McAuley, Courneya, & Verhulst, 2008; Verhaeghe, Bracke, & Bruynooghe, 2008), further buttressing the argument that they are developed together and that the passageways in which these resource caravans travel tend to sustain their aggregation.

Principle 3. Principle 3 is paradoxical. Although resource loss is more potent than resource gain, the salience of gain increases under situations of resource loss (Wells, Hobfoll, & Lavin, 1999). This principle suggests that as people experience more resource loss, resource gain processes accelerate in speed and increase in magnitude of their effect. This paradoxical increase in resource gain saliency is accentuated during traumatic situations, as well as when stress begins to take its toll in the even slower, creeping process of burnout. This transformation in the strength and speed of gain cycles is critical to understanding the process inherent in resiliency efforts. This follows because under conditions of high loss, efforts that result in small gains may nevertheless elicit positive expectancy and hope, and reinforce and encourage further goal-directed efforts. In this manner, resource gains that under less stressful circumstances might be viewed as inconsequential become lifelines for survival and recovery.

New insights in this process are offered through the highly creative emerging work in engagement theory (Schaufeli, Salanova, Gonzalez-Roma, & Bakker, 2002), which I will address later in this chapter in some depth. Engagement may be the companion process to investigations on stress that has been missing since the inception of stress and coping theories. Engagement is certainly implied in some of the pioneering work of Lazarus and Folkman (1984) on coping, but their groundbreaking work may be advanced significantly by an understanding of engagement as both a process and an outcome. Like resiliency, I caution against romanticizing engagement, as it often occurs in conjunction with a difficult coping process that may on balance be more negatively experienced than positive. Nevertheless, it is engagement that may keep people "in the game," especially when major resource loss is experienced or anticipated.

Resource gains and family processes

The vital nature of resource gain can be used next to emphasize the critical role played by families in fostering passageways for resource caravans. The above-detailed argument posits that families are positioned within a certain sociocultural ecology in which the stage is largely set for resources external to the family. Some such ecologies are resource-rich and lend their resources to families generously. Other sociocultural ecologies are poor in social and financial capital and can afford families few resources. Worse, many sociocultural ecologies are dangerous and absorb many of the efforts of families just to stay afloat.

Because resource gains have greater impact amidst resource loss, this suggests that even poor families with few sociocultural resources can play a significant role in creating resource passageways for their children. After the early years when children are mainly home-centered, the tasks that children and adolescents face are how to succeed in school, with peers, with sports, and with moving into the employment world. Families are not the sole influence here by any means, but families play a major role in supporting children for these life tasks and fostering self-esteem, self-efficacy, optimism, and social skillfulness (Cooper, Holman, & Braithwaite, 1983; Frodi, Bridges, & Grolnick, 1985; Grolnick & Ryan, 1989; Openshaw, Thomas, & Rollins, 1984). This central role of families holds true for the adult members of the family as well. In this regard, families filter and translate the meaning of challenges faced in the world. Is a job seen as a sign of success or "not good enough"? Is the money available seen as enough, even if truly never enough, or are financial concerns (shortfalls) seen as a sign of failure? Are the pathways to aging seen as normal, or a sign of decline and invalidity?

These questions are critical to COR theory and are a potential bridge-points between COR theory and appraisal theory (Lazarus & Folkman, 1984). Because much of what occurs to us is ambiguous and many threats are vague, key loved ones (i.e., parents, spouses, adult children) become the translator of meaning. It is far beyond this chapter to discuss the aspects of families that operate here, but they have much to do with the *culture* or *climate* of the family. Is the family optimistic, do they back family members in a supportive, loving manner, are most efforts "good enough," "not good enough," or "great, wonderful"? Key elements of this include family stability, flexibility, positivity, clarity (Henry, 1994; Mathis & Tanner, 1991;

Sokolowski & Israel, 2008; Windle & Jacob, 2007). There is good evidence that families that are characterized by conflict, aggression, coldness, lack of supportiveness, and neglect are vulnerable and have poor stress responding (Repetti, Taylor, & Seeman, 2002), but less is known about how the reverse of these attributes serves to produce resiliency in children who they carry on in their lives.

Here we see the crux of the difficulty for many families. In a chapter several years ago, we argued that the psychological study of hope had little to do with hope (Hobfoll, Briggs-Phillips, & Stines, 2003) but instead was a matter of "betting the odds." What I mean by this is that if things have always gone well and resources are ample, it is not a sign of hope to be hopeful; rather, it is simply betting with the odds. For families who lack resources, the question of whether the future is bright or threatening takes on a completely different meaning. For middle-class children, it is reasonable to believe that with family resources, the future should look bright, or at least positive, given even significant challenges. For many families, however, this is a much more difficult appraisal to make, as the reality of their world may paint a much different picture, making this a much more challenging family culture to create. We still know little about how families shape stress resiliency, but we know much about what resources do need to be shaped, and the study of families and individuals nested in their socioecology would be an area of enormous research potential.

Resource loss and gain spirals

The first two principles of COR theory concerning loss primacy and investment of resources, in turn, lead to two key corollaries pertaining to resource loss and gain spirals (Hobfoll, 1988, 1998). Understanding these principles changes the approach to stress and trauma from a static process to an active process of striving to fulfill important roles, achieve important goals, and offset a sense of despair.

Corollary 2 of COR theory states that not only are those who lack resources more vulnerable to resource loss, but that initial loss begets future loss.

Corollary 3 mirrors Corollary 2, stating that those who possess resources are more capable of gain, and that initial resource gain begets further gain. However, because loss is more potent than gain, loss cycles will be more influential and more accelerated than gain cycles.

Research on stress has tended to look at stressors singularly or additively. COR theory suggests, however, that resource loss cycles tend to occur because stress entails resource loss and because resources must be invested to offset further resource loss. These loss cycles not only are seen as momentous, but also have accelerating speed (Ennis, Hobfoll, & Schroder, 2000; Norris & Kaniasty, 1996). Further, these loss cycles extend across the life cycle for decades and lifetimes (Schumm, Stines, Hobfoll, & Jackson, 2005). These cycles occur both because the emotional impact of major and traumatic stress is long term and because major stress and trauma eat away at key resiliency resources and limit the establishment of new resource reservoirs (Schumm et al., 2005).

These loss cycles can be seen in the lives of women who were abused as children. Not only are these women more likely to suffer from PTSD and depression decades later (Gibb et al., 2001; Schumm et al., 2005), but also they have also been found to be about five times more likely to be raped as adults (Schumm, Hobfoll, & Keogh, 2004). Further, abuse results in a continued loss of key resources, the very resources needed for resiliency (Johnson, Palmieri, Jackson, & Hobfoll, 2007). As adults, they are more likely than women who were not abused to suffer more life stress, and to react more negatively to those stressors (Schumm et al., 2005). Also, those women who had "only" experienced child abuse or adult rape were 6 times more likely to have probable PTSD as adults, whereas women who experienced both child abuse and adult rape were 17 times more likely to have probable PTSD than women who had experienced neither (Schumm et al., 2006), suggesting the multiplicative element of loss cycles. Further, women with PTSD symptoms were found to have over three times the likelihood of incident coronary heart disease than women with no PTSD symptoms (Kubzansky, Koenen, Jones, & Eaton, 2009), illustrating that trauma history cross-cycles into a critical health domain.

Traumatic Growth and Where it Did not Lead Us

In recent years, there has been an increased interest in positive psychology and who might do well amidst stressful environments (Peterson, Park, & Seligman, 2006; Peterson & Seligman, 2003; Seligman & Csikszentmihalyi, 2000). Thus, even where resource loss is omnipresent and where individuals exist within passageways where it is difficult to foster and protect resources, many individuals still do "well enough." To examine the positive impact of resource gains, we began several years ago to explore traumatic growth in our work on war and terrorism with the full expectation that it would be linked to resiliency. We conceptualized post-traumatic growth (PTG) as finding benefits in terms of psychosocial resource gains following exposure to the threat of war and terrorism. PTG is defined as "positive psychological change experienced as a result of the struggle with highly challenging life circumstances" (Tedeschi, 2004, p. 1). PTG is thought to be more than a return to pre-trauma functioning following a traumatic event, but rather to achieving an enhanced level of functioning, sense of meaning or spirituality, and closer relationships than before the traumatic event occurred (Linley & Joseph, 2004).

Using a modified form of the COR-E, we framed our questions similarly to Tedeschi and Calhoun (Calhoun & Tedeschi, 2006; Tedeschi & Calhoun, 1995) in their pioneering work on traumatic growth. We asked respondents, "As a result of the Intifada [terrorist uprising], do you have more . . .: "intimacy with one or more family members," "intimacy with spouse/partner," "intimacy with at least one friend," "hope," "feelings that your life has purpose," and "more confidence in your ability to do things." This short scale essentially captures growth in the three domains of self-perception, interpersonal relationships, and philosophy of life posited by Tedeschi and Calhoun (1995) and has been shown adequate psychometric properties (α = .82) in studies we conducted in Israel (Hobfoll et al., 2006). Further, this scale also correlated at .85 with the full version of the Post-Traumatic Growth Inventory by Tedeschi and Calhoun (Hall & Hobfoll, 2008).

Leading theorists on PTG posited that PTG and psychological distress are orthogonal, and some studies support this viewpoint (Tedeschi, 2004). However, in their own research of war survivors where they argued this orthogonal viewpoint, different factors derived from their scale told a very different story. Specifically, one subscale was positively correlated with PTSD, one was negatively correlated, and one was not correlated (Powell, Rosner, Butollo, & Tedeschi, 2003). Moreover, a recent meta-analysis of many of the best studies on PTG to date found that PTG was related to greater symptoms of PTSD, particularly re-experiencing symptoms (e.g., intrusive thoughts and images) (Helgeson, Reynolds, & Tomich, 2006).

Hence, it is not altogether clear whether PTG has positive benefit, or whether, at least in some instances, it is a defensive attempt to find some good where benefit has not in actuality occurred. As Zoellner and Maerchker (2006) have written, the relationships of PTG to mental health is paramount because "If posttraumatic growth is a phenomenon worthy to be studied in clinical research, it is assumed to make a difference in people's lives by affecting levels of distress, well-being, or other areas of mental health. If it does not have any impact [on these], PTG might just be an interesting phenomenon possibly belonging to the areas of social, cognitive, or personality psychology." (p. 631). As they argued, if PTG does not have adaptive significance it is questionable whether it should be promoted. We find it is reported in a vast majority of those who experience trauma, but that does not mean it is a good thing because we have, by naming it so, described it as beneficial.

In our first study of PTG in Israel, we examined the impact of the Al Aqsa Intifada on Israeli Jews and Arabs (Hobfoll et al., 2006). We nationally sampled Israelis using random digit dialing during September 2003. Our sample included 720 Jewish and 185 Arab citizens of Israel (Arab citizens of Israel constitute 19.6 percent of the Israeli population [not including the West Bank and Gaza]) (Central Bureau of Statistics, 2002). We relied on structured telephone interviews to assess post-traumatic symptoms (PTS), terrorism exposure, the perception of PTG, and several constructs related to outgroup biases, including ethnocentrism, authoritarianism, and support for extreme political violence. We included the political variables as they are potentially important psychological outcomes, at least in terms of how they might relate to support for continuing conflict. We especially wanted to examine how these political attitudes and beliefs related to PTG. We argued that if PTG represented growth as its humanistic theoretical base has framed it (Frankl, 1959), it would be related to a less authoritarian, less ethnocentric, and less aggressively violent approach to the self and the conflict. If, in contrast, it represented a more fundamental, primitive form of coping, it would be positively associated with this violent and retaliatory triad.

We found that those who experienced greater exposure to terrorism also reported greater psychosocial resource loss and greater PTG. In turn, those who experienced greater psychosocial resource loss and greater PTG reported greater PTS and depression symptoms. We further found that greater PTG was related directly or indirectly to greater ethnic exclusionism, greater support for political violence, and greater authoritarianism. Because the study was cross-sectional, it is possible that greater PTG was a response to greater PTS. However, the fact that PTG was related to greater ethnocentrism, authoritarianism, and support for extreme political violence is more difficult to justify as indicating a process of resiliency. Said another way, even if we had found PTG to be related to lower psychological distress, its relation with the promotion of hatred and extreme violence would demand revision of wholly positive models of PTG.

We continued our research during August and September 2004 on a sample of 1,070 Jews and 392 Arab citizens of Israel, essentially replicating our earlier telephone interview methodology (Hobfoll et al., 2008). In this study, we examined several additional questions. Specifically, we examined whether those who were directly exposed to greater terrorism and who reported PTG might experience lower rates of probable PTSD. This was a logical step in our program of research, as directly exposed individuals were more deeply traumatized by events, and therefore might benefit more from PTG. Second, we examined whether our findings for PTG held for both those directly and indirectly exposed to terrorism, as others have argued that PTG has more positive impact for those with high levels of trauma exposure (McMillen, Smith, & Fisher, 1997).

In this study we found that rates of probable PTSD were high for Jews (6.6 percent) and extremely high among Arab citizens of Israel (18 percent). For Jews, we found higher rates of PTSD for those with higher income, traditional religiosity (as opposed to secular or highly religious), greater economic loss due to terrorism, greater psychosocial loss, greater PTG, and less social support. So, once again, PTG was among the vulnerability factors. For Arabs, lower education and greater psychosocial loss were related to higher rates of probable PTSD. Analyses for the entire sample and those directly exposed to terrorism revealed quite similar results. That is, among Jews who were more directly exposed to terrorism, higher PTG was also related to higher rates of probable PTSD. Although few variables in the model were significant for Arabs, many of the same trends existed among Arabs, and would likely have been significant if their sample size was equivalent to that for Jews.

This study supported our prior findings for a positive association of PTG with PTSD diagnosis in models that controlled for other key factors. That PTG was associated with a greater likelihood of probable PTSD diagnosis may indicate that PTG is a response to PTS symptoms, but not one that shows either an orthogonal or a palliative association. Also, because we controlled for exposure, economic resource loss, and psychosocial resource

loss, it cannot be interpreted that the relationship of PTG with PTSD is an artifact of PTG being more common among those more highly exposed.

In the next study, we wanted to explore these questions in a stronger, prospective design and look more carefully at resiliency (Hobfoll et al., 2009). That is, we wanted to examine whether PTG was related to *not* developing symptoms of PTSD and depression or, if developing symptoms, of early recovery. This can be contrasted to what virtually all research on trauma has looked at, which is whether people develop the disorder—that is, high levels of symptoms. We interviewed 709 Israeli Jews and Arabs at two time periods during the Intifada, in 2004 to 2005, in a similar manner to what I have already described. At the time of the initial assessment, terrorism was quite active, whereas at the second time point terrorism had subsided to a significant degree, albeit still to a level that was objectively threatening.

A sizable minority of individuals in this study displayed what we called a resistance trajectory (22.1%), having no more than one symptom of depression and no more than one PTS symptom at either time point. A second group (13.5%) of individuals showed what we termed a resilience trajectory. Specifically, these individuals were not initially resistant, but became relatively free of symptoms over the period of study. Unfortunately, the most common trajectory was that of chronic distress (54.0%), whereby individuals reported experiencing more than one symptom of depression and/or PTS. That is, they were not necessarily in the clinical range of symptoms (although some were), but they had significant symptomatology. Finally, an additional group of individuals displayed what we called a delayed distress trajectory. These individuals were initially resistant (i.e., rather symptom-free), but developed symptoms over the period of study (10.3%).

Thus, our results for resiliency compare well to those of Bleich et al. (Bleich, Gelkopf, & Solomon, 2003), who found that 14.4% of an Israeli sample were resistant, as defined by an absence of symptoms assessed at one time point. They contrast, distinctly, however, with research by Bonanno et al. (Bonanno, Galea, Bucciarelli, & Vlahov, 2006), who found that resistance of Manhattan residents following the World Trade Center attacks, defined by an absence of symptoms assessed at one time point, was not less than 50% for most groups and never fell below one third for even the most exposed groups. This suggests that the more optimistic levels of resiliency found by Bonanno and colleagues may hold for individuals exposed to a single traumatic episode, but that chronic and ongoing exposure of the type found in Israel takes an increasing toll on resiliency.

As COR theory predicted, those who experienced less psychosocial resource loss at either time point were more likely to report being resistant or resilient, and resource loss was the strongest and most consistent predictor of outcomes. Further, men, those with higher income, those with higher education, and those from the majority group (Jews) also were more likely to be in the resilient or resistant trajectory groups. Those who had greater social support from friends also were more likely to be in the resistance and resilience trajectories. As we had also found for PTG in earlier studies, those reporting greater PTG were more likely to be in the chronic or delayed distress groups, and less likely to be in either the resistant or resilient trajectory groups. This means that not only did PTG relate to greater distress, it also related to not becoming relieved from distress, and increasing in distress over time. We further examined the trajectories for those who reported consistent PTG over time, as some have theorized that this is a more genuine form of PTG. The same negative findings held for this group.

Although we had not found PTG to have a positive impact on mental health in several of our studies, we continued to believe that for some, PTG would be a more genuine, salutary process. In line with theorizing of Viktor Frankl (1959) and more recently of Deci and Ryan's self-determination theory (Deci & Ryan, 1985, 1991, 2000), we looked for an opportunity to test what we saw as "action growth." That is, when such individuals reported PTG, it would be represented in a course of action, not just a cognitive view of themselves. We hypothesized that those who could assert PTG cognitively, and act upon their beliefs behaviorally, might find PTG protective.

During 2005, Israel decided upon a policy to disengage from Gaza, directly against the will of the Jews that settled there and had lived "reclaiming the Biblical land of Israel," against a background of constant threat and violence. To enact this policy, the Israeli government was put into the position to have to forcibly remove the settlers in Gaza. For the settlers, this policy was to destroy the dream they had worked so hard for and for which they had risked so much. It was also terribly upsetting because this policy was being enacted by the same leadership that had encouraged and engineered the policy of their settlement, so it was also a betrayal. Those who stayed to resist the forced evacuation could be seen as practicing growth-related actions, as they were taking actions for a cause amidst threat. Further, as a united group, we also argued that their actions fit Frankl's and Deci and Ryan's models by virtue of their actions being collective, thus reinforcing the attachment aspects of PTG.

We conducted telephone interviews with 190 settlers (Hall et al., 2008) in the days prior to the forced evacuation. Placing this in historical context, most settlers, the government, and the media thought it would be a period of marked violence, and included threats of civil war. As might be expected, the rates of probable PTSD increased markedly from 6.5% to 26.3% and probable major depression rose from 3.2% to 27.4%, compared to earlier, separate samples we had from this region. Also, as we had found previously, and supporting COR theory, the highest rates of probable PTSD and depression diagnosis were found among settlers who reported the greatest psychosocial and economic resource loss. In examining the impact of PTG, we found that PTG was related in a stepwise fashion to PTSD diagnosis and depression diagnosis, with each increase in levels of PTG bringing a decrease in disorder. Indeed, an increase in one standard deviation below the mean to one standard deviation above the mean on PTG decreased the relative odds of probable PTSD diagnosis by 63%. We have no other explanation for this difference in these findings from those we found previously, except the differences in the communal action of these settlers, versus the cognitive stance of those in the prior studies.

We have come to believe that rather than PTG being a kind of benefit-finding for the purpose of growth, it may be better explained by terror management theory (Greenberg, Pyszczynski, & Solomon, 1986; Hall, Hobfoll, Canetti-Nisim, Johnson, & Galea, in press). Terror management theory argues that people are sensitive to cues that remind them of the inevitability of their own death and nonexistence (Becker, 1973; Greenberg et al., 1986) and that when these thoughts are evoked, they produce existential terror and anxiety. Cultures counter these anxieties with worldviews that "consist of humanly constructed beliefs about reality shared by individuals in groups that provide a sense that one is a person of value in a world of meaning" (Solomon, Greenberg, & Pyszczynski, 2004, p. 17). In this manner, individuals may lower their sense of anxiety and terror by finding greater meaning in their worldview, but these worldviews are counters to their fears. When the fear is of an enemy or outgroup, then PTG would take the form of affiliation with groups and messages that form a defense against the outgroup; even if that defense is violent and full of hate, the hatred is justified as a good, as hatred of one's enemies is often construed as a form of patriotism. Linked with our finding that in most cases PTG is related to greater PTSD and depression symptoms, and decreased resiliency prospectively, we believe that the evidence is that outside of the possible effects of growth-related actions, at least in the context of war and terrorism, PTG is related to more negative outcomes and more rigid, aggressive coping (Hall et al., in press; Hobfoll et al., 2006).

Engagement and Resiliency

Although we have found little beneficial impact of PTG, our continued interest in positive psychology led us to interest in *engagement* as the inverse of burnout and other distress-indicative processes (Schaufeli et al., 2002). Schaufeli et al.'s (2002) conceptualization of engagement is instructive and informs the potential for understanding the resiliency process, even extending to engagement in the face of traumatic stress. *Engagement* is defined as a persistent, pervasive, and positive affective-motivational state of fulfillment in individuals who are reacting to challenging circumstances (Schaufeli et al., 2002). Engagement is further conceptualized as a product of three dimensions—*vigor, dedication,* and *absorption.*

Dedication is depicted within the engagement framework as the commitment to key life tasks. In the case of major and traumatic stressors, it includes dedication to family, work, organizations, society, and the preservation of the self. *Absorption* is defined as the sense of full involvement and even excitement over life tasks. It also implies a process where one is so absorbed that one loses sense of time. This level of absorption is seen both as satisfying to individuals, as well as aiding the problem-solving process. This raises an important insight from the engagement conceptualization that has often been absent from the stress and coping literature—that is, how successful individuals behave (or function) in the face of stress at accomplishing the life and work tasks that they and life set before them. When people are absorbed in a major challenge, they often lose the sense of time and problem-solving is maximized. This links back to earlier work on test anxiety, which focused both on anxiety and test-taking success (Sarason &

Stoops, 1978). To the extent that people are worried about what might happen or has happened, they become less absorbed in the task before them and likely less capable of performing complex tasks.

Vigor, in turn, refers to high levels of energy and mental resilience when meeting life challenges. Shirom (2006) suggests that vigor is the fundamental element of this process and that, if it occurs, the issues of absorption and commitment are secondary, and even an artifact of vigor. We have argued that when addressing the consequences of terrorism and war, however, absorption and commitment may be more fundamental, as it is critical that individuals and the society at large continue their involvement and sustaining of key life tasks (Hobfoll, Hall, Horsey, & Lamoureux, in press).

The critical nature of loss in engagement

What has so often occurred in the current and prior positive psychology movements is a mirror image of what they criticize—that is, forgetting that both growth and psychopathology are interlinked, co-occur, and affect each other. Moreover, the most interesting phenomenon in positive psychology is the existence of positive, energetic processes amidst difficult challenges where people are often quite distressed. Engagement requires the very resources that are often being lost or are already overcommitted in facing difficult life challenges.

The attendant principle from COR theory for the engagement side of the continuum is that people must have the personal and environmental capacity to invest if they are to navigate and succeed at their engagement while they are dealing with life's everyday or more major vicissitudes. This suggests that they need a strong armamentarium of material, social, personal, and energy resources, and they must have the capacity to attend to the engagement process in terms of time and access. If stressful demands are too high, people often must choose to exit engagement processes in favor of meeting survival demands, or even the demands of a serious challenge. Hence, for example, people often must leave work to care for an ill parent, may not have the money or wardrobe to go to work, or must leave school and stay with a mundane job in order to meet financial responsibilities. Time with potential supporters may need to be sacrificed, not because people want to be socially isolated, but because any free time must be dedicated to addressing stressful environmental circumstances. COR theory also suggests that these steps are taken in a strategic way before resources are drained in order to conserve resources for future demands.

Nevertheless, it is important to highlight that COR theory suggests that gain cycles, as embodied within the engagement framework, also build on themselves. Hence, as people make resource gains and successfully experience the rewards of dedication and absorption, they experience more positive health and well-being and become more capable of further investing resources into the engagement process. With few resource reserves, people will naturally take a conservative investment approach, but as their resource reservoir strengthens they will be more likely to take resource investment risks. But again, as protecting against loss is always more powerful and salient than developing resource gains, this process will remain a conservative one, especially where there is a history of resource loss or where environmental conditions continue to be threatening.

Supportive environments create passageways for engagement

Families, workplaces, schools, and neighborhoods play a crucial role in increasing the likelihood of sustained engagement, especially where individuals may be lacking their own resources or where they have undergone rapid or chronic resource loss. A supportive environment often provides essential conditions for fostering people's engagement. Supportive environments provide such conditions as meaningful goals, share resources that may be lacking, give guidance on how to successfully engage, and potentially include individuals in the shared opportunities for success of the social unit (Csikszentmihalyi, 1997; Sonnentag & Lange, 2002). Hence, organizations that share high levels of work resources are likely to have higher levels of individual and team engagement (Bakker, van Emmerik, & Euwema, 2006).

An example of this comes from the respite literature for families who are caring for an individual who has chronic needs and thus makes chronic demands on the families. Respite care steps in to responsibly provide care, allowing the family to meet other task demands, or just rejuvenate themselves with rest and leisure (Lund, Utz, Caserta, & Wright, 2009). Even for those employees who are high in engagement, the ability to detach from work to "recharge their batteries" during non-work time was related to positive affective states. Often, in high-demand environments, it is the greater social unit that must provide support that is beyond individual or family capacity. For example, following Katrina, the state government of Mississippi took legal action against large insurance companies who

were not responding properly within the terms of their policies with those affected by the disaster. How critical this is can be seen from earlier research by Ironson et al. (1997), who found that time to insurance payment was one of the strongest predictors of mental health outcomes after a hurricane.

There are instances when loss cycles and engagement cycles co-occur, and if the loss cycle is not contained it will undermine the engagement cycle. For example, Bakker, Hakanen, Demerouti, and Xanthopoulou (2007) found that teachers with high resources were engaged whether or not they were coping with high levels of misbehavior in the classroom. In contrast, those with low resources were engaged only if children were well behaved. Engagement was overwhelmed when demand was high and resources low. That these loss and engagement cycles are intertwined is illustrated in a study of platinum mine workers in South Africa (Rothmann & Joubert, 2007). Here it was found that job resources such as autonomy, good communication, and organizational support were related to lower levels of worker burnout and higher engagement, and that burnout undermined worker engagement. Similarly, a recent study in the automotive industry found that an abusive supervisor virtually cancelled out the positive impact of workers' engagement on their work performance (Harris, Kacmar, Zivnuska, & Shaw, 2007).

How these multiple resource loss versus engagement pathways operate is illustrated in one of the few studies that examine stress and engagement over time in an organization (de Lange, De Witte, & Notelaers, 2008). Employees with low resources from work and low autonomy in their job were disengaged and tended to move out of the company. Those with high engagement tended to move into areas of their company with even higher available resources and tended to seek environments that were richer in resources.

In an entirely different context, positive psychological states have been studied in terms of how they affect caregivers' recovery after the death of their partner from AIDS (Moskowitz, Folkman, Collette, & Vittinghoff, 1996). They found that the ability to attain the positive psychological states of productivity and focused attention shortly after bereavement had a significant impact on shortening the course of depressive mood and recovery of positive mood states. As suggested by Fredrickson's (1998) broaden-and-build theory, positive emotions are linked to greater exploration and goal-setting and more flexible thinking and generally broaden thinking. However, as Zautra, Reich, and Gaurnaccia (1990) note, it may be positive events that sustain positive affect—hence the importance of resource gain cycles. COR theory also places secondary emphasis on gain cycles, but would emphasize that positive emotions have difficulty being sustained when resource loss is severe or chronic, especially where other key resources, such as social support, cannot be brought to bear. Further, resource lack or loss over time will impair people's ability to find and sustain positive environments that provide positive affect-enhancing experiences.

Although to date most studies on engagement have occurred within organizational and work environments, it is likely that these findings would extend to other environments where there is high challenge and demand. The link between engagement and positive emotions might then be explored to better understand how some individuals manage to be engaged and experience vigor, dedication, and absorption, leading to sustained problem-solving, and something we know even less about—creative problem-solving of major life challenges. The link to positive emotions and supportive environmental contexts should generalize to other contexts, as Fredrickson found in the aftermath of September 11 (Fredrickson, Tugade, Waugh, & Larkin, 2003) and Moskowitz et al. (1996) noted for caregivers to dying individuals with AIDS.

We have begun to explore this in the high-stress-and-trauma environment of the Palestinian Authority. Israel occupation, internecine warfare, and severe economic and infrastructure destruction have made this a highly stressful environment for decades, and both the Israel response to the Intifada and the increase in internal political struggle have made it worse in recent years. We conducted face-to-face interviews of 1,196 individuals in the West Bank and Gaza from September 16, 2007, to November 1, 2008, in a three-wave panel study. We hoped to explore how trauma exposure and resource loss directly reduced engagement, and how they reduced engagement via their influence on PTS and depression symptoms. At the same time, we wanted to study the more positive pathways, such that social support and self-efficacy might contribute to reduced PTS and depression symptoms and increase engagement.

Our findings (Hobfoll et al., in preparation) were illuminating and support our theorizing in a number of ways. First, many people do continue to be engaged, even amidst the chaos and trauma of this environment. So, engagement was fairly evenly distributed, and as many people were in the high range on the scale as in the low range. The average level of engagement was slightly above what would be the halfway score on the scale, so it can be said that on average more people fell on the engaged end of the continuum than the disengaged. We also found that psychosocial resource loss was the primary predictor of PTS and depression symptoms. Further, psychosocial resource loss directly related to lower-level engagement nearly 2 years later, and resource loss indirectly reduced engagement through its influence on depression. Social support also influenced engagement, as we had theorized, and the effect of social support on engagement was both direct and through its influence on limiting later depression. Notably, engagement was principally a function of depression and the depressive aspects of PTSD and not the other aspects of PTSD.

It was also notable that self-efficacy did not play a significant role in influencing engagement. It is possible that Arabs, having a more communal culture, find self-efficacy less important. However, we found that in severe and chronic circumstances, self-efficacy tended to have a limited influence among Jews in Israel (Palmieri et al., 2008), who are more individualistic in culture. It is possible that self-efficacy is outstripped in circumstances where individualist effort is thwarted by such overwhelming political circumstances. We of course must be cautious about making any conclusions, as we believe this is the first study of these processes.

It is critical to note that depression and engagement were not highly related, with less than 10 percent overlap, suggesting that many people who are depressed remain engaged. This is a critical finding as it indicates how people stay committed and involved in life tasks, even amidst significant trauma exposure and chronically stressful environmental conditions, where many believe there is little hope for this to change. This is quite the opposite of the original hopelessness formulation, and it is interesting that Seligman (2000) has revised his thinking on the hopelessness concept, placing much greater emphasis on optimism.

Conclusions

COR theory emphasizes the real things that occur in people's lives that challenge them, and the real things that result in their accumulation of resource reservoirs. Yet continued emphasis in the stress literature is placed on the perception of stress and on individual differences. It is my belief that this stems largely on the fact that stress, challenge, and resources are measured through questions rather than direct observation. Moreover, these observations would have to be long term, multi-perspective, and from all viewpoints. When we ask people their perceptions that is largely what they will give us, because people are good if imperfect cataloguers of events. One could similarly argue that if we filmed people, that life film is the best predictor of stress. If we solely ask their appraisals, then we will conclude that appraisals are key.

People with different resources will view threats and their likely success in meeting challenges differently. However, as I argued here and elsewhere, the resources upon which such appraisals are based are largely the result of real occurrence in their lives and the caravan passageways that were given them. Those who are optimistic usually have reason to be optimistic based on the realities that mark their lives.

Nevertheless, it is fascinating that some people, given a modicum of support, will continue to remain vigorous, absorbed, and committed to the tasks that face them, even while they are challenged with chronic, traumatic conditions. What interests me in Frederickson's (1998) broaden-and-build theory is not that positive emotions lead to positive ends. Rather, COR theory would ask: To what extent can people who face trauma and generally lack resources remain creative, engaged, and hopeful? The answer here may be that positive emotions will be common among those with the most resources or who have experienced the least resource loss. But it is at least possible that a glimmer of hope and positive emotion may have a germinal effect on creativity, a search for building on that positive emotion, and a reaching out to others.

Of all our recent research, I am most intrigued by that fact that although depression and engagement are correlated, they are not highly correlated. This means that despite experiencing traumatic or major life stress, people are seldom helpless, and helplessness is an unlikely course, even when stress is major and chronic (Folkman, 1997). At some basic level, people have to know that they must be committed to their work, their families, and the tasks that they or life has set before them. A recent novel by Steven Galloway, *The Cellist of Sarajevo*, tells the true story of Vedran Smailovic, the principal cellist of the Sarajevo opera, when the city was under siege in the 1990s.

At 4:00 pm on May 27th, 1992, a long line of starving people waiting in front of the only bakery in Sarajevo that still had enough flour to make bread were shelled. Twenty-two people died as Vedran Smailovic stood at his window a hundred yards away and watched.

The next day hungry people lined up again to beg for bread—certain they would die if they didn't come to the bakery and convinced they could die if they did. Then it happened. Vedran Smailovic arrived. He was dressed in the black suit and white tie in which he had played every night until the opera theater was destroyed. He was carrying his cello and a chair.

Smailovic sat down in the square and, surrounded by debris and the remainders of death and the despair of the living, he began to play the mournful Albinoni "Adagio," the one music manuscript that had been found whole in the city after the carpet bombing of Dresden.

What's more, shelling or no, he came back to the square every day after that for 21 consecutive days (one day for each of the people that had died) to do the same thing, a living reminder that there is a strength in the human spirit that simply cannot be destroyed. Today, where he sat, there is a monument of a man in a chair playing a cello. But the monument is not to his music, as good as it is. It is to his refusal to surrender the hope that beauty could be reborn in the midst of a living hell. Even more important, perhaps, is the fact that that small sound of hope rings on still around the world. (Chittister, 2009).

Author Note

This chapter was made possible, in part, by grants from NIMH (R01 MH073687) and by support of the Judd and Marjorie Weinberg Presidential Chair at Rush Medical College.

I would also like to thank my colleague Brian Hall for his assistance and insightful feedback on the manuscript. I remain responsible for all errors and poorly expressed ideas.

References

Austin, A. (2006). Ivy league price-fixing: Conflict from the intersection of education and commerce. *St. John's University Journal of Legal Commentary, 21*, 1–55.

Bakker, A. B., Hakanen, J. J., Demerouti, E., & Xanthopoulou, D. (2007). Job resources boost work engagement, particularly when job demands are high. *Journal of Educational Psychology, 99*(2), 274–84.

Bakker, A. B., van Emmerik, H., & Euwema, M. C. (2006). Crossover of burnout and engagement in work teams. *Work and Occupations, 33*(4), 464–89.

Becker, E. (1973). *The denial of death.* New York: Simon & Schuster

Benight, C. C., Ironson, G., Klebe, K., Carver, C. S., Wynings, C., Burnett, K., et al. (1999). Conservation of resources and coping self-efficacy predicting distress following a natural disaster: A causal model analysis where the environment meets the mind. *Anxiety, Stress & Coping: An International Journal, 12*(2), 107–26.

Bleich, A., Gelkopf, M., & Solomon, Z. (2003). Exposure to terrorism, stress-related mental health symptoms, and coping behaviors among a nationally representative sample in Israel. *JAMA: Journal of the American Medical Association, 290*(5), 612–20.

Bonanno, G. A., Galea, S., Bucciarelli, A., & Vlahov, D. (2006). Psychological resilience after disaster: New York City in the aftermath of the September 11th terrorist attack. *Psychological Science, 17*(3), 181–6.

Bonanno, G. A., Galea, S., Bucciarelli, A., & Vlahov, D. (2007). What predicts psychological resilience after disaster? The role of demographics, resources, and life stress. *Journal of Consulting and Clinical Psychology, 75*(5), 671–82.

Bowen, W. G., Kurzweil, M. A., & Tobin, E. M. (2005). *Equity and excellence in American higher education.* Charlottesville: University of Virginia Press.

Brissette, I., Scheier, M. F., & Carver, C. S. (2002). The role of optimism in social network development, coping, and psychological adjustment during a life transition. *Journal of Personality and Social Psychology, 82*(1), 102–11.

Brotheridge, C. M., & Lee, R. T. (2002). Testing a conservation of resources model of the dynamics of emotional labor. *Journal of Occupational Health Psychology, 7*(1), 57–67.

Buchwald, P., & Hobfoll, S. E. (2004). Burnout aus ressourcentheoretischer Perspektive. *Psychologie in Erziehung und Unterricht, 51*(4), 247–57.

Calhoun, L. G., & Tedeschi, R. G. (2006). The foundations of posttraumatic growth: An expanded framework. In *Handbook of posttraumatic growth: Research & practice.* (pp. 3–23). Mahwah, NJ: Lawrence Erlbaum Associates.

Center, P. (2009). *Inside the middle class: bad times hit the good life.* Retrieved May 26, 2009, from http://pewsocialtrends.org/pubs/706/middle-class-poll

Central Bureau of Statistics. (2002). *Statistical abstracts.* Jerusalem: Author. [Electronic Version].

Central Intelligence Agency (2009a). *Country Comparisons—Life expectancy at birth* [Electronic Version]. Retrieved May 15, 2009. from https://www.cia.gov/library/publications/the-world-factbook/rankorder/2102rank.html

Central Intelligence Agency (2009b). *Country Comparisons—Infant mortality rate* [Electronic Version]. Retrieved May 15, 2009 from https://www.cia.gov/library/publications/the-world-factbook/rankorder/2091rank.html

Cooper, J. E., Holman, J., & Braithwaite, V. A. (1983). Self-esteem and family cohesion: The child's perspective and adjustment. *Journal of Marriage & the Family, 45*(1), 153–9.

Csikszentmihalyi, M. (1997). *Finding flow: The psychology of engagement with everyday life.* New York: Basic Books.

de Lange, A. H., De Witte, H., & Notelaers, G. (2008). Should I stay or should I go? Examining longitudinal relations among job resources and work engagement for stayers versus movers. *Work & Stress, 22*(3), 201–23.

Deci, E. L., & Ryan, R. M. (1985). The general causality orientations scale: Self-determination in personality. *Journal of Research in Personality, 19*(2), 109–34.

Deci, E. L., & Ryan, R. M. (1991). A motivational approach to self: Integration in personality. In R. A. Dienstbier (Ed.), *Nebraska Symposium on Motivation, 1990: Perspectives on motivation.* (pp. 237–88).

Deci, E. L., & Ryan, R. M. (2000). The "what" and "why" of goal pursuits: Human needs and the self-determination of behavior. *Psychological Inquiry, 11*(4), 227–68.

Diez Roux, A. V., Merkin, S. S., Arnett, D., Chambless, L., Massing, M., Nieto, F. J., et al. (2001). Neighborhood of residence and incidence of coronary heart disease. *New England Journal of Medicine, 345*, 99–106.

Dubner, S. (2008). How big of a deal is income inequality? A guest post. *The New York Times.*

Elias, M. J., & Haynes, N. M. (2008). Social competence, social support, and academic achievement in minority, low-income, urban elementary school children. *School Psychology Quarterly, 23*(4), 474–95.

Ennis, N. E., Hobfoll, S. E., & Schroder, K. E. E. (2000). Money doesn't talk, it swears: How economic stress and resistance resources impact inner-city women's depressive mood. *Special Issue: Minority Issues in Prevention, 28*(2), 149–73.

Fiksenbaum, L. M., Greenglass, E. R., & Eaton, J. (2006). Perceived social support, hassles, and coping among the elderly. *Journal of Applied Gerontology, 25*(1), 17–30.

Finkelstein, D. M., Kubzansky, L. D., Capitman, J., & Goodman, E. (2007). Socioeconomic differences in adolescent stress: The role of psychological resources. *Journal of Adolescent Health, 40*(2), 127–34.

Folkman, S. (1997). Positive psychological states and coping with severe stress. *Social Science and Medicine, 45*(8), 1207–21.

Fowler, W. J., & Walberg, H. J. (1991). School size, characteristics, and outcomes. *Educational Evaluation and Policy Analysis, 13*(2), 189–202.

Frankl, V. (1959). *Man's Search for Meaning.* New York: Touchstone.

Fredrickson, B. L. (1998). What good are positive emotions? *Review of General Psychology, 2*, 300–19.

Fredrickson, B. L., Tugade, M. M., Waugh, C. E., & Larkin, G. R. (2003). What good are positive emotions in crisis? A prospective study of resilience and emotions following the terrorist attacks on the United States on September 11th, 2001. *Journal of Personality and Social Psychology, 84*(2), 365–76.

Freedy, J. R., & Hobfoll, S. E. (1994). Stress inoculation for reduction of burnout: A conservation of resources approach. *Anxiety, Stress & Coping: An International Journal, 6*(4), 311–25.

Freedy, J. R., Saladin, M. E., Kilpatrick, D. G., Resnick, H. S., & et al. (1994). Understanding acute psychological distress following natural disaster. *Journal of Traumatic Stress, 7*(2), 257–73.

Freedy, J. R., Shaw, D. L., Jarrell, M. P., & Masters, C. R. (1992). Towards an understanding of the psychological impact of natural disasters: An application of the conservation resources stress model. *Journal of Traumatic Stress, 5*(3), 441–54.

Frodi, A., Bridges, L., & Grolnick, W. (1985). Correlates of mastery-related behavior: A short-term longitudinal study of infants in their second year. *Child Development, 56*(5), 1291–8.

Gallo, L. C., Bogart, L. M., Vranceanu, A.-M., & Matthews, K. A. (2005). Socioeconomic status, resources, psychological experiences, and emotional responses: A test of the reserve capacity model. *Journal of Personality and Social Psychology, 88*(2), 386–99.

Gallo, L. C., & Matthews, K. A. (2003). Understanding the association between socioeconomic status and physical health: Do negative emotions play a role? *Psychological Bulletin, 129*(1), 10–51.

Geronimus, A. T., Bound, J., Waidmann, T. A., Hillemeier, M. M., & Burns, P. B. (1996). Excess mortality among blacks and whites in the United States. *New England Journal of Medicine, 335*, 1552–8.

Gibb, B. E., Alloy, L. B., Abramson, L. Y., Rose, D. T., Whitehouse, W. G., Donovan, P., et al. (2001). History of childhood maltreatment, negative cognitive styles, and episodes of depression in adulthood. *Cognitive Therapy and Research, 25*(4), 425–46.

Greenberg, J., Pyszczynski, T., & Solomon, S. (1986). The causes and consequences of a need for self–esteem: A terror management theory. In R. F. Baumeister (Ed.), *Public and private self* (pp. 189–212). New York: Springer-Verlag.

Grolnick, W. S., & Ryan, R. M. (1989). Parent styles associated with children's self-regulation and competence in school. *Journal of Educational Psychology, 81*(2), 143–54.

Haber, M. G., Cohen, J. L., Lucas, T., & Baltes, B. B. (2007). The relationship between self-reported received and perceived social support: A meta-analytic review. *American Journal of Community Psychology, 39*(1-2), 133–44.

Halbesleben, J. R. B., & Bowler, W. M. (2007). Emotional exhaustion and job performance: The mediating role of motivation. *Journal of Applied Psychology, 92*(1), 93–106.

Hall, B. J., & Hobfoll, S. E. (2008). *The nature and meaning of posttraumatic growth measures.* Kent State University.

Hall, B. J., Hobfoll, S. E., Canetti-Nisim, D., Johnson, R., & Galea, S. (in press). The defensive nature of benefit finding during ongoing terrorism: An examination of a national sample of Israeli Jews. *Journal of Social and Clinical Psychology.*

Hall, B. J., Hobfoll, S. E., Palmieri, P. A., Canetti-Nisim, D., Shapira, O., Johnson, R. J., et al. (2008). The psychological impact of impending forced settler disengagement in Gaza: Trauma and posttraumatic growth. *Journal of Traumatic Stress, 21*(1), 22–9.

Harris, K. J., Kacmar, K. M., Zivnuska, S., & Shaw, J. D. (2007). The impact of political skill on impression management effectiveness. *Journal of Applied Psychology, 92*(1), 278–85.

Helgeson, V. S., Reynolds, K. A., & Tomich, P. L. (2006). A meta-analytic review of benefit finding and growth. *Journal of Consulting and Clinical Psychology, 74*(5), 797–816.

Henry, C. S. (1994). Family system characteristics, parental behaviors, and adolescent family life satisfaction. *Special Issue: Family processes and child and adolescent development: A special issue, 43*(4), 447–55.

Hobfoll, S. E. (1988). *The ecology of stress.* Washington, DC: Hemisphere.

Hobfoll, S. E. (1989). Conservation of resources: A new attempt at conceptualizing stress. *American Psychologist, 44*(3), 513–24.

Hobfoll, S. E. (1998). *Stress, culture, and community: The psychology and philosophy of stress.* New York: Plenum.

Hobfoll, S. E. (2001). The influence of culture, community, and the nested-self in the stress process: Advancing conservation of resources theory. *Applied Psychology: An International Review, 50*(3), 337–70.

Hobfoll, S. E., Briggs-Phillips, M., & Stines, L. R. (2003). Fact and artifact: The relationship of hope to a caravan of resources. In R. Jacoby & G. Keinan (Eds.), *Between stress and hope: From a disease-centered to a health-centered perspective* (pp. 81–104). Westport, CT: Praeger Publishers/ Greenwood Publishing Group.

Hobfoll, S. E., Canetti-Nisim, D., & Johnson, R. J. (2006). Exposure to terrorism, stress-related mental health symptoms, and defensive coping among Jews and Arabs in Israel. *Journal of Consulting and Clinical Psychology, 74*(2), 207–18.

Hobfoll, S. E., Canetti-Nisim, D., Johnson, R. J., Palmieri, P. A., Varley, J. D., & Galea, S. (2008). The association of exposure, risk, and resiliency factors with PTSD among Jews and Arabs exposed to repeated acts of terrorism in Israel. *Journal of Traumatic Stress, 21*(1), 9–21.

Hobfoll, S. E., & Freedy, J. (1993). Conservation of resources: A general stress theory applied to burnout. In W. B. Schaufeli, C. Maslach & T. Marek (Eds.), *Professional burnout: Recent developments in theory and research* (pp. 115–133).

Hobfoll, S. E., Hall, B. J., Horsey, K. J., & Lamoureux, B. E. (in press). Resilience in the face of terrorism: Linking resource investment with engagement. In M. Friedman, S. Southwick, D. Charney, & B. Litz (Eds.), *Comprehensive textbook on resilience.*

Hobfoll, S. E., Johnson, R. J., Cannetti, D., Hall, B. J., Galea, S., & Palmieri, P. A. (in preparation). A longitudinal study of engagement in the Palestinian Authority.

Hobfoll, S. E., & Lilly, R. S. (1993). Resource conservation as a strategy for community psychology. Journal of Community Psychology, 21(2), 128–48.

Hobfoll, S. E., Palmieri, P. A., Johnson, R. J., Canetti-Nisim, D., Hall, B. J., & Galea, S. (2009). Trajectories of resilience, resistance and distress during ongoing terrorism: The case of Jews and Arabs in Israel. *Journal of Consulting and Clinical Psychology, 77*, 138–48.

Hobfoll, S. E., & Shirom, A. (2001). Conservation of resources theory: Applications to stress and management in the workplace. In R. T. Golembiewski (Ed.), *Handbook of organizational behavior (2nd. ed, rev. and exp. ed.,* pp. 57–80).

Holt, L. J., Bry, B. H., & Johnson, V. L. (2008). Enhancing school engagement in at-risk, urban minority adolescents through a school-based, adult mentoring intervention. *Child & Family Behavior Therapy, 30*(4), 297–318.

Ironson, G., Wynings, C., Schneiderman, N., Baum, A., Rodriguez, M., Greenwood, D., et al. (1997). Posttraumatic stress symptoms, intrusive thoughts, loss, and immune function after Hurricane Andrew. *Psychosomatic Medicine, 59*(2), 128–41.

Ito, J. K., & Brotheridge, C. M. (2003). Resources, coping strategies, and emotional exhaustion: A conservation of resources perspective. *Journal of Vocational Behavior, 63*(3), 490–509.

Jawahar, I. M., Stone, T. H., & Kisamore, J. L. (2007). Role conflict and burnout: The direct and moderating effects of political skill and perceived organizational support on burnout dimensions. *International Journal of Stress Management, 14*(2), 142–59.

Johnson, D. M., Palmieri, P. A., Jackson, A. P., & Hobfoll, S. E. (2007). Emotional numbing weakens abused inner-city women's resiliency resources. *Journal of Traumatic Stress, 20*(2), 197–206.

Kaiser, C. F., Sattler, D. N., Bellack, D. R., & Dersin, J. (1996). A conservation of resources approach to a natural disaster: Sense of coherence and psychological distress. *Journal of Social Behavior & Personality, 11*(3), 459–76.

Kalmijn, M., & Kraaykamp, G. (1996). Race, cultural capital, and schooling: An analysis of trends in the United States. *Sociology of Education, 69*, 22–34.

Kaniasty, K., & Norris, F. H. (1995). In search of altruistic community: Patterns of social support mobilization following Hurricane Hugo. *American Journal of Community Psychology, 23*(4), 447–77.

Kubzansky, L. D., Koenen, K. C., Jones, C., & Eaton, W. W. (2009). A prospective study of posttraumatic stress disorder symptoms and coronary heart disease in women. *Health Psychology, 28*(1), 125–30.

Lazarus, R. S., & Folkman, S. (1984). *Stress, appraisal, and coping.* New York: Springer.

Lee, E., Shen, C., & Tran, T. (2009). Coping with Hurricane Katrina: Psychological distress and resilience among African American evacuees. *Journal of Black Psychology, 35*(1), 5–23.

Lewis, L. S. (1990). *The high-status track.* New York: SUNY Press.

Linley, P. A., & Joseph, S. (2004). Positive change following trauma and adversity: A review. *Journal of Traumatic Stress, 17*(1), 11–21.

Lund, D. A., Utz, R., Caserta, M. S., & Wright, S. D. (2009). Examining what caregivers do during respite time to make respite more effective. *Journal of Applied Gerontology, 28*(1), 109–31.

Luszczynska, A., Gutierrez-Dona, B., & Schwarzer, R. (2005). General self-efficacy in various domains of human functioning: Evidence from five countries. *International Journal of Psychology, 40*(2), 80–9.

Marmot, M. G., Bosma, H., Hemingway, H., Brunner, E., & Stansfeld, S. (1997). Contribution of job control and other risk factors to social variations in coronary heart disease incidence. . *Lancet 350,* 235–9.

Marmot, M. G., Shipley, M. J., & Rose, G. (1984). Inequalities in death: specific explanations of a general pattern? *Lancet 1,* 1003–6.

Mathis, R. D., & Tanner, Z. (1991). Cohesion, adaptability, and satisfaction of family systems in later life. *Family Therapy, 18*(1), 47–60.

McMillen, J. C., Smith, E. M., & Fisher, R. H. (1997). Perceived benefit and mental health after three types of disaster. *Journal of Consulting & Clinical Psychology, 65*(5), 733–9.

Miller, R. K., & McNamee, S. J. (Eds.). (1998). *Inheritance and wealth in America.* New York: Plenum Press.

Miyamoto, R. H., Hishinuma, E. S., Nishimura, S. T., Nahulu, L. B., Andrade, N. N., Goebert, D. A., et al. (2001). Path models linking correlates of self-esteem in a multi-ethnic adolescent sample. *Personality and Individual Differences, 31*(5), 701–12.

Moskowitz, J. T., Folkman, S., Collette, L., & Vittinghoff, E. (1996). Coping and mood during AIDS-related caregiving and bereavement. *Annals of Behavioral Medicine, 18*(1), 49–57.

Neveu, J.-P. (2007). Jailed resources: Conservation of resources theory as applied to burnout among prison guards. *Journal of Organizational Behavior, 28*(1), 21–42.

Norris, F. H., & Kaniasty, K. (1996). Received and perceived social support in times of stress: A test of the social support deterioration deterrence model. *Journal of Personality and Social Psychology, 71*(3), 498–511.

Norris, F. H., Perilla, J. L., Riad, J. K., Kaniasty, K., & Lavizzo, E. A. (1999). Stability and change in stress, resources, and psychological distress following natural disaster: Findings from Hurricane Andrew. *Anxiety, Stress & Coping: An International Journal, 12*(4), 363–96.

Openshaw, D. K., Thomas, D. L., & Rollins, B. C. (1984). Parental influences of adolescent self-esteem. *Journal of Early Adolescence, 4*(3), 259–74.

Palmieri, P. A., Galea, S., Canetti-Nisim, D., Johnson, R. J., & Hobfoll, S. E. (2008). The psychological impact of the Israel-Hezbollah War on Jews and Arabs in Israel: The impact of risk and resilience factors. *Social Science and Medicine 67,* 1208–16.

Payscale. (2009). Retrieved May 15, 2009, from http://www.payscale.com/

Peterson, C., Park, N., & Seligman, M. E. P. (2006). Greater strengths of character and recovery from illness. *Journal of Positive Psychology, 1*(1), 17–26.

Peterson, C., & Seligman, M. E. P. (2003). Character strengths before and after September 11. *Psychological Science, 14*(4), 381–4.

Powell, S., Rosner, R., Butollo, W., & Tedeschi, R. G. (2003). Posttraumatic growth after war: A study with former refugees and displaced people in Sarajevo. *Journal of Clinical Psychology, 59*(1), 71–83.

Repetti, R. L., Taylor, S. E., & Seeman, T. E. (2002). Risky families: Family social environments and the mental and physical health of offspring. *Psychological Bulletin, 128*(2), 330–66.

U.S. News and World Report (2008). Average MBA Starting Salaries at the Top Business Schools. Retrieved May 26, 2009, from http://www.admissionsconsultants.com/mba/compensation.asp

Rogers, L. Q., McAuley, E., Courneya, K. S., & Verhulst, S. J. (2008). Correlates of physical activity self-efficacy among breast cancer survivors. *American Journal of Health Behavior, 32*(6), 594–603.

Rothmann, S., & Joubert, J. H. M. (2007). Job demands, job resources, burnout and work engagement of management staff at a platinum mine in the North West Province. *South African Journal of Business Management, 38,* 49–61.

Rutter, M. (2000). Psychosocial influences: Critiques, findings, and research needs. *Development & Psychopathology, 12*(3), 375–405.

Sarason, I. G., & Stoops, R. (1978). Test anxiety and the passage of time. *Journal of Consulting and Clinical Psychology, 46*(1), 102–9.

Schaufeli, W. B., Salanova, M., Gonzalez-Roma, V., & Bakker, A. B. (2002). The measurement of engagement and burnout: A two sample confirmatory factor analytic approach. *Journal of Happiness Studies, 3*(1), 71–92.

Schumm, J. A., Briggs-Phillips, M., & Hobfoll, S. E. (2006). Cumulative interpersonal traumas and social support as risk and resiliency factors in predicting PTSD and depression among inner-city women. *Journal of Traumatic Stress, 19*(6), 825–36.

Schumm, J. A., Hobfoll, S. E., & Keogh, N. J. (2004). Revictimization and interpersonal resource loss predicts PTSD among women in substance-use treatment. *Journal of Traumatic Stress, 17*(2), 173–81.

Schumm, J. A., Stines, L. R., Hobfoll, S. E., & Jackson, A. P. (2005). The double-barreled burden of child abuse and current stressful circumstances on adult women: The kindling effect of early traumatic experience. *Journal of Traumatic Stress, 18*(5), 467–76.

Schwarzer, R., & Knoll, N. (2007). Functional roles of social support within the stress and coping process: A theoretical and empirical overview. *International Journal of Psychology, 42*(4), 243–52.

Seligman, M. E. P. (2000). Positive psychology. In J. E. Gillham (Ed.), *The science of optimism and hope: Research essays in honor of Martin E. P. Seligman* (pp. 415–29).

Seligman, M. E. P., & Csikszentmihalyi, M. (2000). Positive psychology: An introduction. *American Psychologist, 55*(1), 5–14.

Shirom, A. (2006). Explaining vigor: On the antecedents and consequences of vigor as a positive affect at work. In C. L. Cooper & D. Nelson (Eds.), *Organizational behavior: Accentuating the positive at work*. Thousand Oaks, CA: Sage Publications.

Sokolowski, K. L., & Israel, A. C. (2008). Perceived anxiety control as a mediator of the relationship between family stability and adjustment. *Journal of Anxiety Disorders, 22*(8), 1454–61.

Solomon, S., Greenberg, J., & Pyszczynski, T. (2004). The cultural animal: Twenty years of terror management theory and research. In J. Greenberg, S. Koole, & T. Pyszczynski (Eds.), *The handbook of experimental existential psychology* (pp. 13–34). New York: The Guilford Press.

Sonnentag, S., & Lange, I. (2002). The relationship between high performance and knowledge about how to master cooperation situations. *Applied Cognitive Psychology, 16*(5), 491–508.

Sun, L.-Y., & Pan, W. (2008). HR practices perceptions, emotional exhaustion, and work outcomes: A conservation-of-resources theory in the Chinese context. *Human Resource Development Quarterly, 19*(1), 55–74.

Tedeschi, R. G. (2004). Posttraumatic growth: Conceptual foundations and empirical evidence. *Psychological Inquiry, 15*(1), 1–18.

Tedeschi, R. G., & Calhoun, L. G. (1995). *Trauma and transformation: Growing in the aftermath of suffering*. Thousand Oaks, CA: Sage.

Tomaka, J., Thompson, S., & Palacios, R. (2006). The relation of social isolation, loneliness, and social support to disease outcomes among the elderly. *Journal of Aging and Health, 18*(3), 359–84.

Uchino, B. N., Cacioppo, J. T., & Kiecolt-Glaser, J. K. (1996). The relationship between social support and physiological processes: A review with emphasis on underlying mechanisms and implications for health. *Psychological Bulletin, 119*(3), 488–531.

Verhaeghe, M., Bracke, P., & Bruynooghe, K. (2008). Stigmatization and self-esteem of persons in recovery from mental illness: The role of peer support. *International Journal of Social Psychiatry, 54*(3), 206–18.

Warren, J. S., Jackson, Y., & Sifers, S. K. (2009). Social support provisions as differential predictors of adaptive outcomes in young adolescents. *Journal of Community Psychology, 37*(1), 106–21.

Wells, J. D., Hobfoll, S. E., & Lavin, J. (1999). When it rains, it pours: The greater impact of resource loss compared to gain on psychological distress. *Personality and Social Psychology Bulletin, 25*(9), 1172–82.

Windle, M., & Jacob, T. (2007). Measurement of higher-order family dimensions across self-report and behavioral observational methods. *Psychological Reports, 100*(2), 661–71.

Xanthopoulou, D., Bakker, A. B., Demerouti, E., & Schaufeli, W. B. (2007). The role of personal resources in the job demands-resources model. *International Journal of Stress Management, 14*(2), 121–41.

Zautra, A. J., Reich, J. W., & Gaurnaccia, C. A. (1990). The everyday consequences of disability and bereavement for older adults. *Journal of Personality and Social Psychology, 59*, 550–61.

Zellars, K. L., Perrewe, P. L., Hochwarter, W. A., & Anderson, K. S. (2006). The interactive effects of positive affect and conscientiousness on strain. *Journal of Occupational Health Psychology, 11*(3), 281–9.

Zoellner, T., & Maercker, A. (2006). Posttraumatic growth in clinical psychology: A critical review and introduction of a two component model. *Clinical Psychology Review, 26*(5), 626–53.

Appendix 7.1: COR-Evaluation

We are interested the extent to which you have experienced **actual loss** or **threat of loss** in any of the list of resources listed overleaf in the last 6 months. Resources can include objects, conditions, personal characteristics, or energies.

Actual loss of resources occurs when the resource has decreased in availability to you (e.g., actual loss of personal health or actual loss of intimacy with spouse or partner). If you have experienced "actual loss" in any of the resources in the last six months, you would rate that "actual loss" from 1 to 4 (1 = actual loss to a small degree, to 4 = actual loss to a great degree) and write your response in the "actual loss" column. If the availability of the resource has not changed, or the resource is not applicable, you would rate "actual loss" as 0 (zero = not at all / not applicable).

Threat of loss occurs when you have been threatened with the loss of the resource but no actual loss has occurred (e.g., there has been a chance that you may lose your job and therefore your stable employment has been threatened with loss). If you have experienced "threat of loss" in any of the resources in the last six months, you would rate that "threat of loss" from 1 to 4 (1 = threat of loss to a small degree, to 4 = threat of loss to great degree) and write the number in the "threat of loss" column. If there was no "threat of loss" of the resource, or the resource is not applicable, you would rate "threat of loss" as 0 (zero = not at all / not applicable).

IMPORTANT: DO NOT RATE the availability of the resource to you. We are only interested in the **CHANGE** in the availability of the resource (i.e., actual loss), **OR** if there has been a "threat of loss" to that resource. **FOR EXAMPLE:RESOURCE item 26 - Status / Seniority at work:** If the status / seniority of your job 6 months ago is still the same as today then you write a "0" in the actual loss column. If you had experienced no "threat of loss" in the status / seniority of your job during that time then you would also write a "0" in the threat of loss column. If you had experienced some doubt as to whether you may be demoted in your job, but it hasn't happened yet, then you would rate the "threat of loss" between 1 (threat of loss to a small degree) and 4 (threat of loss to a great degree).

MY RESOURCES

To what extent have I experienced **actual loss** during the past 6 months?

To what extent have I experienced **threat of loss** during the past 6 months?

0 = not at all / not applicable
1 = to a small degree
2 = to a moderate degree
3 = to a considerable degree
4 = to a great degree

	RESOURCES	EXTENT OF ACTUAL LOSS	EXTENT OF THREAT OF LOSS
1.	Personal transportation (car, truck, etc.)	_____	_____
2.	Feeling that I am successful	_____	_____
3.	Time for adequate sleep	_____	_____
4.	Good marriage	_____	_____
5.	Adequate clothing	_____	_____
6.	Feeling valuable to others	_____	_____
7.	Family stability	_____	_____
8.	Free time	_____	_____
9.	More clothing than I need	_____	_____
10.	Sense of pride in myself	_____	_____
11.	Intimacy with one or more family members	_____	_____
12.	Time for work	_____	_____
13.	Feelings that I am accomplishing mygoals	_____	_____
14.	Good relationship with my children	_____	_____
15.	Time with loved ones	_____	_____
16.	Necessary tools for work	_____	_____
17.	Hope	_____	_____
18.	Children's health	_____	_____
19.	Stamina/endurance	_____	_____
20.	Necessary home appliances	_____	_____
21.	Feeling that my future success depends on me	_____	_____
22.	Positively challenging routine	_____	_____
23.	Personal health	._____	_____
24.	Housing that suits my needs	_____	_____
25.	Sense of optimism	_____	_____
26.	Status/seniority at work	_____	_____
27.	Adequate food	_____	_____
28.	Larger home than I need	_____	_____

29.	Sense of humour	_____	_____
30.	Stable employment	_____	_____
31.	Intimacy with spouse or partner	_____	_____
32.	Adequate home furnishings	_____	_____
33.	Feeling that I have control over my life	_____	_____
34.	Role as a leader	_____	_____
35.	Ability to communicate well	_____	_____
36.	Providing children's essentials	_____	_____
37.	Feeling that my life is peaceful	_____	_____
38.	Acknowledgement of my accomplishments	_____	_____
39.	Ability to organise tasks	_____	_____
40.	Extras for children	_____	_____
41.	Sense of commitment	_____	_____
42.	Intimacy with at least one friend	_____	_____
43.	Money for extras	_____	_____
44.	Self-discipline	_____	_____
45.	Understanding from my employer/boss	_____	_____
46.	Savings or emergency money	_____	_____
47.	Motivation to get things done	_____	_____
48.	Spouse/partner's health	_____	_____
49.	Support from co-workers	_____	_____
50.	Adequate income	_____	_____
51.	Feeling that I know who I am	_____	_____
52.	Advancement in education or job training	_____	_____
53.	Adequate financial credit	_____	_____
54.	Feeling independent	_____	_____
55.	Companionship	_____	_____
56.	Financial assets (stocks, property, etc.)	_____	_____
57.	Knowing where I am going with my life	_____	_____
58.	Affection from others.	_____	_____
59.	Financial stability	_____	_____
60.	Feeling that my life has meaning/purpose	_____	_____
61.	Positive feelings about myself	_____	_____
62.	People I can learn from	_____	_____
63.	Money for transportation	_____	_____

64.	Help with tasks at work	_____	_____
65.	Medical insurance	_____	_____
66.	Involvement with church, synagogue, etc	_____	_____
67.	Retirement security (financial)	_____	_____
68.	Help with tasks at home	_____	_____
69.	Loyalty of friends	_____	_____
70.	Money for advancement or self-improvement (education, starting a business, etc.)	_____	_____
71.	Help with child care	_____	_____
72.	Involvement in organisations with others who have similar interests	_____	_____
73.	Financial help if needed	_____	_____
74.	Health of family/close friends	_____	_____

We are also interested if you have experienced **gain** in any of the following resources in the last 6 months.

Gain of resources occurs when the availability of a particular resource has increased for you (e.g., you and your family have spent more time together in the last 6 months so you have experienced gain in the resource of "time with loved ones"). If you have experienced "gain" in any of the resources in the last 6 months, you would rate that "gain" from 1 to 4 (1 = gain to a small degree to 4 = gain to a great degree) and write your response in the "gain" column. If the availability of the resource is unchanged to you, or the resource is not applicable, you would rate "extent of gain" as 0 (zero = not at all / not applicable).

IMPORTANT: DO NOT RATE THE AVAILABILITY OF THE RESOURCE. We are only interested in the **GAIN** you have experienced in the resource. FOR EXAMPLE: **RESOURCE item 4 – Good Marriage**: If you had a good marriage 6 months ago and you still do now, then you would rate the extent of the gain as "0".

MY RESOURCES

To what extent have I **gained** them during the past 6 months?	0 = not at all / not applicable 1 = to a small degree 2 = to a moderate degree 3 = to a considerable degree 4 = to a great degree

RESOURCES	EXTENT OF GAIN
1. Personal transportation (car, truck, etc.)	____
2. Feeling that I am successful	____
3. Time for adequate sleep items continue as on the list of resource loss	____
4. . . .items continue as on the list of resource loss	

Coping with Bereavement

Margaret S. Stroebe

Abstract

Although bereavement is a normal part of life, it is associated with detrimental mental and physical health consequences and is thus an important topic in the context of stress, coping, and health. Research on the relationship between bereavement and physical and mental health is reviewed. Ways that persons cope are likely to interact with diverse risk factors (circumstances of death, intra- and interpersonal variables, etc.) to co-determine excesses in ill health or poor adaptation. Thus, close attention is given to empirical and theoretical contributions to understanding the relative effectiveness of different coping strategies. In addition to summarizing the state of knowledge in the field in the above areas, new directions for the field are considered.

Keywords: bereavement, grief, mental health, physical health, coping, Dual Process Model

Bereavement—the loss of a significant person due to that person's death—is a normal part of life, one that most of us can expect to experience personally sooner or later. Yet, there are many different reasons why it can be counted as one of the most stressful life events that can happen to someone, the impact of which may be felt for months or even years. The death of a loved one frequently means the loss of an attachment figure, a person to whom one has had (and still has) a deeply significant emotional bond. Permanent separation brings with it a myriad of reactions, including excruciating loneliness, protest, and despair. Sometimes death occurs suddenly or in terrible circumstances, leaving emotions such as shocked disbelief, horror, or intense anger in its wake. In addition, many bereaved people are faced with life situations that cause anxieties beyond their grief. For example, following the death of a young spouse, the widow or widower may have to cope with simultaneous disruptions and secondary stressors, for example, bringing up young children alone; severe financial hardship due to the death; having to master tasks that the deceased had taken care of, maybe in addition to loss of social status/integration and primary support networks. Such deficits can lead to tremendous worries about being able to cope and doubts about one's own ability to do so adequately - associated, for example, with a drastic lowering of self-esteem. All of these life changes related to bereavement can add enormously to the bereaved person's distress.

People cope with the death of a close person and all that goes with it in very different ways, with some managing more effectively than others. Likewise, health outcomes among bereaved people vary from extremely negative to far more positive ones over the course of time. Taken together, these differences raise important questions for scientists about potential links between processes (ways of coping) and outcomes (e.g., health consequences). What is "adaptive coping" with bereavement, and how have theoreticians explained the links with health outcomes? How can differences in adjustment between bereaved persons be understood? These questions are central in this chapter, the basic aim of which is to provide a review of contemporary scientific understanding of processes of coping with bereavement and their relationship to adaptation to this stressful life event.

First, research on the relationship between bereavement and physical and mental health is reviewed. Research on so-called "risk factors," which increase vulnerability of some bereaved persons to poor health outcomes, is then considered within our Integrative Risk Factor Framework (Stroebe, Folkman, Hansson, & Schut, 2007a). Given that coping processes have been postulated to contribute to bereavement outcome, a coping category is incorporated within the risk factor framework, and—given the scope of this chapter—this category is selected for particular attention. However, it is important to realize that coping takes place within the context of other risk factors, and that the latter have an impact on coping. Empirical evidence on (mal)adaptive ways of coping with bereavement is evaluated. Limitations in this body of research and the need for theoretical understanding are noted. Thus, attention turns in the final major part of this chapter to theoretical contributions to understanding (mal)adaptive coping. Finally, suggestions are made for future directions in research on coping with bereavement.

Health Consequences of Bereavement

What psychological and physical effects does loss through death of a loved person have on survivors? Is the risk of succumbing to health disorders greater in bereaved than non-bereaved counterparts? In this section, the range of health consequences following bereavement is reviewed, with indications of the prevalence of different health outcomes, where possible. Researchers have investigated a broad range of physical and psychological health consequences of bereavement (see Stroebe, Schut & Stroebe, 2007b, for an extended review), from mortality and physical debilities, to mental disorders and complicated grief. The main patterns to emerge from this extensive body of research are outlined next. As will become clear, bereaved persons are indeed at higher risk of suffering from various health problems than non-bereaved controls (i.e., persons of the same age, gender, and other sociodemographic characteristics).

Mortality

In one sense, the severest consequence of bereavement is mortality of the bereaved person him- or herself. The death of a loved one increases the mortality risk of the surviving person, understood popularly as dying of a broken heart. Longitudinal studies including non-bereaved controls and controlling for confounders such as socioeconomic and lifestyle factors have generally indicated an early excess risk of mortality, with some studies finding that risk persists for longer than 6 months after bereavement (Stroebe et al., 2007b). Most of these studies have been on spousal bereavement, where excesses for widowers are frequently, though not always, found to be higher than those among widows (e.g., Lillard & Waite, 1995). In a rare large-scale investigation of the mortality of parents after the death of their child conducted in Denmark, Li, Precht, Mortensen and Olsen (2003) found increased mortality from natural and unnatural causes among mothers, extending over the 18-year period of the investigation, while for fathers, the excess risk was more confined to the early years of bereavement and was mainly from unnatural causes. Death from both natural and unnatural causes has been documented in other studies too (see Stroebe et al., 2007b), with some, for example, looking specifically at heart disease (e.g., Parkes, Benjamin & Fitzgerald, 1969), others at suicide (Agerbo, 2005), and recording excesses among the bereaved in each of these cases. For instance, men who had lost a partner to suicide had a highly excessive risk of dying from suicide themselves, more excessive than death from other causes (which were still excessive compared with the non-bereaved), and more excessive than women's (whose excesses nevertheless followed the same general pattern: deaths from suicide among widows were higher than from other causes).

Although one can conclude from such findings that people can indeed die of a broken heart, mortality is a relatively rare occurrence: in terms of absolute numbers, few bereaved people die. In a category of males over 54 years, about 5 in 100 widowers compared with 3 in 100 married men would die in the first 6 months of bereavement (Stroebe, Stroebe, & Schut, 2001). Thus, excess rates cannot be expected to show up among small samples of bereaved people.

Physical health detriments

If one looks at less extreme, but still serious, physical health outcomes, it becomes evident that health problems do occur in larger proportions of bereaved people, particularly those who have been recently bereaved. Bereaved persons report more physical health symptoms and ailments than non-bereaved counterparts, and they also have higher rates of illness and disability, medication use, and hospitalization than the non-bereaved. To take just a few examples: In a study including fathers following the violent death of their child, there was an indication of physical health deterioration over time: 14 percent said they were in poor health 4 months after bereavement, while as many as 24 percent reported ill health at 24 months (Murphy et al., 1999). In another study, among younger bereaved spouses, 20 percent of the widowed (compared with 3 percent married) were above the cutoff point for severe physical symptomatology 4 to 6 months post-loss. After 2 years, the rate among the widowed declined to 12 percent (Stroebe & Stroebe, 1993). Excesses have also been reported among more elderly bereaved spouses, including their rates for illness and use of medication: The odds of a new or worsened illness was estimated at 1.4 times the risk for the non-bereaved at 2 months post-loss, and self-reported medication use was estimated to be 1.73 times greater (Thompson, Breckenridge, Gallagher, & Peterson, 1984).

Such health effects are associated with changes in physiological mechanisms: Research has begun to show biological links between bereavement and increased risks of physical illnesses. For example, research has examined how bereavement affects the immune system and leads to changes in the endocrine, autonomic nervous, and cardiovascular systems, and helps to account for increased vulnerability to external agents (see Gerra et al., 2003; Stroebe, Stroebe, & Hansson, 1993; Stroebe, Hansson, Stroebe & Schut, 2001).

Finally, there is concern about the receipt of medical treatment among the bereaved: There is, worryingly, some evidence that bereaved persons with intense grief may not consult doctors when they need to for physical health disorders (Prigerson et al., 2001), suggesting that there may be underestimation of physical health problems within this group. In this context, it is important to note that emotional loneliness (the feeling of utter aloneness even in the presence of others) mediates between the stressful event of bereavement and poor outcome (Stroebe, Stroebe, & Abakoumkin, 2005b). Following this, it seems likely that persons who are profoundly lonely, grieving intensely, and deeply missing the presence of their loved one may simply not take good care themselves, or not make an effort with respect to their own physical health. In fact, there are indications that this is the case (see Parkes, 1996). Physical consequences are clearly intricately linked with psychological reactions, to which I turn next.

Psychological symptoms and psychiatric disorders

Bereaved persons also suffer from psychological symptoms and ailments (Table 8.1), such that bereavement is said to be a complex emotional syndrome, with reactions ranging across, but not necessarily always including, loneliness, despair, guilt, yearning, suicidal ideation, and social withdrawal, and varying from mild and comparatively short-lived to extreme and long-lasting symptoms over months and even years of bereavement. Thus, there is mental suffering among persons considered to be "normally" (in the sense of uncomplicated) grieving. There is also an increase in the prevalence of psychiatric disorders, including post-traumatic stress disorder (PTSD), anxiety disorders, and clinical depression. Five years after the violent death of their child, 27.7 percent of mothers, compared with 9.5 percent of non-bereaved mothers, suffered from PTSD, while among fathers, the respective percentages were 12.5 percent compared with 6.3 percent (Murphy, Johnson, Chung, & Beaton, 2003). Among spouses during their first 2 years of bereavement, 50 percent reached criteria for PTSD symptomatology at one of four points of measurement, while 9 percent did so at all four measurement points (Schut, de Keijser, van den Bout, & Dijkhuis, 1991). Anxiety disorders are also found excessively among bereaved persons, and it has been suggested that they are more prevalent than clinical depression (Raphael, Minkov, & Dobson, 2001), although to my knowledge prevalences have not been established among reasonably sized samples. Clinical depression among bereaved spouses has been documented for 24 to 30 percent 2 months post-loss, compared with 16 percent at 1 year (Zisook & Shuchter, 2001). In one study specifically among the elderly, 12 percent of widowers (compared with 0 percent non-bereaved) suffered clinical levels of depression at 6 weeks post-loss (Byrne & Raphael, 1999); similarly, in another

Table 8.1   Reactions to bereavement

Affective	Depression, despair, dejection, distress
	Anxiety, fears, dread
	Guilt, self-blame, self-accusation
	Anger, hostility, irritability
	Anhedonia (loss of pleasure)
	Loneliness
	Yearning, longing, pining
	Shock, numbness
Cognitive	Preoccupation with thoughts of deceased, intrusive ruminations
	Sense of presence of deceased
	Suppression, denial
	Lowered self-esteem
	Self-reproach
	Helplessness, hopelessness
	Sense of unreality
	Memory, concentration problems
Behavioral	Agitation, tenseness, restlessness
	Fatigue
	Overactivity
	Searching
	Weeping, sobbing, crying
	Social withdrawal
Physiological/ Somatic	Loss of appetite
	Sleep disturbances
	Energy loss, exhaustion
	Somatic complaints
	Physical complaints similar to deceased
	Immunologic and endocrine changes
	Susceptibility to illness, disease

study, among elderly widows, 12 percent (compared with 3 percent non-bereaved) did so (Carnelley, Wortman, & Kessler, 1999). Although these figures suggest that distress/depression may be lower among the elderly, this should not be taken as an indication of less suffering among older people (both their reactions and their concerns are different, the impact of loss tending to be long-drawn-out; see Hansson & Stroebe, 2007).

Complicated grief

Complications in the grief process itself, currently labeled prolonged grief disorder (which is not yet a separate diagnostic category in the *Diagnostic and Statistical Manual of Mental Disorders*, APA, 1994, see Parkes, 2005; Prigerson, Vanderwerker, & Maciejewski, 2008), also occur among bereaved persons. Not surprisingly, given such differences between samples and studies, such as those concerning the type (from loss of a child or spouse to more remote persons), and characteristics of the bereavement situation (such as duration of loss, cause of death), estimates for complicated grief vary considerably. One review reported that prevalences among studies ranged from 33 percent to 5 percent reaching criteria for complicated grief among acutely bereaved persons (Middleton, Raphael, Martinek, & Misso, 1993). Prigerson and Jacobs (2001) established an upper 20 percent criterion for "caseness" of complicated or prolonged grief among a large community sample (given that this threshold had emerged as the best for distinguishing individuals at risk for functional impairments), thus falling within the prevalence range found by Middleton et al. (1993).

The above prevalences indicate that quite substantial minorities of bereaved persons suffer from severe health consequences. There may be comorbidity: A bereaved person may suffer from different debilities, either at the same time or at different times during bereavement. This pattern of prevalences is consistent with research on resilience among bereaved persons, which has similarly shown that the majority recover from their loss, emotionally and physically, over time (e.g., Bonanno, 2008; Bonanno, Boerner & Wortman, 2008; Stroebe, in press), without the aid of professional help (Currier, Neimeyer, & Berman, 2008; Schut & Stroebe, 2005). Some bereaved persons even gain from the experience (Davis, 2008; Schaefer & Moos, 2001; Tedeschi & Calhoun, 2004). Nevertheless, it must be remembered that bereavement itself is not a rare phenomenon, with, for example, even as many as 3.4 percent of children under 18 years of age experiencing the death of a parent (Christ, Siegel, & Christ, 2005), while, among elderly populations, the percentage of non-institutionalized persons who are widowed rises from 20 percent for 65- to 74-year-olds to 63 percent among the 85-plus-year-olds (Hansson & Stroebe, 2007). Thus, while representing only a minority of all bereaved persons, in terms of actual numbers, many people will be experiencing negative health consequences of bereavement in our society. There are good reasons to target this subgroup for potential intervention (Schut, Stroebe, van den Bout, & Terheggen, 2001), Scientists have endeavored to find out who among the bereaved are at risk for these health debilities and have some useful leads.

Risk Factors for Bereavement Outcome

The main question to be addressed next is what makes some persons vulnerable while others remain resilient. Elsewhere, we have identified different categories of so-called risk factors—the situational, intrapersonal, and interpersonal characteristics associated with increased vulnerability to the range of bereavement outcomes—and developed an integrative risk factor framework to enhance understanding of individual differences in adjustment to bereavement and to help to establish pathways in the adaptation process (Stroebe, Folkman, Hansson & Schut, 2006; Figure 8.1). The framework was derived from two models that will be described later in this chapter, namely the generic cognitive stress, appraisal, and coping model (Lazarus & Folkman, 1984; Folkman, 2001) and a compatible bereavement-specific stress model, the Dual Process Model of Coping with Bereavement (DPM; Stroebe & Schut, 1999, 2008). As can be seen in Figure 8.1, the risk factor framework incorporates an analysis of stressors, intra- and interpersonal risk or protective factors, and appraisal and coping processes, all of which are postulated to have an impact on outcome. It is beyond the scope of this chapter to cover all the five interlinked elements in the framework that combine to describe and determine sources of individual differences in adjustment to bereavement (for a detailed review see Stroebe et al., 2006; 2007). Our focus will be on the coping and appraisal category, but first, a few words about risk factor research in general are in order.

Risk factor research: Shortcomings

There are a number of reasons why one must be cautious in drawing conclusions about risk factors (see also van der Houwen et al., 2010; Stroebe et al., 2007a & b; W. Stroebe & Schut, 2001). First, different types of factors contribute to determining the outcome of bereavement in complex ways; for example, there are interactions between factors. To illustrate, sudden death is likely to have the most effect on vulnerable people, such as those with low self-esteem and those who are personally less well prepared (Barry, Kasl, & Prigerson, 2002; Ong,

Bergman, & Bisconti, 2005). Furthermore, there are discrepancies in findings. For example, while earlier findings indicated that poor relationships led to difficulties in bereavement (Parkes & Weiss, 1983), there are discrepancies in the more recent literature (see Stroebe et al., 2007b). This is probably due to the lack of clarity concerning various features of relationships. For example, one would need to identify different concepts represented among those measuring "closeness," such as overdependence versus healthy reliance, or lack of harmony versus autonomy. Clearly, such dimensions may be differentially related to adjustment (e.g., according to attachment theory, see Mikulincer, 2008).

In connection with this point, risk factor research frequently proceeds atheoretically. To use the example of marital relationships again: While much research fails to justify predictions theoretically, research that is steeped in attachment theory suggests particular ways in which the quality or nature of the lost relationship may influence the outcome (Bowlby, 1980; Stroebe, Schut & Stroebe, 2005a; Parkes, 2006). Thus, such a theoretical perspective can help researchers specify hypotheses and operationalize relevant concepts more precisely. Another shortcoming of risk factor research is simply the lack of controlled studies investigating variables (e.g., on personality or predisposing vulnerabilities), or more particularly, of studies investigating these in combination, so that the relative contribution of different factors in accounting for variance can be established. Wrong conclusions have been drawn when factors have been researched in isolation (see van der Houwen et al., 2010; Wijngaards-de Meij et al., 2005). And without non-bereaved control groups, it is impossible to say whether a given variable is a generic risk factor that affects a bereaved sample any differently than it would the general population. Finally, due to the lack of adequate research, little is known about how risk factors relate precisely to different health outcomes—that is, why one person will succumb to mental health disorders while another might suffer from physical complaints or disorders. With these cautions about the quality of research in mind, we can turn to examination of coping variables in the context of establishing risk for poor bereavement outcome.

(Mal)adaptive coping and appraisal as risk or protective factors in bereavement

As indicated already, it is important to include the coping process in an analysis of individual differences in adjustment to bereavement, not least

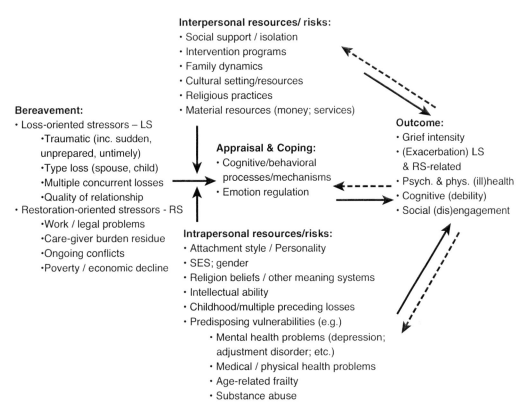

Interpersonal resources/ risks:
- Social support / isolation
- Intervention programs
- Family dynamics
- Cultural setting/resources
- Religious practices
- Material resources (money; services)

Bereavement:
- Loss-oriented stressors – LS
  - Traumatic (inc. sudden, unprepared, untimely)
  - Type loss (spouse, child)
  - Multiple concurrent losses
  - Quality of relationship
- Restoration-oriented stressors - RS
  - Work / legal problems
  - Care-giver burden residue
  - Ongoing conflicts
  - Poverty / economic decline

Appraisal & Coping:
- Cognitive/behavioral processes/mechanisms
- Emotion regulation

Outcome:
- Grief intensity
- (Exacerbation) LS & RS-related
- Psych. & phys. (ill)health
- Cognitive (debility)
- Social (dis)engagement

Intrapersonal resources/risks:
- Attachment style / Personality
- SES; gender
- Religion beliefs / other meaning systems
- Intellectual ability
- Childhood/multiple preceding losses
- Predisposing vulnerabilities (e.g.)
  - Mental health problems (depression; adjustment disorder; etc.)
  - Medical / physical health problems
  - Age-related frailty
  - Substance abuse

Fig. 8.1 The integrative risk factor framework for prediction of bereavement outcome. (Copyright 2001, reprinted with permission of American Psychological Association.)

because evidence has suggested that coping strategies mediate between the confrontation with stressful situations or events such as bereavement and the consequences for health and well-being (Aldwin & Revenson, 1987), as depicted in Figure 8.1: To understand *processes* of adjustment, we need to include coping. Coping is also one of the few factors influencing bereavement outcomes that is amenable to brief interventions (Folkman, 2001). Nevertheless, one needs to be modest about expectations because, as Folkman (2001) also cautioned: "coping may have a relatively small influence on adjustment and recovery compared to factors such as the timing and nature of the death, history, and personality" (p. 564).

EMPIRICAL EVIDENCE

What evidence is there that differences in coping account for individual differences in the health consequences of bereavement? Through most decades of the 20th century, researchers and clinicians generally accepted that adaptive coping entailed *grief work*—the process of emotionally confronting the reality of loss, of going over events that occurred

before and at the time of the death, and of focusing on memories and working toward detachment or separation from the deceased (cf. Freud, 1917; Bowlby, 1980; for a review see Stroebe, 1992). Following this line of reasoning, grief work is essential for overcoming the impact of bereavement and adapting well to one's loss (the so-called "grief work hypothesis"; Stroebe, 1992). However, empirical support for the efficacy of "working through" as a strategy for overcoming grief has been equivocal (and additional concerns have been raised in Stroebe's [1992] and Wortman & Silver's [2001] reviews). For example, some research has shown that people who do not work through their grief frequently recover as well as, if not better than, those who do so (Bonanno, 2001; Wortman & Silver, 2001).

The concepts of *emotional disclosure* and *social sharing* are closely related to that of grief work, given that they necessitate confrontation with some aspect of the bereavement experience (grief work can also be done alone). Findings of studies on the benefits of emotional disclosure or social sharing have provided little support for the grief work notion: somewhat surprisingly, disclosure and sharing have not emerged as strong predictors of bereavement outcome (Pennebaker, 1997; Pennebaker, Zech, & Rimé, 2001; M. Stroebe, Stroebe, Schut, Zech, & van den Bout, 2002; W. Stroebe, Schut, & Stroebe, 2005).

The seeking of *social support*—a variable that is evidently related to disclosure and sharing—can be considered part of the coping process, in that it implies the use of interpersonal resources to help with emotional, instrumental, companionship, or information aspects/deficits associated with bereavement (W. Stroebe et al., 2005; Zettel & Rook, 2004). One would expect social support to buffer individuals against the negative health outcomes of bereavement. However, this assumption has not been well founded empirically (W. Stroebe & Schut, 2001; W. Stroebe et al., 2005; Stroebe et al. 2007a & b). Inadequate social support is a general risk factor, one that affects the health and well-being of non-bereaved people as much as those who are bereaved. *Continuing bonds* could likewise be considered a coping strategy, the idea being that retaining the tie with the deceased person would help the bereaved person to adapt. Klass, Silverman, and Nickman (1996) made a strong case in favor of the positive impact in their volume *Continuing Bonds: New Understandings of Grief*, but failed to provide rigorous empirical evidence for this claim. Subsequent research, however, has not only provided little evidence that retaining bonds is associated with good adaptation, but has also revealed associations with poor adaptation (see Field, 2008, for a review). Interestingly, findings of a study by Lalande and Bonanno (2006) indicated that the adaptiveness of continuing bonds may be culture-related: in a prospective study, they reported positive relationships between continuing bonds at 4 months and adaptation at 18 months in China, but the opposite pattern in the United States, where higher levels of continuing bonds were related to poorer adjustment later on.

The concept of continuing bonds needs closer specification. For example, some items in continuing bonds scales cover aspects that are clearly related to yearning and pining, and such items are also included on grief scales—which are used as outcome variables (Boelen, Schut, Stroebe, & Zijerveld, 2006a; Schut, Stroebe, Boelen, & Zijerveld, 2006). As the work of Prigerson and her colleagues has demonstrated, high levels of yearning for the deceased are a major criterion for grief complications (Prigerson, Vanderwerker, & Maciejewski, 2008).

Thus, in some of the continuing bonds studies (reviewed by Field, 2008), the coping strategy of retaining the tie to the deceased is confounded with the outcome of grief. It is not surprising, then, that a scale including such items would be associated with poor outcome. The precise type of bond needs to be specified too (in relationship to prediction of adjustment): Continuing the bond through yearning for the deceased, or if it reflects non-acceptance of the fact that the deceased has gone forever (e.g., "I still expect him to walk through the door"), which in our view is a fundamental indicator of poor adjustment (see Stroebe et al., 2007), would not be expected to be associated with or lead to good outcomes, while referring to the deceased as a model for decision-making would be more likely to.

In contrast with the variables reviewed so far, which have yielded rather equivocal findings, additional, fine-grained examinations of coping processes have provided useful leads. Some researchers have investigated a number of more specific coping strategies and examined whether they lead to a reduction in the negative psychosocial and physical health consequences or to a lowering of grief. For example, studies have suggested the importance of positive and negative cognitions.

With respect to *positive cognitions*, a study by Moskowitz, Folkman, and Acree (2003) showed that, controlling for depression, positive affect (which is strongly associated with a coping process known as positive reappraisal) leads to lower levels of depressed mood over time. It has even been shown that the occurrence of smiling and laughter during the grieving process is positively related to subsequent adjustment (Bonanno & Keltner, 1997). Being able to find positive meaning in bereavement-related stressful events brings about or enhances positive affect and reduces distress. Positive emotional states, even laughter, emerge as part of the effective coping process (cf. Folkman & Moskowitz, 2000). Again, the same stringent methodological requirements, with baseline controls, have been included in the research that backs up these interpretations (cf. Bonanno, 2001, Bonanno & Kaltman, 1999; Folkman, 1997, 2001).

With respect to *negative cognitions*, Nolen-Hoeksema and Larson (1999) have shown that a ruminative coping style (that is, focusing on distressing aspects and meanings in a repetitive and passive manner) was associated with poorer adaptation to bereavement (particularly, higher depression rates) over time. These were also carefully designed studies, which controlled for levels of grief or depression early on. In general, this body of research has demonstrated that people whose style is to confront and talk about negative aspects of their loss over time do not do as well as those who refrain (more) from this type of disclosure (e.g., Nolen-Hoeksema & Larson, 1999; Nolen-Hoeksema, 2001; Nolen-Hoeksema, Parker & Larson, 1994), and there is support from other researchers: Bonanno and colleagues, (e.g., Bonanno, 2001; Bonanno & Eddins, 2000) showed that disclosure of negatively valanced emotions was associated with increased distress and somatic complaints.

Recent research has confirmed and further explored the impact of such processes on bereavement outcomes. For example, Boelen and colleagues examined the role that negative cognitions (about the self, life, etc.) play in emotional difficulties after bereavement (e.g., Boelen, van den Bout, & van den Hout, 2006). Negative cognitions were positively related to current and prospective symptomatology. The authors suggested the need for further scrutiny of these cognitive processes (e.g., to address conceptual overlap between cognitive variables and symptomatology).

Related to this focus on cognitions, researchers have empirically explored *meaning-making* as instrumental in furthering adaptation and drawn the conclusion that there are indeed benefits in finding meaning related to the loss (e.g., Bower, Kemeny, Taylor, & Fahey, 1998; Davis, Nolen-Hoeksema, & Larson, 1998; Murphy, 2008). For example, Murphy (2008) reported that parents who found meaning in the deaths of their children 5 years post-death reported better health and higher levels of marital satisfaction than those who had not found meaning 5 years after the loss, suggesting that this had to do with two meaning-related tasks that are addressed by survivors: (a) minimizing the terror of a meaningless world and (b) maximizing value in their own lives (cf. Janoff-Bulman & Frantz, 1997). Not only will it be necessary for researchers to continue to specify meaning-making precisely, as Murphy (2008) did, but causal relationships between types of meaning-making and adjustment to bereavement need to be further established. Too often, assumptions about causality of meaning-making in the adjustment process are made without proper empirical testing (which requires longitudinal designs). Research exploring the role of attributions (interpretations with which people make sense of what is happening to them) is likely to contribute to this endeavor (e.g., Boelen, 2005).

One of the most important coping dimensions in relationship to (mal)adaptive adjustment to bereavement, in my view, has to do with confrontation-avoidance, and here, too, research so far has suggested the need for further specification and clarification of relationships with outcome. For example, while Nolen-Hoeksema (see, e.g., 2001) showed that those with a *distractive* style became less depressed over time (e.g., "I got busy with other things to keep my mind occupied"), Boelen et al. (2006) found that strategies of *avoidance* (e.g., of reminders of the deceased) were positively related to current and prospective symptomatology, and, in a separate investigation, that misinterpretations were related to increases in the negative effect of avoidance behavior among bereaved persons (Boelen & van den Hout, 2008). Similarly, Shear et al. (2008) identified avoidance as a key element in the development of complicated grief, and Smith, Tarakeshwar, Hansen, Kochman, and Sikkema (2009) found that avoidant coping mediated the impact of intervention on depression and grief among HIV-positive bereaved persons. Decreases in avoidant coping in their intervention group were associated with decreases in depression and grief. However, denial, repression, or avoidance may not always be detrimental. Bonanno and colleagues (see Bonanno, 2001; Bonanno, Papa, Lalande, Zhang, & Noll, 2005) did not find support for the claim that *avoidance* or *repression* has negative effects. Bonanno, Keltner, Holen, and Horowitz (1995; Bonanno, 2001) also reported a dissociation between physiologically measured arousal and indices of psychological upset among bereaved men who were placed in an "empty chair" situation. High physiological arousal but low psychological confrontation were associated with good outcome (measured at a later time point). Thus, it could be that, while too complete a denial may be associated with pathological forms of grieving (e.g., Jacobs, 1993), some degree of avoidance may be healthy.

Evidence in support of some possible benefits of denial has come from other sources, including the benefits of keeping secrets (Kelly & McKillop, 1996) and, in certain circumstances, suppressing extremely traumatic experiences (Kaminer & Lavie, 1993). These studies point to the possibility that at times it is potentially adaptive to "keep grief within" and regulate grieving. "Involuntary" nondisclosure may, however, have negative consequences: Lepore, Silver, Wortman, and Wayment (1996) found that bereaved mothers who perceived their social environments as constraining (i.e., as hindering their possibilities for disclosure), and who had high initial levels of intrusive thoughts about their loss, were more depressed in the long term. Possibly, personal control over the regulation (confrontation-avoidance) of grieving may be critical. Research (cf. Boelen, 2005) has begun to explore the role of *emotion regulation processes* (processes that people use to modify aspects of their emotions), a promising line for future research, especially since there are good theoretical grounds to argue for its importance (these will become evident later on).

Taking the above lines of research on confrontation and avoidance together, one can infer that emotion regulation is likely to be critical to adaptation. Bereaved individuals need to confront pain and work through loss, which is an effortful process. Yet, they also need to fight against the reality of loss (cf. Janoff-Bulman, 1992). On the other hand, denial is also effortful. What empirical studies so far also seem to indicate is that too much confrontation or too much avoidance is detrimental to adaptation. Both processes may be linked with detrimental health effects if undertaken relentlessly, possibly causing exhaustion. Further scientific research needs to clarify when precisely avoidant or confrontational coping is protective versus maladaptive in the coping process, and to work toward further conceptual clarification (e.g., avoidance vs. denial, repression, distraction). Scientific analysis also needs to explore and represent the tendency, even necessity, to confront combined with the tendency to avoid, deny, or suppress aspects of grieving as part of the adaptive coping process. As will be seen later on, such emotion regulation needs to, and can be, built into a model of coping with bereavement.

Coping Research: Current Status and Remaining Concerns

Taken together, it becomes evident that different types of coping processes are associated, even causally, with adaptation to bereavement. But the picture is far from clear: Despite promising beginnings, it will have become evident that the investigation of the role of coping processes in bereavement outcome is still in its infancy, due to some extent to gaps in scientific investigation and lack of methodologically sound research. Another source of difficulty has to do with the nature of the bereavement experience: Coping with the loss of a loved person is an extremely complex, multifaceted phenomenon. It is to be expected that such a multidimensional life event will require a variety of ways of coping to manage different aspects of the stressful situation and the negative emotional reaction of grief. At this point in time, researchers are still grappling with the identification of coping strategies and appraisal processes that lead to adaptation to bereavement, and indeed, few categories of coping have received adequate research attention (cf. the lists of coping categories reviewed by Skinner, Edge, Altman, & Sherwood, 2003). Not only does research still need to clarify these relationships, it also needs to investigate how the ways that persons cope interact with diverse factors (circumstances of death, intra- and interpersonal variables, etc.) to co-determine excesses across various categories of ill health or poor adaptation.

Some concerns about the quality of existing research have come up already in this section, and these need to be taken into account in forthcoming research. Additional matters for improvement include assessment and measurement issues in research on coping with bereavement (for a review, see van Heck & de Ridder, 2001). For example, there are major shortcomings in currently existing coping scales, and there are very few well-validated bereavement-specific measures available. Other features (to do with coping specifically with bereavement) contribute to difficulties in the assessment of adaptive coping strategies or styles. Different coping strategies may be more effective at different durations of bereavement or for coping with different aspects of the bereavement experience; a strategy may be useful in the shortterm but harmful in the long term; it may positively affect physical health but increase distress. Methodologically, too, many studies have shortcomings. Assessments are not frequently made longitudinally (e.g., coping strategy at the first measurement point predicting outcome at the second), and sometimes have even been conducted retrospectively. Finally, definitions of coping strategies or styles often include outcome as well as process variables. For example, some of the scales used to assess emotion-focused coping contain items that confound coping strategy with coping outcome (e.g., including questions about distress or low self-esteem among those on controlling emotions).

In addition to the need for these conceptual and methodological improvements, there are also good reasons to argue the importance of incorporating theoretical approaches, to further progress in understanding (mal)adaptive coping with bereavement. Just as the Integrative Framework of Risk Factors helps us to categorize the wide variety of variables and postulate pathways between them, so can theories help us to understand why (sets of) variables would be expected to have a positive or negative impact on outcomes. On the one hand, a theoretical approach helps us to focus research investigation on those coping strategies that are likely to affect bereavement outcomes; on the other hand, empirical results on (mal)adaptive strategies may or may not be consistent with our theoretical propositions, which may guide us toward refining our theoretical propositions. For example, in one of our own research studies, social support (a coping resource) did not buffer bereaved widows and widowers against depression (W. Stroebe et al., 1996). This led us to seek alternative theoretical guidelines (our results turned out to be more compatible with attachment theory). Sometimes, no explicit mention is made of adaptive coping in theoretical formulations, nor is any empirical exploration of this undertaken, but the theory in question clearly has implications that could be explored.

Thus, in the following section of this chapter, attention is given to exploring how general and bereavement-specific theories can guide us toward establishing the nature of adaptive coping with bereavement, and how such a theoretical base can stimulate empirical investigation on the role of coping in bereavement outcome. The extent to which the empirical findings described above fit within one or the other theoretical framework, providing support for, or disproof of, certain theoretical tenets, will also be discussed. A summary of the main principles of adaptation in coping reviewed in this last section, that have been postulated in bereavement theories and models, either explicitly or at least implicitly, is given in Table 8.2.

Adaptive Coping with Bereavement: Theoretical Approaches[1]

As can be seen in Table 8.2, the scientific literature has yielded a number of potentially useful theoretical approaches for understanding adaptive coping with bereavement. These can be classified as either general psychological theories or grief-specific models. These different categories of theories have resulted in independent lines of research on adaptive coping with bereavement. The general theories may, explicitly or implicitly, include an analysis of coping as part of their framework. Within the grief-specific category, some of the models are designed to explain the broad range of manifestations and processes of grief, including but not limited to ways of coping. Others are specific to coping with bereavement, which (again, explicitly or implicitly) try to distinguish and elucidate adaptive versus maladaptive ways of grieving.

Each of these theoretical approaches can be examined to try to identify principles of (mal)adaptive coping. The extent to which the empirical results described in the previous section provide support for the different perspectives will become evident. Different ideas on adaptive coping emerge from the various perspectives, although at times there is compatibility and even concordance with respect to predictions about adaptive coping strategies. It will also become evident that the same applies to the theories themselves: There is sometimes compatibility between their constructs, while at other times there are conflicting claims.

Generic theories
TRAUMA THEORIES
To begin with the generic theories: trauma theories have been more confined to deeply disturbing, even horrendous, life events than other theories included in Table 8.2 and discussed below. Clearly, bereavement is sometimes, but not always, a traumatic event. Three trauma perspectives have had a major impact within the bereavement field.

Stress response syndrome
Horowitz's (1986) analysis of stress response syndromes was a landmark in the scientific study of trauma. He described the normal manifestations of human reactions following traumatic events, which may reach an intensity and frequency to an extent that can be diagnosed as PTSD (Kleber & Brom, 1992). Of particular importance here, Horowitz (1986) described the antithetical reactions of intrusion–avoidance as distinctive features of traumatic reactions. Intrusion is the compulsive re-experiencing of feelings and ideas surrounding the event, including sleep and dream disturbance and hypervigilance. Avoidance signifies a denial process, including reactions such as amnesia, inability to visualize memories, and evidence of disavowal.

It is important to note that Horowitz's purpose was to determine how much impact the traumatic event had, intrusion–avoidance[2] being a "symptomatic" process useful for classification of pathology. By contrast, the current interest in adaptive coping leads to the question whether intrusion–avoidance strategies lead to adjustment to the event, perhaps paralleling the confrontation–avoidance dimension discussed in the previous section. Horowitz did not present intrusion–avoidance as a dynamic coping process but as an indicator of disturbance in reactions, although, below a specified clinically relevant level, intrusion–avoidance represents a normal coping

Table 8.2   Coping with bereavement: Main principles of adaptation in theories and models

I.   *GENERAL THEORY*

- Trauma theory

  - Stress Response Syndromes (Horowitz, 1976)[3]   *Cognitive regulation (intrusion/avoidance)*

  - Emotional Disclosure & Sharing (Pennebaker, 1997)   *Communication about the loss*

  - Assumptive World Views   *Revision of assumptions/meanings*

- Psychoanalytic Theory (Freud, 1917)   *Grief work*

- Attachment Theory (Bowlby, 1980)   *Grief work & affect regulation*

- Cognitive Stress Theory (Lazarus & Folkman, 1984)   *Emotion- and problem-focused coping; confrontation-avoidance; appraisal processes*

II.   *BEREAVEMENT MODELS: GENERAL*

- Psychosocial Transition Model (Parkes, 1996)   *Revision of assumptions; working through*

- Two-Track Model (Rubin, 1981)   *Two-track processing (leading to transformation of attachment & recovery)*

III.   *BEREAVEMENT MODELS: COPING-SPECIFIC*

- Task Model (Worden, 1982)   *Four tasks (working through)*

- Social Construction/ Meaning-Making Models (Neimeyer, 2001)   *For example, six principles to shape adaptation*

- Incremental Grief Model (Cook & Oltjenbruns, 1998)   *Symmetry & congruence within bereaved (family) groups*

- New Model of Grief (Walter, 1996)   *Biography (re)construction in (family) groups*

- Integrative Model (Bonanno & Kaltman, 1999)   *Appraisal/evaluation processing & changed representations as part of emotion regulation (dissociation of negative; enhancement of positive)*

- Dual Process Model (Stroebe & Schut, 1999)   *Confrontation–avoidance of loss vs. restoration-oriented stressors; positive-negative meaning (re)construction; oscillation (emotion regulation)*

---

process. Another difficulty for the bereavement stressor is that this process is only measured in relation to the traumatic event itself, while it will already have become clear that many additional (secondary) aspects to do with bereavement act as stressors too. A distinctive feature of intrusion–avoidance reactions to traumatic deaths of loved ones is that they are likely to incorporate comparatively higher levels of involuntary processing (lack of personal control) than non-traumatic bereavements.

Although reactions to traumas in general and bereavements in particular share certain features (see Stroebe et al., 2001b), to understand the latter, we need a more differentiated analysis of the nature of the stressor and the cognitions involved in intrusion–avoidance. It is noteworthy, though, that both of the theoretical perspectives described so far include a confrontation–avoidance dimension in reactions to stressful life events, an aspect that is far less apparent in the general bereavement models. However, it is a feature that can be picked up in developing an integrative perspective, as will be shown later.

Emotional disclosure

The theme of disclosure has been central to the body of research produced by Pennebaker and his colleagues (e.g., Pennebaker, 1989, 1993; Pennebaker, Zech, & Rimé, 2001). Empirical evidence has shown that engaging in experimental disclosure about traumatic events and the personal upset of these experiences is beneficial to psychological health, physical health, and overall functioning (for a recent meta-analytic review, see Fratarolli, 2006). In general, participants for whom this sort of intervention is helpful tend to be those with a health problem or with a history of trauma and who disclose events that had not yet been fully processed (Frattarolli, 2006).

Pennebaker's theoretical and empirical work, and that of a number of other research teams too, has attempted to unravel the social and cognitive dynamics associated with the health benefits of disclosure. Different theories about the mechanisms underlying the impact of disclosure have been proposed and, to different extents, empirically tested. These include disinhibition theory, cognitive-processing theory, self-regulation theory, social integration theory, and exposure theory (see Frattarolli, 2006). Frattarolli (2006) reported that most support was found for exposure theory, which argues that confronting, describing, and reliving the thoughts and experiences about a negative experience will lead to extinction of those thoughts and feelings.

Bereavement would clearly fall within the type of life event for which experimental disclosure would be expected to be effective, and exposure theory would seem a plausible explanation in this case too. However, as described in the last section, recent studies have not found convincing evidence that writing about feelings associated with bereavement assists in coping (Stroebe et al., 2002; W. Stroebe et al., 2005). Research on the related area of social sharing has produced similarly negative results: Contrary to lay beliefs, sharing the experience with others does not lead to emotional recovery (see Pennebaker, Zech, & Rimé, 2001).

The results for experimental exposure particularly are puzzling, in view of the positive results for other life events. Future research needs to explore subgroup differences and features to do with the writing paradigm more thoroughly, to try to establish for whom and in what manner disclosure might work.

Assumptive world views

Janoff-Bulman and her colleagues (e.g., Janoff-Bulman, 1992; Janoff-Bulman & Berg, 1998) provided a theoretical framework for understanding the role of meaning in coming to terms with traumatic life events, arguing that the fundamental assumptions that people hold about themselves, the world, and the relation between these two are shattered by traumatic events such as the death of a loved one. Three core assumptions were postulated, namely that we are worthy, that the world is benevolent, and that what happens to us "makes sense" (e.g., Janoff-Bulman, 1992). Normally, such assumptions go unchallenged, but when a loved one dies, particularly if the death circumstances were traumatic, these basic assumptions are shattered, and the bereaved person struggles to integrate the experience of the event into these meaning structures.

According to this framework, coping involves the rebuilding of the inner world to reestablish meaning, to adjust old assumptions, or (partly at least) to accept new ones. Over time, most bereaved people reestablish an assumptive world that is not so completely threatening. One would surmise that effective coping would entail searching for meaning and integration of the event into more positively meaningful structures (rather than focusing on negative aspects, such as malevolence). A key question here would be how to distinguish between bereaved persons who do this effectively, and those who do not. Defining "finding meaning" following bereavement is difficult, and, as mentioned before, identifying a causal pathway from meaning-making to outcome is difficult. For example, if one finds negative meaning ("the world is malevolent"), it would not seem surprising if this were closely associated with adjustment (e.g., in terms of distress), but it is less clear whether distress has led to the negative assumption, or vice versa. Nevertheless, as illustrated in the review of empirical evidence, researchers have linked certain types of meaning-making with positive bereavement outcomes (see also Davis, 2008).

In fact, in general this theoretical perspective focuses more on describing and understanding trauma reactions than on adaptive versus maladaptive coping. Nevertheless, as will become evident, the meaning variables identified here can be integrated into a bereavement coping framework and subjected to further empirical testing.

PSYCHOANALYTIC THEORY

In his theoretical paper on mourning and melancholia, Freud (1917/1957) had a huge influence on ideas about adaptive coping with bereavement, one that lasted across the whole of the last century and that retains its mark today. Freud proposed that when a loved one dies, the bereaved person is faced with the struggle to sever ties with and detach energy from the deceased person. The psychological function of grief is to free the individual of his or her bond to the deceased, achieving a gradual detachment by means of reviewing the past and dwelling on memories of the deceased. Grief work brings about a severance of the "attachment to the non-existent object" (Freud, 1917/1957, p. 166).

The concept of "grief work," introduced in the last section, has been fundamental to the psychoanalytic perspective on adaptive coping, and indeed, this theory has been the driving force behind empirical investigation of this principle of coping. Successful adaptation is understood to involve working through the loss, without which grief cannot be overcome. Freud described "the work which mourning performs" (1917/1957, p. 253) and explained how bereaved people undertake "reality testing," through which they gradually come to realize that the person no longer exists.

Although the grief work concept retains its theoretical and practical significance even today, in addition to the lack of much empirical support, it has also received much critical examination as a concept (Bonanno, 1998; Bonanno & Kaltman, 1999; Stroebe, 1992; Wortman & Silver, 1987, 1989, 2001). However, like meaning-making, it can usefully be incorporated into other perspectives. The first extensive effort to do this was made by Bowlby (e.g., 1980), to which I turn next.

ATTACHMENT THEORY

Within the attachment theory framework, working through grief is important for the purpose of rearranging representations of the deceased person and of the self (Bowlby, 1980; for detailed reviews see Archer, 1999; Mikulincer & Shaver, 2008; Shaver & Tancredy, 2001). It takes place through a sequence of overlapping, flexibly occurring phases: shock, yearning and protest, despair, and recovery. According to Bowlby, working through these phases enables detachment (labeled reorganization in his later work) or the breaking of affectional bonds (Bowlby, 1979). It is also understood to further the continuation of the bond, implying a relocation of the deceased so that adjustment can gradually be made to the physical absence of this person in ongoing life (Fraley & Shaver, 1999; Shaver & Tancredy, 2001).

Attachment theory differs from psychoanalytic theory with respect to the function that grief work was said to serve. Here it reflects not severance, but a characteristic response of many species following the disruption of a strong affectional bond—namely, to try to recover proximity. In the case of separation through death, proximity cannot be reestablished, resulting in protest and despair. The biological function of grieving—to end separation—is then dysfunctional.

While, as noted earlier, there is rather equivocal evidence for the value of grief work, it remains a theoretically meaningful concept and analytic tool for understanding the way people adapt to bereavement. It captures at least part of the essence of coming to terms with loss, at least in our own culture. It has to be recognized too that the writings of the major theorists such as Bowlby (1980) reflect awareness of greater complexity, while considering grief work fundamental to adaptive grieving. Fortunately, theoretical analyses of finer-grained processes relating to grief work (and empirical investigation of them) have recently been undertaken.

Notably, the work of Mikulincer and his colleagues has been heavily guided by attachment theory (e.g., Mikulincer, 2008; Mikulincer & Shaver, 2008). Mikulincer (e.g., 2008) has explored processes of *affect regulation*, which come into play when the attachment figure is not available (as in bereavement). These so-called secondary strategies are of two kinds: hyperactivation and deactivation (Mikulincer & Shaver, 2003). Hyperactivation is characterized by cognitive and behavioral efforts to reestablish proximity, while deactivation refers to inhibition of proximity-seeking inclinations and suppression of threats. In the case of separation through bereavement, proximity-seeking does not work, so these secondary strategies come into play. Reorganization of attachment, through which security is restored (said to be fundamentally important following loss), requires both hyper- and deactivation. However, this does not always take place, with some bereaved persons showing high hyperactivation and others far more deactivation in their strategies. Hyperactivation is associated with yearning and preoccupation with the loss—closely related to a ruminative coping style, rendering a person vulnerable to chronic grieving and depression. Rather the opposite takes place in the case of deactivation: A person will avoid feelings related to the loss and attempt to dismiss the importance of the lost relationship—related to a dismissive, avoidant coping style (Mikuliner, 2008). Both these strategies can produce difficulties in the case of deep attachments and are related to poor bereavement outcome (chronic vs. absent grieving, cf. Bowlby, 1980).

Despite its usefulness, the attachment theory perspective focuses consideration on relationship aspects, particularly in our case on the relationship between the bereaved and deceased person. By contrast, as will become evident in the following section, cognitive stress theory provides a framework that enables examination of the manifestations and phenomena of bereavement in much broader context, enabling systematic investigation of a variety of variables.

COGNITIVE STRESS THEORY
Cognitive stress theory (Lazarus & Folkman, 1984) is a generic theory that can easily be applied to bereavement; in fact, Folkman (2001) described such application in detail. This theory provides a framework for the fine-grained definition of characteristics of the stressor (bereavement), the coping process and outcomes, from which cause-and-effect relationships can be derived (cf. Figure 8.1). The global stressor of bereavement involves a number of simultaneous, ongoing, specific stressors, such as those to do with the loss of an attachment figure, and those relating to secondary stressors such as financial and skill losses. The model acknowledges that different stressors can coexist, though it does not describe a process of concurrent appraisal and coping with the different stressors, which is particularly relevant in the case of bereavement. Rather, it details appraisal and coping with one stressor at a time (e.g., Folkman et al., 1991).

Given the different stressors associated with bereavement, the duration-related changes in bereavement reactions, and the number and variety of empirically derived coping strategies, it is not easy to derive predictions about strategies of effective coping within this framework; indeed, Folkman (2001) noted that the coping processes which are used will be mixed and change over time. However, problem- and emotion-focused coping are especially relevant (as are positive and negative appraisal processes, to which we turn later). These were postulated as instrumental in dealing with stressful situations in general.

Some changeable aspects of the bereavement situation may be better dealt with in a problem-focused manner, since this is aimed at managing and changing the problem causing distress (Folkman, 2001; Lazarus & Folkman, 1984), such as earning money to repair the finances. Others may be better dealt with in an emotion-focused manner, because they are unchangeable (the deceased cannot be brought back), but it is hard to differentiate between adaptive and maladaptive emotion-focused coping, since in the case of bereavement, emotion-focused coping cuts across categories such as working through versus avoidance, including rumination, suppression, and denial: emotion-focused coping includes both control of emotions and expression of them. Despite such difficulties, successful coping would appear to require both problem- and emotion-focused coping strategies, and this is in line with the theoretical propositions.

Difficulties in deriving predictions about adjustment to bereavement from this theory have a lot to do with the multifaceted nature of this stressful life event. Nevertheless, cognitive stress theory has much to offer in understanding adaptive coping. For example, on a general level, it can be used to develop a much finer-grained analysis than is provided in theories that focus on the phenomenon of "grief work," described earlier. A more specific advantage is that cognitive stress theory pinpoints the mediating role of cognitive processes such as positive affect and appraisal. Folkman (1997, 2001) described pathways to explain why positive affect led to good adjustment in her *revised cognitive-stress model*, which was specified for bereavement. On the basis of her empirical findings, Folkman identified three types of processes. First, negative psychological states may motivate people to search for and create positive psychological states in order to gain relief (coping as a response to distress). Second, meaning-based processes (e.g., positive reappraisals) lead to positive psychological states. Third, positive psychological states lead back to appraisal and coping, so that coping efforts are sustained. Research from other sources has suggested that the occurrence of positive emotions *per se* may not be sufficient to affect outcomes: positive affect alone may not be efficacious in adaptive coping (cf. Pennebaker, Mayne & Francis, 1997). Rather, it may be especially the first aspect identified by Folkman that is particularly critical: positive meaning construction and reconstruction that represents adaptive coping.

Somewhat mirroring the research on positive appraisal and affect, and compatible with a cognitive stress approach, Nolen-Hoeksema (2001; see also Nolen-Hoeksema & Jackson, 1996) suggested pathways whereby *ruminative coping* may lead to a lengthening and worsening of the impact of loss: first, through enhancing the effects of depressed mood on thinking; second, through interfering with everyday instrumental behavior (reducing motivation to act that would normally increase the sense of control and lift mood); third, through interfering with effective problem-solving (because they think negatively about themselves and their lives); and fourth, through reducing necessary social support (perhaps because persistent ruminations violate social norms of coping). Following this, adaptation would be associated with more active, problem-solving, distractive, outgoing styles of coping.

Bereavement models: General

BEREAVEMENT AS A PSYCHOSOCIAL TRANSITION

Parkes's (1996) psychosocial transition model is compatible with attachment theory, a theory that Parkes (e.g., 2006) based much of his reasoning on as well. It is also comparable to Janoff-Bulman's (1992) analysis of traumas as disruptions of assumptive world views. However, Parkes provided a specific description of what types of assumptions actually change in bereavement, noting, for example, that: "When somebody dies a whole set of assumptions about the world that relied upon the other person for their validity are suddenly invalidated. Habits of thought which have been built up over many years must be reviewed and modified, a person's view of the world must change . . . it inevitably takes time and effort" (Parkes, 1996, p. 90).

According to this model, a gradual changing of assumptions is needed following a loss through death. This is difficult to achieve and takes time, since assumptions are deeply bound up with one's "internal model" of the world and of the self within it. Continued resistance to changing one's assumptions will inhibit adaptation, although in the early days and weeks it may be functional, since—given that new or revised assumptions are as yet absent—change needs to be interpreted in terms of old, familiar assumptions. Parkes (1996) accepted that grief work was an essential part of adaptive grieving. He went further than previous theorists in his specification of component, interdependent parts of the grief work process. First, he maintained, there is preoccupation with thoughts of the lost person. Second, there is painful, repetitive recollection of the loss experience, or "worry work," enabling the bereaved person

to come to acceptance of the irrevocability of loss. Third, there is an attempt to make sense of the loss, to fit it into one's set of assumptions about the world (one's "assumptive world") or to modify those assumptions if need be.

THE TWO-TRACK MODEL

Rubin's (1981; Rubin & Malkinson, 2001; Rubin & Schechter, 1997) two-track model of bereavement was formulated to enhance understanding of the bereavement process and its outcome. It can be classified as a general model as it seeks to understand ongoing functioning and the importance of the relationship to the deceased (the ways in which the deceased person is conceptualized and remembered). Like Parkes' psychosocial transition model that has just been described, it does not focus on the coping process per se, but has relevance for understanding of adaptive coping. Rubin focused his analysis on the phenomena of bereavement following the loss of a child, an area where much of his own research and clinical experience lies. The two tracks that were postulated in this model are Track I, an outcome track, describing the biopsychosocial reactions to bereavement, and Track II, which was focused on the attachment to the deceased, describing ways that this becomes transformed and a new still-ongoing relationship to the deceased is established. Track I focuses on functioning, including such aspects as anxiety and depression; family relationships; self-esteem and meaning structure; and work and investment in life tasks (Rubin & Malkinson, 2001). Track II focuses on the relationship to the deceased and includes such dimensions as imagery and memory; emotional distance; positive versus negative affect respecting the deceased; conflict; and memorialization.

These two tracks make up a dual-axis paradigm whereby the intense preoccupation with the deceased (Track II) sets in motion the bereavement response (Track I) (cf. Rubin, 1993). Different types of stressors are clearly indicated in this model, as well as different coping dimensions (e.g., emotional distancing), but, in contrast to cognitive stress theory (e.g., Folkman et al., 1991), the model was not intended to provide a detailed analysis of cognitive processes or structures. However, importantly, it highlights the central role of the nature of the relationship not only to the deceased (in Track II), but also to others in ongoing life (in Track I) in adaptation to bereavement. Likewise, it suggests a dynamic mechanism associated with the attachment bond, through its identification and clear distinction of the two tracks.

Bereavement models: Coping-specific

The general bereavement models described above do not offer a fine-grained analysis of the coping process along the lines that cognitive stress theory does. The coping-specific bereavement models to be discussed next do go further toward specifying coping dimensions and are also typically quite compatible with cognitive stress theory. As is the case for the above perspectives, there is frequently a lack of empirical testing of the coping-specific bereavement models, some being derived more from clinical wisdom and experience than from rigorous research investigation.

THE TASK MODEL

Within a framework that clearly incorporates (and refines) the notion of grief work as a coping strategy, Worden (1982/1991/2002/2009) described "tasks" that the bereaved person has to perform in order to adjust to bereavement. Such a model represents coping as a more dynamic process than the "phases" or "stages" described above under attachment theory. Within the task model, the griever is presented as actively working through grief (rather than more passively experiencing it), which seems to mirror the reality that most grievers report. The grief process is viewed to encompass four tasks: (1) accepting the reality of loss; (2) experiencing the pain of grief; (3) adjusting to an environment without the deceased; and (4) "relocating" the deceased emotionally. In his revisions over the years, Worden made slight adjustments to these tasks. Most notably, in his most recent revision (Worden, 2009) the fourth task is now "To find an enduring connection with the deceased in the midst of embarking on a new life."

Although it is sometimes misrepresented, it is clear that Worden did not claim that all grievers undertake these tasks, or in the set order outlined above. Nevertheless, according to this perspective, completion of the work associated with each task should facilitate adaptation. This formulation also incorporates an implicit "time" dimension: different coping tasks are appropriate at different durations of bereavement (e.g., task 1 would rather naturally come before task 4 above), which is a useful consideration in making predictions about adaptive coping.

However, additional tasks need to be performed, such as working toward acceptance of the changed world, not just the reality of loss. One needs to take time out from grieving, as well as experiencing pain. The subjective environment itself (not just adjustment to the environment) needs to be reconstructed. Finally, we need to specify that bereaved people work toward developing new roles, identities, and relationships, not just relocating the deceased and "moving on." As argued further on, integrating such aspects could increase the predictive potential of coping models.

SOCIAL CONSTRUCTION AND MEANING-MAKING MODELS

A significant development in the scientific study of bereavement has been the recognition of grieving as a process of meaning reconstruction. This builds on the work of Janoff-Bulman (e.g., Janoff-Bulman & Berg, 1998) on assumptive world views described earlier, and it also has its roots in symbolic interactionism and in family systems theory (see Rosenblatt, 1993, 2001). This type of research has focused on grief as a social (construction) process. In fact, there are good reasons to assume that the way one bereaved person copes and adapts will be strongly influenced by the way that others around him or her do so. Following this assumption, meaning is understood to be constructed or "negotiated," often between grieving family members, and the process of coming to terms with bereavement is an ongoing (social) effort. Assumptions about the relationship to the deceased are actively explored and adjusted, rather than static, entrenched phenomena. Bereaved people develop "narratives" about the nature of the deceased's life and death, and these "social constructions" themselves can affect the outcome of grief. However, not all investigators have been specifically interested in the relationship between social constructions and adaptive coping (cf. Nadeau, 1998, 2001; Rosenblatt, 2001).

Neimeyer's meaning-making approach (1998, 2001; Neimeyer, Keesee & Fortner, 1998) emphasized the extent to which one's adaptation to loss is shaped by personal, familial, and cultural factors. He suggested that meaning reconstruction is the central process of grieving (along similar lines here, then, to Walter). More specifically, though, he proposed six principles or "propositions" that would help in the construction of a more adequate theory of coping with bereavement. The first proposition concerned the (in)validation of beliefs, or experience for which there are no existing constructions; the second involved the personal nature of grief (our sense of who we are); the third, "grieving is something we do, not something that is done to us" (p. 101); the fourth requires reconstructing the personal world of meaning; the fifth focused on the functions (not just symptomatology) of grief feelings as signals of meaning-making efforts. Finally, the sixth places the griever in social context: we (re)construct our identities in negotiation with others.

According to this perspective, the process of adaptation would entail confronting and exploring these six concerns relating to loss. It involves an ongoing process of confrontation of the meaning of the deceased person for the bereaved, and articulation of the personal construction of the relationship. Coping effectively with grief entails meaning reconstruction, or rebuilding of previously held beliefs, and negotiation and renegotiation over time. Lack of adaptation will occur if the bereaved person cannot explore and articulate his or her ongoing construction of the relationship with the deceased.

INCREMENTAL GRIEF MODEL

The social construction and meaning-making approaches described above have made clear that bereaved people do not grieve alone, but with others who have also suffered the loss of the loved one, and that it is necessary to extend analysis beyond the intrapersonal to interpersonal perspectives. Another interpersonal model—rather different in nature than those described so far—that deserves further expansion and recognition is the so-called incremental grief model.

Basic to Cook and Oltjenbrun's (1998) model of incremental grief is the understanding that one loss can often trigger another loss. Consequently, there is a magnification of grief occurring with each added loss. Importantly here, these investigators describe the "dissynchrony of grief" among bereaved persons (particularly families), as different persons grieving together over the loss of a loved one exhibit discrepant coping styles. Asymmetry and incongruence in grieving is said to lead to secondary loss, meaning a change between the grievers in their relationship. The latter is an additional source of stress for the survivors. The argument, then, is that loss of a child (primary loss) would trigger change in the relationship with one's partner (secondary loss), and precipitate yet another loss, possibly divorce (tertiary loss). Thus, "incremental loss" denotes "the additive factor of grief due to multiple related losses" (Cook & Oltjenbruns, 1998, p. 160). In this manner, Cook and Oltjenbruns (1998; Oltjenbruns, this volume) place individual coping reactions within the context of the surrounding social environment.

It seems fair to assume that poor adaptation to grief would be predicted in cases where incremental grieving takes place. More specifically, one would predict that the outcome would be poor in cases of asymmetry and incongruence. In contrast, couples coping "congruently" might be expected to adjust more easily. These analyses, then, introduce an important new dimension in understanding processes of adaptive coping, and complement the more intrapersonal, cognitive-level perspectives. Still needed, however, are operationalizations of "(in)congruence" and investigations of relationships to health detriments/benefits.

NEW MODEL OF GRIEF

While not strictly a "coping model," Walter's (1996) new model of grief—also an interpersonal model in some respects—described the process of grief in such a way that hypotheses about adaptive coping can be derived. Walter (1996) proposed that the purpose of grief is to grasp the reality of the death. This is accomplished through "the construction of a durable biography that enables the living to integrate the memory of the dead into their ongoing lives" (p. 7). This is achieved principally through talking to others who knew the deceased. According to Walter, even if talking does not help adjustment in terms of recovery from distress, it does help in the process of biography construction, the dimension along which adjustment should, he says, be measured. Walter argued that grieving is done when a durable biography has been constructed that enables the living to integrate the memory of the deceased into their ongoing lives. The emphasis is on talking rather than feeling, and on a non-medical outcome of grieving, namely the relocation of the deceased. Following this line of argument, adaptive coping would necessitate talking to people. Only if this is done can a durable biography be derived, and the deceased can move on and stop grieving, having found a ongoing place for the deceased.

INTEGRATIVE PERSPECTIVE ON BEREAVEMENT

Exceptionally, Bonanno and Kaltman (1999) derived their integrative perspective from a variety of empirically tested sources. They considered bereavement in terms of four components. The first of these is the *context of the loss*, which refers to risk factors such as type of death, age, gender, social support, and cultural setting. The second factor is *the continuum of subjective meanings associated with loss*, ranging from appraisals and evaluations of everyday matters and problems as well as existential concerns about the meaning of life and death. The third is *the changing representations of the lost relationship over time*, which plays an important role in the grieving process: "there appears to be an optimal or manageable level of grief that allows for the reorganization of the bereaved survivor's representational world into a supportive and ongoing bond with the deceased" (p. 770). Finally, most important for current concerns, *the role of coping and emotion-regulation processes* highlights the range of coping strategies that may "potentially mollify or exacerbate the stress of loss" (p. 770). This fourth component draws on the cognitive stress perspective described above, and on emotion theory. Importantly, according to the latter perspective, "emotion is not a unitary phenomenon but, rather, manifests in multiple channels, including experiential, expressive, and physiological responses" (Bonanno & Kaltman, 1999, p. 771). They further argue that emotion regulation research can be used to show ways to draw these perspectives together, by showing how regulation of emotion may at times involve deliberate or strategic processing and at others, more spontaneous or automatic regulatory processing and thereby not available to conscious awareness—or easily captured by self-report instruments.

Bonanno and Kaltman (1999) identified an important aspect of emotion regulation in bereavement that would enhance adjustment, namely the regulation or even dissociation of negative emotions and the enhancement of positive emotions: "these processes foster adjustment to loss because they help maintain relatively high levels of functioning, and thus contribute to retrospective reappraisals that the pain of loss can be coped with and that life can go on after the death of a loved one" (p. 771).

A unique aspect of Bonanno and Kaltman's (1999) model is the focus on emotion theory and on the identification of spontaneous or automatic processes. There is also some empirical support for this approach (e.g., Bonanno & Keltner, 1997; Bonanno et al, 1995). Adaptive ways of grieving may be better understood, then, if such processes are included in the analysis. Furthermore, this perspective adds weight to the argument that positive emotions foster adjustment. It also supports Folkman's (1997, 2001) analysis of positive appraisal pathways, and her contention that negative emotion exacerbates grief. Similarly, it is consistent with Nolen-Hoeksema's analysis of ruminative pathways (Nolen-Hoeksema, 2001; Nolen-Hoeksema & Jackson, 1996).

THE DUAL PROCESS MODEL

Many of the above perspectives have influenced the formulation of our own DPM (Stroebe & Schut, 1999, 2001b, 2008), most particularly cognitive stress and attachment theories. As such, the DPM represents an attempt to integrate existing ideas, rather than an altogether new model, although, as will become evident, it does incorporate unique features. It was designed to address a number of limitations of previous perspectives. For example, as noted earlier, we found that little empirical evidence was actually available for the grief work notion, which is such a fundamental concept in many of the perspectives (Stroebe & Schut, 1999). Clearly, conceptual refinement of this construct was needed. We were also concerned about the applicability of some of the coping models in different cultural settings: Other societies have very different ways of going about dealing with bereavement. Furthermore, some models seemed to neglect the existence of multiple stressors in bereavement, a feature that cognitive stress theory clearly recognized. Related to the last point, there seemed too little acknowledgement of the dynamic nature of coping with bereavement and too little consideration of the fact that emotion regulation must be part and parcel of dealing with loss.

The following taxonomy was thus developed. The DPM defines two broad types of stressors. In grieving, people have to deal with a number of diverse stressors, which can be classified into those that are loss- versus restoration-oriented. "Loss orientation" refers to the bereaved person's processing of some aspect of the loss experience itself. The focus of attachment theory on the nature of the lost relationship would be consistent with this, as would the integration of grief work in this orientation. "Restoration orientation" refers to the focus on secondary stressors that are also consequences of bereavement. This is in accordance with cognitive stress theory, since the latter perspective assumes that a range of sub-stressors may occur. Both orientations are sources of stress, are burdensome and are associated with distress and anxiety. Both are, then, involved in the coping process, and are attended to in varying degrees (according to individual and cultural variations).

Confrontation versus avoidance of these two types of stressors is formulated as dynamic and fluctuating, and also as changing over time. The DPM specifies a dynamic coping process (the regulatory process of "oscillation") that distinguishes it from other models. It is proposed that a bereaved person will alternate between loss- versus restoration-oriented coping. At times the bereaved will confront aspects of loss and at other times will avoid them, and the same applies to the tasks of restoration. Sometimes, too, there will be "time out," when grieving is left alone. What emerges is a more complex regulatory process of confrontation and avoidance than that described above in the models of confrontation (disclosure, etc.) versus avoidance (denial, etc.). The DPM postulates that oscillation between the two types of stressor is necessary for adaptive coping. The introduction of this regulatory process of oscillation in the DPM amends previous grief work conceptions, and it includes facilitative functions of periodic withdrawal from grieving, as emphasized by Rosenblatt (1983). The structural components are depicted in Figure 8.2.

The DPM provides an analysis of cognitions related to the confrontation–avoidance process. Following the analyses of Folkman (2001) and Nolen-Hoeksema (2001), there are good reasons to argue the need for oscillation between positive and negative affect and (re)appraisal as an integral part of the coping process. Persistent negative affect enhances grief, yet working through grief, which includes rumination, has been identified as important in coming to terms with a bereavement. On the other hand, positive reappraisals sustain the coping effort. Yet, if positive psychological states are maintained relentlessly, grieving is neglected. Folkman's (1997, 2001) integration of positive meaning states in the revision of stress-coping theory can be incorporated into the DPM. Following the work of Nolen-Hoeksema (2001; Nolen-Hoeksema & Jackson, 1996), integration of negative appraisals is also needed. This leads to pathways, as shown in Figure 8.3. Following this model, adaptive coping would require oscillation between positive and negative (re)appraisal in relationship not only to loss but also restoration orientation. This cognitive analysis provides a framework for addressing the types of assumptive worlds, meaning systems, or life narratives of bereaved people that other theorists had identified as critical to adaptive coping.

The DPM is also broadly applicable. For example, it lends itself to the analysis of between- and within-cultural group differences in ways of coping with grief; pathological grief manifestations; and duration of bereavement changes in adaptive coping (see Stroebe & Schut, 1999). Furthermore, although the analysis so far has been essentially intrapersonal, an interpersonal framework can be superimposed (cf. Stroebe & Schut, 2008). For example, individuals (and groups) differ in the extent to which they are loss- or restoration-oriented. Women tend to be more loss-oriented in their grieving than men (cf. Wijngaards de Meij et al., 2008). The "profile"

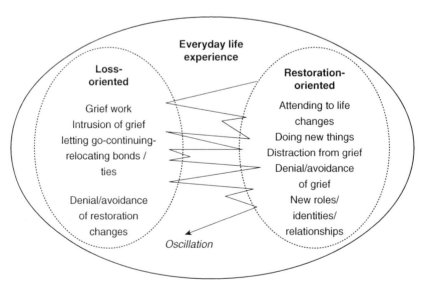

Fig. 8.2 The Dual Process Model of coping with bereavement.

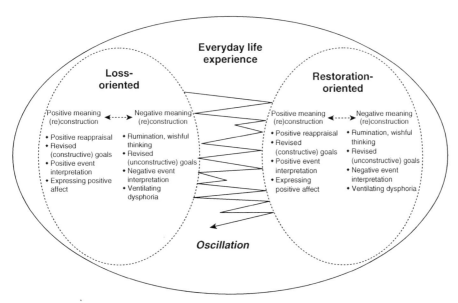

Fig. 8.3 Appraisal processes in the Dual Process Model.
(Copyright 2001, reprinted with permission of American Psychological Association.)

of coping with grief as represented in Figures 8.2 and 8.3 would be different for men and women. Since bereaved people typically grieve in families or other small groups, it would be predicted that lack of congruence in ways of grieving could lead to conflicts and poorer adaptation of the grievers (cf. Cook & Oltjenbruns, 1998). Furthermore, although the DPM was originally developed as a framework for understanding partner loss, it has application to other types of bereavement (e.g., parents grieving over the loss of their child; see Wijngaards et al., 2008).

Although the DPM looks straightforward, it is difficult to test its parameters and relate the coping processes to bereavement outcomes. Nevertheless, several research teams have begun to explore the validity of DPM constructs (e.g., Caserta & Lund, 2007; Richardson & Balaswamy, 2001; Shear, Frank, Houck & Reynolds, 2005; Wijngaards de Meij et al., 2008). For example, Shear et al. (2005) used the DPM as a guideline for designing an intervention program and evaluated the efficacy of this program against an established one. DPM tasks were described to clients with complicated grief. The need to focus on restoration as well as loss tasks was emphasized and directly addressed in therapy sessions. The DPM-type intervention was more effective (even) than the standard therapy. This research provides preliminary evidence that confronting and coping with both types of stressors can

indeed lead to adaptation to bereavement (among those with complicated forms of grief).

There are good reasons to argue the need for a bereavement-specific rather than general model of adaptive coping with grief, not least because manifestations of bereavement are complex and largely idiosyncratic to this particular stressor. Nevertheless, as has become evident, useful guidelines for the development of a model such as the DPM can be derived from the more general theories. Further refinement and testing of this and other models is a task for the future.

General Conclusions

The empirical studies on coping with bereavement and the theoretical approaches reviewed above demonstrate that coping processes play a role in the well-established relationship between the stress of bereavement and illness or health. The scientific knowledge base reviewed in this chapter has indeed illustrated how important it is to understand the ways that people cope, both on a concrete level of day-to-day dealing with bereavement (e.g., with loss and restoration stressors) and at the more abstract level of assumptions and appraisals. Clearly, as Folkman (2001) pointed out, the influence of coping on adjustment needs to be compared with that of other factors, such as the cause and type of death, an individual's personal history of loss, personality characteristics, and so on. Focusing on the coping dimension alone will not provide sufficient explanation for the variance in persons' recovery from loss. Nevertheless, as studies of the efficacy of intervention programs have shown, even though one cannot change the harrowing reality of the death of a loved one, it is possible to influence the ways that bereaved persons cope with and appraise their loss, and intense suffering can thereby perhaps be lessened.

Looking to the future, what focus do we need to take in order to advance understanding of coping with bereavement? Several lines for future investigation and conceptual refinement have already been suggested in the preceding sections of this chapter. As will also have become evident, in my view, research on coping with bereavement can most profitably proceed from a sound theoretical base, with systematic attempts made to obtain empirical evidence to back up conceptual propositions. There are several reasons why a scientific model of coping with bereavement is needed, some of which have been touched on already.

First, a scientific perspective provides a useful basis for testing the validity of assumptions that people have about the coping process. For example, lay assumptions about the importance of "grief work" have varied between the poetical notion that one must "give sorrow words" and the belief that one must "keep grief within." Without a systematic analysis based on theoretical principles (why one needs to confront grief; what precisely confronting or "grief work" is, or what function it serves), it is difficult to establish which assumption is valid, or whether people's beliefs about what is best for them, actually is (cf. Wortman & Silver, 2001).

Second, theories of coping can provide guidelines for the process of collecting valid data. Questionnaires for measuring coping used to be developed on the basis of clinical experience or intuition and were subject to extremely negative evaluation (e.g., Coyne & Gottlieb, 1996). Currently, theoretical models are deemed important for the development of assessment instruments: "rational, theory-driven strategies are to be recommended over inductive, empirical approaches which run the risk of coincidental solutions" (van Heck & de Ridder, 2001). For example, Caserta and Lund (2007) have developed a coping questionnaire based on the DPM, which puts parameters of this model to empirical test.

Third, theories can clearly guide the actual planning of research. The task of scientists is to search for regularities, so that predictions can be made

(e.g., about the likelihood of poor adjustment). For example, attachment theory suggests different ways of coping according to the security of one's relationships with loved persons. Research has in fact found associations between anxious and avoidant attachment and poor bereavement outcome (Mikulincer & Shaver, 2008; M. Stroebe, Schut, & Stroebe, 2005a; Wijngaards et al., 2007). Establishment of these patterns can be used to develop therapy protocols for those experiencing complicated grief (cf. Shorey & Snyder, 2006). In connection with this, there are applied as well as scientific reasons for a theoretical approach to adaptive coping. In understanding how people come to terms with loss, we learn much about the nature of grief itself, but we also need answers to questions about effective coping in order to help those who suffer extremely.

Following the last point above, an equally important concern for future scientific endeavor is the translation of research into practice, and vice versa: Research on coping with bereavement needs to be fuelled, for example, by questions that arise from healthcare professionals encountering bereaved clients in difficulties, or by bereaved clients themselves; and research findings (e.g., on (in)effective coping strategies) need to be fed back into practice to improve care for acutely grieving clients who are in trouble. Key questions need to be addressed: How can scientific knowledge about coping with bereavement be applied in planning support, and can types of intervention be designed and implemented according to patterns that have emerged from scientific research? Does it really help to focus on scientifically established maladaptive coping processes in intervention? Examples of studies that address such questions are already becoming available in the literature. As reported earlier, Shear et al. (2005) "translated" the DPM into an effective therapy program for persons with complicated grief. Somewhat conversely, indicating the impact of study participants' feedback on the research process, Folkman (2001) described how their reports on sustained positive affect during the pre-bereavement caregiving period led to the revision of cognitive stress theory.

It has become amply evident in this chapter that the concept of coping has had an enormous impact on the bereavement research field so far, not least in guiding scientists and practitioners beyond the grief work notion toward specification of the ways that people go about dealing (mal)adaptively with bereavement. Adopting a theoretical approach to empirical investigation and furthering links with practice, as suggested above, should lead to better understanding of the difficulties encountered by bereaved people in coming to terms with the loss of a loved one.

Notes

1 Parts of this section have been adapted from M. Stroebe & Schut (2001a).

2 Later, an additional dimension, namely hyperarousal, was added (see Weiss & Marmar, 1997).

3 Key/original references only are given in this table.

References

Agerbo, E. (2005). Midlife suicide risk, partner's psychiatric illness, spouse and child bereavement by suicide or other modes of death: a gender specific study. *Journal of Epidemiology and Community Health, 59,* 407–12.

Aldwin, C., & Revenson, T. (1987). Does coping help? A reexamination of the relationship between coping and mental health. *Journal of Personality and Social Psychology, 53,* 337–48.

American Psychiatric Association. (1994). *Diagnostic and statistical manual of mental disorders* (4th ed.). Washington, DC: Author.

Archer, J. (1999). *The nature of grief: The evolution and psychology of reactions to loss.* London: Routledge.

Barry, L., Kasl, S., & Prigerson, H. (2002). Psychiatric disorders among bereaved persons: The role of perceived circumstances of death and preparedness for death. *American Journal of Geriatric Psychiatry, 10,* 447–57.

Boelen, P. (2005). *Complicated grief: Assessment, theory, and treatment.* Enscede/Amsterdam: Ipskamp.

Boelen, P., van den Bout, & van den Hout, M. (2006). Negative cognitions and avoidance in emotional problems after bereavement: A prospective study. *Behavior Research and Therapy, 44,* 1657–72.

Boelen, P., & van den Hout, M. (2008). The role of threatening misinterpretations and avoidance in emotional problems after loss. *Behavioural and Cognitive Psychotherapy, 36, 71–88.*

Boelen, P., Schut, H., Stroebe, M., & Zijerveld, A. (2006a). Continuing bonds and grief: A prospective analysis. *Death Studies,* 30, 767–76.

Bonanno, G. (1998). The concept of "working through" loss: A critical evaluation of the cultural, historical, and empirical evidence. In A. Maercker, M. Schuetzwohl, & Z. Solomon (Eds.), *Posttraumatic stress disorder: Vulnerability and resilience in the life-span* (pp. 221–47). Gottingen, Germany: Hogrefe & Huber.

Bonanno, G. (2001). Grief and emotion: A social-functional perspective. In: M. S. Stroebe, R. O. Hansson, W. Stroebe, & H. A. W. Schut (Eds.), *Handbook of bereavement research: Consequences, coping and care* (pp. 493–515). Washington, DC: American Psychological Association Press.

Bonanno, G. (2004). Loss, trauma, and human resilience: have we underestimated the human capacity to thrive after extremely aversive events? *American Psychologist, 59,* 20–8.

Bonanno, G. (2008). Grief, trauma, and resilience. *Grief Matters: The Australian Journal of Grief and Bereavement,* 11, 11–7.

Bonanno, G., Boerner, K., & Wortman, C. (2008). Trajectories of grieving. In M. S. Stroebe, R. O. Hansson, H. Schut, & W. Stroebe (Eds.) *Handbook of bereavement research and practice: Advances in theory and intervention* (pp. 287–307). Washington, DC: American Psychological Association.

Bonanno, G., & Kaltman, S. (1999). Toward an integrative perspective on bereavement. *Psychological Bulletin, 125,* 760–76.

Bonanno, G. A., & Keltner, D. (1997). Facial expressions of emotion and the course of conjugal bereavement. *Journal of Abnormal Psychology, 106,* 126–37.

Bonanno, G. A., Keltner, D., Holen, A., & Horowitz, M. J. (1995). When avoiding unpleasant emotions may not be such a bad thing: Verbal-autonomic response dissociation and midlife conjugal bereavement. *Journal of Personality and Social Psychology, 69,* 975–89.

Bonanno, G., Papa, A., Lalande, K., Zhang, N., & Noll, J. (2005). Grief processing and deliberate grief avoidance: A prospective comparison of bereaved spouses and parents in the United States and the People's Republic of China. *Journal of Consulting and Clinical Psychology,* 73, 86–98.

Bower, J., Kemeny, M., Taylor, S., & Fahey, J. (1988). Cognitive processing, discovery of meaning, CD4 decline, and AIDS-related mortality among bereaved HIV-seropositive men. *Journal of Consulting and Clinical Psychology, 66,* 979–86.

Bowlby, J. (1979). *The making and breaking of affectional bonds.* London: Tavistock.

Bowlby, J. (1980). *Attachment and loss. Vol. 3. Loss: Sadness and depression.* London: Hogarth.

Byrne, G., & Raphael, B. (1999). Depressive symptoms and depressive episodes in recently widowed older men. *International Journal of Geriatric Psychiatry, 12,* 241–51.

Carnelley, K., Wortman, C., & Kessler, R. (1999). The impact of widowhood on depression: Findings from a prospective survey. *Psychological Medicine, 29,* 1111–23.

Caserta, M., & Lund, D. (2007). Toward the development of an inventory of daily widowed life (IDWL): Guided by the Dual Process Model of coping with bereavement. *Death Studies, 31,* 505–35.

Christ, G., Siegel, K., & Christ, A. (2005). Adolescent grief: "It never really hit me until it actually happened." *Journal of the American Medical Association, 288,* 1269–79.

Cook, A., & Oltjenbruns, K. (1998). *Dying and grieving: Lifespan and family perspectives.* Fort Worth: Harcourt and Brace.

Coyne, J., & Gottlieb, B. (1996). The mismeasure of coping by checklist. *Journal of Personality, 64,* 959–91.

Currier, J., Neimeyer, R., & Berman, J. (2008). The effectiveness of psychotherapeutic interventions for the bereaved: A comprehensive, quantitative review. *Psychological Bulletin, 134,* 648–61.

Davis, C. (2008). Redefining goals and redefining self: A closer look at posttraumatic growth following loss. In: M. Stroebe, R. O. Hansson, H. Schut, & W. Stroebe (Eds.), *Handbook of bereavement research and practice: Advances in theory and intervention* (pp. 309–25). Washington, DC: American Psychological Association Press.

Davis, C., Nolen-Hoeksema, S., & Larson, J. (1998). Making sense of loss and benefitting from the experience: Two construals of meaning. *Journal of Personality and Social Psychology, 75,* 561–74.

Folkman, S. (1997). Positive psychological states and coping with severe stress. *Social Science and Medicine, 45,* 1207–21.

Folkman, S. (2001). Revised coping theory and the process of bereavement. In: Stroebe, M., Hansson, R. O., Stroebe, W., & Schut, H. (Eds.). *Handbook of bereavement research: Consequences, coping, and care* (pp. 563–84). Washington, DC: American Psychological Association Press.

Folkman, S., Chesney, M., McKusick, L., Ironson, G., Johnson, D., & Coates, T. (1991). Translating coping theory into an intervention. In J. Eckenrode (Ed.), *The social context of coping* (pp. 239–60). New York: Plenum.

Fraley, R. C., & Shaver, P. (1999). Loss and bereavement: Attachment theory and recent controversies concerning "grief work" and the nature of detachment. In: J. Cassidy & P. R. Shaver (Eds.), *Handbook of attachment: Theory, research, and clinical applications* (pp. 735–59). New York: Guilford.

Frattarolli, J. (2006). Experimental disclosure and its moderators: A meta-analysis. *Psychological Bulletin, 132,* 823–65.

Freud, S. (1917/1957). Mourning and melancholia. In J. Strachey (Ed. & Trans.), *Standard edition of the complete psychological works of Sigmund Freud.* London: Hogarth.

Friborg, O., Hjemdal, O., Rosenvinge, J., Martinussen, M., Aslaksen, P., & Flaten, M. (2006). Resilience as a moderator of pain and stress. *Journal of Psychosomatic Research, 61,* 213–9.

Hansson, R. O., & Stroebe, M. S. (2007). *Bereavement in later life: Coping, adaptation, and developmental influences.* Washington, DC: American Psychological Association Press.

Heck, G. van, & Ridder, D. de (2001). Assessment of coping with loss: Dimensions and measurement. In: Stroebe, M., Hansson, R. O., Stroebe, W. & Schut, H. (Eds.), *Handbook of bereavement research: Consequences, coping, and care* (pp. 449–69). Washington, DC: American Psychological Association Press.

Horowitz, M. (1976, 1st Ed.). *Stress response syndromes.* Northvale, NJ: Aronson.

Houwen, K. van der, Stroebe, M., Stroebe, W., Schut, H., van den Bout, J., & Wijngaards-de Meij, L. (2010). Risk factors for bereavement outcome: A multivariate approach. *Death Studies, 34,* 195–220.

Jacobs, S. (1993). *Pathologic grief: Maladaptation to loss.* Washington, DC: American Psychiatric Press.

Janoff-Bulman, R. (1992). *Shattered assumptions: Towards a new psychology of trauma.* New York: Free Press.

Janoff-Bulman, R., & Berg, M. (1998). Disillusionment and the creation of value: From traumatic losses to existential gains. In J. H. Harvey (Ed.), *Perspectives on loss: A sourcebook* (pp. 35–47). Philadelphia: Taylor & Francis.

Janoff-Bulman, R., & Frantz, C. (1997). The impact of trauma on meaning: From meaningless world to meaningful life. In M. Power & C. Brewin (Eds.), *The transformation of meaning in psychological therapies* (pp. 91–106). New York: Wiley.

Kaminer, H., & Lavie, P. (1993). Sleep and dreams in well-adjusted and less-adjusted Holocaust survivors. In M. Stroebe, W. Stroebe, & R. O. Hansson (Eds.), *Handbook of bereavement: Theory, research and intervention* (pp. 331–45). New York: Cambridge University Press.

Kelly, A. E., & McKillop, K. J. (1996). Consequences of revealing personal secrets. *Psychological Bulletin, 120,* 450–65.

Kleber, R., & Brom, D. (1992). *Coping with trauma: Theory, prevention, and treatment.* Amsterdam: Swets & Zeitlinger.

Lazarus, R., & Folkman, S. (1984). *Stress, appraisal and coping.* New York: Springer.

Lepore, S. J., Silver, R., Wortman, C., & Wayment, H. A. (1996). Social constraints, intrusive thoughts, and depressive symptoms among bereaved mothers. *Journal of Personality and Social Psychology, 70,* 271–82.

Li, J., Precht, D., Mortensen, P., & Oldsen, J. (2003). Mortality of parents after death of a child in Denmark. *Lancet, 361,* 363–7.

Lillard, L., & White, L. (1995). Till death do us part—marital disruption and mortality. *American Journal of Sociology, 100,* 1131–56.

Middleton, W., Raphael, B., Martinek, N., & Misso, V. (1993). Pathological grief reactions. In: M. Stroebe, W. Stroebe, & R. O. Hansson (Eds.), *Handbook of bereavement* (pp. 44–61). New York: Cambridge University Press.

Mikulincer, M. (2008). An attachment perspective on disordered grief reactions and the process of grief resolution. *Grief Matters: The Australian Journal of Grief and Bereavement, 11,* 34–7.

Mikulincer, M., & Shaver, P. (2003). The attachment behavioral system in adulthood: Activation, psychodynamics, and interpersonal processes. In M. Zanna (Ed.), *Advances in experimental social psychology* (Vol. 35, pp. 53–152).

Mikulincer, M., & Shaver, P. (2008). An attachment perspective on bereavement. In M. S. Stroebe, R. O. Hansson, H. Schut, & W. Stroebe (Eds.), *Handbook of bereavement research and practice: Advances in theory and intervention* (pp. 87–112). Washington, DC: American Psychological Association.

Moskowitz, J., Folkman, S., & Acree, M. (2003). Do positive psychological states shed light on recovery from bereavement? *Death Studies, 27,* 471–500.

Murphy, S. (2008). The loss of a child: Sudden death and illness perspectives. In M. S. Stroebe, R. O. Hansson, H. Schut, & W. Stroebe (Eds.), *Handbook of bereavement research and practice: Advances in theory and intervention* (pp. 375–95). Washington, DC: American Psychological Association.

Murphy, S., Lohan, J., Braun, T., Johnson, L., Cain, K., Beaton, R., & Baugher, R. (1999). Parents' health, health care utilization, and health behaviors following the violent deaths of their 12- to 18-year-old children: a prospective, longitudinal analysis. *Death Studies, 23,* 589–616.

Murphy, S., Johnson, L., Chung, I., & Beaton, R. (2003). The prevalence of PTSD following the violent death of a child and predictors of change 5 years later. *Journal of Traumatic Stress, 16,* 17–25.

Nadeau, J. (1998). *Families making sense of death.* Thousand Oaks, CA: Sage.

Nadeau, J. (2001). Meaning making in family bereavement: A family systems approach. In: M. Stroebe, R. O. Hansson, W. Stroebe, & H. Schut (Eds.), *Handbook of bereavement research: Consequences, coping, and care* (pp. 329–47). Washington, DC: American Psychological Association Press.

Neimeyer, R. (1998). *The lessons of loss: A guide to coping.* Raleigh, NC: McGraw Hill.

Neimeyer, R. (2001). *Meaning reconstruction and the experience of loss.* Washington, DC: American Psychological Association Press.

Neimeyer, R., Keesee, N., & Fortner, B. (1998). Loss and meaning reconstruction: Propositions and procedures. In S. Rubin, R. Malkinson, & E. Witztum (Eds.), *Traumatic and non-traumatic bereavement.* Madison, CT: International Universities Press.

Nolen-Hoeksema, S. (2001). Ruminative coping and adjustment to bereavement. In: M. S. Stroebe, R. O. Hansson, W. Stroebe, & H. A. W. Schut (Eds.), *Handbook of bereavement research: Consequences, coping and care* (pp. 545–62). Washington, DC: American Psychological Association Press.

Nolen-Hoeksema, S., & Jackson, B. (1996). *Ruminative coping and the gender differences in depression.* Paper presented at the American Psychological Association Meeting, Toronto, August 10.

Ong, A., Bergeman, C., & Bisconti, T. (2005). Unique effects of daily perceived control on anxiety symptomatology during conjugal bereavement. *Personality and Individual Differences, 38,* 1057–67.

Parkes, C. M. (1996). *Bereavement: Studies of grief in adult life* (3rd ed.). Harmondsworth/London: Penguin/Routledge.

Parkes, C. M. (2005). Symposium on complicated grief. *Omega: Journal of Death and Dying, 52,* whole issue.

Parkes, C. M. (2006). *Love and loss: the roots of grief and its complications.* Hove, UK: Routledge.

Parkes, C., Benjamin, B., & Fitzgerald, R. (1969). Broken heart: A statistical study of increased mortality among widowers. *British Medical Journal, 1,* 740–3.

Parkes, C. M., & Weiss, R. (1983). *Recovery from bereavement.* New York: Basic Books.

Pennebaker, J. (1989). Confession, inhibition and disease. In L. Berkowitz (Ed.), *Advances in Experimental Social Psychology, 22,* 211–44. New York: Academic Press.

Pennebaker, J. (1993). Putting stress into words: Health, linguistic, and therapeutic implications. *Behavior Research & Therapy, 31,* 539–48.

Pennebaker, J. (1997). *Opening up: The healing power of expressing emotions.* (Rev. ed.). New York: Guilford Press.

Pennebaker, J., Mayne, T. J., & Francis, M. E. (1997). Linguistic predictors of adaptive bereavement. *Journal of Personality and Social Psychology, 72,* 863–71.

Pennebaker, J., Zech, E., & Rimé, B. (2001). Disclosing and sharing emotion: Psychological, social, and health consequences. In M. S. Stroebe, R. O. Hansson, W. Stroebe, & H.A.W. Schut (Ed.), *Handbook of bereavement research: Consequences, coping and care* (pp. 517–43). Washington, DC: American Psychological Association Press.

Prigerson, H., & Jacobs, S. (2001). Traumatic grief as a distinct disorder: A rationale, consensus criteria, and a preliminary empirical test. In M. Stroebe, R. O. Hansson, W. Stroebe, & H. Schut (Eds.), *Handbook of bereavement research: Consequences, coping and care* (pp. 613–45). Washington, DC: American Psychological Association Press.

Prigerson, H., Silverman, G., Jacobs, S., Maciejewski, P., Kasl, S., & Rosenheck, R. (2001). Traumatic grief, disability, and the underutilization of health services: A preliminary look. *Primary Psychiatry, 8,* 61–9.

Prigerson, H., Vanderwerker, L. & Maciejewski, P. (2008). A case for inclusion of prolonged grief disorder in DSM-IV. In M. S. Stroebe, R. O. Hansson, H. Schut, & W. Stroebe (Eds.), *Handbook of bereavement research and practice: Advances in theory and intervention* (pp. 165–86). Washington, DC: American Psychological Association.

Raphael, B. (1983). *The anatomy of bereavement.* New York: Basic Books.

Raphael, B., Minkov, C., & Dobson, M. (2001). Psychotherapeutic and pharmacological intervention for bereaved persons. In M. Stroebe, R. O. Hansson, W. Stroebe, & H. Schut (Eds.), *Handbook of bereavement research: Consequences, coping and care* (pp. 587–612). Washington, DC: American Psychological Association Press.

Richardson, V., & Balaswamy, S. (2001). Coping with bereavement among elderly widowers. *Omega, 43,* 129–44.

de Ridder, D. (1997). What is wrong with coping assessment? A review of conceptual and methodological issues. *Psychology and Health, 12,* 417–31.

Rosenblatt, P. (1993). Grief: The social context of private feelings. In M. Stroebe, W. Stroebe, & R. O. Hansson (Eds.), *Handbook of bereavement: Theory, research and intervention* (pp. 102–11). New York: Cambridge University Press.

Rosenblatt, P. (2001). A social constructionist perspective on cultural differences in grief. In M. Stroebe, R. O. Hansson,

W. Stroebe, & H. Schut (Eds.), *Handbook of bereavement research: Consequences, coping, and care* (pp. 285–300). Washington, DC: American Psychological Association Press.

Rubin, S. (1981). A two-track model of bereavement: Theory and application in research. *American Journal of Orthopsychiatry, 51,* 101–9.

Rubin, S., & Malkinson, R. (2001). Parental response to child loss across the life cycle: Clinical and research perspectives. In M. Stroebe, R. O. Hansson, W. Stroebe, & H. Schut (Eds.), *Handbook of bereavement research: Consequences, coping, and care* (pp. 219–40). Washington, DC: American Psychological Association Press.

Rubin, S., & Schechter, N. *(1997).* Exploring the social construction of bereavement: Perceptions of adjustment and recovery for bereaved men. *American Journal of Orthopsychiatry, 67,* 279–89.

Schaefer, J., & Moos, R. (2001). Bereavement experiences and personal growth. In M. Stroebe, R. O. Hansson, W. Stroebe, & H. Schut (Eds.), *Handbook of bereavement research: Consequences, coping, and care* (pp. 145–67). Washington, DC: American Psychological Association Press.

Schut, H., Keijser, J. de, Bout, J. van den, & Dijkhuis, J. (1991). Posttraumatic stress symptoms in the first years of conjugal bereavement. *Anxiety Research, 4,* 225–34.

Schut, H., & Stroebe, M. *(2005). Interventions to enhance adaptation to bereavement.* Journal of Palliative Medicine, 8, S140–7.

Schut, H., Stroebe, M., Boelen, P., & Zijerveld, A. (2006). Continuing relationships with the deceased: Disentangling bonds and grief. *Death Studies, 30,* 757–66.

Schut, H., Stroebe, M., van den Bout, J., & Terheggen, M. (2001). The efficacy of bereavement interventions: Determining who benefits. In M. Stroebe, R. O. Hansson, W. Stroebe, & H. Schut (Eds.), *Handbook of bereavement research: Consequences, coping, and care.* Washington, DC: American Psychological Association Press.

Shaver, P., & Tancredy, C. (2001). Emotion, attachment, and bereavement: A conceptual commentary. In M. Stroebe, R. O. Hansson, W. Stroebe, & H. Schut (Eds.), *Handbook of bereavement research: Consequences, coping, and care* (pp. 63–88). Washington, DC: American Psychological Association Press.

Shear, K., Frank, E., Houck, P., & Reynolds, C. (2005). Treatment of complicated grief: A randomized controlled trial. *Journal of the American Medical Association, 293,* 2601–8.

Skinner, E., Edge, K., Altman, J., & Sherwood, H. (2003). Searching for the structure of coping: A review and critique of category systems for classifying ways of coping. *Psychological Bulletin, 129,* 216–69.

Smith, N., Tarakeshwar, N., Hansen, N., Kochman, A., & Sikkema, K. (2009). Coping mediates outcome following a randomized group intervention for HIV-positive bereaved individuals. *Journal of Clinical Psychology, 65,* 319–35.

Stroebe, M. (1992). Coping with bereavement: A review of the grief work hypothesis. *Omega: Journal of Death and Dying, 26,* 19–42.

Stroebe, M. (in press). From vulnerability to resilience: Is the pendulum swing in bereavement research justified? *Bereavement Care.*

Stroebe, M., & Schut, H. (1999). The Dual Process Model of Coping with Bereavement: Rationale and description. *Death Studies, 23,* 197–224.

Stroebe, M., & Schut, H. (2001a). Models of coping with bereavement: A review. In M. Stroebe, R. O. Hansson, W. Stroebe, & H. Schut (Eds.), *Handbook of bereavement research: Consequences, coping, and care* (pp. 375–403). Washington, DC: American Psychological Association Press.

Stroebe, M., & Schut, H. (2001b). Meaning making in the Dual Process Model. In R. Neimeyer (Ed.), *Meaning reconstruction and the experience of loss.* Washington, DC: American Psychological Association Press.

Stroebe, M., Folkman, S., Hansson, R. O., & Schut, H. (2006). The prediction of bereavement outcome: Development of an integrative risk factor framework. *Social Science and Medicine, 63,* 2446–51.

Stroebe, M. S., Hansson, R. O., Schut, H., & Stroebe, W. (Eds.) (2008). *Handbook of bereavement research and practice: Advances in theory and intervention.* Washington, DC: American Psychological Association.

Stroebe, M., & Schut, H. (2008). The Dual Process Model of Coping with Bereavement: Overview and update. *Grief Matters: The Australian Journal of Grief and Bereavement, X,* 1–4.

Stroebe, M., Schut, H., & Finkenauer, C. (2001b). The traumatization of grief: A conceptual framework for understanding the trauma-bereavement interface. *Israeli Journal of Psychiatry, 38,* 185–201.

Stroebe, M., Schut, H., & Stroebe, W. (2005a). Attachment in coping with bereavement: A theoretical integration. *Review of General Psychology, 9,* 48–66.

Stroebe, M., Stroebe, W., & Abakoumkin, G. (2005b). The broken heart: Suicidal ideation in bereavement. *American Journal of Psychiatry, 162,* 2178–80.

Stroebe, M., Stroebe, W., & Schut, H. (2001). Gender differences in adjustment to bereavement: An empirical and theoretical review. *Review of General Psychology, 5,* 62–83.

Stroebe, M., Stroebe, W., Schut, H., Zech, E. & van den Bout, J. (2002). Does disclosure of emotions facilitate recovery from bereavement? Evidence from two prospective studies. *Journal of Consulting and Clinical Psychology, 70,* 169–78.

Stroebe, M., Stroebe, W., & Schut, H. (2007b). Health consequences of bereavement: A review. *The Lancet, 370,* 1960–73.

Stroebe, W., & Schut, H. A. W. (2001). Risk factors in bereavement outcome: A methodological and empirical review. In M. S. Stroebe, R. O. Hansson, W. Stroebe, & H. A. W. Schut (Eds.), *Handbook of bereavement research: Consequences, coping and care* (pp. 349–72). Washington, DC: American Psychological Association Press.

Stroebe, W., Schut, H., & Stroebe, M. (2005). Grief work, disclosure and counseling: Do they help the bereaved? *Clinical Psychology Review, 25,* 395–414.

Stroebe, W., & Stroebe, M. (1993). Determinants of adjustment to bereavement in younger widows and widowers. In M. Stroebe et al. (Eds.), *Handbook of bereavement* (pp. 208–26). New York: Cambridge University Press.

Stroebe, W., Stroebe, M., Abakoumkin, G., & Schut, H. (1996). Social and emotional loneliness: A comparison of attachment and stress theory explanations. *Journal of Personality and Social Psychology, 70,* 1241–9.

Tedeschi, R., & Calhoun, L. (2004). Posttraumatic growth: Conceptual foundations and empirical evidence. *Psychological Inquiry, 15,* 1–18.

Thompson, L., Breckenridge, J., Gallagher, D., & Peterson, J. (1984). Effects of bereavement on self-perceptions of physical health in elderly widows and widowers. *Journal of Gerontology, 39,* 309–14.

Walter, T. (1996). A new model of grief: Bereavement and biography. *Mortality, 1,* 7–25.

Walter, T. (1999). *On bereavement: The culture of grief.* Buckingham: Open University Press.

Weiss, D., & Marmar, C. (1997) The impact of event scale revised. In J. Wilson & T. Kearne (Eds.), *Assessing psychological trauma and PTSD* (pp. 399–411). New York: Guilford.

Wijngaards-de Meij, L., Stroebe, M., Schut, H., Stroebe, W, van den Bout, J., Heijmans, P., & Dijkstra, I. (2005). Couples at risk following the death of their child: Predictors of grief versus depression. *Journal of Consulting and Clinical Psychology, 73,* 617–23.

Wijngaards-de Meij, L, Stroebe, M., Schut, H, Stroebe, W., van den Bout, J. van der Heijden, P., & Dijkstra, I. (2007). Neuroticism and attachment insecurity as predictors of bereavement outcome. *Journal of Research in Personality, 41,* 498–505.

Wijngaards, L., Stroebe, M., Stroebe, W., Schut, H., van den Bout, J., van der Heijden, P., & Dijkstra, I. (2008). Parents grieving the loss of their child: Interdependence in coping. *British Journal of Clinical Psychology, 47,* 31–42.

Worden, W. (1982/1991/2002/2009 1st–4th Eds.). *Grief counseling and grief therapy: A handbook for the mental health practitioner.* New York: Springer.

Wortman, C. B., & Silver, R. C. (1987). Coping with irrevocable loss. In G. R. Vandenbos & B. K. Bryant (Eds.), *Cataclysms, crises and catastrophes: Psychology in action* (pp. 189–235). Washington, DC: APA.

Wortman, C. B., & Silver, R. C. (1989). The myths of coping with loss. *Journal of Consulting and Clinical Psychology, 57,* 349–57.

Wortman, C., & Silver, R. (2001). The myths of coping with loss revisited. In M. S. Stroebe, R. O. Hansson, W. Stroebe, & H. A. W. Schut (Eds.), *Handbook of bereavement research: Consequences, coping and care* (pp. 405–29). Washington: American Psychological Association Press.

Zettel, L., & Rook, K. (2004). Substitution and compensation in the social networks of older widowed women. *Psychology and Aging, 19,* 433–43.

Zisook, S., & Shuchter, S. (2001). Treatment of the depressions of bereavement. *American Behavioral Scientist, 44,* 782–97.

Resilience: The Meanings, Methods, and Measures of a Fundamental Characteristic of Human Adaptation

Alex J. Zautra *and* John W. Reich

Abstract

Moving from a disease model of stress and coping to the more integrative model of positive influences represents a fundamental shift in our understanding of how people adapt to and grow in their environment. This new paradigm has raised stress and coping approaches into a framework that models the extent to which personal strengths and other psychosocial resources contribute to the prediction of resilience, independent of the catalog of risks and vulnerabilities identified within the person and his or her social network. We describe this resilience paradigm and review current evidence for its utility in this chapter. In doing so, we point out how the work of Susan Folkman presaged the current attention to models of resilience by calling attention to the importance of coping and positive adaptations to stressful life experience. Three features predominate in scientific discourse on resilience: recovery, sustainability, and growth. These features are inherent to virtually any type of organized entity, from a simple biological system to a person, an organization, a neighborhood, a community, a city, a state, or even a nation. We illustrate further how variables such as "trust," thought to be central to resilience, are best understood as multi-level constructs, with meanings, measures, and potential interventions at the biological, psychosocial, organizational, and community level. In conclusion, we see this paradigm shift to resilience to be a valuable direction for future research, a highly appealing framework for the design of clinical and community interventions, and a refreshing new perspective that offers exciting new directions for public health and public policy.

Keywords: resilience, positive adaptation, stress, adversity, recovery, sustainability, growth, positive emotion, social capital, multi-level, job enrichment, community psychology, positive mental health, positive psychology, coping

"I lose and find myself in the long water;
I am gathered together once more;
I embrace the world."
From "Long Waters" in *The Far Field* by Theodore Roethke (1964)

A historical shift in conceptualizing human adaptation has occurred throughout the social sciences. This new orientation has a distinct focus both conceptually and empirically on *the positive*. From an earlier near-complete domination of focus on pathology, mental illness, risk factors, and "social problems," a sea change has now opened up new horizons by bringing to the fore conceptualizations and measurement of the strengths of people and their societies rather than attending solely to their weaknesses. *Resilience* is arguably the most valuable of those strengths, and the topic of this chapter.

The early work of Susan Folkman and her collaborators ranks as among the most influential in setting the foundations for the explosive growth of this new way of thinking in the science and practice of psychology. An early landmark publication by Folkman and Lazarus (1980) introduced a new theme in the study of stressful life events. In contrast to the prior exclusive focus on upending life events and their health consequences, their study of stress and coping was broadly integrative; it allowed incorporation of cognitive and affective responses and social relations in the search for understanding how people adapt successfully to stressful events.

That same year saw the publication of Lazarus, Kanner, and Folkman's (1980) paper on the assessment of daily events. With this work, assessment attention was expanded to the assessment of daily hassles and uplifts and significantly influential daily experiences related to psychological well-being. Indeed, they "uplifted" our own interests in developing a means of assessing the positive side of everyday life, presaging our own paper that introduced an inventory of everyday life events (Zautra, Guarnaccia, Reich, & Dohrenwend, 1986).

Folkman went on to introduce the study of positive emotions in the stress process as a domain of investigation not accounted for by the mere absence of distressing emotions: a body of work that greatly informed our own efforts along similar lines (Zautra & Reich, 1983). Beginning in the mid-1990s, Folkman and her colleagues and students (Folkman, 1997; Folkman, Chesney, & Christopher-Richards, 1994; Folkman, Moskowitz, Ozer, & Park, 1997; Moskowitz, Folkman, Collette, & Vittinghof, 1996; Park & Folkman, 1997) began their seminal work on coping and adaptation to HIV/AIDS. It is perhaps here that Folkman offered the greatest lesson for us studying resilience: that life (and certain death) brings more than sorrow and other troubling emotions to the heart. She found and reported on co-occurring positive emotions even for those most troubled by their illness, emotions that catch hold within the person to enhance well-being and brighten social relations in spite of ubiquitous "worse-case" scenarios. Folkman and Moskowitz (2000a) and more recently Rabkin, McElhiney, Moran, Acree, and Folkman (2008) have surveyed their own work and the work of others showing clearly that positive affect can co-occur with distress, it can facilitate and strengthen capacity for adaptive coping and it can ameliorate the negative effects of stressful experiences. Her work has now contributed to cutting-edge therapeutic interventions to further adaptation to HIV (e.g., Chesney, Chambers, Taylor, Johnson, & Folkman, 2003; Chesney & Folkman, 2007), end-of-life care (Mohr, Moran,

Kohn, Hart, Armstrong, Dias, Bergsland, & Folkman, 2003), and cancer (Folkman & Greer, 2000).

The shift of focus toward positive aspects of the human psyche is now a well-established tradition in both the science and practice in psychology as well as other social sciences. This historical shift can best be interpreted in the conceptual framework of a "paradigm shift" in the sense initially proposed by Kuhn (1962). Moving from a disease model of stress and coping to the more integrative model of positive influences represents a fundamental shift in our understanding of how people adapt to, and grow in, their environment. This new paradigm has raised stress and coping approaches into a framework that models the extent to which personal strengths and other psychosocial resources contribute to the prediction of resilience, independent of the catalog of risks and vulnerabilities identified within the person and his or her social network. We refer to this as a *resilience model* of well-being, and it is the focus of this chapter.

The Kuhnian paradigm shift model is particularly appropriate for the rise in interest in resilience thinking about adjustment. As Masten (2001) and Masten and Wright (2010) have noted, a number of investigators were finding that the traditional risk factors/disease model was missing something significant in observations of individual differences in adaptation to stress. In longitudinal studies of youth at high risk for later developmental problems because of a family history of psychiatric problems and disadvantaged environments, Masten (2000) nevertheless found that positive adaptation and low antisocial behavior were surprisingly prevalent. These early observations led to a shift of focus to the factors providing resilience in the face of such stressors. Ryff and Singer (1998) have called attention to "the contours of positive human health" as a new approach to adaptation, one based on positive aspects of experience and adaptation. This chapter provides a review of the main developments in this area, with a focus on adult resilience. Masten and a number of other investigators have already established a strong body of research on child resilience (e.g., Garmezy, 1987; Masten, 2001; Rutter, 1987), but the concepts are relatively new to the realm of adult adjustment and well-being and are reviewed here.

Definitions of Resilience

There is a surprising degree of agreement on at least the basic parameters of what is involved when systems are being characterized as resilient.

Zautra, Hall, and Murray (2008) have identified two primary features of resilience in their definition: *recovery* that is swift and thorough, and *sustainability* of purpose in the face of adversity. One of the salient outcomes of resilience under the terms defined by Zautra et al. (2008) is new learning, often referred to as growth. Masten and Wright (2010) succinctly encapsulate this outcome in the following definition: "Human resilience refers to the processes or patterns of positive adaptation and development in the context of significant threats to an individual's life or function." In sum, three features predominate in scientific discourse on resilience: recovery, sustainability, and growth.

Our attention to these three features of resilience is best seen through the dynamic lens of coping and adaptation to stress. Indeed, the concept of stress is inherently tied to the definition, indicating that resilience has to be seen in the context of events in which the person is challenged to respond effectively, and there is some cost of not doing so. Folkman and Moskowitz (2000b) remind us that coping has to be contextualized, and here we follow their lead in our discussions of resilience. A fundamental Person × Environment (P × E) model is to be assumed *a priori*. This has important conceptual and methodological implications that will guide the review presented in this chapter.

Origins of Resilience Thinking: "Ordinary Magic"

Moving from a risk-factors approach to a resilience perspective has led researchers to attend closely to the specific types of stressors experienced and the extent of distress responses to those stressors. One of the most important perspectives in this new approach is what Masten (2001) has called "ordinary magic." Bonanno (2005) showed that more than half of a sample of bereaved persons did not differ significantly in distress from a non-bereaved sample in the months following the loss. Over a quarter of parents who lost a child from sudden infant death syndrome showed only minimal levels of grief over time (Silver & Wortman, 1987), while even greater frequencies of minimal grief reactions were found in samples of conjugal loss: 57% (Bournstein et al., in press) and 65% (Zisook & Schuchter, 1986). Even in catastrophic events such as the terrorist attack on New York City, at least a third of those who lost a loved one or a close friend reported either no or only one PTSD symptom (Bonanno, Galea, Bucciarelli, & Vlahov, 2007). These and other similar findings (Reich, Zautra, &

Hall, 2010) have now firmly established the everyday nature of resilience as a characteristic response to stressful experiences. From this foundation has come new research on the properties of resilience and techniques whereby it may be enhanced. We will review this literature below.

Classes of Resilience-Related Variables

Coping concepts and techniques introduced by Folkman provide an integrative framework for approaching adaptation processes under stress. The literature to date has implicated relatively stable personality and trait variables (Block & Block, 1980) and social network capabilities (Carpiano, 2006) as well as such basic variables as education level and income. While these static features are important, other lines of reasoning have suggested that a process approach may be more fruitful (Bonanno, 2004; Luthar, Cicchetti, & Becker, 2000). Resilient processes are those that lead to successful resolution of stressful situations. Indeed, Bonanno (2004) and Zautra et al. (2008) have suggested that resilience might best be considered an outcome, the product of successful adaptive functioning in the presence of adverse events.

In proposing variables that make up individual resilience, whether researchers speak of these variables are processes or outcomes, they share the common perspective that resilience is to be seen as more than the absence of a distress reaction to unfavorable life circumstances. This approach introduces a range of variables, from positive traits such as ego-resiliency (Block & Kremen, 1996) and optimism (Carver, Smith, Antoni, Petronis, Weiss, & Derhagopian 2005) to measures of affect and emotion. The selection of measures depends on theoretical frameworks such as the broaden-and-build model of Fredrickson (2001), and models of positive mental health (e.g., Ryff & Singer, 1998).

Dimensions of Resilience Processes: A Two-Factor Model

In our research on daily life experience we have argued for the importance of assessing both positive and negative domains of life experience in any comprehensive model of coping and adaptation. Such early studies as those by Zautra and Simons (1979), Block and Zautra (1980), and Zautra and Reich (1982) reported compelling data about the independent effects of positive events in a person's daily life over and above the effects of stressful negative events. Lazarus, Kanner, and Folkman (1980) also argued convincingly that they require separate treatment. This issue became melded into a larger research tradition on the structure of emotions and emotional well-being.

The nature of the dimensionality of emotional space has been a source of a great deal of theoretical and empirical interest (Cacioppo & Berntson, 1994; Russell & Carroll, 1999; Watson, Clark, & Tellegen, 1988). The proper labeling of the two-dimensional axes depends on the perspective taken by the researcher. For the examination of the influence of life changes, which represent moderately to highly arousing events, there is uniform agreement among investigators and ample empirical evidence to support the view that desirable events influence the positive affective domains of well-being, independent of the influence of concurrent stressful events on negative emotions (see Guarnaccia & Zautra, 1998; Ong & Bergeman, 2004; Reich, Zautra, & Davis, 2003; Zautra, Potter, & Reich, 1997).

Application to Affect Models of Resilience

The key elements of resilience can be mapped onto these separate affective domains. Recovery refers to a return to homeostasis following (affective) disturbance. Sustainability of purpose revealed in positive affective outcomes is linked with features such as control and efficacy expectations. It is useful to chart these effects as arising from two fundamentally different motivational systems: the need to defend against harm, and the need to move forward, learn, and grow (Berntson, Cacioppo, & Gardner, 1999). Resilient responding relies on the successful execution of each of these underlying motivational substrates to permit recovery, sustainability, and growth.

The distinctiveness of these general dimensions of response and outcome does not, however, necessarily require them to be functionally independent. For instance, Ong, Bergeman, Bisconti, and Wallace (2006) have shown that trait resilience's effects in reducing negative reactions to daily stressful events are fully mediated by positive emotions. Moskowitz, Folkman, and Acree (2003) found that even though people suffering the loss of a partner reported higher levels of negative emotions than non-bereaved samples, they also reported more positive emotions. Tugade and Fredrickson (2004) showed that although higher levels of trait resilience were related to quicker cardiovascular recovery from a manipulated (laboratory) stressor, that effect was mediated by positive affect. Thus, although the most effective models of resilience are based on the assumption

of, and data showing, separable dimensions of resilience, it is clear that both should be seen in interaction and not assessed as strictly functioning independently. Growth itself as a resilient response to a stressor appears transformative. At first glance, the person in a highly stressful situation would appear motivated to defend against the threat. However, the capacity to also see the threat as a challenge and as a source for new learning engages approach motivations. The product of these efforts to cope, when successful, then could lead to growth from adversity. Although these complexities put the burden on the investigator to employ a comprehensive approach to assessment of these processes, the gain in richness and representativeness of the true state of the person and the environment is a more productive model to pursue.

Levels of analysis: The Broad Range of Applicability of the Resilience Construct

One of the outstanding features of the construct of resilience is that it can be thought of as a systemic process (or processes) inherent to virtually any type of organized entity, from a simple biological system to a person, an organization, a neighborhood, a community, a city, a state, or even a nation. Although the content and particular units of analysis of a given entity may vary in size, scope, or complexity, nevertheless any entity that is organized to function as a unit can be viewed as having characteristics of recovery and sustainability following an encounter with events that disturb equilibrium. This gives the concept great unifying power. It also offers the potential of having great heuristic value, in that analyses of an entity at one level may well be enlightened by considerations of resilience operating at another level.

With that in mind, the following section provides a brief review of some research literature on resilience concepts currently being actively applied at various levels of analysis. Given space limitations, we can provide only a brief but we hope a representative view of the utility of the concept at various levels of analysis. We have provided a more detailed treatment of resilience at many levels in a forthcoming volume, *Handbook of Adult Resilience* (Reich, Zautra, & Hall, 2009, 2010).

Psychobiological resilience

A large body of literature has been devoted to the stress reactions from the perspective of the concept of allostasis (Sterling & Eyer, 1968), a dynamic process of physiological adaptation to stressors that can maintain homeostatic stability. The key to resilient responding is rapid resolution of the stress response, with a resultant (re)balancing of neurohumoral subsystems (Charney, 2004). Adaptation to chronic stress, however, may engender heterostatic processes referred to as "allostatic load" (McEwen & Wingfield, 2003). Elevated hypothalamic-pituitary-adrenal (HPA) axis activation that fails to return to resting levels, creating strains on physiological adaptation, is one example. In this case, adaptation depletes resources and can lead to longer-term systemic damage.

Genetic influences play a significant role in resilience. Heritability studies have shown significant genetic influences on positive emotions, cognitive flexibility, and active coping (Southwick, Vythilingam, & Charney, 2005), positive emotions and resilience (Boardman, Blalock, & Button, 2008), mental toughness (Vernon, Martin, Schermer, & Mackie, 2008), and psychological well-being (Kessler, Gilman, Thornton, & Kendler, 2004), to name only a few resilience-promoting processes investigated to date. Inheritance studies are now being backed up by molecular genetics research. Genes thought to be related to various aspects of resilience are the COMT gene involved in dopamine processing (Boulton & Eisenhofer, 1998; Heinz & Smolka, 2006), the 5-HTTPLR gene related to depression (Caspi, Sugden, Moffitt, Taylor, Craig, Harrington, et al., 2003), and the BNDF and NPY genes related to anxiety disorders (Chen, Jing, Ieraci, Khan, Siao, et al., 2006; Zhou, Zhu, Hariri, Enoch, Scott, Sinha, et al., 2008). These genetic markers are just the "tip of the iceberg." Much more work is underway that will further delineate genetic predispositions to resilience.

The danger of genetic approaches in such a brief treatment is that they tend to be regarded as "main effects." But molecular processes are complex to begin with, and an accounting of the environment to which the organism is exposed initially and over the longer term must also be considered. (Kim-Gold & Cohen, 2009). Rutter (2006) has pointed out that the same genetic variations can be considered both as risk factors and as protective factors, depending on developmental history and the nature of the stressful challenge. Luecken and Lemery (2004) have reviewed studies showing that stressful early environments can alter neurotransmitter systems, leading to hypersensitivity to stressful experiences. Thus, gene–environment interaction tests are essential to achieve accurate and replicable evidence of genetic influences on resilience. Thus far, this work has focused on elements of the stress response most closely aligned with recovery. The genetic contributions to sustainability and growth under threat and challenge are rarely explored.

Developmental Processes

Resilience research arose in the area of child development. The early research by Garmezy, Masten, and Tellegen (1984; Masten, 1989), Rutter (1987), and Werner and Smith (1982), among others, investigated the extent to which adverse childrearing environments (e.g., poverty, parental maladjustment, poor community environments) influenced child adjustment. The key finding was that the rate of child maladjustment was significantly lower than what might be expected from a standard risk factors model. Then came the classic phrase, "ordinary magic" (Masten, 2001), shifting the focus from risk factors for psychopathology to psychosocial resources associated with resilience such as healthy parental attachment, strong peer relationships, and language competence (Luthar, 2006). Research in this area has moved from the initial concern with a basic description of the properties of resilient children, to more recent concerns with genetic factors (e.g., Cicchetti & Curtis, 2007; Kim-Cohen, Moffitt, Caspi, & Taylor, 1994) and social environments that increase the likelihood of resilience. There are also a number of empirically supported interventions designed to increase resilient processes, such as positive parenting (e.g., Wolchik, Sandler, Millsap, Plummer, Greene, Anderson, et al., 2002) and school engagement (e.g., Hawkins, Catalano, Kosterman, Abbott, & Hill, 1999). These latter models incorporate multiple levels of analysis into a comprehensive picture of developmental processes (Masten, 2007).

Recently, other investigators have attempted to organize the literature on resilience in adolescents and young adults (e.g., Luecken & Gress, in press; Zimmerman & Brenner, in press) and older adults (Reich, Zautra, & Hall, in press). These developments seem promising for establishing a genuine lifespan approach to resilience (Mancini & Bonnano, in press).

Organizational Resilience

Continuing with our cross-level review of resilience concepts, the literature on organizational development is recently turning to analyses of capacities for adaptive management of stress and challenge through structural changes in the workplace and attention to leadership. The organizational level of analysis moves resilience thinking beyond the level of biological and individual-psychological variables and into a qualitatively different realm of discourse. While biological and psychological systems are in some important way "natural," organizations are created around social variables, the aim of which is to create an entity designed to meet certain goals, such as manufacturing a product, solving social problems, instituting military action, creating a government, etc. As such, what we might call structural/functional goals guide the development of the organization, and it is on these rational grounds that an organization is initiated and maintained.

Organizational theory and research has been devoted to understanding the underlying principles of organizations, their structure and modes of functioning. As expected, finding the variables that best predict lasting financial success has been the dominant theme. Indeed, economic vitality is a critical feature of organizational resilience. The "case history" method of organizational training and consulting has developed an extensive literature on how organizational success in meeting intended goals can be achieved, while a contrasting literature has been devoted to failures of adaptation (e.g., Weick & Sutcliffe, 2007). Traditional organizational theory espoused a clear and stable hierarchical structure, a division of labor, communication moving downward with expertise concentrated at the top, and formal rules and regulations for functioning (Gerth & Mills, 1946).

Historically, it became obvious that such desiderata, although often common in organizations, nevertheless did not prevent financial disasters from occurring. There are numerous examples of organizations falling into dysfunctional modes of operation, often leading to complete financial collapse, in spite of demonstrating classical structural characteristics (Weick & Sutcliffe, 2007). From that perspective, the question became to determine whether the standard characteristics failed in practical applications, or whether they failed for a more fundamental reason, that they were not structured and functioning appropriately for meeting the contingencies of a fast-changing marketplace, workforce changes, and global competitive pressures stressing rigid, inflexible structural characteristics.

While there are no simple answers to these questions, it is clear that organization theory and research has made a major shift in its thinking, and principles of resilience as we have been discussing them here have been brought to the fore. Indeed, one leading organizational theorist is deliberately attempting to infuse the principles of positive psychology into organizational thinking (Luthans, 2002). Contemporary analyses now are concerned with organizational capacities and functional principles that should be built into the organizational structure for times of normal functioning as well as times of stress and disaster. Flexibility and interconnectedness rather than a rigid hierarchical structure are now the hallmarks of an adaptable organization.

Early efforts to enhance employee motivation through structural changes in the design of work were suggested. Herzberg (1966) proposed particularly useful ways of building flexible and responsive organizations. Job enrichment increases the level of expertise, authority, and motivation in the workplace, and in so doing it enhances organizational resilience by moving from a hierarchical structure to a more interconnected and horizontal one.

Wildavsky (1988) suggests the value of creating a degree of instability in the organization's subsystem components rather than structured stability in order to make the overall organization adept at handling change. His underlying model is that the system need not use up resources to try to prevent problems but to anticipate that there will be unexpected problems and to build capacity for flexible responding as needed. Weick and Sutcliffe (2007) suggest the value of *mindfulness,* a condition of internal communication in which all facets of organizational functioning are continually monitored for responsiveness to changing conditions. They particularly suggest that this capacity be built into the system such that it is a preexisting condition, enabling ongoing scrutiny and, consequently, appropriate responsiveness to any unexpected system stressors.

Command structures in organizations such as the armed services need to be rethought in this new framework. Although traditionally expertise and command power are supposed to be at higher levels of the organization, a resilience model such as suggested by Eisenhart (1989) would distribute monitoring and decision-making such that command comes from the most expert entity at the time it is most needed. Sutcliffe and Vogus add that, "An entity not only survives threats by positively adjusting to current adversity, but also, in the process of responding, strengthens its compatibilities to make future adjustments" (2003, p. 97).

Neighborhood and Community Resilience

In recent years there has been an outcropping of research that studies positive dimensions of community health. At the forefront of this research, extensive examinations of *social capital* have underscored the importance of social trust, reciprocity, neighborhood efficacy, and civic engagement in many aspects of community life (Coleman, 1990; Portes, 2000; Putnam, 2000; Putnam, Felstein, & Cohen, 2003; Putnam, Leonardi, & Nanetti, 1993). Social connectedness and cohesion have been linked to greater vitality and stability in communities (Langdon, 1997).

The bridge from culture to health is built across neighborhoods and communities that connect individuals who share common space as well as common ground to support collective hope and efficacy (Duncan, Duncan, Okut, Strycker, & Hix-Small, 2003). Yet, studies that have examined the relations between community-level factors like social capital and person-level variables like health have had mixed results (Carpiano, 2006; Portes, 2000; Ziersch, Baum, Macdougall, & Putland, 2005), suggesting we have only begun to understand the boundaries of influence of the social domain on individuals.

When thinking of a community's resilience, the distinction between recovery and sustainability is apparent. For many, an effectively managed community would be one that operates like clockwork. The trains run on time, regardless of what is happening, and people shuffle forward, as expected, undeterred by calamity. Indeed, an effective plan for recovery for a community following a natural disaster is one that arranges resources in such a way that the response is as swift and automatic as possible. During the disaster, the community hopes everyone knows what he or she is to do without question. Residents may be guided to safety by set programs, modified in process by only a select few engineers with authority at the top. Yet from experience we know that a substantial transfusion of cooperation as a result of disaster can sometimes be the key ingredient in community recovery.

Sustainability of community life requires thinking and planning of a different kind, one that relies on raising awareness and participation of the whole, not just investment in the skills of a few. Fundamental to elevation of awareness to purposeful collective action are democratic processes that promote awareness, informed choice, and citizen participation. Here is where Sarason's concept "psychological sense of community" is most applicable. Without a shared sense of purpose within the community, there may be "bricks and mortar," but for purposes not defined by those who live and work there. Citizen engagement and empowerment are resilience-promoting processes that further sustainability by enhancing the meaning and collective value of community development.

There are ways that these purposes can be misguided, and there is ample history of communities being manipulated through false advertising and political campaigns. There is no community to protect from such influences, however, unless the members who reside there are free to think, plan, discuss, and vote.

Each of these levels of inquiry invites comparisons with the standard paradigm of risk and vulnerability In Table 9.1, we provide an illustration of how inquiries regarding resilience are different from those that focus only on risk across levels of inquiry, from the biological to organizational/community life. The table does not attempt to be exhaustive; rather, we offer the items as an invitation for others to expand upon in our work with their own innovative approaches.

Methods of Inquiry Appropriate for Studying Resilience

Formal methods for studying resilience, its antecedents, properties, and consequences, require some special considerations over and above a simple one-time assessment. Referring back to the definition, it is critical that the role of stressful events be considered, in that resilience has to be seen in light of stressful encounters (Bonanno, 2005). This suggests the necessity of a Person × Environment approach. At a minimum, then, the following desiderata are suggested for optimal measurement of resilience.

Longitudinal design

Two of the key foundational studies of resilience that set its basic framework were both longitudinal studies of child development. Werner and Smith (1982) in the Kauai study followed a sample of Hawaiian children from infancy through adulthood. After 40 years from pre- to post-assessment, the researchers found that individual characteristics such as self-esteem and purpose in life were significant correlates of adult well-being. Family variables such as maternal caregiving and extended family support also were important correlates. A number of studies have similar findings (cf. Luthar, 2006, for a comprehensive review). In the 1970s Garmezy initiated a project investigating antecedents of psychopathology in Minneapolis children and their families; continuing reassessment of these children over the following decades led to the formal labeling of the investigation as Project Competence (Garmezy, Masten, & Tellegen, 1984). The title reflects the consistent finding that most children showed good adaptation. Those who had higher

Table 9.1 Risk and resilience resource indices

Risk factor index	Resilience resource index
Biological	
Blood pressure: diastolic >90, systolic >140	Heart rate variability
Cholesterol >240, fasting glucose >124, BMI >25	Regular physical exercise, healthy diet
Genetic factors associated with anxiety	Genetic factors associated with stress resilience
High C-reactive protein and/or other elevations in inflammatory processes	Immune responsivity and regulation
Individual	
History of mental illness	Positive emotional resources
Depression/helplessness	Hope/optimism/agency
Traumatic brain injury	High cognitive functioning, learning/memory & executive functioning
Interpersonal/family	
History of childhood trauma/adult abuse	Secure kith/kin relations
Chronic social stress	Close social ties, synchrony
Community/organizational	
Presence of environmental hazards	Green space and engaging in the natural environment through community gardening
Violent crime rates	Volunteerism
Stressful work environment	Satisfying work life

levels of family stability and cohesion, for instance, later showed higher academic achievement and social adjustment.

A longitudinal perspective is particularly valuable because, across the lifespan, developmental tasks change as the child moves into maturity while the child's own knowledge, skills, and capabilities evolve; conclusions about resilience at one age may have to be modified as the changing child interacts with a changing environment (Masten, Burt, & Coatsworth, 2006). Also, across-time assessment allows a window of opportunity for children not succeeding at age-appropriate developmental tasks (Havighurst, 1972) at one age level to later appear as late-bloomers, now fully competent when positive change has had a chance to appear (Masten, Obradovic, & Burt, 2006).

Given that resilience is best captured following the occurrence of stressors, a longitudinal model is important because it allows for the detection and mapping of a recovery trajectory following the stressor. Bonanno, Galea, Bucciarelli, and Vlahov

(2006) studied samples of New Yorkers' posttraumatic stress disorder (PTSD) symptoms following the attack on the Twin Towers and used the prevalence of PTSD symptoms 6 months after the attacks to establish a reliable measure of resilience. Taking extended measurements makes it possible to distinguish between recovery over a longer period of time, whereas resilience would be demonstrated by a shorter time course of adaptation (Bonanno, 2004).

When resilience researchers examine evidence of positive adaptations following stress, "pre" as well as "post" stress assessments are even more important to rule out possible demand characteristics of these natural experiments. Many people may report to investigators something akin to the colloquialism, "That which does not kill you, makes you stronger." Only with measures of resilience outcomes prior to as well as following the stressor can we be assured that positive changes have actually occurred. A recent study of post-traumatic growth (Frazier, Tennen, Gavian, Park, Tomich, & Tashiro, 2009) provides an illustration. The authors measured perceptions of post-traumatic growth (PTG) reported by college student participants after encountering the stressor. Wisely, the authors collected data prior to and after the stressors on the same dimensions of growth on the PTG questionnaire. By differencing the "pre" from the "post," they estimated actual growth across time. There was no correlation between perceptions of growth and actual change registered "pre" to "post" on the same dimensions.

Multilevel analysis

Humans do not reside in a vacuum, and stressful experiences often affect the person and his or her social environment, often coming from the larger sociocultural context of living. Accordingly, resilience processes can be best understood by multi-level statistical analytic techniques incorporating data from biological, psychological, and social/organizational and community levels (McIntyre, Ellaway, & Cummins, 2002; Subrumanian, 2004). Given two-factor models of resilience, then tests of both risk and resilience factors are possible (Zautra, Hall, & Murray, 2010). Specifically, multi-level modeling allows estimates of influence of within- and between-person or community processes.

We will use the concept of multilevel analysis to demonstrate the power of one resilience-sustaining variable. The construct of "trust" is a fundamental building block of resilience, particularly when examined across multiple levels simultaneously. In Table 9.2 we use "trust" to illustrate how a variable changes across levels yet retains its utility to capture a key component of resilient processes at each level of inquiry. Of interest among social scientists is the degree to which measures of a construct taken at one level predict the scores at another level. Indeed, "trust" at different levels takes on new meanings and new relationships with resilient outcomes, fostering neighborliness at the community

level, openness in close ties, and parasympathetic/sympathetic balance in the nervous system of the individual.

Interventions to Enhance Resilience

The history of therapeutic "treatments" for people who have problems in living has for decades emphasized (1) the expertise of the therapist, (2) analysis of the "problem," and (3) applying the therapist's expertise to remove the problem *for* the patient. Resilience interventions, based generally if not explicitly on a two-factor approach, shift the focus from the negative state of the person to an elicitation of that person's own capabilities, skills, and strengths, as seen by the person.

From the early era of resilience studies that were focused on children, there has been an abiding interest in moving basic research into the practice of enhancing resilience (Masten, Herbers, Cutuli, & Lafavor, 2008). Thus, there has been a continuing focus not only on reducing chances of psychopathology, but on fostering capabilities for achieving age-relevant developmental tasks (Masten, Burt, & Coatsworth, 2006). Several major examples of this approach are reflected in the Seattle Social Development Project (Hawkins, Kosterman, Catalano, Hill, & Abbott, 2005), the Strength-Based School Counseling movement (Akos & Galassi, 2008), and the movement in child welfare practice, Looking After Children (Flynn, Dudding, & Barber, 2006).

A focus on positive adaptation has parallels in the behavioral tradition, and its emphasis on reinforcing behaviors. Fordyce (1981) tested an intervention in which adults were guided in engaging in basic methods for increasing happiness (e.g., spend more time socializing, keeping busy and becoming more active, etc.). Compared to controls, adults engaging in these activities reported significantly

Table 9.2 The study of trust at different levels of observation

Level of analysis	Sample constructs	Research approaches
Biological	Oxytocin, parasympathetic response	Experimental designs, lab assessments, physiological markers
Individuals	Interpersonal trust, synchrony	Daily diary studies, studies of responses between pairs
Families	Family cohesion, mutuality, and trust	Cross-sectional, family, and genetic studies
Communities	Collaborative ties, reciprocity, fairness	Epidemiological/community samples, social indicator research

higher levels of happiness. This effect continued to hold up to 18 months after the intervention (Fordyce, 1983). More recently, the positive psychology emphasis has provided additional methods of intervention for adults that may be thought to benefit both recovery and sustainability (Seligman & Csikszementmihalyi, 2003). Techniques fostering positive engagement and "flourishing" have shown promise (Keyes & Haidt, 2002), as has instruction to engage in forgiveness in the context of family stress (McCullough, Pargament, & Thoresen, 2000). Cognitive manipulations such as having people write about three positive things that happened and using "signature strengths" are related to higher reports of happiness and lower ratings of depression (Seligman, Steen, Park, & Peterson, 2005). In a "gratitude" manipulation, Lubomirsky, Sheldon, and Schkade (2005) had students "count their blessings" once a week. Results showed that they reported significantly increased feelings of positive affect. Mindfulness, intentionally focusing attention, and non-judgmental awareness of one's thoughts and experiences has been shown to lead to higher positive affect and lower negative affect (Brown & Ryan, 2003).

Interventions based more directly on emotional states are also showing impressive effects. As we noted earlier, Folkman's research has shown that positive affect plays a salubrious role among cancer patients (Folkman & Moskowitz, 2000). Interventions aimed at increasing positive emotions led to a more rapid return to physiological baseline after the induction of negative affect (Fredrickson & Levenson, 1998). Instructing people to actively increase the frequency of positive daily events in their lives led to a concomitant increase in positive emotions and, under conditions of higher stressful events, more reduction of psychological distress (Reich & Zautra, 1981).

Our intervention work with arthritis patients demonstrates that participants need not be disease-free to benefit from these kinds of interventions. We compared a standard pain management intervention with one we crafted from our work in mindfulness and emotion regulation in two dimensions: positive affect enhancement and negative affect reframing. Both were contrasted with education-only controls. Not only did we demonstrate improvements in positive affect and coping efficacy in the mindfulness condition (Zautra et al., 2008), but we have recently uncovered strong evidence of better sustainability of positive emotion on stressful days and quicker recovery among those who received the mindfulness and emotion-regulation intervention (Davis & Zautra, 2009).

Epilogue

The early work of Susan Folkman and her colleagues on analyzing positive and negative experiences was a substantial advancement even at the time it initially occurred. Two modern research traditions can clearly be traced back to that early work. The positive psychology emphasis has sought to shift the focus to more positive aspect of adjustment and well-being. Second, in this chapter we have attempted to make the case that resilience models of well-being are also traceable to Folkman's early work. The resilience model has two major features of relevance here. First, it is comprehensive, as we have shown, extending from the molecular scale of genetic and biological influence to molar concepts that define resilience within organizational and community life. Second, it is highly integrative, in modeling irreducible interactive relationships between the person, the setting, and positive and negative dimensions of life's events. Finally, the resilience approach suggests an entirely new universe of theory, research, and application operating comfortably within a consistent framework for thinking about system effectiveness.

It is difficult to predict the direction of research and theory that a new set of thoughts can take. Some ideas go on to a further development, while others sometimes fail to get carried forward. At this stage of the development of a general resilience approach to human welfare, it is clear that strong and reliable basic science data have been established for both children and adults. Furthermore, the data of interventions based on the resilience model are beginning to show evidence that these change programs can be significantly influential in furthering the three primary outcomes of resilient functioning: recovery, sustainability, and growth. In our view, the resilience approach meets the criteria for a Kuhnian paradigm shift and provides a model development in the human sciences that will inform our understanding of human capacities for many years to come.

The future is difficult to forsee for new paradigms, particularly given the rapid advancements in the social sciences of late. Although predicting where a science will go is always difficult, and sometimes impossible, tracing resilience thinking back to its "early days" is not. There is a distinct line of inheritance in our modern "phenotype" from the fundamental "genotype" contributions of Professor Susan Folkman. Her contributions are timeless.

References

Akos, P., & Galassi, J. P. (2008). Special issue: Strengths-based school counseling. *Professional School Counseling, 12.*

Berntson, G. C., Caccioppo, J. T., & Gardner, W. L. (1999). The affect system has parallel and integrative processing components: Form follows function. *Journal of Personality and Social Psychology, 76,* 839–55.

Block, J. H., & Block, J. (1980). The role of ego-control and ego-resilience n the organization of behavior. In W. A. Collins (Ed.), *The Minnesota Symposium on Child Psychology* (Vol. 13, pp. 39–101). Hillsdale, NJ: Erlbaum.

Block, J., & Kremen, A. M. (1996). IQ and ego-resiliency: Conceptual and empirical connections and separateness. *Journal of Personality and Social Psychology, 79,* 349–61.

Block, M., & Zautra, A. (1980). Satisfaction and distress in a community: A test of the effects of life events. *American Journal of Community Psychology, 9,* 165–80.

Boardman, J. D., Blalock, C. L., & Button, T. M. M. (2008). Sex differences in the heritability of resilience. *Twin Research and Human Genetics, 11,* 12–27.

Bonanno, G. A. (2004). Loss, trauma, and human resilience; Have we underestimated the human capacity to thrive after extremely aversive events? *American Psychologist, 59,* 20–8.

Bonanno, G. A. (2005). Resilience in the face of potential trauma. *Current Directions in Psychological Science, 14,* 135–8.

Bonanno, G. A., Galea, S., Bucciarelli, A., & Vlahov, D. (2007). What predicts psychological resilience after disaster? The role of demographics, resources, and life stress. *Journal of Consulting and Clinical Psychology, 75,* 671–82.

Boulton, A. A., & Eisenhofer, G. (1998). Catecholamine metabolism: From molecular understanding to clinical diagnosis and treatment. Overview. *Advanced Pharmacology, 42,* 273–92.

Bournstein, P. E., Clayton, P. J., Halikas, J. A. Maurice, W. L., & Robins, E. (1973). The depression of widowhood after thirteen months. *British Journal of Psychiatry, 122,* 561–6.

Brown, K. W., & Ryan, R. M. (2003). The benefits of being present: Mindfulness and its role in psychological well-being. *Journal of Personality and Social Psychology, 84,* 822–48.

Cacioppo, J. T., & Berntson, G. G. (1994). Relationship between attitudes and evaluative space: A critical review, with emphasis on the separability of positive and negative substrates. *Psychological Bulletin, 115,* 401–23.

Carver, C. S., Smith, R. G., Antoni, M. H., Petronis, V. M., Weiss, S., & Derhagopian, R. P. (2005). Optimistic personality and psychosocial well-being during treatment predict psychosocial well-being among long-term survivors of breast cancer. *Health Psychology, 24,* 508–16.

Caspi, A., Sugden, K., Moffitt, T. E., Taylor, A., Craig, I. W., Harrington, H., et al. (2003). Influence of life stress on depression: Moderation by a polymorphism in the 5-HTTP gene. *Science, 3021,* 386–39.

Charney, D. S. (2004). Psychobiological mechanisms of resilience and vulnerability: Implications for successful adaptation to extreme stress. *American Journal of Psychiatry, 161,* 195–216.

Chen, Z. Y., Jing, D., Bath, K. G., Ieraci, A., Khan, T., Siao, C. J., et al. (2008). Genetic variant BNDF (Val66Met) polymorphism alters anxiety-related behavior. *Science, 314,* 140–3.

Chesney, M. A., Chambers, D. B., Taylor, J. M., Johnson, L. M., & Folkman, S. (2003). Coping effectiveness training for men living with HIV: Results from a randomized clinical trial testing a group-based intervention. *Psychosomatic Medicine, 65,* 1038–46.

Chesney, M. A., & Folkman, S. (2007). The CHANGES project: Coping effectiveness training for HIV+ gay men. Web site: www.caps.ucsf.edu/projects/CHANGES

Cicchetti, D., & Curtis, W. (Eds.) (2007). Special issue: A multilevel approach to resilience. *Development and Psychopathology, 19.*

Eisenhart, K. M. (1989). Make fast strategic decisions in high-velocity environments. *Academy of Management Journal, 32,* 543–76.

Fredrickson, B. L. (1998). The role of positive emotions in positive psychology. *American Psychologist, 56,* 218–26.

Lazarus, R. S., Kanner, A. D., & Folkman, S. (1980). Emotions: A cognitive-phenomenological analysis. In R. Plutchik & H. Kellerman (Eds.), *Theories of emotion* (pp. 189–217). New York: Academic Press.

Flynn, R. J., Dudding, P. M., & Barber, J. G. (Eds.) (2006). *Promoting resilience in child welfare.* Ottawa, Canada: University of Ottawa Press.

Folkman, S. (1997). Positive psychological states and coping with severe stress. *Social Science and Medicine, 45,* 1207–21.

Folkman, S., Chesney, M.A., & Christopher-Richards, A. (1994). Stress and coping in partners of men with AIDS. *Psychiatric Clinics of North America, 17,* 35–55.

Folkman, S., & Greer, S. (2000). Promoting psychological well-being in the face of serious illness: When theory, research, and practice inform each other. *Psycho-Oncology, 9,* 11–9.

Folkman, S., & Moskowitz, J. T. (2000a). Positive affect and the other side of coping. *American Psychologist, 55,* 647–54.

Folkman, S., & Moskowitz, J. T. (2000b). The context matters. *Personality and Social Psychology Bulletin, 26,* 150–1.

Folkman, S., Moskowitz, J. T., Ozer, E. M. & Park, C. L. (1997). Positive meaningful events and coping in the context of HIV/AIDS. In B. H. Gottlieb (Ed.), *Coping with chronic stress* (pp. 293–314). New York: Plenum.

Fordyce, M. W. (1981). *The psychology of happiness. Fourteen fundamentals.* Fort Myers, FL: Cypress Lake Media.

Fordyce, M. W. (1983). A program to increase happiness: Further studies. *Journal of Counseling Psychology, 30,* 483–98.

Frazier, P., Tennen, H., Gavian, M., Park, C., Tomich, P., & Tashiro, T. (2009). Does self-reported posttraumatic growth reflect genuine positive change? *Psychological Sciences, 20,* 912–9.

Fredrickson, B. L., & Levenson, R. W. (1998). Positive emotions speed recovery from the cardiovascular sequelae of negative emotions. *Cognition and Emotion, 12,* 191–220.

Garmezy, N., Masten, A. S., & Tellegen, A. (1984). The study of stress and competence in children: A building block for developmental psychology. *Child Development, 55,* 97–111.

Gerth, H. H., & Mills, C.W. (1946). *From Max Weber: Essays in sociology.* New York: Oxford. Press.

Heinz, A., & Smolka, M. N. (2006). The effects of catechol-O-methyltransferase genotype on brain activation elicited by affective stimuli and cognitive tasks. *Reviews in the Neurosciences, 17,* 359–67.

Keyes, C. L., & Haidt, J. (2002). *Flourishing: Positive psychology and the life well-lived.* Washington, DC: American Psychological Association.

Kim-Cohen, J., & Gold, A. I. (2009). Measured gene-environment interactions and mechanisms promoting resilient development. *Current Directions in Psychological Science, 18,* 138–42.

Kim-Cohen, J., Moffitt, T. E., Caspi, A., & Taylor, A. (1994). Genetic and environmental processes in young children's resilience and vulnerability to socioeconomic deprivation. *Child Development, 75,* 651–68.

Kessler, R.C., Gilman, S. E., Thornton, L.M., & Kendler, K. S. (2004). Health, well-being, and social responsibility in the MIDUS twin and sibling subsamples. In O. G. Brim, C. D. Ryff, & R. C. Kessler (Eds.), *How healthy are we? A national study of well-being at midlife* (pp. 124–52). Chicago: University of Chicago Press.

Havighurst, R. J. (1972). *Developmental tasks and education* (3rd ed.). New York: MacKay.

Hawkins, J. D., Catalano, R. F., Kosterman, R., Abbott, R. D., & Hill, K. G. (1999). Preventing adolescent health-risk behavior by strengthening protection during childhood. *Archives of Pediatrics and Adolescent Medicine, 153,* 226–34.

Kuhn, T. S. (1962). *The structure of scientific revolutions.* Chicago: University of Chicago Press.

Lewinsohn, P. M., & Graf, M. (1973). Pleasant activities and depression. *Journal of Consulting and Clinical Psychology, 41,* 261–8.

Lewinsohn, P. M., Sullivan, M., & Grosscup, S. J. (1980). Changing reinforcing events: An approach to the treatment of depression. *Psychotherapy: Theory, Research, and Practice, 17,* 322–34.

Luecken, L. J., & Gress, J. (2010). Early adversity and resilience in emerging adulthood. In J. W. Reich, A. J. Zautra, & J. S. Hall (Eds.), *Handbook of adult resilience* (pp. 238–57). New York: Guilford.

Luthans, F. (2002). The need for and meaning of positive organizational behavior. *Journal of Organizational Behavior, 23,* 695–706.

Luthar, S. S. (2006). Resilience in development: A synthesis of research across five decades. In D. Cicchetti & D. Cohen (Eds.), *Developmental psychopathology. Vol. 3. Risk, disorder, and adaptation* (2nd ed., Vol. 3). New York: Wiley.

Luthar, S. S., Cicchetti, D., & Becker, B. (2000). The construct of resilience: A critical evaluation and guidelines for future work. *Child Development, 71,* 543–62.

Lyubomirsky, S., Sheldon, K. M., & Schkade, D. (2005). Pursuing happiness: The architecture of sustainable change. *Review of General Psychology, 9,* 111–31.

Macintyre, S., Ellaway, A., & Cummins, S. (2002). Place effects on health: How can we conceptualize, operationalize and measure them? *Social Science and Medicine, 55,* 125–39.

Mancini, A. D., & Bonanno, G. A. (2010). Resilience to potential trauma: Toward a lifespan approach. In J. W. Reich, A. J. Zautra, & J. S. Hall (Eds.), *Handbook of adult resilience* (pp. 258–82). New York: Guilford.

Masten, A. S. (1989). Resilience in development: Implications of the study of successful adaptation for developmental psychopathology. In D. Cicchetti (Ed.), *The emergence of a discipline: Rochester Symposium on Developmental Psychopathology* (Vol. 1, pp. 261–94. Hillsdale, NJ: Erlbaum.

Masten, A. S. (1994). Resilience in individual development: Successful adaptation despite risk and adversity. In M. C. Wang & E. W. Gordon (Eds.), *Educational resilience in inner-city America: Challenges and prospects* (pp. 3–25). Hillsdale, NJ: Erlbaum.

Masten, A. (2001). Ordinary magic: Resilience processes in development. *American Psychologist, 56,* 227–38.

Masten, A. S. (2007). Resilience in developing systems: Progress and promise as the fourth wave rises. *Development and Psychopathology, 19,* 921–30.

Masten, A. S., Burt, K. B., & Coatsworth, J. D. (2006). Competence and psychopathology in development. In D. Cicchetti & D. Cohen (Eds.), *Developmental Psychopathology. Vol. 3. Risk, disorder and psychopathology* (2nd ed., pp. 696–738). New York: Wiley.

Masten, A. S., Herbers, J. E., Cutuli, J. J., & LaFavor, T. L. (2008). Promoting competence and resilience in the school context. *Professional School Counseling, 12,* 76–84.

Masten, A. S., & Obradovic, J. (2006). Competence and resilience in development. *Annals of the New York Academy of Science, 1094,* 13–27.

Masten, A., S., & Wright, M. O. (2010). Resilience over the lifespan: Developmental perspectives on resistance, recovery, and transformation. In J. W. Reich, A. J. Zautra, & J. S. Hall (Eds.), *Handbook of adult resilience* (pp. 213–37). New York: Guilford.

McCullouch, M. E., Pargament, K. I., & Thoreson, C. E. (2000). *Forgiveness: Theory, research, and practice.* New York: Guilford Publications.

McEwen, B. S., & Wingfield, J. C. (2003). The concept of allostasis in biology and biomedicine. *Hormones and Behavior, 43,* 2–15.

Mohr, D.C., Moran, P., Kohn, C., Hart, S., Armstrong, K., Dias, R., Bergsland, E., & Folkman, S. (2003). Couples therapy at end-of-life. *Psycho-oncology, 12,* 620–7.

Moskowitz, J. T., Folkman, S., & Acree, M. (2003). Do positive psychological states shed light on recovery from bereavement? Findings from a 3-year longitudinal study. *Death Studies, 27,* 471–500.

Moskowitz, J., Folkman, S., Collette, L., & Vittinghoff, E. (1996). Coping and mood during AIDS-related care giving and bereavement. *Annals of Behavioral Medicine, 18,* 49–57.

Ong, A. D., & Bergeman, C. S. (2004). The complexity of emotions in later life. *Journal of Gerontology: Psychological Sciences and Social Sciences, 59B,* P117–P122.

Ong, A. D., Bergeman, C. S., Bisconti, T. L., & Wallace, K. (2006). Psychological resilience, positive emotions, and successful adaptation to stress in later life. *Journal of Personality and Social Psychology, 91,* 730–49.

Park, C. L., & Folkman, S. (1997). Meaning in the context of stress and coping. *Review of General Psychology, 2,* 115–44.

Rabkin, J. G., McElhiney, M., Moran, P., Acree, M., & Folkman, S. (2009). Depression, distress and positive mood in late-stage cancer. *Psycho-Oncology, 18,* 79–86.

Reich, J. W., & Zautra, A. J. (1981). Life events and personal causation: Some relationships with satisfaction and distress. *Journal of Personality and Social Psychology, 41,* 1002–12.

Reich, J. W., Zautra, A. J., & Davis, M. (2003). Dimensions of affect relationships: Models and their integrative implications. *Review of General Psychology, 7,* 66–83.

Reich, J. W., Zautra, A. J., & Hall, J. S. (Eds.) (2010). *Handbook of adult resilience.* New York: Guilford.

Rutter, M. (1987). Psychosocial resilience and protective mechanisms. *American Journal of Orthopsychiatry, 57,* 316–31.

Russell, J. A., & Carroll, J. M. (1999). On the bipolarity of positive and negative affect. *Psychological Bulletin, 125,* 3–30.

Rutter, M. (2006). *Genes and behavior: nature-nurture interplay explained.* Malden, MA: Blackwell.

Ryff, C. D., & Singer, B. H. (1998). The contours of positive human health. *Psychological Inquiry, 9,* 1–28.

Seligman, M. E. P., & Csikzmentmihalyi, M. (Eds.) (2000). Special issue: Positive psychology. American Psychologist, 55.

Seligman, M. E. P., Steen, T. A., Park, N., & Peterson, C. (2005). Positive psychology progress: Empirical validation of interventions. *American Psychologist, 60,* 410–21.

Southwick, S. M., Vythlingam, M., & Charney, D. S. (2005). The psychobiology of depression and resilience to stress: Implications for prevention and treatment. *Annual Review of Clinical Psychology, 1,* 255–91.

Sterling, P., & Eyer, J. (1988). Allostasis, a new paradigm to explain arousal pathology. In S. Fisher, J. Reason, & S. Fisher (Eds.), *Handbook of life stress, cognition and health.* New York: Wiley.

Subrumanian, S. V. (2004). The relevance of multilevel statistical methods for identifying causal neighborhood effects. *Social Science and Medicine, 58,* 1961–7.

Tugade, M. M., & Fredrickson, B. L. (2004). Resilient individuals use positive emotions to bounce back from negative emotional experiences. *Journal of Personality and Social Psychology, 86,* 320–33.

Vernon, P. A., Martin, R. A., Schermer, J. A., & Mackie, A. (2008). A behavioral genetic investigation of humor styles and their correlations with the Big Five personality dimensions. *Personality and Individual Differences, 44,* 1116–25.

Watson, D., Clark, L. A., & Tellegen, A. (1988). Development and validation of brief measures of positive and negative affect: The PANAS scale. *Journal of Personality and Social Psychology, 54,* 1063–70.

Weick, K., & Sutcliffe, K. (1997). The devil in the dynamics: Adaptive management on the front lines. In L. H. Gunderson & C. S. Holling (Eds.), *Panarchy.* Washington Inland Press, 333–60.

Werner, E. E., & Smith, R. S. (1992). *Overcoming the odds: High-risk children from birth to adulthood.* Ithaca, NY: Cornell University Press.

Wildavsky, A. (2003). *Searching for safety.* New Brunswick, NJ: Transaction Publishers.

Wolchik, S. A., Sandler, I. N., Millsap, R. E., Plummer, B. A., Greene, S. M., Anderson, E. R., et al (2002). Six-year follow-up of preventive interventions for children of divorce. A randomized controlled trial. *Journal of the American Medical Association, 288,* 1874–81.

Zautra, A. J., Hall, J. S., & Murray, K. E. (2010). Resilience: A new definition of health for people and communities. In J. W. Reich, A. J. Zautra, & J. S. Hall (Eds.), *Handbook of adult resilience* (pp. 3–34). New York: Guilford.

Zautra, A. J., Potter, P. T., & Reich, J. W. (1997). The independence of affects is context-dependent: An integrative model of the relationship between positive and negative affect. *Annual Review of Gerontology and Geriatrics, 17,* 75–103.

Zautra, A. J., & Reich, J. W. (1983). Life events and perceptions of life quality: Developments in a two-factor approach. *Journal of Community Psychology, 11,* 121–32.

Zautra, A. J., & Simons, L. S. (1978). An assessment of a community's mental health needs. *American Journal of Community Psychology, 6,* 351–62.

Zhou, Z., Shu, G., Hariri, A. R., Enoch, M A., Scott, D., Sinha, R., et al. (2008). Genetic variation in human NPY expression affects stress response and emotion. *Nature, 452,* 997–1001.

Zimmerman, M. A., & Brenner, A. B. (2010). Resilience in adolescence: Overcoming neighborhood disadvantage. In J. W. Reich, A. J. Zautra, & J. S. Hall (Eds.), *Handbook of adult resilience* (pp. 126–45). New York: Guilford.

Zisook, S., & Shuchter, S. R. (1986). The first four years of widowhood. *Psychiatric Annals, 16,* 288–94.

Positive Emotions and Coping: Examining Dual-Process Models of Resilience

Michele M. Tugade

Abstract

This chapter reviews dual-process models of resilience. One model of resilience considers the importance of investigating the intersections between positive and negative emotions (e.g., Folkman, 1997, 2001; Folkman & Moskowitz, 2000). Indeed, maintaining and enhancing positive emotions yields important advantages when coping with stress. Another dual-process model of resilience focuses on the interplay between automatic and controlled processes. Most prior research on resilience has centered mainly on *deliberate, response-focused* processes, which may be costly to an individual due to the conscious effort involved in cultivating positive emotions in times of stress. This literature, however, has excluded another important aspect of resilience: the *automatic* activation of positive emotions. The automatic activation of positive emotions is pervasive in everyday life, and may have far-reaching consequences for individuals' abilities to cope with stressors. Automatic processes of resilience might operate with less cost to the individual, as they are executed relatively effortlessly. The theoretical underpinnings of these models will be examined and recent research will be reviewed, showing that dual-process models of resilience may lay the groundwork for important new directions in research on positive emotions, stress, and coping.

Keywords: positive emotion, coping, resilience, dual-process models

Within the landscape of our emotional lives, we generally experience positive emotions with greater frequency and intensity than negative emotions (Carstensen, Pasupathi, Mayer, & Nesselroade, 2000; Zelinski & Larsen, 2000). Although empirical research has traditionally tipped the scale in favor of studies on negative emotions, in recent years a greater balance has begun to emerge. Given the mosaic of our emotional lives, it seems important to investigate the dynamic interplay among all of our valenced experiences. The literature on psychological resilience provides a useful lens through which to examine the associations between positive

and negative emotions, especially with respect to coping behavior.

Resilience is defined as the psychological quality of resetting oneself after significant setbacks, and of returning from adversity relatively unscathed, and perhaps even stronger. A "deceptively simple construct" (Kaplan, 2007, p. 39), resilience is a dynamic and multidimensional concept that can inform research across multiple levels of analysis. With the goal of gaining a deeper understanding about the construct of resilience, scholars often raise several questions: What are the roots of resilience? How does one develop important protective factors to help recover from adversity? What are the pathways to adaptation and wellness? Recently, researchers have identified that one important factor that contributes to successful coping and resilience is the capacity to experience positive emotions in the midst of stressful circumstances.

The aim of the present chapter is to examine *how* and *why* positive emotions are useful in the coping process. Towards this aim, this chapter reviews dual-process models associated with resilience. One such model considers the importance of investigating the intersections between positive and negative emotions (e.g., Folkman, 1997, 2001; Folkman & Moskowitz, 2000). Indeed, maintaining and enhancing positive emotions yield important advantages when coping with stress. There are also individual differences in this capacity, with high-trait-resilient people being especially proficient at using positive emotions to cope (Tugade & Fredrickson, 2002, 2004). Another dual-process model identifies two types of regulatory processes: automatic and controlled processes. Most prior research on resilience has centered mainly on *deliberate, response-focused* processes, which may at times be costly to an individual due to the conscious effort involved in cultivating positive emotions in times of stress. The literature, however, has excluded another important aspect of resilience: the *automatic* activation of positive emotions. The automatic activation of positive emotions is pervasive in everyday life and may have far-reaching consequences for individuals' abilities to cope with stressors. Automatic processes might operate with less cost to the individual, as they are executed relatively effortlessly. The theoretical underpinnings of these models will be examined and recent research will be reviewed, showing that dual-process models of resilience may lay the groundwork for important new directions in research on positive emotions, stress, and coping.

State and Trait Resilience

Resilience is characterized by effective coping and adaptation despite significant loss, hardship, or adversity in one's life (Block & Kremen, 1996; Cicchetti & Tucker, 1994; Luthar, 2003; Masten, 2001). Studies on resilience have burgeoned in the past decade, with growing attention spanning multiple disciplines in psychology (e.g., developmental, psychopathology, social/personality, behavioral genetics, affective neuroscience). Much of the earlier work on the construct of resilience began in the field of developmental psychology. Early studies focused on identifying protective factors that help individuals function well and even thrive in later adulthood despite exposure to early childhood hardships such as poverty, maltreatment or abuse, parental divorce, family mental illness, parental alcoholism, or exposure to violence (cf., Cicchetti & Tucker, 1994; Luthar, Cicchetti, & Becker, 2000; Masten, 2001).

Many scholars consider psychological resilience to be both a state and a trait construct. When faced with downturns and disturbances, "low-resilient individuals" are more easily derailed, seemingly unable to return to normative levels of functioning in their daily lives. In contrast, "high-resilient individuals" have an ability to bounce back and remain steadily on course when mildly disrupted or faced with significant adversity. Scholars emphasize that it is a misconception that high-resilient individuals are "invulnerable" to stress, or that they have an absence of negative affect in their lives (cf., Luthar et al., 2000). Rather, for these individuals, negative affect is experienced but it does not endure. Moreover, when they do experience negative affect, there are fewer long-term negative consequences for them. Indeed, trait-resilient individuals have a unique ability to react to stress in an adaptive (vs. maladaptive) way, across a wide array of environments, even though they have experienced adversity. How do they do it? A number of hypotheses have been explored. Some researchers theorize that, starting at a young age, high-resilient individuals take an active role in seeking and receiving the experiences that are developmentally appropriate for them (Cicchetti & Tucker, 1994). Others theorize that high-resilient individuals have a heightened ability to use the information provided by negative emotions, and learn from the experience to help guide their future behavior (Davidson, 2000). Still others posit that the ability to harness positive emotions in the midst of negative experiences explains patterns of resilient coping (Tugade & Fredrickson, 2004). To investigate which factors predict the ability to fare well under stress, researchers have examined cognitive, emotional, and physiological response patterns of low- and high-resilient individuals.

Neural correlates of resilience

One feature of psychological resilience is the capacity to respond flexibly and appropriately with respect to changing situational demands. Three regions of interest in the brain were recently examined with the aim of discovering the neural mechanisms of resilience. The *amygdala* is activated in response to emotionally salient stimuli; the *insula* is activated in anticipation of impending anxiety; and the *orbito-frontal prefrontal cortex* (OFC) is activated when one expects threat, and is deactivated when the threat doesn't actually occur or is no longer present. Together, these neural regions are important for understanding emotional flexibility, which is a characteristic often associated with individual differences in trait resilience (Waugh, Fredrickson, & Taylor, 2008).

To investigate the neural correlates of resilience, low- and high-resilient individuals were identified based on self-reports on the ego-resiliency scale (Block & Kremen, 1996). This scale measures the extent to which people can modify their responses to meet the demands of changing circumstances, and has been used in a host of studies that investigate individual differences in trait resilience (Fredrickson et al., 2004, 2008; Waugh et al., 2007, 2008). This measure has also been shown to have ecological validity, as evidenced in a study that used this measure to investigate positive emotions and resilience in the midst of a national disaster, such as the September 11 terrorist attacks on the United States (Fredrickson et al., 2003). To investigate the neural correlates of resilience, participants passively viewed a series of aversive or neutral pictures that were each preceded by threat (aversive) or no-threat (neutral) cues. When under threat, low-resilient individuals exhibited prolonged activation in the anterior insula and amygdala in response to both the aversive and neutral pictures. In contrast, high-resilient individuals exhibited insula and amygdala activation only in response to the aversive pictures. The orbito-prefrontal cortex (OFC) was also shown to be an important region to investigate with respect to anticipatory coping and release of anticipation after a threat is no longer relevant. Both low- and high-resilient people showed heightened activation in the posterior OFC in response to threat versus non-threat cues (reflecting expectation of threat). Only high-resilient people, however, showed activation in the anterior OFC (reflecting expectation of safety when the threat was removed) (Waugh et al., 2008).

Together, these findings provide neural evidence that in threatening situations, high-resilient people exhibit greater emotional flexibility to meet changing situational demands. Specifically, high-resilient individuals (vs. low-resilient individuals) engage in appropriate emotional and physiological coping responses when threat is present, and likewise engage in non-emotional responses when threat is not present (Waugh et al., 2008). These results are in line with previous research showing that high- (vs. low-) resilient individuals appraise upcoming stressors as a challenge to be met and overcome rather than a debilitating threat, and consequently they recover more quickly once the threat has passed (Tugade & Fredrickson, 2004). In all, these findings add support to theoretical views that resilient individuals display greater emotional flexibility, recruiting important and appropriate behavioral responses to match the demands of the situation, which can change frequently and unpredictably. Future research in the neuroscience of resilience may benefit from investigating the role of positive emotions in facilitating emotional flexibility in the midst of changing situational demands. These future lines of work may help to discover the neural bases of the affective capacities that enable resilience.

Autonomic correlates of resilience

Theoretically, resilience is defined as the ability to "bounce back" from stressful experiences quickly and effectively. Until recently, however, few studies provided empirical support for this definition. Researchers have investigated the autonomic correlates of psychological resilience by examining patterns of cardiovascular recovery from negative emotional arousal (Tugade & Fredrickson, 2004). If high-resilient individuals are theorized to rebound efficiently in the face of stressful experiences, then it was hypothesized that this ability to recover from stress should be reflected physiologically as well. To test this hypothesis, researchers identified low- and high-resilient individuals based on self-reported responses to the ego-resiliency scale (Block & Kremen, 1996). Researchers then experimentally induced experiences of anxiety by asking low- and high-resilient participants to prepare a speech to be delivered in front of a videocamera for evaluation (in fact, no participants actually delivered their prepared speeches). As expected, the speech preparation instructions induced cardiovascular arousal as well as subjective reports of anxiety as intended, with no differences between low- and high-resilient individuals. Differences in trait resilience, however, emerged in two important ways. First, high-resilient (vs. low-resilient) individuals were more likely to report experiencing positive emotions, such as interest, alongside their self-reported anxiety. Second, high-resilient participants evidenced faster cardiovascular recovery from the arousal generated by the anxiety-inducing task, reflecting the ability to physiologically "bounce back" from stress. Mediational analyses revealed that the experience of positive emotions contributed, in part, to high-resilient participants' abilities to achieve efficient emotion regulation, demonstrated by accelerated cardiovascular recovery from negative emotional arousal. These findings indicate that high-resilient individuals are characterized by using positive emotions to cope with stress (Tugade & Fredrickson, 2004; Tugade et al., 2004).

Positive Emotions: Form and Function

Why are positive emotions, such as love, interest, joy, or gratitude, useful in the coping process? The broaden-and-build theory details the adaptive function of positive emotions (Fredrickson, 1998, 2001). This theory posits that positive emotions hold evolutionary significance beyond simply the hedonic experience of pleasantness. Indeed, positive emotions signal safety to an individual, cueing one that it is safe to roam and explore one's environment or sit quietly still without vigilance. Fredrickson's theory states that positive emotions function to broaden people's momentary thoughts and actions. For instance, experiences of gratitude function to increase the awareness of the social connection people have with their benefactors. When feeling grateful, people think about the many ways their benefactors are important in their life, and they consider creative and meaningful ways to express their appreciation (cf., Fredrickson, 2004). The outgrowth of positive emotions, like gratitude, is more expansive thinking and a greater breadth of action that helps one to build personal resources (e.g., cognitive, social, intellectual, and coping resources).

The broadening function of positive emotions may be useful for developing a repertoire of coping strategies to be kept in store until needed to cope with stress. Research shows, for example, that positive emotions produce more expansive options for behavioral action. After being experimentally induced to experience positive emotions (contentment, amusement), negative emotions (fear, anxiety), or neutrality, participants were asked to consider different activities they would like to pursue at that very moment. Findings indicated that those induced to experience positive emotions listed significantly more activities, compared to those induced to experience neutral or negative emotions (Fredirickson & Branigan, 2005). Considering a broader array of possible actions can have important benefits for coping. One advantage is that it might increase emotion knowledge, allowing one to consider different behaviors and actions important for responding to a stressful situation with the aim of determining the most efficient or appropriate action when the situation calls for coping (Tugade et al., 2004). To the extent that positive emotions broaden coping resources, they are also useful in strengthening people's social resources by developing and maintaining social relationships. Indeed, interventions to increase positive emotional experiences (e.g., cognitive-behavioral interventions, mindfulness meditation) are associated with health-enhancing outcomes in part because these interventions strengthen and enhance social connections (Chesney et al., 2005).

Another function of positive emotions is the "undoing" function, which is especially relevant to coping. The undoing effect illustrates the complementary effects of positive and negative emotions on the cardiovascular system. Negative emotions such as fear, anger, or anxiety have an alarm function; they produce sympathetic arousal that physiologically prepares the body to fight or flee. In contrast, positive emotions, such as contentment, joy, or interest, have a quieting function; they reduce the sympathetic arousal generated by negative emotions, helping to bring physiological reactivity back to levels prior to the onset of the stressor. To empirically test the undoing effect, continuous measures of cardiovascular responding were collected from participants who were induced to experience a high-arousal negative emotion (e.g., anxiety), after which participants were randomly assigned to experience either positive emotion, negative emotion, or neutrality. Findings revealed that participants induced to experience positive emotion (e.g., contentment, mild joy) had faster cardiovascular recovery from negative emotional arousal compared to participants induced to experience negative emotion or neutrality (Fredrickson et al., 2004; see also Fredrickson & Levenson, 2001). In the realm of coping, then, it appears that positive emotions function to help down-regulate negative emotional experiences, giving individuals the opportunity to pursue a wider array of thoughts or actions. These findings also lend support to theories indicating that positive emotions give individuals short "breathers" from stressful experiences (Lazarus & Folkman, 1984), giving them the momentary pause necessary to restore and replenish lost resources after experiencing stress.

Positive Emotions and Physical Health Outcomes

Within the past decade, accumulating research evidence points to the physical health benefits of positive emotions. Experiences of positive emotion have been shown to speed recovery from coronary artery bypass surgery (Scheier, Matthews, Owens, Schulz, Bridges, Magovern, & Carver, 1999) and reduce the risk of disability, stroke, and cardiovascular mortality in older adults (Danner, Snowdon & Friesen, 2001; Ostir et al., 2000; Richman et al., 2005).

Recent research has investigated the role of positive emotion in predicting resilient outcomes for individuals from disadvantaged social groups. Ostir and his colleagues (2006) investigated the relation between positive emotions and blood pressure levels among Mexican Americans, a minority group that is faced with disadvantages in health care access, lower income, and greater risk for obesity and diabetes, compared to non-Hispanic White Americans in the United States. Greater experiences of positive emotion were associated with lower blood pressure despite experiencing stressors associated with minority status. Specifically, for participants who were not taking antihypertensive medication, greater reports of positive emotions were associated with lower levels of systolic and diastolic blood pressure. For participants taking antihypertensive medication, higher levels of positive emotion were associated with lower systolic blood pressure (Ostir, Berges, Markides, & Ottenbacher, 2006). In related research on the importance of positive emotion on cardiovascular health outcomes, Ostir and his colleagues found that increases in reports of positive emotion were associated with a lower incidence of stroke among older White and Black Americans (Ostir, Markides, Peek, & Goodwin, 2001) and higher motor, cognitive, and overall functional status 3 months following a stroke, even after adjusting for relevant health risk factors (Ostir, Berges, Ottenbacher, Clow, & Ottenbacher, 2008). Together, these findings suggest that assessments of positive emotions during and following the onset of acute health events may aid our understanding of disease prevention, progression, and recovery.

Experiences of positive emotions also predict lower susceptibility to the common cold. Researchers asked participants to rate their positive emotions (lively, happy, cheerful) and negative emotions (depressed, nervous, angry) over a 2-week period. After the 2 weeks, participants were given nose drops of rhinovirus, which resulted in the flu for over 33% of the participants. Notably, those who reported greater positive emotions prior to exposure to the virus were less likely to develop the flu. In contrast, there was no significant relation between negative emotions and flu symptoms (Cohen, Doyle, Turner, Alper, & Skoner, 2003).

Positive emotions experienced over time may be most useful for predicting long-term benefits on health. Previous research reported no association between baseline positive affect and morbidity or mortality among HIV-positive individuals. Measuring positive affect only at one time point (baseline) may not tell the whole story, however. When positive affect is assessed across several time points prior to death, findings reveal the importance of chronic positive emotions on health. In one study, HIV-positive gay men completed measures of the Center for Epidemiologic Studies Depression Scale (CES-D; Radloff, 1977), which comprises four subscales: positive affect, negative affect, somatic, and interpersonal relations. The positive affect subscale measures the frequency of feeling happiness, hope, and joy. None of the CES-D subscales predicted AIDS-related mortality, except for the positive affect scale. HIV-positive gay men who reported greater cumulative positive affect prior to death had lower AIDS-related mortality compared to those who reported lower positive affect throughout the study, even when controlling for other markers of disease progression (Moskowitz, 2003). These findings advance research on positive affect and health for two important reasons. First, the results demonstrate that positive affect is uniquely associated with mortality due to AIDS. Second, they suggest that survival rates may depend on chronic (vs. episodic) positive affect when considering AIDS-related mortality.

Positive Emotions, Coping, and Health in Everyday Life

When are positive emotions most likely to confer their benefits on coping? The daily diary methodology is a useful technique for tracking the fluctuations of both positive and negative emotional experiences over time. One theoretical model, called the Dynamic Model of Affect (DMA; Zautra, Affleck, Tennen, Reich, & Davis, 2005), employs diary techniques and proposes that daily experiences of positive emotion are important for the regulation of negative emotions (Zautra, Johnson, & Davis, 2005; Zautra et al., 2005).

Empirical support for the DMA has been shown in research demonstrating the role of daily positive emotional experiences among elderly individuals coping with the challenges and stresses of late adulthood (Ong, Bergeman, Bisconti, & Wallace, 2006).

Examining patterns of emotional reactivity and recovery in the daily lives of elderly widows, Ong and his colleagues posit that positive emotions are useful in the coping process for two reasons. First, positive emotions may interrupt the ongoing stress response. Second, positive emotions may accelerate one's ability to adapt to subsequent stressors (Ong et al., 2006). In line with previous research (Tugade & Fredrickson, 2004; Tugade et al., 2004), trait resilience accounted for meaningful differences in the coping process. High-resilient widows in their sample were more likely to experience both positive and negative emotions throughout their bereavement process. Importantly, the researchers reported that daily experiences of positive emotion moderated stress reactivity and mediated stress recovery. These results indicate that those with greater daily positive emotions had lower overall stress reactivity, compared to those with lower daily positive emotions. In addition, daily positive emotions aided stress recovery for the high-resilient widows (Ong et al., 2006). Over time, then, the experience of positive emotions functions to assist high-resilient individuals in their ability to recover effectively from daily stress. These findings are in line with other research showing that daily positive emotions accelerate recovery from stress (Moskowitz, Folkman, & Acree, 2003), which may be especially useful for individuals in late adulthood (Carstensen & Mikels, 2005). Older adults are at greater risk of cardiovascular illness, and thus examining their emotional responses to changes in health status is particularly important. Indeed, reports of higher positive emotion are associated with lower blood pressure in older adults (Ostir et al., 2006), as well as lower levels of symptom distress, fewer depressive symptoms, higher daily activity scores, and higher perceived physical and mental health-related quality of life (Hu & Gruber, 2008). Emerging evidence also reveals that tracking the emotional well-being of older adults can be predictive of their recovery following cardiovascular illness, such as heart attack or stroke (Ostir et al., 2008).

Additional support for the DMA has been found in a host of daily diary studies, showing that experiences of positive emotions are useful for coping, especially on days when one experiences elevated levels of stress (Ong, Bergeman, & Bisconti, 2004; Zautra et al., 2005). Using the DMA as a theoretical model, researchers found that resilient bereaved individuals show weaker positive-to-negative affect correlations (demonstrating greater emotional

complexity) compared to less-resilient bereaved individuals. This greater emotional complexity predicted better adjustment after bereavement. Importantly, this effect remained even after controlling for self-reported distress (Coifman, Bonanno, & Rafaeli, 2007). Thus, the DMA is a useful theoretical model for demonstrating the beneficial function of emotional complexity (positive emotions generated in the midst of negative affect) for resilient individuals in the aftermath of aversive life events.

Resilience in the Face of Adversity

The idea that positive emotions can arise in the face of adversity and produce healthy outcomes for individuals is sometimes met with skepticism. Some suggest that this pattern of responding is maladaptive, reflecting defensive denial that will result in the delayed onset of grief (e.g., Bowlby, 1980).

Other researchers argue that no empirical evidence to date supports the idea that experiencing positive emotion in the midst of adversity will result in the delayed onset of grief (Bonanno, 2004; Wortman & Silver, 1989). Challenging the long-standing view that the ability to function well despite loss reflects repression, denial, or pathology, Bonanno and his colleagues have conducted a host of longitudinal studies to show that having the capacity to generate positive emotions in the face of adversity reflects resilience (Bonanno, 2004). Resilient trajectories are those that maintain a steady and stable equilibrium over time. Specifically, resilience is operationalized as a trajectory of response over time that reflects healthy physical and psychological functioning despite highly disruptive events in one's life, including the death of a loved one, illness, violence, national disaster, or caregiving for a loved one with chronic illness (e.g., Bonanno, 2008; Bonanno et al., 2002; Bonanno, Papa, & O'Neill, 2001).

There is growing evidence for the salutary nature of positive emotions in the bereavement process. Experiences of positive emotions are transformative and have long-lasting consequences for individuals, even if the positive emotions themselves are rather mild and short-lived. For example, behavioral markers of positive emotional experience, such as smiling and laughing while discussing a recent loss of a loved one, have been shown to be associated with better adjustment over time and stronger social relationships (Bonanno & Keltner, 1997; Keltner & Bonanno, 1997). These behaviors are generally subtle and spontaneous, and they are rather common responses to grief. Researchers state that resilience is not a rare or extraordinary response in the face of stress. All people, not just a subset of individuals, have the capacity to experience positive emotions, even in the face of extreme life circumstances (Bonanno, 2008; cf., Masten, 2001). Together, these studies show that the ability to experience even mild forms of positive emotions in the midst of adversity contributes to resilient trajectories.

The Resilience Response

Thus far, I have reviewed research and theory that examine how, when, and why positive emotions fuel resilience in the face of adversity. To date, the existing research has not differentiated between automatic and controlled processes of resilience. In the sections that follow, I propose a new model of resilience that explores the dual-process nature of generating positive emotions in the service of coping.

Dual-process theories are prevalent in social and personality psychology (Barrett, Tugade, & Engle, 2004; Chaiken & Trope, 1999). The central tenet in these theories is that thoughts, feelings, and behaviors are driven by two separate though complementary processes: automatic and controlled. Automatic and controlled processes are characterized by four important qualities (Bargh, 1994): *awareness* (whether you are consciously aware that a process is happening), *efficiency* (the extent to which you expend cognitive or attentional resources), *intention* (whether you see yourself as having agency in your thoughts, feelings, or behavior), and *control* (whether you are able to modify the behavior in any way). Dual-process theories can be applied to resilience by examining how positive affect is generated via automatic or controlled processes in the service of managing stress.

Controlled processes of resilience

Research shows that positive emotions can be either increased or decreased via controlled processes of emotion regulation (Tugade & Fredrickson, 2007). For example, people may actively seek a means to momentarily lift their spirits or to maintain good feelings and pleasantness. Research on using humor to cope sheds light on the role of cultivating positive emotion to manage a stressful experience. People often intentionally maximize experiences of amusement for a number of reasons. An individual may make efforts to think about a humorous aspect of a stressful experience (deliberate "up-regulation") to cope with the situation. Subjective experience, behavior (smiling, laughing), and autonomic physiology (including heart rate, respiration, and sympathetic nervous system activation) are enhanced in accordance with cognitive "up-regulation" processes (Giuliani, McRae, & Gross, 2008). There are also neural activation patterns unique to the conscious up-regulation of positive emotion (Kim & Hamann, 2007).

Other controlled processes of positive emotion generation involve actively increasing and enhancing one's positive emotional experiences. These are considered "top-down" strategies that require cognitive control and effortful processing because they involve explicit goals that are consciously initiated. Benefits accrue from actively cultivating positive emotions in everyday life (see Fredrickson, 2000, for a review) as well as in response to negative circumstances. One study examined the extent to which people used different strategies to elicit positive emotions in the face of different stressors, including daily hassles such as boredom, social stress, personal failure, or physical discomfort. Findings revealed that actively cultivating positive emotions increased with the severity of stressors. More specifically, the use of coping strategies that elicited positive sensory experiences (e.g., seeking pleasant scents, sounds, or sights) increased with the severity of a stressor over the course of a week. Interestingly, even strategies that are more cognitively demanding (e.g., positive reappraisal) were used with more frequency as the severity of the stressor increased (Shiota, 2006).

Although engaging in positive reappraisal may be cognitively taxing when coping with short-term stressors, this same strategy has important long-term benefits on well-being. When examining personal narratives, researchers have discovered individual differences in how people interpret negative circumstances and challenges in their life. Some individuals are able to find *positive resolution*. Their narratives reflect a sense of personal growth following important challenges in life. Narratives characterized by positive resolution are those that reflect a "coherent and complete story of a difficult event that ends positively, conveying a sense of emotional resolution or closure" (Pals, 2006, p. 1082). Similarly, longitudinal research indicates that personal narratives that reflect sequences of *redemption* have important implications for personality development. A common theme in American personal narratives, *redemption* is a narrative sequence in which one transforms suffering, adversity, or pain into a more positive experience (McAdams, 2008). People with narratives characterized by redemption evidence increases in life satisfaction, eudaimonic well-being, resiliency, and physical health reported over time (Bauer, McAdams, & Pals, 2008; Pals, 2006).

Another important strategy that requires cognitive effort but has long-term benefits for individuals involves trying to find positive meaning in negative events. This strategy has been found to produce positive emotions that help buffer against stress (Folkman & Moskowitz, 2000). Three paths to meaning-making have been identified: (1) positive reappraisal (i.e., finding a "silver lining"), (2) problem-focused coping (i.e., efforts directed at solving or managing the problem causing distress), and (3) infusing ordinary events with positive meaning (e.g., appreciating a compliment).

Although it may seem like a trivial act, infusing ordinary events with positive meaning is linked to striking advantages in coping. When a negative event occurs, the individual psychologically creates a positive event or reinterprets a commonplace event more positively, as a way of buffering from distress. In their research on caregivers of people with AIDS, for example, Folkman and Moskowitz (Folkman, 1997; Moskowitz et al., 1996) found that even in the midst of their distress, over 99% of their participants were able to find positive meaning in ordinary events (e.g., appreciating friendship when one lends a helping hand; noticing the beauty of a flower on one's path) (Folkman, 1997; Folkman & Moskowitz; 2000). Notably, it is likely that the ability of the caregivers in their study to find positive meaning in "run-of-the-mill" events did not occur accidentally (Folkman & Moskowitz, 2000). Rather, these caregivers may have *intentionally* looked to positive aspects of their lives as a way of coping with their distress. These deliberately cultivated positive emotions play an important role in the coping process: Positive reappraisal generates experiences of positive emotion even amidst stress. In turn, these positive emotional experiences can provide the needed psychological lift to help people continue and move forward in their lives (Folkman & Moskowitz, 2000).

Benefit-finding in the midst of adversity allows individuals to find meaning in important life challenges. Mounting research evidence shows that being able to find benefits in chronic illness or pain can be protective against cardiovascular illness (e.g., high blood pressure and other cardiovascular ailments). There is a distinction between benefit-finding and benefit-reminding, although both processes work hand-in-hand (Affleck & Tennen, 1996; Tennen & Affleck, 1999). Benefit finding is the process of considering good things that can arise from one's misfortunes (e.g., growth, wisdom, competence, strengthened values). A related coping strategy, benefit-reminding, is described as the cognitive strategy marked by an *intentional* reminding of previously found benefits. Both strategies have been shown to predict important health outcomes, such as less rheumatoid arthritis pain and lower psychological distress (Danoff-Burg & Revenson, 2005), lower depression scores, greater social support, more physical activity among HIV-positive men and women (Littlewood, Vanable, & Carey, 2008), and decreased chronic pain (Tennen, Affleck, & Zautra, 2006).

Do positive emotions facilitate benefit-finding and benefit-reminding, or do these coping strategies produce positive emotions in the midst of important life challenges? Bower and her colleagues proposed an integrative model that describes psychological pathways to explain the relation between benefit-finding and health (Bower, Low, Moskowitz, Sepah, & Epel, 2007). One pathway focused on the important role of positive affect. The authors suggested that positive affect increases as one tries to find benefits in adversity, thereby producing advantages in health (e.g., lower rates of mortality). They also suggest that benefit-finding might help to buffer against future stressors, allowing people to adapt to future stressors more adaptively, flexibly, and effectively. In line with this idea, research shows that positive affect buffers the effect of high pain and high interpersonal stress among women with fibromyalgia and osteoarthritis (Zautra, Johnson, & Davis, 2005). Other supportive evidence can be found in studies showing that positive affect may buffer physiological reactivity. Individuals who are rated as happier have lower daily cortisol levels and lower ambulatory heart rate (Steptoe, Wardle, & Marmot, 2005). In an experience-sampling study, greater daily positive affect was associated with lower blood pressure (Ong & Alliare, 2005).

Automatic processes of resilience

Much of the empirical research on the nature of coping has been focused on deliberate, or controlled processes; however, recent research shows that aspects of emotion-regulation that are activated via automatic processes may be just as pervasive (e.g., Bargh & Williams, 2007; Mauss, Bunge, & Gross, 2007). This section will focus on automatic processes of resilience, with specific focus on the automatic activation of positive emotion in the service of coping with stress. Indeed, although it may often involve conscious processes, emotion regulation does not always require awareness or explicit strategies (Gross & Muñoz, 1995), and therefore can be unconscious and automatic.

Automatic processes of resilience can operate in two ways. First, positive affect can be automatically activated in one's environment in the midst of a stressful experience, helping to down-regulate the negative experience. In this view, automatically activated affective responses serve as an organizing force, thereby disrupting whatever other processes may be operating at the time. When undergoing a stressful experience, certain sensory experiences can activate positive affect in the service of coping, even outside of one's conscious awareness. For example, the feel of warmth from a cup of tea can soothe an individual; the smile from a passerby can trigger feelings of social connectedness and support; or the smell of the ocean air that reminds one of a pleasant vacation can elicit feelings of contentment. As each of these examples illustrates, perception can introduce the idea of action, which has important implications for affective response (Chartrand & Bargh, 1996; Chartrand et al., 2006) and social behavior (Bargh & Chartrand, 1999). Through the automatic process of perception, sensory experiences can activate positive affect outside of one's conscious awareness, thereby interrupting the trajectory of the stressful episode before it can fully unfold.

In a sense, these "bottom-up" processes of perception can activate responses in systems that are typically associated with emotional responding (e.g., autonomic changes, behavioral action, facial action; Barrett, Mesquita, Ochsner, & Gross, 2007). As such, the information from valenced environmental stimuli can be computed rapidly and can influence subsequent behavior and experience (Barrett et al., 2007). This has important implications for the coping process. Indeed, automatically activated positive emotion can fuel recovery from stress with minimal effort, freeing up important resources to use for coping with the stressful situation.

A second way that automatic processes of coping can occur is via implicit goals for coping, which can be automatically initiated and enacted outside of one's conscious awareness (Bargh, 1989). Empirical research demonstrates how goals can be automatically activated to influence behavior. For example, participants who are subliminally primed with the goal to form an impression about someone have been shown to successfully complete the goal (effective recall of behaviors and clear organization of information in memory) without the ability to articulate

why they behaved that way or even *that* they behaved that way (Chartrand & Bargh, 1996).

Research on automatic emotion regulation (Mauss et al., 2007) shows that it is possible for an implicit goal to alter one's emotional experience in a given situation automatically. In other words, the goal to modify an aspect of one's emotional experience can occur without making a conscious decision to do so, without expending attentional resources, and without deliberate control. For instance, when the goal to control one's anger (vs. express it) is subliminally primed, participants report lower levels of felt anger. Moreover, there is no evidence of physiological cost to an individual for controlling versus expressing one's anger (Mauss et al., 2007). These findings indicate that implicit goals to cope (in this case, to control one's emotion) can indeed be automatically activated in the service of minimizing stressful experiences. These automatically activated coping goals involve minimal costs to individuals and therefore can produce beneficial outcomes for well-being and psychological health.

Recent research has investigated the automatic and controlled processes of resilience. Participants were experimentally induced to experience sadness via a mental visualization exercise. Immediately following the sadness induction, participants were randomly assigned to experience positive emotion via automatic or controlled possessing. The automatic processing task included a supraliminal priming task (unscrambling words to form a sentence, with one of the embedded words serving as a positive emotion prime). The controlled processing task involved positive reappraisal (asking participants to find positive meaning in the sadness they just experienced). Participants then completed a cognitive flexibility task (Stroop, 1935). Cognitive flexibility is important for selecting the optimal coping strategy at the appropriate time (e.g., Sapolsky, 2004) and thus is important for resilient responding in the face of stress. Continuous measures of cardiovascular responding were collected throughout the experimental session.

Findings indicated that participants induced to experience positive emotion via automatic processes showed greater cognitive flexibility compared to those induced to experience positive emotion via controlled processes. Automatic and controlled processes also differentially predicted physiological recovery following the stressor, with automatic processes producing faster cardiovascular recovery from sadness compared to controlled processes (Tugade & Alpern, 2010). Because of the cognitive effort usually required to use problem-focused coping, positive reappraisal may be difficult in the midst of an immediate, short-term stressor. In these challenging situations, having positive emotions easily accessible to an individual may produce greater coping efficacy. It is important to note that positive emotions generated via automatic processes may confer their benefits in response to *short-term* stressors. As reported previously in this chapter, positive emotions generated via controlled processing have important benefits for *long-term* coping (Bauer, McAdams, & Pals, 2008; Pals, 2006).

Intersections Between Automatic and Controlled Processes

Two distinct though interacting dual-process models of coping are the focus of the present chapter. One model focuses on the intersections between positive and negative emotions in the coping process. Growing attention is focused on this model, which shows that positive emotional experiences have important functions in down-regulating distressing experiences. Along these lines, research indicates that there are individual differences in the capacity to use positive emotions to cope. The second model discussed in this chapter focuses on the interplay between automatic and controlled processes to better understand how positive emotions are generated in the service of coping. A newer model in the stress and coping literature, this explores the mechanisms that promote resilience in the midst of short-term and long-term stressors in one's life.

At the crux of these dual-process models is the dynamic and multifaceted nature of resilience. As the findings reviewed in this chapter indicate, positive emotions can be deliberately cultivated cognitively (e.g., positive reappraisal) or behaviorally (e.g., smiling while feeling sad) to help down-regulate negative emotional experiences. Over time, as with other controlled processes, these deliberate coping strategies can become automatized. For resilient individuals, cultivating positive emotions when coping with stress can become an automatic behavior, just like any other behavior or complex action sequence can become automatized with repetition (Bargh & Chartrand, 1999; Norman & Shallice, 1986). Automatic skill acquisition (like emotion regulation) depends on the frequent and consistent pairing of internal responses with external events (Shiffrin & Dumais, 1981; Shiffrin & Schneider, 1977). Supportive evidence can be found in research on the positivity effect, which shows that as one ages, automatic processes of coping are more likely to be enacted (Carstensen & Mikels, 2005). For instance, older (vs. younger) adults quickly shift attention away from negative stimuli to positive emotional stimuli (Isaacowitz, Wadlinger, Goren, & Wilson, 2006a, 2006b; Mather & Carstensen, 2005). This coping strategy may have begun as a deliberate process, but became automatized with age after repetition across different situations throughout one's life. Emotion regulation skills begin to develop as early as infancy (Posner & Rothbart, 1998). It is possible that one can consistently use coping strategies that elicit positive emotions (e.g., positive reappraisal, benefit-finding, infusing ordinary events with positive meaning). Over time, these strategies can emerge independent of conscious intention (Bargh & Chartrand, 1999) and facilitate effective outcomes of coping with stress.

The intersections between automatic and controlled processes of resilience can also be found in research on meditation practices. Empirical research shows that novice individuals can be trained to use two types of meditative practices (mindfulness, loving-kindness meditation), which reap important benefits in physical and psychological functioning. Mindfulness-based stress reduction (MBSR; Kabat-Zinn, 2005) involves techniques that cultivate greater awareness of the mind and body. Novice meditators who were trained on MBSR techniques over the course of 8 weeks evidenced greater left-hemispheric brain activation, a region consistently shown to be associated with positive affect (Davidson et al., 2003). Another meditation practice, loving-kindness meditation (LKM), involves actively cultivating positive emotions in order to learn about the nature of one's emotional experiences. In a field study, Fredrickson and her colleagues trained working adults to practice LKM in their daily lives over the course of 9 weeks. Findings indicated that those who practiced LKM evidenced increased daily experiences of positive emotions, which in turn helped to build personal resources, including resilience (Fredrickson et al., 2008). Together, these findings indicate that meditation may at first be a deliberative practice; however, over time the emotional and bodily awareness that result from meditation may produce increases in daily positive emotion, which in turn may interrupt the stressor before it fully unfolds and help to buffer against future stressors.

Indeed, attention to one's own affective experiences can promote positive emotion knowledge (Tugade et al., 2004), which is important for coping and resilience.

Conclusions and Recommendations for Future Research

Several areas of future research on positive emotions and resilience bring exciting possibilities for building on existing paradigms in stress, health, and coping research. For instance, future research may benefit from considering the cultural proscriptions associated with the expression and experience of positive emotion. The Affect Valuation Theory (AVT; Tsai, Knutson, & Fung, 2006) is useful in understanding cultural differences in the positive emotions that people ideally want to feel (i.e., "ideal affect"). For instance, compared to Hong Kong Chinese, European Americans place more value on high-arousal positive emotions (e.g., excitement) and less value on low-arousal positive emotions (e.g., calmness) (Tsai et al., 2006). Future studies may be aimed toward investigating whether the AVT can help explain the different types of positive emotions that are useful for health and coping across different cultural groups. The AVT might also be useful investigating whether low- or high-arousal positive emotions are more easily accessible among people of different cultures.

Future research might also capitalize on methodological advances in science to investigate the intersections between positive/negative emotion and automatic/controlled processes associated with resilience. Experience-sampling methodology (ESM) has been used effectively in stress, coping, and health research to investigate within-person patterns of emotional experience as they pertain to stress and health (e.g., Conner, Tugade, & Barrett, 2004; Ong & Allaire, 2005; Ong et al., 2004; Zautra et al., 2005a,b). Beyond assessing whether positive emotions are experienced during stressful circumstances, forthcoming studies might use ESM to investigate whether actively cultivating positive emotions in the midst of stress can become automatically activated over time. ESM might also be useful in investigating which positive emotions are more easily activated under stressful circumstances.

Different positive emotions may confer their benefits onto stress and health in distinct ways. Advances in research might focus on the differentiation of positive emotions in the coping process. To illustrate, recent research has shown that general positive affect is associated with a lower risk of mortality among chronically ill individuals with diabetes, even when controlling for negative affect and other risks of mortality (Moskowitz, Epel, & Acree, 2008). In a comparison sample of not chronically ill participants, positive affect did not predict mortality risk. When teasing apart different experiences of positive affect (as assessed by four items on the CES-D positive affect subscale; Radloff, 1977), a somewhat different pattern emerges. For chronically ill individuals, certain positive affects (measured by the items "enjoyed life" and feeling "happy") continued to predict lower risk of mortality, whereas other items (measured by "self esteem" and feeling "hopeful") were no longer significant predictors (Moskowitz et al., 2008). Other research examined the associations between two positive affective dispositions (trait hope and trait curiosity) on the prevalence and incidence of hypertension, diabetes, and respiratory tract infections over a 2-year period. Higher levels of trait hope were associated with a lower prevalence of hypertension and diabetes and a lower incidence of respiratory tract infections. In contrast, higher levels of trait curiosity were associated with a lower prevalence of diabetes and a lower incidence of hypertension (no association with respiratory tract infection; Richman et al., 2005). Together, these studies demonstrate that distinct positive emotions (joy, pride, happiness, hope, interest/curiosity) are differentially associated with physical health outcomes. Future studies that systematically investigate how a larger range of positive emotions may be associated with health outcomes and research that investigates the potential mechanisms that underlie these associations would help advance current research in important ways.

Summary

The research reported in this chapter suggests that strategies that elicit positive emotions are important for establishing beneficial coping outcomes, especially for resilient individuals. Resilient people may initially use positive emotions strategically while coping with a stressful situation, actively cultivating positive emotions to down-regulate distress. To the extent that this same strategy is enacted over time, the conscious strategy can become automatized (Bargh & Chartrand, 1999). Using positive emotions to cope, then, may be likened to mastering a skill. With repeated practice, the skill becomes automatic, requiring only minimal attention or cognitive effort. These benefits can be valuable for coping in the short run and can also have long-lasting benefits for an individual.

Author Note

Preparation of this chapter was supported in part by the Lucy Maynard Research Fund (Vassar College) and the Thomas Meloy Foundation. The author thanks Jannay Morrow, Abigail Baird, and members of the Vassar College Emotions and Psychophysiology Laboratory for their insightful comments on an earlier draft of this chapter.

References

Affleck, G., & Tennen, H. (1996). Construing benefits from adversity: Adaptational significance and dispositional underpinnings. *Journal of Personality, 64*, 899–922.

Bargh, J. A. (1989). Conditional automaticity: Varieties of automatic influence in social perception and cognition. In J. S. Uleman, & J. A. Bargh (Eds.), *Unintended thought* (pp. 3–51). New York: Guilford Press.

Bargh, J. A. (1994). The four horsemen of automaticity: Awareness, intention, efficiency, and control in social cognition. In R. S. Wyer Jr. & T. K. Srull (Eds.), *Handbook of social cognition, vol. 1: Basic processes; vol. 2: Applications (2nd ed.)* (pp. 1–40). Hillsdale, NJ: Lawrence Erlbaum Associates, Inc.

Bargh, J. A., & Chartrand, T. L. (1999). The unbearable automaticity of being. *American Psychologist, 54*(7), 462–479.

Bargh, J. A., & Williams, L. E. (2007). The nonconscious regulation of emotion. In J. J. Gross (Ed.), *Handbook of emotion regulation* (pp. 429–445). New York: Guilford Press.

Barrett, L. F., Mesquita, B., Ochsner, K. N., & Gross, J. J. (2007). The experience of emotion. *Annual Review of Psychology, 58*, 373–403.

Bauer, J. J., McAdams, D. P., & Pals, J. L. (2008). Narrative identity and eudaimonic well-being. *Journal of Happiness Studies, 9*, 81–104.

Block, J., & Kremen, A. M. (1996). IQ and ego-resiliency: Conceptual and empirical connections and separateness. *Journal of Personality and Social Psychology, 70*(2), 349–361.

Bonanno, G. A. (2004). Loss, trauma, and human resilience: Have we underestimated the human capacity to thrive after extremely aversive events? *American Psychologist, 59*(1), 20–28.

Bonanno, G. A., & Keltner, D. (1997). Facial expressions of emotion and the course of conjugal bereavement. *Journal of Abnormal Psychology, 106*(1), 126–137.

Bonanno, G. A., Papa, A., & O'Neill, K. (2001). Loss and human resilience. *Applied and Preventive Psychology, 10*, 193–206.

Bonanno, G. A., Wortman, C. B., Lehman, D. R., Tweed, R. G., Haring, M., Sonnega, J., et al. (2002). Resilience to loss and chronic grief: A prospective study from pre-loss to 18 months post-loss. *Journal of Personality and Social Psychology, 83*, 1150–1164.

Bower, J. E., Low, C. A., Moskowitz, J. T., Sepah, S. & Epel, E. (2007) Benefit finding and physical health: Positive psychological changes and enhanced allostasis. *Social and Personality Psychology Compass, 2*, 223–244.

Bowlby, J. (1980). *Loss: Sadness and depression: Vol. 3. Attachment and loss.* New York: Basic Books.

Carstensen, L. L., & Mikels, J. A. (2005). At the intersection of emotion and cognition: Aging and the positivity effect. *Current Directions in Psychological Science, 14*(3), 117–121.

Carstensen, L. L., Pasupathi, M., Mayr, U., & Nesselroade, J. R. (2000). Emotional experi- ence in everyday life across the adult life span. *Journal of Personality and Social Psychology, 79*, 644–655.

Chaiken, S., & Trope, Y. (Eds.). (1999). *Dual-process theories in social psychology.* New York: Guilford Press.

Chartrand, T. L., & Bargh, J. A. (1996). Automatic activation of impression formation and memorization goals: Nonconscious goal priming reproduces effects of explicit task instructions. *Journal of Personality and Social Psychology, 71*(3), 464–478.

Chartrand, T. L., van Baaren, R. B., & Bargh, J. A. (2006). Linking automatic evaluation to mood and information processing style: Consequences for experienced affect, impression formation, and stereotyping. *Journal of Experimental Psychology: General, 135*(1), 70–77.

Chesney, M. A., Darbes, L. A., Hoerster, K., Taylor, J. M., Chambers, D. B., & Anderson, D. E. (2005). Positive emotions: Exploring the other hemisphere in behavioral medicine. *International Journal of Behavioral Medicine, 12*(2), 50–58.

Cicchetti, D., & Tucker, D. (1994). Development and self-regulatory structures of the mind. *Development and Psychopathology. Special Issue: Neural Plasticity, Sensitive Periods, and Psychopathology, 6*(4), 533–549.

Cohen, S., Doyle, W. J., Turner, R. B., Alper, C. M., & Skoner, D. P. (2003). Emotional style and susceptibility to the common cold. *Psychosomatic Medicine, 65*, 652–657.

Coifman, K. G., Bonanno, G. A., & Rafaeli, E. (2007). Affect dynamics, bereavement and resilience to loss. *Journal of Happiness Studies, 8*(3), 371–392.

Conner, T., Tugade, M. M., & Barrett, L. F. (2004). Ecological momentary assessment. In N. Anderson (Ed.), *Encyclopedia of health and behavior* (pp. 291–292). Thousand Oaks, CA: Sage.

Danner, D., Snowdon, D., & Friesen, W. (2001). Positive emotion in early life and longevity: findings from the nun study. *Journal of Personality and Social Psychology, 80*, 804–813.

Danoff-Burg, S., & Revenson, T. A. (2005). Benefit-finding among patients with rheumatoid arthritis: Positive effects on interpersonal relationships. *Journal of Behavioral Medicine, 28*, 91–103.

Davidson, R. J. (2000). Affective style, psychopathology, and resilience: Brain mechanisms and plasticity. *American Psychologist, 55*(11), 1196–1214.

Davidson, R. J., Jackson, D. C., & Kalin, N. H. (2000). Emotion, plasticity, context, and regulation: Perspectives from affective neuroscience. *Psychological Bulletin, 126*, 890–909.

Davidson, R. J., Kabat-Zinn, J., Schumacher, J., Rosenkranz, M., Muller, D., Santorelli, S. F., et al. (2003). Alterations in brain and immune function produced by mindfulness meditation. *Psychosomatic Medicine, 65*(4), 564–570.

Folkman, S. (1997). Positive psychological states and coping with severe stress. *Social Science & Medicine, 45*(8), 1207–1221.

Folkman, S., & Moskowitz, J. T. (2000). Positive affect and the other side of coping. *American Psychologist, 55*(6), 647–654.

Folkman, S., & Moskowitz, J. T. (2000). Stress, positive emotion, and coping. *Current Directions in Psychological Science, 9*(4), 115–118.

Fredrickson, B. L. (1998). What good are positive emotions? *Review of General Psychology. Special Issue: New Directions in Research on Emotion, 2*(3), 300–319.

Fredrickson, B. L. (2001). The role of positive emotions in positive psychology: The broaden-and-build theory of positive emotions. *American Psychologist, 56*, 218–226.

Fredrickson, B. L. (2004). Gratitude, like other positive emotions, broadens and builds. In R. A. Emmons & M. E. McCullough (Eds.), *The psychology of gratitude* (pp. 145–166). New York: Oxford University Press.

Fredrickson, B. L., & Branigan, C. (2005). Positive emotions broaden the scope of attention and thought-action repertoires. *Cognition & Emotion, 19*(3), 313–332.

Fredrickson, B. L., Cohn, M. A., Coffey, K. A., Pek, J., & Finkel, S. M. (2008) Open hearts build lives: Positive emotions, induced through loving-kindness meditation, build consequential personal resources. *Journal of Personality and Social Psychology, 95,* 1045–62.

Fredrickson, B. L., Mancuso, R. A., Branigan, C., & Tugade, M. M. (2000). The undoing effect of positive emotions. *Motivation and Emotion, 24*(4), 237–258.

Fredrickson, B. L., & Levenson, R. W. (1998). Positive emotions speed recovery from the cardiovascular sequelae of negative emotions. *Cognition and Emotion, 12,* 191–220.

Fredrickson, B. L., Tugade, M. M., Waugh, C. E., & Larkin, G. (2003). What good are positive emotions in crises? A prospective study of resilience and emotions following the terrorist attacks on the United States on September 11th, 2001. *Journal of Personality and Social Psychology, 84,* 365–376.

Giuliani, N. R., McRae, K., & Gross, J. J. (2008). The up- and down-regulation of amusement: Experiential, behavioral, and autonomic consequences. *Emotion, 8*(5), 714–719.

Gross, J. J., & Munoz, R. F. (1995). Emotion regulation & mental health. *Clinical Psychology: Science and Practice, 2,* 151–164.

Hu, J., & Gruber, K. (2008). Positive and negative affect and health functioning indicators in older adults with chronic illnesses. *Issues in Mental Health Nursing, 29,* 895–911.

Isaacowitz, D. M., Wadlinger, H. A., Goren, D., & Wilson, H. R. (2006). Is there an age-related positivity effect in visual attention? A comparison of two methodologies. *Emotion, 6*(3), 511–516.

Isaacowitz, D. M., Wadlinger, H. A., Goren, D., & Wilson, H. R. (2006). Selective preference in visual fixation away from negative images in old age? an eye-tracking study. *Psychology and Aging, 21*(1), 40–48.

Kabat-Zinn, J. (2005). *Coming to our senses: Healing ourselves and the world through mindfulness.* New York: Hyperion.

Kaplan, H. B. (2007). Understanding the concept of resilience. In S. Goldstein & R. B. Brooks (Eds.), *Resilience in children* (pp. 39–47). New York: Springer Publishing.

Keltner, D., & Bonanno, G. A. (1997). A study of laughter and dissociation: Distinct correlates of laughter and smiling during bereavement. *Journal of Personality and Social Psychology, 73*(4), 687–702.

Kim, S. H., & Hamann, S. (2007). Neural correlates of positive and negative emotion regulation. *Journal of Cognitive Neuroscience, 19*(5), 776–798.

Lazarus, R. S., & Folkman, S. (1984). *Stress, appraisal, and coping.* New York: Springer.

Littlewood, R. A., Vanable, P. A., Carey, M. P., & Blair, D.C. (2008). The association of benefit finding to psychosocial and health behavior adaptation among HIV+ men and women. *Journal of Behavioral Medicine, 31,* 145–55.

Luthar, S. S. (Ed.). (2003). *Resilience and vulnerability: Adaptation in the context of childhood adversities.* New York: Cambridge University Press.

Luthar, S. S., Cicchetti, D., & Becker, B. (2000). Research on resilience: Response to commentaries. *Child Development, 71*(3), 573–575.

Masten, A. S. (2001). Ordinary magic: Resilience processes in development. *American Psychologist, 56*(3), 227–238.

Mather, M., & Carstensen, L. L. (2005). Aging and motivated cognition: The positivity effect in attention and memory. *Trends in Cognitive Sciences, 9*(10), 496–502.

Mauss, I. B., Bunge, S. A., & Gross, J. J. (2007). Automatic emotion regulation. *Social and Personality Psychology Compass, 1*(1), 146–167.

McAdams, D. P. (2008). American identity: The redemptive self. *The General Psychologist, 43,* 20–27.

Moskowitz, J. T. (2003). Positive affect predicts lower risk of AIDS mortality. *Psychosomatic Medicine, 65,* 620–626.

Moskowitz, J. T., Epel, E. S., & Acree, M. (2008). Positive affect uniquely predicts lower risk of mortality in people with diabetes. *Health Psychology, 27,* S73–S82.

Moskowitz, J. T., Folkman, S., & Acree, M. (2003). Do positive psychological states shed light on recovery from bereavement? Findings from a 3-year longitudinal study. *Death Studies, 27*(6), 471–500.

Moskowitz, J. T., Folkman, S., Collette, L., & Vittinghoff, E. (1996). Coping and mood during AIDS-related caregiving and bereavement. *Annals of Behavioral Medicine, 18*(1), 49–57.

Norman, D. A., & Shallice, T. (1986). Attention to action: Willed and automatic control of behaviour (pp. 1–18; Revised reprint of Norman and Shallice, 1980). In R. J. Davidson, G. E. Schwartz, & D. Shapiro, *Consciousness and self-regulation: Advances in research and theory.* New York: Plenum Press.

Ong, A., & Allaire, J. C. (2005). Cardiovascular intraindividual variability in later life: The influence of social connectedness and positive emotions. *Psychology and Aging, 20,* 476–485.

Ong, A. D., Bergeman, C. S., & Bisconti, T. L. (2004). The role of daily positive emotions during conjugal bereavement. *The Journals of Gerontology: Series B: Psychological Sciences and Social Sciences, 59B*(4), P168–P176.

Ong, A. D., Bergeman, C. S., Bisconti, T. L., & Wallace, K. A. (2006). Psychological resilience, positive emotions, and successful adaptation to stress in later life. *Journal of Personality and Social Psychology, 91*(4), 730–749.

Ostir, G. V., Berges, I. M., Markides, K. S., & Ottenbacher, K. J. (2006). Hypertension in older adults and the role of positive emotions. *Psychosomatic Medicine, 68,* 727–733.

Ostir, G. V., Berges, I. M., Ottenbacher, M. E., Clow, A., & Ottenbacher, K. J. (2008). Associations between positive emotion and recovery of functional status following stroke. *Psychosomatic Medicine, 70,* 404–9.

Ostir, G. V., Markides, K. S., Black, S.A., Y Goodwin, J.S. (2000). Emotional well-being predicts subsequentt functional independence and survival. *Journal of the American Geriatric Society, 48,* 473–8.

Ostir, G. V., Markides, K. S., Peek, M. K., & Goodwin, J. S. (2001). The association between emotional well-being and the incidence of stroke in older adults. *Psychosomatic Medicine, 63,* 210–215.

Pals, J. L. (2006). Narrative identity processing of difficult life experiences: Pathways of personality development and positive self-transformation in adulthood. *Journal of Personality, 74*(4), 1079–1110.

Posner, M. I., & Rothbart, M. K. (1998). Attention, self-regulation, and consciousness. *Philosophical Transactions of the Royal Society of London, B, 353,* 1915–1927.

Radloff, L. S. (1977). The CES-D scale: A self-report depression scale for research in the general population. *Applied Psychological Measurement, 1,* 385–401.

Richman, L. S., Kubzansky, L., Maselko, J., Kawachi, I., Choo, P., & Bauer, M. (2005). Positive emotion and health: Going beyond the negative. *Health Psychology, 24,* 422–429.

Sapolsky, R. M. (2004). *Why zebras don't get ulcers.* New York: Henry Holt & Company.

Scheier, M. F., Matthews, K. A., Owens, J. F., Schulz, R., Bridges, M. W., Magovern, G. J., Jr., & Carver, C. S. (1999). Optimism and rehospitalization following coronary artery bypass graft surgery. *Archives of Internal Medicine 159,* 829–835.

Shiffrin, R. M., & Schneider, W. (1977). Controlled and automatic human information processing: II. perceptual learning, automatic attending and a general theory. *Psychological Review, 84*(2), 127–190.

Shiffrin, R. M., & Dumais, S. T. (1981). The development of automatism. In J. Anderson (Ed.), *Cognitive skills and their acquisition* (pp. 111–40). Hillsdale, NJ: Erlbaum.

Shiota, M. N. (2006). Silver linings and candles in the dark: Differences among positive coping strategies in predicting subjective well-being. *Emotion, 6*(2), 335–339.

Steptoe, A., Wardle, J., & Marmot, M. (2005) Positive affect and health-related neuroendocrine, cardiovascular, and inflammatory processes. *Proceedings from the National Academy of Sciences of the United States, 102,* 6508–6512.

Stroop, J. R. (1935). Studies of interference in serial verbal reactions. *Journal of Experimental Psychology, 18,* 643–662.

Tennen, H., Affleck, G., & Zautra, A. (2006). Depression history and coping with chronic pain: A daily process analysis. *Health Psychology, 25,* 370–379.

Tennen, H., & Affleck, G. (1999). Finding benefits in adversity. In C. R. Snyder (Ed.), *Coping: The psychology of what works* (pp. 279–304). New York: Oxford University Press.

Tsai, J. L., Knutson, B., & Fung, H. H. (2006). Cultural variation in affect valuation. *Journal of Personality and Social Psychology, 90,* 288–307.

Tugade, M. M., & Alpern, A. (2010). The resilience response: Examining automatic and controlled processes of positive emotion. Manuscript submitted for publication.

Tugade, M. M., & Fredrickson, B. L. (2002). Positive emotions and emotional intelligence. In L. F. Barrett, & P. Salovey (Eds.), *The wisdom in feeling: Psychological processes in emotional intelligence* (pp. 319–340). New York: Guilford Press.

Tugade, M. M., & Fredrickson, B. L. (2004). Resilient individuals use positive emotions to bounce back from negative emotional experiences. *Journal of Personality and Social Psychology, 86*(2), 320–333.

Tugade, M. M., & Fredrickson, B. L. (2007). Regulation of positive emotions: Emotion regulation strategies that promote resilience. *Journal of Happiness Studies, 8*(3), 311–333.

Tugade, M. M., Fredrickson, B. L., & Barrett, L. F. (2004). Psychological resilience and positive emotional granularity: Examining the benefits of positive emotions on coping and health. *Journal of Personality. Special Issue: Emotions, Personality, and Health, 72*(6), 1161–1190.

Waugh, C. E., Fredrickson, B. L., & Taylor, S. F. (2008). Adapting to life's slings and arrows: Individual differences in resilience when recovering from an anticipated threat. *Journal of Research in Personality, 42*(4), 1031–1046.

Waugh, C. E., Wager, T. D., Fredrickson, B. L., Noll, D. C., & Taylor, S. F. (2008). The neural correlates of trait resilience when anticipating and recovering from threat. *Social Cognitive and Affective Neuroscience, 3*(4), 322–332.

Wortman, C. B., & Silver, R. C. (1989). The myths of coping with loss. *Journal of Consulting and Clinical Psychology, 57,* 349-357.

Zautra, A. J., Affleck, G. G., Tennen, H., Reich, J. W., & Davis, M. C. (2005). Dynamic approaches to emotions and stress in everyday life: Bolger and Zuckerman reloaded with positive as well as negative affects. *Journal of Personality. Special Issue: Advances in Personality and Daily Experience, 73*(6), 1511–1538.

Zautra, A. J., Johnson, L. M., & Davis, M. C. (2005). Positive affect as a source of resilience for women in chronic pain. *Journal of Consulting and Clinical Psychology, 73*(2), 212–220.

Zelenski, J. M., & Larsen, R. J. (2000). The distribution of emotions in everyday life: A state and trait perspective from experience sampling data. *Journal of Research in Personality, 34,* 178–197.

Hedonic Adaptation to Positive and Negative Experiences

Sonja Lyubomirsky

Abstract

Empirical and anecdotal evidence for hedonic adaptation suggests that the joys of loves and triumphs and the sorrows of losses and humiliations fade with time. If people's goals are to increase or maintain well-being, then their objectives will diverge depending on whether their fortunes have turned for the better (which necessitates slowing down or thwarting adaptation) or for the worse (which calls for activating and accelerating it). In this chapter, I first introduce the construct of hedonic adaptation and its attendant complexities. Next, I review empirical evidence on how people adapt to circumstantial changes, and conjecture why the adaptation rate differs in response to favorable versus unfavorable life changes. I then discuss the relevance of examining adaptation to questions of how to enhance happiness (in the positive domain) and to facilitate coping (in the negative domain). Finally, I present a new dynamic theoretical model (developed with Sheldon) of the processes and mechanisms underlying hedonic adaptation. Drawing from the positive psychological literature, I propose ways that people can fashion self-practiced positive activities in the service of managing stress and bolstering well-being.

Keywords: hedonic adaptation, happiness, subjective well-being, positive emotions, aspiration level, variety, surprise

> "Man is a pliant animal, a being who gets accustomed to anything."
> — *Fyodor Dostoyevsky*

The thrill of victory and the agony of defeat abate with time. So do the pleasure of a new sports car, the despondency after a failed romance, the delight over a job offer, and the distress of a painful diagnosis. This phenomenon, known as hedonic adaptation, has become a hot topic lately among both psychologists and economists (e.g., Diener, Lucas, & Scollon, 2006; Easterlin, 2006; Frederick & Loewenstein, 1999; Kahneman & Thaler, 2006; Lucas, 2007a; Lyubomirsky, Sheldon, & Schkade, 2005; Wilson & Gilbert, 2007). It has been invoked to explain the relatively strong temporal stability of well-being (e.g., Costa, McCrae, & Zonderman, 1987) and why people tend to "recover" from both positive and negative life events (e.g., Suh, Diener,

& Fujita, 1996). People have been found to be notoriously bad at forecasting its effects (Wilson & Gilbert, 2003, 2005), and the possibility of its power has even cast a pall on optimistic predictions that everyone can become happier simply by changing his or her life for the better (Lyubomirsky, 2008; Lyubomirsky, Sheldon, et al., 2005).

Hedonic adaptation occurs in response to both positive and negative experiences. Not surprisingly, however, if individuals' overarching goals are to increase or maintain well-being, then their objectives will diverge depending on whether their fortunes have recently turned for the better or for the worse. The negative domain calls for activating and accelerating adaptation. The positive domain necessitates slowing down or thwarting it. In this chapter, I first introduce the construct of hedonic adaptation and several complexities surrounding it. Next, I review empirical evidence on how people adapt to circumstantial changes, and speculate about why the rate and course of adaptation differ in response to favorable versus unfavorable life changes. I then discuss the relevance of examining adaptation to questions of both how to enhance happiness (in the positive domain) and to facilitate coping (in the negative domain). Finally, I present a new dynamic theoretical model of the processes and mechanisms underlying hedonic adaptation, and, drawing from the positive psychological literature, the means by which adaptation may be managed in the service of managing stress and bolstering well-being.

The Hedonic Adaptation to Positive and Negative Experiences (HAPNE) model, developed in collaboration with Ken Sheldon, posits that adaptation proceeds via two separate paths, such that initial well-being gains or drops corresponding to a positive or negative life change (e.g., relationship start-up vs. break-up) are eroded over time. The first path specifies that the stream of positive or negative emotions resulting from the life change (e.g., joy or sadness) may lessen over time, reverting people's happiness levels back to their baseline. The second, more counterintuitive path specifies that the stream of positive or negative events resulting from the change may shift people's expectations about the positivity (or negativity) of their lives, such that the individual now takes for granted circumstances that used to produce happiness or is inured to circumstances that used to produce unhappiness.

Notably, the HAPNE model has significant implications for strategies that people can use to intervene in the adaptation process, thereby facilitating coping with stressors and making the most of triumphs. These implications are derived from three critical variables proposed by the model to affect the rate of adaptation. Specifically, people will adapt more slowly to a particular change in their lives if they attend to the historical contingency and transience of the change, and if that change produces a stream of experiences that are variable and unexpected. I draw from the literature in positive psychology, as well as empirical support from my own laboratory, to propose ways that people can exploit understanding of these factors to fashion self-practiced positive activities that will ultimately help them increase well-being in the face of positive events and facilitate coping and resilience in the face of painful or traumatic ones.

The What, How, and Why of Hedonic Adaptation

Hedonic adaptation is the psychological process by which people become accustomed to a positive or negative stimulus, such that the emotional effects of that stimulus are attenuated over time (Frederick & Loewenstein, 1999; see also Helson, 1964; Parducci, 1995). The "stimulus" can be a circumstance (new mansion in the hills), a single event (a pink slip), or a recurring event (thrice-weekly dialysis), and it must be constant or repeated for adaptation to occur. The homeowner will experience hedonic adaptation as long as her mansion remains unchanged, the worker as long as he is unemployed, and the kidney patient as long as disease progression is kept at bay. If the new mansion is renovated to include a tennis court, the employee is offered a new job 2 weeks from Monday, or the dialysis treatment is extended, a brand new adaptation process will unfold.

A question that is yet unresolved concerns whether the stimulus to which one adapts must be an actual situation (e.g., the situation of driving a particular car or being in a particular marriage or experiencing a particular offense) or the *knowledge* or recognition of that situation (e.g., "I own a hybrid" or "I am married to an alcoholic" or "She fired me"). It is undoubtedly difficult, if not impossible, to disentangle these two aspects—for example, to separate being married (i.e., the complex stream of experiences that make up a marriage) from one's identity and self-labeling as a married person, and researchers have yet to do so. Another unresolved question is whether reductions in emotional responses over time represent evidence of true adaptation or merely relabeling—that is, giving a different label to the same perception. As an illustration, both before and after moving away from her family, a woman may rate her overall life satisfaction as a 6 on a 10-point scale. The second rating may indicate hedonic adaptation to the move (i.e., her original 6 initially dropped to a 4 but in due course rebounded back to 6), *or* it may reflect changes in her interpretation and use of the scale. For example, if her new reference group (her new-found colleagues and neighbors) is less happy as a whole, then her new 6 may be a result of her implicitly rating her happiness (or unhappiness) against this group instead of the old, happier reference group.

Multiple mechanisms are presumed to underlie hedonic adaptation, including cognitive processes (e.g., attention, goals and values, perceptions, aspirations, explanations, and social and temporal comparisons), behavioral efforts (e.g., avoiding particular situations or seeking solace from friends), and physiological processes (such as opponent processes of emotion; Solomon, 1980). However, it is disputable whether hedonic adaptation must be passive and automatic (i.e., the person eventually adjusts to a disability without actively "doing" something about it or without any particular preference or intention) or whether active coping strategies (like intentionally trying to find the silver lining in the disability or reprioritizing family over work) are part and parcel of the adaptation process (cf. Warr, Jackson, & Banks, 1988). Because people do not have an incentive to hasten adaptation to positive experience, this question appears to apply to hedonic adaptation only in the negative domain.

Theorists agree that hedonic adaptation is adaptive (Frederick & Loewenstein, 1999; cf. Carver & Scheier, 1990; Frijda, 1988). If people's emotional reactions did not weaken with time, they would not be able to discriminate between more and less significant stimuli (i.e., new events that offer new information) and less significant stimuli (i.e., past events that should fade into the background). This property is important for the emotional system to function efficiently, as people must have the capacity, first, to safeguard themselves from physiologically arousing (and potentially destructive) long-lasting and intense affective reactions; and, second, to retain sensitivity to the signal value of subsequent events (e.g., an opportunity for a new relationship or the danger of a snake underfoot). Indeed, in a world without hedonic adaptation, human beings would be overwhelmed by their emotions and lose the vital ability to be attuned to changes (rather than to absolute magnitudes) in stimuli or circumstances (Kahneman & Tversky, 1979). To quote a line from the film *Before Sunset* (2004), if passion did not fade, "we would end up doing nothing at all with our lives." The same can be said for anger, anxiety, and grief.

Previous Empirical Findings in the Negative and Positive Domains

Empirical work on hedonic adaptation aims to determine the effect of a particular stimulus, event, or circumstance on the individual's emotional response. Studies have used a variety of "hedonic" measures, including scales of life satisfaction, positive affect, negative affect, psychological adjustment, and single-item indicators of happiness. Although there is debate about whether different components of well-being (e.g., its cognitive and affective aspects) are unitary or, instead, show different trajectories over

time (e.g., Diener et al., 2006), I will assume that the well-being measures used in the research herein are reasonably well correlated (e.g., Busseri, Sadava, & Decourville, 2007; see Diener, 1994, for a review) and would likely produce similar results if interchanged.

Negative experiences
A growing body of research has explored the indicators and consequences of hedonic adaptation to negative circumstances and events. The first such studies used cross-sectional designs, yet nonetheless offered suggestive evidence that people adapt to some negative experiences but not to others. For example, 1 month to 1 year after becoming paralyzed, accident victims reported being significantly less happy than a control group (Brickman, Coates, & Janoff-Bulman, 1978); 16 months after the building of a new freeway, residents were still not adjusted to the noise (Weinstein, 1982); but 1 to 60 months after surgery for breast cancer, the majority of patients reported that their lives had been altered for the better (Taylor, Lichtman, & Wood, 1984). Without a pre-event baseline, however, researchers cannot determine whether and how much adaptation had actually taken place.

Prospective longitudinal studies, recently pioneered by Lucas and his colleagues, are much more instructive. In a 19-year investigation of representative German residents, Lucas (2007b) found that those who had experienced a government-certified disability during the course of the study showed a significant and sustained drop in their level of well-being from before to after the onset of disability, even after income and employment were controlled. Participants from the same data set who were followed up from 15 to 18 years reported significantly reduced well-being years after becoming unemployed (Lucas, Clark, Georgellis, & Diener, 2004), divorced (Lucas, 2005), and widowed (Lucas, Clark, Georgellis, & Diener, 2003). Notably, in all these studies, whether individuals had experienced disability, unemployment, widowhood, or divorce (all extremely negative experiences in the domains of health, work, and interpersonal relationships), their levels of well-being took a "hit" from the event and, on average, never fully recovered.[1]

Positive experiences
Compared to the negative domain, the literature on hedonic adaptation to positive circumstances and events is relatively scarce, with only a small number

of published cross-sectional studies and even fewer longitudinal ones. Interestingly, every one of these investigations evidences fairly rapid and apparently complete adaptation to positive events. The most widely-cited study is that of Brickman and his colleagues (1978), who reported that winners of $50,000 to $1,000,000 (in 1970s dollars) in the Illinois State Lottery were no happier from less than 1 month to 18 months after the news than those who had experienced no such windfall. Findings that increases in citizens' average incomes have not been accompanied by increases in average well-being—for example, that Americans' mean happiness scores shifted slightly from 7.5 (out of 10) in 1940 to 7.2 in 1990, a time period when incomes more than tripled (Lane, 2000)—have also been interpreted to indicate the work of hedonic adaptation.

Much more persuasive research showed that German residents who had married sometime during the 15-year period of their prospective longitudinal investigation initially obtained a significant boost in their happiness levels, but reverted to their baseline after 2 years on average (Lucas et al., 2003; see also Lucas & Clark, 2006). Another relevant longitudinal study followed high-level managers for 5 years to track their job satisfaction before and after a voluntary job change (Boswell, Boudreau, & Tichy, 2005). Much like what was observed with marriage, the managers experienced a burst of satisfaction immediately after the move (labeled the *honeymoon* effect), but their satisfaction plummeted within a year (the so-called *hangover* effect, but actually evidence of adaptation). In contrast, managers who chose not to change jobs during the same time period showed relatively stable job satisfaction levels. Furthermore, evidence from my laboratory suggests that feelings of enhanced well-being—triggered by receiving positive, self-relevant feedback 5 days in a row—dissipate in a near-linear fashion within 2 weeks (Boehm & Lyubomirsky, 2008). To my knowledge, although a few longitudinal studies have assessed satisfaction with a particular event (such as acquiring breast implants) for months or years after the procedure (e.g., Cash, Duel, & Perkins, 2002), no investigations other than the two described above have tracked well-being both before and after the significant positive circumstantial change occurred, and hardly any have compared the well-being trajectory of individuals who experienced major life events with that of matched controls who did not experience such events.

Why is hedonic adaptation faster to positive experiences?

Although researchers know a great deal more about hedonic adaptation than they did merely 10 years ago, the vast majority of theory and empirical work to date has addressed adaptation to *negative* circumstances and events. Consequently, recent conclusions about the effects and processes underlying hedonic adaptation—for example, that it is often not complete (Diener et al., 2006; Lucas, 2007a)—apply primarily to negative experiences. Interestingly, the empirical research to date suggests that hedonic adaptation is faster—and more likely to be "complete"—in response to positive than negative experiences. I propose that the primary mechanism underlying this difference involves the robust finding that, in Baumeister and colleagues' eloquent words, "bad is stronger than good" (Baumeister, Bratslavsky, Finkenauer, & Vohs, 2001; see also Taylor, 1991). Numerous investigations offer evidence for an asymmetry in positive and negative experiences and in positive and negative emotions. To begin, many cognitive effects are weaker for positive than negative stimuli, including those illustrated by priming (Smith et al., 2006), Stroop (e.g., Pratto & John, 1991), memory (e.g., Bless, Hamilton, & Mackie, 1992; Ohira, Winton, & Oyama, 1997; Porter & Peace, 2007), and emotion detection (e.g., Oehman, Lundqvist, & Esteves, 2001) tasks. For example, a series of studies using the emotional Stroop procedure showed that negative words interfere with color naming (i.e., attract more attention) more than do positive words; that 85% of participants exhibit this effect; and that negative words are twice as likely to be recalled (Pratto & John, 1991). Furthermore, people are relatively more likely to monitor negative feedback than positive feedback (e.g., Graziano, Brothen, & Berscheid, 1980), more likely to remember it (e.g., Mischel, Ebbesen, & Zeiss, 1976), and more likely to be influenced by it (e.g., Coleman, Jussim, & Abraham, 1987; Leary, Tambor, Terdal, & Downs, 1995).

Negative information has also been found to be stronger (i.e., weighted more heavily) than positive information in first impressions (e.g., Peeters & Czapinski, 1990; Skowronski & Carlston, 1989), nonverbal messages (e.g., Frodi, Lamb, Leavitt, & Donovan, 1978), interpersonal interactions (e.g., Gottman & Krokoff, 1989), and evaluative categorization (Ito, Larsen, Smith, & Cacioppo, 1999). Finally and perhaps most important, daily diary studies have shown that the impact of everyday negative events is more powerful and longer-lasting than that of positive events (e.g., Lawton, DeVoe, & Parmelee, 1995; Nezlek & Gable, 2001; Sheldon, Ryan, & Reis, 1996; see also Oishi, Diener, Choi, Kim-Prieto, & Choi, 2007). For example, after a bad day, students reported lower well-being the following day, but, after a good day, their positive well-being did not carry over (Sheldon et al., 1996).

An intriguing line of research that may also shed light on the "bad is stronger than good" phenomenon is exploring the *positivity* (good-to-bad) ratios that distinguish flourishing individuals, couples, and groups; such ratios generally range from 3-to-1 to 5-to-1 (Fredrickson, 2009; Fredrickson & Losada, 2005). For example, happily married couples are characterized by ratios of approximately 5-to-1 in their verbal and emotional expressions to each other, as compared to very unhappy couples (who display ratios of less than 1-to-1; Gottman, 1994). Tellingly, the exact same optimal good-to-bad ratios (5-to-1) characterize the verbal utterances of profitable and productive versus less profitable and productive business teams (Losada, 1999). Additional evidence comes from daily diary studies. In an 8-day study, healthy community-residing men aged 35 to 55 exhibited a ratio of 2.7 good daily events to 1 bad one (David, Green, Martin, & Suls, 1997; see also Nezlek & Gable, 2001), and comparable ratios (ranging from 2.1 to 3.4) were found for flourishing undergraduates in a 28-day study (Fredrickson & Losada, 2005). Although it is premature to conclude that negative experiences are three times as bad as positive experiences, these findings at a minimum suggest that the "punch" of one bad emotion, utterance, or event can match or outdo that of three or more good ones. My speculation is that if bad were *not* stronger than good, then healthy, happy, or flourishing individuals would show ratios closer to 1:1.

In sum, although much of the evidence is indirect, it highlights the predominance of negative over positive experience. In this way, the positive–negative asymmetry data support the possibility that people are made much more unhappy by a negative event than they are made happy by an equivalent positive event, the same pattern indicated by prospect theory's value function (Kahneman & Tversky, 1984) and referred by others as the negativity bias (Ito & Cacioppo, 2005; Rozin & Royzman, 2001; see also Strahilevitz & Loewenstein, 1998).

Recently, in a new model of hedonic adaptation (AREA), Wilson and Gilbert (2008) proposed that people engage in the sequential process of attending, reacting, explaining, and ultimately adapting to events. Their model is consistent with the hypothesis that adaptation is easier and more rapid in response to pleasant stimuli, and the breakdown of hedonic adaptation into three antecedent processes makes it clear how. First, people are less likely to attend to positive rather than negative events. Second, they have weaker emotional reactions to positive events. And finally, it is less difficult and less time-consuming to explain or make sense of positive than negative events. For these three reasons, people are more likely to hedonically adapt to positive experiences (see also Frijda, 1988). The three asymmetries—in attention, reaction, and explanation—are supported by ample evidence (see Baumeister et al., 2001, for an excellent review) and consistent with functional approaches to emotion (Clore, 1994; Frijda, 1994; Tooby & Cosmides, 1990). In other words, positive affect signals to individuals that things are going well and that they may continue engaging with their environment. Negative affect, by contrast, warns people of potential danger or unpleasantness in the environment to which they must respond (e.g., attack, flee, conserve resources, expel). Because survival is arguably much more dependent on urgent attention to potential dangers than on passing up opportunities for positive experiences, it is thereby more adaptive for "bad to be stronger than good" (Baumeister et al., 2001).

That hedonic adaptation to positive circumstances and events is relatively rapid and complete leads to the intriguing hypothesis that such adaptation may be a formidable barrier to raising happiness. That hedonic adaptation to negative circumstances and events is relatively slow and curtailed raises the concern that such adaptation may critically interfere with successful coping. These two ideas—which I discuss in turn below—underscore the importance of studying hedonic adaptation in order to enhance researchers' understanding of how people can optimize well-being and manage stress and adversity.

Hedonic Adaptation to Positive Events

"Happy thou art not, for what thou hast not, still thou striv'st to get, and what thou hast, forget'st."
— *William Shakespeare* (1564/1616)

Although the desire for happiness has existed since antiquity, its pursuit is more vigorous than ever in today's society, both in Western nations like the

U. S. and increasingly around the globe (Diener, 2000; Diener, Suh, Smith, & Shao, 1995; Freedman, 1978; Triandis, Bontempo, Leung, & Hui, 1990). Moreover, well-being appears to be a worthwhile goal, because happiness not only "feels" good, but also has tangible benefits for individuals, as well as for their friends, families, and communities, and even society at large. Specifically, happiness and positive emotions have been found to be associated with and to promote numerous successful life outcomes, including superior physical and mental health, enhanced creativity and productivity, higher income, more prosocial behavior, and stronger interpersonal relationships (see Lyubomirsky, King, & Diener, 2005, for a meta-analysis). Furthermore, positive emotions (feelings like joy, contentment, serenity, interest, vitality, and pride), which are the very hallmark of happiness (Diener, Sandvik, & Pavot, 1991; Urry et al., 2004), are also advantageous during the process of recovery from negative experiences (Fredrickson, 2001; Fredrickson & Cohn, 2008).

Is it possible to enhance and sustain happiness? In other words, how can an individual preserve well-being in the face of stressful or traumatic life events and maintain boosts in well-being following positive ones? For the average person not beset by poverty or trauma, one of the biggest challenges to striving to maintain and increase happiness is undoubtedly the magnitude of his or her genetically determined happiness "set point" (or temperament; Lykken & Tellegen, 1996; Lyubomirsky, Sheldon, et al., 2005). Behavioral genetic studies show that about 50% of the variance in people's levels of well-being can be accounted for by genes (e.g., Braungart, Plomin, DeFries, & Fulker, 1992; Tellegen et al., 1988; see also Hamer, 1996; Williams & Thompson, 1993). This set point or baseline may partially explain why happiness is remarkably cross-situationally consistent (e.g., Diener & Larsen, 1984) and stable over time (Costa et al., 1987; Headey & Wearing, 1989), despite notable life changes. For example, fully 76% of Fujita and Diener's (2005) longitudinal sample followed from 1984 to 2000 did not show a significant change in their baseline well-being from the first 5 years of their study to the last 5 years. Furthermore, a 2-year longitudinal study found that significant life events, such as being accepted into graduate school, becoming an uncle, experiencing the death of a close friend, having financial problems, and getting promoted, influenced well-being for 3 to 6 months and no longer (Suh et al., 1996). These studies suggest that

trying to increase happiness is an effort that is doomed from the start, as people cannot help but return to their set point, or baseline, over time.

To address this pessimistic hypothesis, Sheldon, Schkade, and I developed a model that identified the most important determinants of the chronic happiness level as (1) the set point (accounting for about 50% of the observed variance in well-being), (2) life circumstances (accounting for about 10%), and (3) intentional activity (accounting for the remaining 40%). Accordingly, we argued that the assumption of a fixed, genetically determined set point does not logically lead to the conclusion that well-being cannot be changed, as even the existence of the set point leaves much "room" for improvement, as well as for resilience (Lyubomirsky, Sheldon, et al., 2005; Sheldon & Lyubomirsky, 2004). Specifically, up to 40% of the individual differences in happiness appear to be determined by what people *do*. In other words, our model suggests that, with intentional efforts, people can both preserve happiness and become sustainably happier. The individual's goals and happiness-supportive activities must differ, however, depending on whether his or her circumstances are changing for the better or for the worse. I first discuss the mechanisms underlying hedonic adaptation to positive events— and implications for how to bolster happiness and manage coping—and then the mechanisms and implications of adaptation to negative events.

Hedonic adaptation as a barrier to sustainable well-being

As noted earlier, I propose that relatively rapid and complete hedonic adaptation to positive events and to improvements in life circumstances is one of the biggest obstacles to raising and sustaining happiness. This obstacle, it is worth noting, may conceivably relate to or interact with the set point or temperament; indeed, the rate of adaptation may itself be genetically determined (Lykken, 2000; Lykken, Iacono, Haroian, McGue, & Bouchard, 1988). The bottom line, however, is that if an individual adapts to all things positive, then no matter what thrilling, meaningful, and wonderful experiences await her, these experiences will not make her any happier, but, instead, may drive her to acquire ever more new and thrilling things and risk placing herself squarely on a futile and desperate hedonic treadmill (Brickman & Campbell, 1971). The good news, however, is that people appear to vary in their rates of hedonic adaptation in both positive and negative domains, and that a sizeable proportion become reliably happier over time. The chief reason, I submit, is that people have the capacity to control the speed and extent of adaptation via intentional, effortful activities.

Consequently, I argue that one of the secrets to achieving increased and sustainable well-being lies in strategies that prevent, slow down, or impede the positive adaptation process. That such practices can be successful is suggested, albeit speculatively, by three types of data—the first showing that people's happiness can lastingly improve, the second indicating that people vary in how well and how rapidly they adapt to positive events, and the third demonstrating that specific adaptation-thwarting activities can bolster happiness.

PEOPLE'S HAPPINESS CAN IMPROVE

The fact is that happiness can and does change over time. For example, a 22-year study that followed approximately 2,000 healthy veterans found that life satisfaction increased over these men's lives, crested at age 65, and did not start significantly declining until age 75 (Mroczek & Spiro, 2005). A positive correlation between age and well-being measures has also been found in a 23-year longitudinal study of four generations of families (Charles, Reynolds, & Gatz, 2001) and in a cross-sectional study of adults aged 17 to 82 (Sheldon & Kasser, 2001). In the 1984–2000 longitudinal study described earlier by Fujita and Diener (2005), although 76% of the respondents remained unchanged in their well-being, 24% reported significant shifts (though, unfortunately, most of these were for the worse, not for the better). Lucas (2007c) contends that stability estimates for well-being bottom out at around .30 and .40, pointing up the possibility of real change. Although these data are merely suggestive, they intimate the possibility that true changes in well-being may be related to people's capacity to resist adaptation.

PEOPLE VARY IN ADAPTATION RATES

As several theorists have noted (e.g., Diener et al., 2006; Lucas, 2007a), longitudinal studies of hedonic adaptation reveal variability in the extent to which people's happiness changes (and/or returns to baseline) following important life events. For just two examples, in the 15-year investigation of marital transitions, some individuals got much happier after getting married and then stayed happier, while others' well-being began dropping even before their wedding day (see Figure 2 in Lucas et al., 2003). Furthermore, whereas some widows' and widowers'

happiness plummeted (and never recovered) after their spouses' deaths, others actually became happier and remained that way (see Figure 4 in the same paper). The mechanisms underlying this variability are undoubtedly complex, random, or dependent on people's unique situations; for example, some of the "happy widows" may have experienced terrific caregiving responsibilities and experienced a natural sense of relief when their spouses passed away. However, I suggest that these mechanisms are also coherent and systematic across individuals. Specifically, I propose that the primary source of individual differences in rates of adaptation (and in capacity to experience positive shifts in happiness over time) involves differences in *intentional efforts* that people can undertake in order to slow down adaptation to positive events and speed up adaptation to (i.e., cope with) negative ones. With the HAPNE model, I hope to elucidate these common processes and effects.

Hedonic Adaptation to Negative Events

> "Life is not always what one wants it to be, but to make the best of it as it is, is the only way of being happy."
> – Jennie Jerome Churchill

No life is without stress, adversity, or crisis. The possibilities are endless: deaths of loved ones, illnesses, accidents, victimizations, natural disasters, abusive relationships, financial crises, stigmatizations, divorces, and job losses. Close to half of U.S. adults will experience one severe traumatic event during their lifetimes (Ozer & Weiss, 2004), and almost everyone will occasionally endure moderate to severe daily stress. In the wake of such challenges, many become depressed, anxious, or confused. They may find it difficult to concentrate on the daily tasks of living, and they may not be able to sleep or eat or function well. Some have such intense and long-lasting reactions to a trauma that they are unable to return to their previous ("normal") selves for many months or even years. Indeed, as revealed by the literature on hedonic adaptation, over time, people adapt to some negative experiences completely but show protracted or only partial adaptation to others.

To preserve well-being and foster emotional adjustment, an important objective of individuals facing aversive, threatening, or traumatic situations is to endure and prevail in such a way that they are able to return to their previous "selves," before the event occurred. In other words, the goal is to speed up adaptation. A large literature has accumulated on the strategies and processes underlying coping—that is, on how people manage stressful demands, or what they do to alleviate the hurt, distress, or suffering caused by a negative event or situation (e.g., Carver, 2007; Compas, Connor-Smith, Saltzman, Thomsen, & Wadsworth, 2001; Lazarus, 2000; Skinner, Edge, Altman, & Sherwood, 2003). Although coping is one general label one might affix on how people can act to hasten adaptation in the negative domain, this chapter focuses on strategies rooted in positive psychology—that is, positive activities that people can engage in that generate positive thoughts, positive emotions, and positive events, as opposed to practices that simply regulate negative states. I argue that lessons learned from how people can avert adaptation to positive experiences can be applied to how people can accelerate adaptation to negative ones.

How can People Shape Adaptation to Positive and Negative Experiences? Adaptation-Forestalling and Adaptation-Accelerating Mechanisms

As highlighted by the HAPNE model, described below, adaptation-thwarting and adaptation-hastening processes share a number of properties that help them retain their potency and efficacy. Notably, it appears that the same mechanisms will thwart adaptation to positive and negative circumstances, which suggests that people should seek to learn how to activate or maximize these mechanisms in the positive domain and how to block or minimize them in the negative domain. One key adaptation-thwarting property is attention—that is, once we stop paying attention to a life change (e.g., stop appreciating it if positive or stop ruminating on it if negative), we have adapted. Furthermore, the types of both pleasant and unpleasant experiences that are best able to maintain attention are those that are (a) varied and dynamic and (b) novel and surprising. Although some of these properties undoubtedly interact with one another, I describe them separately in the three sections that follow. It is also worth noting that adaptation-forestalling (and adaptation-accelerating) activities and processes can be engaged in effortfully and intentionally, or automatically and habitually.

Attention enticing

William James once made a remarkable and rather radical proposition: "My experience is what I agree to attend to." Indeed, what people pay attention to is their experience; it *is* their life. What grabs attention? That which people chew on, remember, emotionally react to, and factor into their judgments and decisions. If a thing, attribute, person, or idea fails to capture attention, one can be said to have adapted to it. When an individual suddenly obtains more disposable income than she ever had before, the shift in financial status is captivating and novel. She cannot help but be aware of all the extra money she has to spend and may think about it constantly. Importantly, she recognizes (1) that she has not always had this added income and (2) that the surplus may not endure forever. With time, however, the change in income will cease to be novel or surprising and other conquests, failures, uplifts, and hassles will elicit emotional reactions, drawing attention away from the financial change and thereby compelling it to fade into the psychological background (cf. Kahneman & Thaler, 2006). Similarly, after an individual unexpectedly loses a large proportion of his life savings in a Ponzi scheme, he will have recurrent and intrusive thoughts, memories, and worries related to the financial setback. In due time, however, these ruminations, and their associated negative emotions, will slowly recede. However, any object that continues to captivate attention—that is, any object of which people are continually aware or that frequently and perhaps even unintentionally pops into their minds—will be less prone to hedonic adaptation. For example, owners of luxury sedans are no happier during car trips than owners of compact two-door coupes, *unless* their cars' attributes are on their minds while driving (Schwarz, Kahneman, & Xu, in press); and people who continue to be aware of a positive activity change in their lives are less likely to adapt to it (Sheldon, & Lyubomirsky, in press). Similarly, individuals who have lost loved ones experience bouts of sadness each time their attention is drawn to the loss (Bonnano & Keltner, 1997). Thus, adaptation-forestalling activities and processes have this very attention-grabbing capability.

Dynamic and varied

In his widely quoted classic book, *The Joyless Economy*, Scitovsky (1976) argued that focusing on "comforts" (read: circumstantial changes) is joyless, because individuals eventually adapt to them. Instead, people should spend their money on joyful things, which yield continual fascination, challenge, and fulfillment, like the "pleasures" of meeting good friends or backpacking through a gorgeous landscape (cf. Van Boven, 2005). The so-called pleasures

Scitovsky described, which deliver partial and intermittent (rather than continuous) satisfaction, are parallel to the intentional activities that I propose people can engage in to thwart or slow down adaptation in the positive domain. What such activities have in common is that they are dynamic and episodic—that is, variable and intermittent—and thereby share the critical attribute of supplying changeable and dynamic experiences. After all, when it comes to their activities, people do not persist in doing only one thing and doing it the same way each time. Of course, as applied to negative life changes, precisely those ones that give rise to varied and intermittent negative events (such as the diagnosis of a chronic illness yielding a series of blows, fears, and hassles) will be those to which people will find it hardest to adapt.

To address this attribute of adaptation-thwarting strategies and processes in the positive domain, Sheldon and I have conducted four longitudinal field studies, three correlational (Sheldon & Lyubomirsky, 2006a) and one experimental (Sheldon & Lyubomirsky, in press). This work was motivated by the argument that circumstantial changes are particularly prone to adaptation, because they are generally one-time improvements that represent relatively static "facts" about one's life (e.g., "I live in Beverly Hills," "I am married to my second husband," "I was promoted"). Building on the notion that hedonic adaptation occurs in response to constant stimuli, we hypothesized that increasing and sustaining happiness must involve partaking in dynamic *activities*, which entail persistent effort and engagement in an intentional, self-directed process. Such efforts have the property that they can be varied and episodic and can produce a fluid and diverse set of positive experiences, opportunities, and possibilities. Consequently, positive changes in such activities should presumably produce bigger and more sustained increases in well-being relative to positive changes in life circumstances.

Supporting this argument, Sheldon and I found that undergraduates reported that positive changes in their dynamic activities (e.g., deciding to study harder, learning a new language, cultivating a friendship, or trying to climb the world's highest peaks) were more "variable" and that they were less likely to become "accustomed" to them, relative to positive changes in their circumstances (e.g., acquiring a better dorm room or more financial aid; Sheldon & Lyubomirsky, 2006a; Study 1). Furthermore, two longitudinal studies showed that both changes in activities *and* changes in circumstances made participants happier 6 weeks after the start of a study, but only changes in activities continued to make them happier 12 weeks later (Studies 2 and 3). By the 12th week, students appeared to have already adapted emotionally to improvements in their circumstances, but not to their intentional activities. This result was replicated in a 6-week long study in which people were prompted to make dynamic and variable changes versus static, one-time changes in their lives (Sheldon & Lyubomirsky, in press). Interestingly, among participants who took up a new dynamic activity, the effects on well-being were strongest for those who reported that the change added variety to their lives *and* who reported remaining aware of the change—that is, the two factors interacted to predict the most sustained change. These findings are consistent with Van Boven's (2005) argument that people are made happier by obtaining experiences rather than possessions.

As these earlier studies suggest, experiences that are variable and dynamic can serve to inhibit adaptation, a conclusion that applies to both the positive and negative domain. With respect to positive events, the dynamic and varied nature of activity suggests that its impact can be maximized by attending to its timing—that is, an optimal frequency of engagement that permits the activity to remain novel, consequential, and positive. Indeed, studies from my laboratory have shown that how frequently and close together an individual commits acts of kindness (five acts in a single day vs. spread across the week) and "counts his blessings" (once vs. three times per week) determines the extent to which his happiness is boosted over time (Lyubomirsky, Sheldon, et al., 2005). Analogous recommendations can be made with respect to negative events. For example, a schedule of medical treatments can be devised in such a way that the individual becomes accustomed and "jaded" to its frequency.

Adaptation-forestalling activities not only can be timed in optimal ways; they can be varied—mixed up, spiced up—in optimal ways as well that permit a positive experience to remain fresh, meaningful, and pleasant. Recall that, by definition, adaptation occurs only in response to constant or repeated stimuli, not to changing and dynamic ones. Variety, in both thoughts and behaviors, appears to be innately stimulating and rewarding (Berlyne, 1970; Pronin & Jacobs, 2008; Rolls et al., 1981; see Ebstein, Novick, Umansky, Priel, & Osher, 1996; Suhara et al., 2001, for links to dopamine activity), probably because it generates an inflow of diverse positive experiences. It is not surprising, then, that people seek variety in their behavior (e.g., Ratner, Kahn, & Kahneman, 1999) and habituate more slowly to pleasurable stimuli that vary (Leventhal, Martin, Seals, Tapia, & Rehm, 2007). An activity that is practiced with variety (or a life change that naturally yields variety) is more likely to remain rewarding and meaningful over time and thus less prone to hedonic adaptation.

Indirect evidence for this hypothesis comes from a 10-week intervention that found that individuals who performed different acts of kindness every week (e.g., did an extra household chore, sent e-cards to family members, gave their pet a special treat, or made breakfast for their partners) displayed an upward trajectory for happiness during the intervention and 4 weeks after, relative to those who performed similar acts of kindness each week (e.g., making breakfast for someone again and again; Boehm, Lyubomirsky, & Sheldon, 2008). By analogy, if the goal is to accelerate adaptation to negative events, then one needs to find ways to reduce variety and promote repetition. Accordingly, unpleasant dinners, dental procedures, or project deadlines are more easily endured when they are predictable and unvarying.

Novel and surprising

A beautiful and plush new sofa can provide the buyer with hours of satisfaction. The comfort of its fabric and the colors of its design supply a burst of pleasure at first use, but the novelty wears off and the sofa retains few, if any, more surprises for the person occupying it. The same cannot as readily be said about a new friend, lover, or career. As described above, relationships, work, and many activities have the property that they yield novel and often surprising experiences and opportunities, which are likely to capture people's attention and trigger frequent memories and thoughts (Wilson, Centerbar, Kermer, & Gilbert, 2005; Wilson & Gilbert, 2008). One's partner may reveal a side of him one never knew; an unforeseen career path may be suggested by a colleague; new wealth can pay for new adventures; and an act of kindness or a shared gratitude may prompt an unexpected change in one's identity. Accordingly, the activities that will be most effective in reducing adaptation are those that generate novel and unexpected (and hence varied) moments, which are likely to engender relatively strong emotional reactions (Ortony, Clore, & Collins, 1988). To wit, when it comes to positive experiences, it is challenging to maintain surprise and novelty, and, hence, one must muster effort to inject it or be open to it

when possible, or to choose activities that have the potential to yield relatively more frequent novel moments (e.g., new travels, hobbies, or relationships vs. new possessions or routines). By contrast, when it comes to negative experiences, one will seek to tone down surprises and attempt to inject repetition and even "boredom."

Notably, surprising events often prompt a search for understanding ("why did this happen?"), and the emotional punch of surprising events may diminish when understanding is reached. Wilson and Gilbert's (2008) AREA model (attend, react, explain, adapt) illustrates that surprise and understanding are in a sense two poles of the same continuum; to be surprised is to face what is not expected or not yet understood. Indeed, Wilson and Gilbert proposed that "lack of understanding" is a general principle that accounts for the adaptation-thwarting effects of many other properties of events—not only surprise but also variety, novelty, and certainty.

Stream of emotions and events

As it concerns the positive domain, all of the features of adaptation-forestalling strategies described above appear to have the consequence of yielding (or preserving) a persistent stream of positive events, thoughts, and emotions. Such efforts as viewing one's future in an optimistic light, becoming a more generous person, reading all the classics, or starting a new fitness regimen all have the property of providing varied and novel experiences, which invite one's attention, savoring, and appreciation. Hence, after a positive change, they are most likely to produce a sustainable boost in one's happiness, keeping one in the upper portion of one's set range of happiness potential.

With respect to the negative domain, however, those stressors, setbacks, and traumas that entice attention and rumination, and that continue to vary and surprise, are precisely the ones likely to generate an inflow of *negative* emotions, thoughts, and events. Accordingly, if individuals suffer declines in well-being after such upheavals, the stream of negative events will help sustain those declines, keeping them in the lower part of their happiness set range.

Hedonic Adaptation to Positive and Negative Events (HAPNE) Model

In a nutshell, people generally adapt, and do so rather quickly, to most positive changes in their circumstances—to an apartment with a view, a face-lift, recovery from illness, a new job, a 15% higher salary, a bigger house, and even getting married. People also adapt, though less rapidly and less completely, to many negative circumstantial changes and events, including chronic diseases, widowhood, ends to relationships, layoffs, and moves from larger homes to smaller ones. What is the process underlying this adaptation, and how can people intervene in it, such that they can forestall it in the case of positive events (Fig. 11.1) and speed it up in the case of negative ones (Fig. 11.2)? In other words, what we should do more of for positive events (to maintain well-being gains) is what we should do less of for negative events (to prevent maintaining well-being drops). Sheldon's and my HAPNE model was developed to address these questions.

How do people adapt?

Imagine first a hypothetical individual who has experienced a discrete *positive change*, like moving into a nice new house, finding a new love, starting a new hobby, buying a work of art, or having plastic surgery. According to the model, the life change, when large enough, triggers a boost in well-being (WB; labeled *+a*) and produces a stream of (more or

less discrete) *positive events.*[2] This process is displayed in Figure 11.1.

Next imagine a hypothetical individual who has experienced a *negative change*, like downsizing to an apartment after foreclosure, suffering a breakup, totaling the car, or gaining weight. In an analogous process (shown in Fig. 11.2), that change triggers a drop in WB (labeled *−a*) and generates a stream of *negative events*.

In line with my earlier theoretical articles (Lyubomirsky, Sheldon, et al., 2005; Sheldon & Lyubomirsky, 2007), I define WB in terms of both cognitive and emotional components—namely, as high life satisfaction and positive affect, and low negative affect (Diener, Suh, Lucas, & Smith, 1999). My primary question is, how do people ultimately adapt to the positive or negative change? In other words, what precise mechanisms erode the positive boost (*+a*) or negative decrement (*−a*), prompting it to revert to zero, and thus returning the person to her original levels of happiness or well-being (back to *T1 WB*)?

With respect to both the positive and negative domains, Sheldon and I propose two paths to

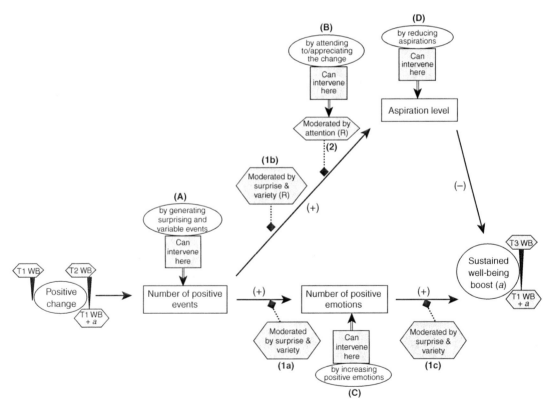

Fig. 11.1 Hedonic Adaptation to Positive and Negative Events (HAPNE) Model: The positive domain.

adaptation, though, of course, the positive path will unfold more rapidly than the negative. The first, bottom-up route is through declines in the number or frequency of experienced emotions (see the bottom path in Fig. 11.1, *number of positive emotions*, and in Fig. 11.2, *number of negative emotions*). That is, the emotions that the individual will initially derive from the change will become less and less frequent over time and may cease altogether. For example, one may experience many positive events after buying a Prius, but those occasions will become less and less numerous, and the positive emotions (excitement, happiness, pride, relief at the reduced gas bill, etc.) will recur less and less over time. Similarly, experiences of negative emotions after losing a beloved pet (pain, sadness, longing) will become more and more sporadic over time.

However, I also argue that it is possible to adapt even when one *continues* to enjoy positive events and positive emotions as a result of positive life changes, or when negative events and negative emotions persist following negative life changes. So, after losing weight, a person's social life might *continue* to be improved and regularly yield her positive episodes and emotions, but she'll begin to feel that those experiences are simply part of her new life, becoming her new norm or standard, and she will desire even more. For an extreme example, after *Thriller* became the biggest-selling album of all time, Michael Jackson reportedly declared wanting his next album to sell twice as much. Notably, the reverse may happen after gaining weight. In other words, the person's aspiration level regarding the expected quality of her life has now shifted either higher or lower (see the top path, *aspiration level*, in both figures).

The idea of an aspiration-level path to adaptation, especially in the positive domain, is very similar to Kahneman's (1999) notion of the operation of a "satisfaction treadmill" or "aspiration treadmill," which arises when the standard with which experiences are judged is itself changed. Kahneman suggested that people can essentially adapt to their new level of positive experience and thus *require* that new level simply to maintain their baseline happiness. Changes in aspiration level can provide a top-down route to changes in global well-being, by shifting how ongoing positive (or negative) experiences are framed and contextualized. Notably, then, the HAPNE model incorporates both bottom-up

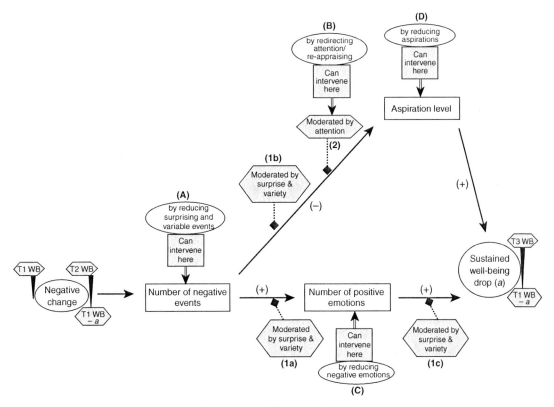

Fig. 11.2 Hedonic Adaptation to Positive and Negative Events (HAPNE) Model: The negative domain.

(via the accumulation of small positive or negative experiences) and top-down (via changes in standards or expectations) influences on well-being (Diener, 1984).

How do people forestall or hasten adaptation?

Now I turn to the implications of the model for how to thwart or slow down hedonic adaptation after positive life changes and to accelerate it after negative ones. Figures 11.1 and 11.2 also highlight several important variables (shown in numbered hexagons) that Sheldon and I propose moderate these two paths towards adaptation, such that they help forestall or expedite it.

The first set of moderators suggest that, in the case of positive changes, the more *variable and surprising* one's positive events (see Fig. 11.1), the more likely they'll produce frequent positive emotions (see moderator *1a*) and the less likely they'll raise one's aspiration level (see moderator *1b; R = reverse*). Analogously, in the case of *negative* changes (see Fig. 11.2), the more *variable and surprising* one's negative events, the more likely they'll produce frequent negative emotions (again see moderator *1a*) and the less likely they'll lower one's aspiration level (again see moderator *1b; R = reverse*). In addition, the more *variable and surprising* one's positive or negative emotions, the more likely they will maintain well-being gains or drops (see moderator *1c* in both figures). These predictions, as discussed above, are supported by research on the consequences of variety (e.g., Boehm et al., 2008; Leventhal et al., 2007) and surprise (e.g., Wilson & Gilbert, 2008). It should be noted that although variety and surprise can be distinguished theoretically (e.g., experiences can be varied but not surprising), they often co-occur.

To consider an example in the positive domain, after purchasing a work of art, the events that the owner experiences regarding that object (e.g., friends admiring it, relishing it in his home, having ideas for where to place it) may eventually become fairly expected and similar to one another over time. As a result, he will become used to the positive events, deriving fewer and fewer positive emotions from them; at the same time, his aspirations will increase, such that he will desire an even greater number of such positive events. This is a perilous combination for sustained happiness. A parallel process will occur in response to negative changes, such as financial setbacks. The individual's emotional reactions will become more predictable over time, leading her to become accustomed to the negative events (e.g., bill payments missed, inability to buy her child a toy), which would thereby trigger fewer and less intense negative emotions over time, while simultaneously lowering her desires regarding the positivity of her life. In contrast to the positive domain, this may be a desirable outcome, if one's objective is to revert to earlier levels of well-being.

As a second moderator, the HAPNE model specifies that continued *attention* to the life change—purchase of new house versus foreclosure, new weight loss versus weight gain—can forestall rising aspirations in the case of positive events or forestall declining aspirations in the case of negative ones (and thus thwart adaptation in both cases) (e.g., Kahneman & Thaler, 2006; Lyubomirsky et al., 2008). As discussed earlier, by recognizing that the change producing a person's inflow of positive or negative experiences may never have come to pass and that its future is uncertain, the person keeps the change "fresh" in her mind. As long as those experiences remain feeling "new," aspirations will be maintained; the moment they get "old," one starts getting used to them and/or taking them for granted and aspirations rise. As discussed earlier, attention to positive changes is also likely to trigger gratitude or appreciation, and attention to negative changes is likely to trigger negatively biased ruminations. To extend my earlier examples, appreciation of how his life experiences have improved after the art purchase (cf. Wilson, & Ross, 2001)—e.g., that this improvement is neither inevitable nor permanent—will prevent a person from taking for granted the positive events associated with the art and from desiring even more. Similarly, maintaining awareness of how her life has worsened after an income plunge will prevent a person from becoming inured to the negative events following that event (see moderator *2*).

The remainder of the HAPNE model (see ovals A, B, C, and D in both figures) suggests ways that individuals can consciously and deliberately *intervene* in (i.e., slow down or avert vs. speed up or activate) adaptation to life changes. Because people essentially hold opposite goals depending on whether they are confronting good or bad experiences, the first way to intervene in the adaptation process is to actively try to generate—or be open to—unexpected and variable experiences following a positive life change and to actively try to reduce unexpected and variable experiences following a negative life change (see *A*). For example, one might deliberately plan to do different things in one's new house or with one's new iPhone or with one's new spouse, or to try new opportunities and activities after losing weight or beginning a new hobby. Supportive evidence for such positive strategies comes from research showing that couples who engage together in novel and arousing activities (Aron, Norman, Aron, McKenna, & Heyman, 2000; Reissman, Aron, & Bergen, 1993) show greater improvements in the quality of their relationships.

By contrast, after gaining weight or losing the ability to engage in a favorite hobby, the goal is to curtail the variety of activities and experiences associated with the unfortunate turn of events—for example, by avoiding situations that evoke painful feelings, such as visiting hobby websites, trying on clothes that no longer fit, or spending time with people who evoke unfavorable comparisons. When such experiences are repeated over and over, however, the individual's negative emotional response to them is likely to weaken over time, which helps promote adaptation.

Second, one can intentionally try to maintain attention and awareness of one's positive change (e.g., new job, car, hobby, facelift) and the daily positive events it yields (e.g., learning a new skill at work) (see B in Fig. 11.1). Positive attention *per se* is associated with increased well-being and reduced adaptation (Schwarz et al., in press; Sheldon & Lyubomirsky, 2007). Also, as described earlier, studies that have induced people to appreciate and express gratitude for the things and people in their lives have revealed significant benefits for well-being (Emmons & McCullough, 2003; Lyubomirsky, Dickerhoof, Boehm, & Sheldon, 2008; Lyubomirsky, Sheldon, et al., 2005; Seligman et al., 2005). The act of attention is aimed at maintaining one's awareness that (1) one has good things in one's life that were not always there and (2) those good things may not continue. Indeed, Koo, Algoe, Wilson, and Gilbert (2008) found that mentally subtracting positive events led to bigger improvements in mood than simply reviewing them. Of course, if one's attempts at attention lead one to consider *negative* implications (e.g., "What if it's taken away?" "Are my friends jealous?") or to explain or understand the change (Wilson & Gilbert, 2008), this would likely be problematic.

A parallel recommendation applies to ways to intervene with respect to attention to *negative* changes. After one is forced to trade in a luxurious car for a junker, one can deliberately try *not* to ruminate about the downgrade (see B in Fig. 11.2) and *not* to mentally subtract them (Koo et al., 2008).

Research suggests that this goal can be accomplished through distractions—namely, cognitions and behaviors that help divert one's attention away from the negative life change and turn it to pleasant or benign thoughts and activities that are absorbing and engaging (Nolen-Hoeksema, 1991, 2004; Nolen-Hoeksema, Wisco, & Lyubomirsky, 2008; cf. Csikszentmihalyi, 1990). This can essentially be achieved via any activity that turns attention away from the negative change, and from its associated negative emotions and negative events—for example, concentrating on a project at work, going for a hike or bike ride, or seeing a film with friends.

The third way to intervene in the adaptation process is to directly increase the number of positive emotions that one experiences in response to a positive life change and to decrease the number of negative emotions that one experiences in response to an adverse one (see C in both figures). A multitude of strategies can be used to accomplish this, with recommendations found in literatures on positive mood inductions (e.g., Coan & Allen, 2007; Gerrards-Hesse, Spies, & Hesse, 1994), positive activity interventions (e.g., Fredrickson, 2009; Lyubomirsky, 2008; Seligman et al., 2005), and cognitive-behavioral therapy (e.g., Hollon, Haman, & Brown, 2002).

Finally, an individual can take steps to reduce his or her aspirations regarding a positive change and to keep them low after a negative change (see D in both figures). In Aristotle's words, "Bring your desires down to your present means. Increase them only when your increased means permit." This may be the most challenging way to thwart adaptation, necessitating the full arsenal of psychological tools at the individual's disposal, including most of the recommendations described above. For example, a person who has just obtained a hefty raise might remind himself of what life was like before (Liberman, Boehm, Lyubomirsky, & Ross, in press) and limit his spending habits to match earlier patterns; and a person who has recently been furloughed might resign herself to the loss of income and instead focus on productive ways to use her new-found extra time. Because my goal is to describe the process by which well-being boosts and drops can be sustained, the question of whether reduced aspirations are adaptive in the long term with respect to future performance and goal success will be set aside as falling outside the scope of this chapter. However, following the logic of Heath, Larrick, and Wu (1999), I speculate that people may seek to regulate their aspirations dynamically and optimally to fit their idiosyncratic goals and situations—for example, by raising aspirations immediately before attempting to realize a goal (i.e., feeling confident that one will win a tournament) but downgrading them *after* the tournament is over (thereby feeling satisfied with whatever one's performance).

Intervening in the Adaptation Process: Empirical Evidence Regarding Positive Activities

A primary assumption of this chapter is that people can control the extent and speed of their hedonic adaptation and thus, by developing and practicing the relevant skills, they can both surmount one of the biggest challenges to increasing happiness (in the positive domain) and foster coping and resilience (in the negative domain). How precisely one can go about doing so comes in part from the small but growing work on "happiness interventions," which is showing that effortful strategies and practices can instill new ways of thinking and behaving and thereby preserve well-being in the context of stress and trauma, and produce potentially lasting increases in well-being in their absence. Although dozens, even hundreds, of such strategies arguably exist (see Lyubomirsky, 2008, for a review), only a few will be described here for purposes of illustration. It is worth noting that what all the strategies have in common is that, first, they direct the individual's attention to positive aspects and away from negative aspects of experiences; second, they keep positive experiences "fresh" (i.e., dynamic, varied, novel, or surprising); and, third, they produce (or preserve) a stream of positive emotions, positive thoughts, and positive events, thereby serving as a foil to negative states (Fredrickson & Levenson, 1998; Fredrickson, Mancuso, Branigan, & Tugade, 2000). Feelings of joy, satisfaction, interest, serenity, or pride can help people view their lives with a larger perspective and provide a "psychological time-out" in the midst of stress or hardship, thus lessening the sting of any particular unpleasant experience. Thus, even brief or minor positive emotions, positive thoughts, and positive events marshaled in the face of adversity can build resilience by helping people bounce back from stressful experiences (Fredrickson, 2001; Keltner & Bonnano, 1997; Ong, Bergeman, Bisconti, & Wallace, 2006).

Gratitude, savoring, and positive thinking
POSITIVE DOMAIN
I begin with a discussion of the cultivation of gratitude, because it is a strategy that essentially involves appreciative attention—namely, a particular *kind* of attention, albeit a positive kind. Appreciative attention—in the form of gratefulness, as well as "savoring" (Bryant & Veroff, 2006), in which one consciously attends to an activity's enjoyment potential—is believed to impede adaptation to positive circumstances and events both directly *and* indirectly. Expressing gratitude involves noticing and reappreciating the good things in one's life, both concrete and abstract – a comfortable house, a kind friend, strong arms, a thrilling European vacation, the exquisiteness of a Caravaggio painting – and re-evaluating them as gifts or "blessings." The concomitants and consequences of grateful thinking appear to include bolstered resources for coping with adversity, enhanced self-worth, reduced materialism, fortified social bonds, and the countervailing of negative feelings like envy, bitterness, avarice, and irritation (Emmons, 2007).

The practice of gratitude may *directly* forestall adaptation by prompting people to extract the maximum possible enjoyment and satisfaction from their life circumstances, thereby helping them to relish these things and keep them from being taken for granted. Indeed, to appreciate a positive life change is to recognize that it may never have occurred (cf. Koo et al., 2008) and that it can be taken away. The genuine expression of gratitude may achieve this in large part because it helps combat two important mechanisms underlying hedonic adaptation—namely, escalating expectations and social comparisons (Layard, 2005). The joy of moving to a tonier address subsides after the person becomes "spoiled" by the view, garden, pool, and famous neighbors, desiring an even better location, and after she begins to notice that everyone else on the block drives an even more expensive car and throws fancier parties. Pausing to appreciate the positives in one's life—to focus on what one has today, as opposed to what other people have or what one could potentially have—is a step toward inhibiting or reducing the impact of the rising aspirations and upward comparisons that result from positive circumstantial changes (cf. Tversky, & Griffin, 1991). Other ways to accomplish this are by savoring the here-and-now and by maintaining a positive and optimistic perspective. When a person relishes his garden, mentally transports himself to his happiest day, luxuriates in the sound of his new speakers, or truly lives in the present moment, he is not taking his daily life for granted. When an individual perceives the silver lining in her situation ("I don't have the biggest house in the neighborhood, but it's just right for me"), she is not becoming jaded to the house's pleasures.

A number of experiments from my laboratory, as well as those of others, have demonstrated that the regular practices of gratitude, optimism, and savoring, performed over the course of anywhere from 1 to 12 consecutive weeks, bring about significant increases in well-being. For example, the intentional and effortful expression of gratitude, whether through "counting one's blessings" once a week (Emmons & McCullough, 2003; Lyubomirsky, Sheldon, et al., 2005) or penning gratitude letters to individuals who have been kind and meaningful (Lyubomirsky et al., 2008; Seligman, Steen, Park, & Peterson, 2005), has been shown to produce increases in happiness for as long as 9 months relative to control groups. Furthermore, experiments that have prompted individuals to express optimistic thinking by visualizing the realization of their very best hopes and dreams have demonstrated subsequent increases in physical health (King, 2001), happiness (Lyubomirsky et al., 2008), and positive affect (Sheldon & Lyubomirsky, 2006b). Although a much less studied topic, effortful attempts at savoring the present and the past have also been shown to boost feelings of well-being (Bryant, Smart, & King, 2005; Seligman, Rashid, & Parks, 2006). These studies do not provide direct evidence for the efficacy of gratitude, optimism, savoring, or any happiness-enhancing strategy for that matter in foiling adaptation to positive aspects of a person's life. Nevertheless, to date, they offer the only available data consistent with the notion that such activities may defy positive adaptation.

NEGATIVE DOMAIN

As discussed above, growing research supports the power of positive thinking, especially in the form of gratitude and savoring, to direct attention to positive life changes and prevent the individual from taking them for granted. However, the empirical evidence also underscores that the very same strategies can help people cope with stress and trauma and deter negative emotions. In other words, the capacity to appreciate one's life circumstances may be an adaptive coping method by which the individual is able to positively reinterpret stressful or aversive life experiences (Fredrickson, Tugade, Waugh, & Larkin, 2003). For example, traumatic memories are less likely to come to the surface, and are less intense when they do, in individuals who are regularly grateful (Watkins, Grimm, & Kolts, 2004). Interestingly, many people instinctively express gratitude when confronted with adversity. For example, Fredrickson and colleagues (2003) found that in the days immediately after the 9/11 terrorist attacks on the United States, gratitude was found to be the second most commonly experienced emotion (after sympathy).

In sum, practicing gratefulness, savoring, and optimism during adversity can help people adjust, move on, and perhaps begin anew. For example, positive thinking appears to be incompatible with negative emotions and may actually diminish or inhibit such feelings as anger, bitterness, and greed (McCullough, Emmons, & Tsang, 2002). Furthermore, those individuals who tend to savor and reminisce about the past—for example, summing up happy times, rekindling joy from happy memories—are best able to buffer stress (Bryant, 2003). Finally, research on optimism suggests that optimistic thinking prompts people to engage in active and effective coping (Nes & Segerstrom, 2006; Scheier, Weintraub, & Carver, 1986). Indeed, optimists routinely maintain relatively high levels of well-being and mental health during times of stress: Optimistic women are less likely to become depressed subsequent to childbirth than women who are less optimistic, and optimistic college freshmen are less likely to experience distress 3 months after enrolling in college (see Scheier & Carver, 1993).

Stop making sense
POSITIVE DOMAIN

Wilson and Gilbert (2005, 2008) have proposed that attempts to understand and make sense of positive experiences facilitate hedonic adaptation by transforming such experiences from something novel, attention-grabbing, emotion-eliciting, and extraordinary to something pallid, predictable, and ordinary. The implication of their model is that people should not try to think too much about and make sense of their successes, windfalls, and love affairs. In other words, one should savor but not explain. For example, in three studies, the participants' pleasure was prolonged when they remained uncertain about the source of an unexpected act of kindness (Wilson et al., 2005). Another implication of their model is that one strategy to inhibit adaptation to a positive experience is to keep reminding oneself *not* to think about the experience, as this practice would likely produce the ironic (but desired) consequence of the positive event popping back into consciousness and doing so often (Wegner, 1994). Future studies to test these ideas will be instructive.

NEGATIVE DOMAIN

Interestingly, the opposite recommendation applies to the domain of negative events, as research suggests that it is actually valuable to systematically analyze and come to terms with stresses, traumas, and hurt feelings—for example, by writing "expressively" about them (e.g., Lyubomirsky, Sousa, & Dickerhoof, 2006; Pennebaker, 1997). As Pennebaker and his colleagues have persuasively shown, writing is inherently a structured process that forces a person to organize and integrate her thoughts, to reflect on what causes what, to create a coherent narrative about herself, and to consider systematic, step-by-step solutions (e.g., Pennebaker, Mayne, & Francis, 1997; Pennebaker & Seagal, 1999). Thus, writing is an effective strategy when one needs to cope with negative experiences because it appears to reduce how often and how intensely a person experiences intrusive thoughts about them, by helping her make sense of them, find meaning in them, and get past them. (In contrast, one does not aim to "get past" positive experiences.)

A large and still growing literature in this area reveals that such "expressive writing" about past negative or traumatic events has many beneficial consequences. For example, compared with control groups, people who spend 3 days exploring their deepest thoughts and feelings in a journal about ordeals or traumas make fewer visits to a doctor in the months following the writing sessions, show stronger immune function, report less depression and distress, obtain higher grades, and are more likely to find new jobs after unemployment (see Frattaroli, 2006; Pennebaker, 1997, for reviews).

Investing in relationships, practicing kindness

POSITIVE DOMAIN

Efforts to be a helpful and charitable person may deliver a cascade of personal and social consequences —for example, insights into oneself, appreciation of one's own good fortune, new or strengthened relationships, a distraction from troubles, and more compassionate views of one's community (Lyubomirsky, 2008). Each of these consequences has the potential to bring about sustained positive experiences, thereby impeding hedonic adaptation to day-to-day existence. After all, when any event or circumstance or person stops generating positive or meaningful experiences, then one can be said to have adapted to it.

Two studies have shown that simply asking people to practice acts of kindness for several weeks produces increases in well-being, as long as those acts are committed with optimal timing (e.g., not too infrequently; Lyubomirsky, Sheldon, et al., 2005) and optimal variety (e.g., consistently bestowing different kindnesses rather than the same ones from week to week; Boehm et al., 2008). These findings are not surprising, given that philanthropy has been shown to stimulate two areas of the brain associated with pleasure, euphoria, trust, and cooperation (Moll et al., 2006).

Notably, the activity of trying to commit acts of kindness is closely related to that of nurturing interpersonal relationships, as both build social bonds and bolster self-efficacy and self-esteem. Most would agree that one does not adapt as swiftly (if at all) to other people as to objects or possessions. Apparently, money can't buy love, and most of what it can buy is prone to hedonic adaptation. Cultivating interpersonal relationships appears to be a reliable way to inhibit adaptation by working to create a stream of positive and varied experiences. Easterlin (2005) has shown, for example, that relative to aspirations for material goods, people's desires for happy marriages and children do not decline as they successfully attain them. Undoubtedly there is something special and unique about relationships, and actively strengthening, nourishing, and enjoying them may ward off adaptation. To take marriage as an example, whereas the average person may derive just a 2-year boost in happiness after getting married (Lucas et al., 2003), the person who *acts* within the marriage to improve and cherish it may cause that boost to last significantly longer. The effect of marriage doesn't "wear off" for him or her. My speculation is that those respondents in the German marriage study who showed essentially no hedonic adaptation 5 years into their marriages were the ones who were intentionally and effortfully working towards keeping their relationships fresh, vibrant, meaningful, and loving.[3]

Many theorists, armchair psychologists, and authors of marriage manuals have considered the ways that intimate relationships and friendships can be buttressed and strengthened. These techniques include making time to just be together and talk, communicating (i.e., truly listening and conveying admiration, appreciation, and affection), managing conflict, being supportive and loyal, and sharing an inner life, such as dreams, rituals, and responsibilities (Gottman & Silver, 1999; McGinnis, 1979; cf. Lyubomirsky, 2008). As just one illustration, research suggests that flourishing relationships are distinguished not by how the partners respond to each other's disappointments, losses, and reversals but how they react to *good* news. The closest, most intimate, and most trusting relationships have been found to be those in which the couple responds "actively and constructively"—that is, with interest and delight—to each other's windfalls and successes (Gable, Reis, Asher, & Impett, 2004). Appreciating, validating, and "capitalizing" on a partner's good news thus appears to be an effective strategy to bolster the relationship and thereby to intensify the pleasure and satisfaction one obtains from it— in short, to preclude hedonic adaptation. One study showed that people who strove to show genuine enthusiasm, support, and understanding of their partner's good news, however small—and did so three times a day over a week—became happier and less depressed (Schueller, 2006).

NEGATIVE DOMAIN

Practicing kindness and thoughtfulness towards others can also counteract the negative thoughts and negative emotions sustained in the wake of adverse life changes. As suggested above, doing kindness leads people to view others from a more positive and more charitable perspective and engenders a heightened sense of interdependence and cooperation in their neighborhoods and communities. Being generous and thoughtful often relieves guilt or discomfort over others' ordeals and troubles and triggers appreciation for one's own good fortune. In other words, assisting others makes people feel advantaged (and grateful) by comparison (e.g., "I'm thankful that my life is comfortable"). Indeed, providing help or consolation to other people can deliver a welcome distraction from one's own miseries and ruminations, as it shifts the focus from oneself onto somebody else. Surveys of volunteers, for example, show that volunteering is associated with an alleviation of depressive symptoms and increases in feelings of happiness, self-regard, mastery, and control (Piliavin, 2003).

Finally, and perhaps most important, committing acts of kindness can satisfy a basic human need for human connection and thereby galvanize a cascade of positive social consequences. An individual who delivers help and comfort to other people will experience shows of liking, smiles, appreciation, gratitude, and valued friendship in return. Evidence for this dynamic was obtained in one of my laboratory's "kindness interventions" (Boehm et al., 2008). Participants were assessed not only on how helpful they were and how much their happiness increased over 10 weeks but also on the extent to which they perceived gratitude in those they helped. The results showed that this "perceived gratitude" significantly mediated the relationship between helping and increased well-being. In other words, a chief reason that being kind to others made the participants happier is that it led them to recognize how much the recipients appreciated their kind acts. It is not surprising, then, that their generosity today may lead the recipients to reciprocate in the givers' time of need tomorrow (Trivers, 1971).

Pursuing important and intrinsic personal goals

POSITIVE DOMAIN

All the adaptation-forestalling activities described above could be, in some sense, lumped under the umbrella of working toward significant life goals— that is, one could conceivably have as one's goal to "be a more helpful person" or to "keep experiences fresh." In contrast, I wish to distinguish this particular category by focusing on the typical and familiar life goals that the majority of people seem to share (Kaiser & Ozer, 1997). Indeed, committed goal pursuit is a vital strategy in and of itself, because it involves the infinite variety of projects, schemes, plans, tasks, endeavors, ventures, missions, and ambitions, both large and small, that people can undertake in their daily lives. Although the *achievement* of goals can potentially lead to adaptation, escalating expectations, and even letdown, if people "enjoy the struggle along the way" (Csikszentmihalyi, 1990, p. 10), they will derive pleasure and satisfaction by simply pursuing or working on the goal. They will ideally stretch their skills, discover novel opportunities, grow, strive, learn, and become more competent and expert. They will attain a sense of purpose in their lives, feelings of efficacy over their progress, and mastery over their time, and, perhaps most important, they will likely frequently engage with others. Although a person can become adapted to the knowledge that she has attained a particular goal or subgoal, she may avoid adaptation in several ways—by savoring the accomplished goal, by continually moving on from accomplished goals to new ones, and, instead of focusing too much on the finish line in the first place, by focusing on carrying out the multiple steps necessary to make progress.

Numerous studies have shown that people who strive to realize important goals are happier, especially when such goals are intrinsic (e.g., Kasser & Ryan, 1996), realistic (e.g., McGregor & Little, 1998), culturally valued (e.g., Cantor & Sanderson, 1999), self-determined (e.g., Sheldon & Elliot, 1999), and harmonious (e.g., Emmons & King, 1988).

For example, students who pursue and attain self-generated personal goals over the course of a semester are happier at the end of the semester, in part because they accumulate positive daily experiences along the way (see Sheldon, 2002, for a review). Notably, the pursuit of goals also helps individuals satisfy their basic human needs for autonomy, competence, and relatedness (Deci & Ryan, 2000) and thereby increase their well-being (e.g., Reis, Sheldon, Ryan, Gable, & Roscoe, 2000; Sheldon & Elliot, 1999; Sheldon, Elliot, Kim, & Kasser, 2001).

NEGATIVE DOMAIN

How does goal pursuit help people manage stress and negative emotions in the wake of negative life changes? For many of the same reasons that it fosters well-being during the good times. First, committed goal pursuit offers people a sense of purpose and a feeling of control over their lives (Cantor, 1990)—both invaluable resources during efforts to cope. Whether the valued activity is becoming an inventor or raising a child, it gives the individual something to work for and to look forward to. Second, possessing meaningful goals bolsters people's self-efficacy and self-worth. Indeed, the accomplishment of every step (on the way to the bigger goal) is yet another opportunity for an emotional and ego boost. Third, goal pursuit imparts structure and meaning to people's daily lives, creating obligations, deadlines, and timetables, as well as opportunities for mastering new skills and for interacting with others. Finally, although it may be challenging to continue striving toward significant life goals during times of stress or crisis, research suggests that commitment to goals during such times may help people cope more effectively with problems. Of course, sometimes traumatic or negative situations may require giving up goals that are no longer tenable. A grave injury or severe financial crisis may lead people to reconsider whether they should surrender their dream of becoming a dancer or obtaining a law degree. Sustained well-being requires that people bring themselves to substitute new goals for old ones.

Future Directions

I have argued that one can become happier by thwarting hedonic adaptation to positive life changes, but cannot one also become happier *in spite of* such adaptation? To be sure, a person could conceivably be fortunate or exceptional enough to have one wonderful circumstance thrust upon him after another; a person could somehow—psychologically or biologically—be "predisposed" not to adapt to positive experience or to adapt relatively swiftly to negative experiences; and a person could conceivably develop the capacity to require less and less positive emotion to experience the same levels of satisfaction as before (Kahneman, 1999). These examples illuminate how difficult it is to posit ways that sustained increases in happiness can be achieved without the need to actively combat adaptation (in the positive domain) or to actively speed up adaptation (in the negative domain). Future studies that follow people's experiences and reactions over long periods of time may be able to identify some of these ways, as well as to describe potential individual differences—and their sources—in adaptation rates.

This chapter has focused primarily on activities and strategies that are desirable and adaptive when the person's aim is to intervene in hedonic adaptation to positive and negative events. The choice to focus here on intentional behaviors (rather than life events) was not arbitrary, as people have a fair amount of control over their behavior, and thus, are potentially able to heed specific happiness-enhancing recommendations arising from the literature on hedonic adaptation. However, people can also control to some degree the life changes that take place (cf. Diener, Suh, Lucas, & Smith, 1999; Headey & Wearing, 1989; Scarr & McCartney, 1983). Thus, an area ripe for future research concerns the question of what kinds of life changes generate more positive events and emotions than others, thus buffering negative states and cumulating to enhanced global well-being. A potential target of investigation are positive events based on *intrinsic* (rather than *extrinsic*) life changes. Kasser and colleagues (Kasser & Ryan, 1993; Kasser, 2002; Sheldon & Kasser, 2008) have shown that intrinsic values and goals (community, growth, intimacy) produce greater well-being than do extrinsic ones (popularity, wealth, physical attractiveness), because the former better satisfy innate psychological needs (Deci & Ryan, 2000; Niemiec, Ryan, & Deci, in press).

Directly pertaining to the HAPNE model, future studies could test whether the *type* of life change that occurs (intrinsic vs. extrinsic) moderates the effects of downstream positive events on both experienced emotions and rising aspiration levels. Concerning positive emotions, research suggests that positive extrinsic events deriving from a particular life change (e.g., getting a compliment on one's new car) do not deliver as much happiness as positive intrinsic events (e.g., serving as a Big Brother; Dunn, Aknin, & Norton, 2008; Kasser, 2002). Thus, positive events based on intrinsic life changes should produce more actual positive emotions, and be better able to neutralize negative emotions, compared to positive events based on extrinsic changes. Concerning aspirations, extrinsic experiences do not satisfy basic needs and instead are likely to lead to ever-increasing desires for psychologically unfulfilling objects (Myers, 2000), much like an addiction (Koob & Le Moal, 2001). In contrast, building close interactions or seeking novel self-discoveries activates feelings of satisfaction and contentment, which are more likely to be appreciated and less likely to be taken for granted.

Another question raised by the work described in this chapter concerns the role of possible individual differences or cultural factors. For example, do individualists benefit more from experiencing such emotions as enthusiasm and pride (as opposed to serenity and contentment) than collectivists? And, do those with more stable lives or who are higher in sensation-seeking benefit more from variety and surprise? One possibility is that although a person with a chaotic life might in some ways prefer predictability and familiarity (and, indeed, some amount of familiarity mixed in with novelty may be optimal in general [Bell, 1913; Berlyne, 1971]), when she does experience a positive change, that change should have longer-lasting effects when it conforms to the tenets of the HAPNE model. Conversely, if a stressed person is being dragged down by too many negative events, the model should reveal how he might more quickly adapt to those events, such that he is more receptive to positive life changes that he might subsequently experience or even seek out.

As this chapter makes clear, relatively little is still known about adaptation in the positive domain. Future prospective, longitudinal, and experimental studies, with appropriate control groups, would further inform researchers about the mechanisms—cognitive, behavioral, motivational, and physiological—by which positive adaptation operates. For example, people's emotional responses in advance of, during, and following a naturally occurring positive event (e.g., upgrading to a bigger home, getting engaged, winning an Oscar) or an induced positive event (e.g., learning that they are destined to succeed professionally or that they have won $100 or that they were selected for a date by an attractive peer) could be followed across time and compared to responses of those who did not experience the same event. Furthermore, experimental intervention studies that prompt people to directly resist or slow down adaptation to positive experiences (whether induced or naturalistic) could seek to establish the efficacy of this process, as well the moderators and mediators that underlie it. Ideally, a variety of measures should be used in such investigations, including global scales of happiness and satisfaction, "objective" assessments of daily and momentary affect (e.g., Csikszentmihalyi & Larson, 1987; Kahneman, Krueger, Schkade, Schwarz, & Stone, 2004), and behavioral indicators (e.g., mental and physical health care utilization, peer reports, and Duchenne smiles; Harker & Keltner, 2001; Sandvik, Diener, & Seidlitz, 1993), as well as physiological and neural ones (e.g., asymmetric frontal function; Urry et al., 2004).

Conclusion

The sports car manufacturer Porsche has a print ad showing a Boxster speeding down a rural highway. The caption says, "Every time you drive it, it puts a smile on your face. How much is that worth?" Not much, according to a great deal of research, because the bursts of pleasure one may reap from powering up the car are destined to last even less long than from a non-material circumstantial change, like moving cross-country or beginning a new job. One might be tempted to conclude that sustained happiness cannot be bought with Porsches or any other material possessions. I actually believe that that conclusion is wrong. Hedonic adaptation *can* be resisted, even to material objects, but only with conscious, active efforts. If the Porsche owner strives to overcome his auto-ennui by appreciating his enormously good fortune, if he uses his sports car as a vehicle for pleasurable renewable experiences and for strengthening relationships (e.g., road tripping with friends, loaning to a family member), if he puts effort into savoring the stereo system and the speed (e.g., reveling in the wind in his face, luxuriating in the music), he will continue to derive happiness from his purchase.

The good news is that the same processes that make it easy to adapt to material gains also make it easy to adapt to material losses. In due course, the individual's attention is captured less and less by the contrast between the old and new standard of living, and unpleasant experiences become more and more rare. Accordingly, when it comes to managing the slings and arrows of life's misfortunes (when one's aim is to speed up rather than inhibit adaptation), similar strategies are likely to be effective—namely, appreciating what one has rather than yearning for what one would like to have, searching for opportunities to generate positive experiences, cultivating a sense of connection with others, building competence and expertise, and looking outside of oneself to contribute to others.

If swift hedonic adaptation to positive experiences and slow-going adaptation to negative ones are the enemies of lasting happiness, then self-determined, dynamic, and attention-capturing positive activities are the weapons to surmount it. Such activities can serve as part of a broader strategy to accelerate adaptation when things go awry, but they can also serve to *act on* static circumstances (like the Boxster, an ocean view, or one's good health) in order to preclude adaptation to those circumstances and forestall adaptation to one's job, marriage, friends, and leisure, and to daily life in general.

Notes

1 It is worth noting that all but one of Lucas and colleagues' influential longitudinal studies have used the same 10-point life satisfaction question from the German dataset—namely, "How happy are you at present with your life as a whole?" This question arguably calls respondents to reference the significant events and circumstances that they are currently facing in their lives when gauging their levels of satisfaction (cf. Kahneman et al., 2004). As a result, responses to this question may reflect relatively enhanced (rather than attenuated) effects of such events as marriage, unemployment, and disability.

2 The HAPNE model makes a distinction between one large event (or life change)—the seminal change—and the discrete daily/weekly events—the downstream episodes—that it produces. Although this distinction can sometimes blur, researchers typically study adaptation to discrete life changes or circumstantial changes (e.g., changes in income, job status, health status, relationships, and education), and that is what the model seeks to examine as well.

3 Alternatively, it is possible that those individuals who did not show adaptation to their married life may have simply been more fortunate or skilled in their selections of superior or better-matched spouses. The character and ubiquitousness of hedonic adaptation, however, suggest that even the most positive circumstances, instigated by the luckiest and ablest persons, can come to yield less and less pleasure and satisfaction over time.

References

Baumeister, R. F., Bratslavsky, E., Finkenauer, C., & Vohs, K. D. (2001). Bad is stronger than good. *Review of General Psychology, 5*, 323–70.

Bell, C. (1913). *Art.* London: Putnam.

Berlyne, D. (1970). Novelty, complexity, and hedonic value. *Perception and Psychophysics, 8*, 279–86.

Berlyne, D. E. (1971). *Aesthetics and psychobiology.* New York: Appleton-Century-Crofts.

Bless, H., Hamilton, D. L., & Mackie, D. M. (1992). Mood effects on the organization of person information. *European Journal of Social Psychology, 22*, 497–509.

Boehm, J. K., & Lyubomirsky, S. (2008). *The course of hedonic adaptation to a stream of positive events: Exploring moderators and mediators.* Unpublished data, Department of Psychology, University of California, Riverside.

Boehm, J. K., Lyubomirsky, S., & Sheldon, K. M. (2008). *Spicing up kindness: The role of variety in the effects of practicing kindness on improvements in mood, happiness, and self-evaluations.* Manuscript in preparation.

Bonnano, G. A., & Keltner, D. (1997). Facial expressions of emotion and the course of conjugal bereavement. *Journal of Abnormal Psychology, 106*, 126–37.

Boswell, W. R., Boudreau, J. W., & Tichy, J. (2005). The relationship between employee job change and job satisfaction: The honeymoon-hangover effect. *Journal of Applied Psychology, 90*, 882–92.

Braungart, J. M., Plomin, R., DeFries, J. C., & Fulker, D. W. (1992). Genetic influence on tester rated infant temperament as assessed by Bayley's Infant Behavior Record: Nonadoptive and adoptive siblings and twins. *Developmental Psychology, 28*, 40–7.

Brickman, P., & Campbell, D. T. (1971). Hedonic relativism and planning the good society. In M. H. Appley (Ed.), *Adaptation-level theory* (pp. 287–302). New York: Academic Press.

Brickman, P., Coates, D., & Janoff-Bulman, R. (1978). Lottery winners and accident victims: Is happiness relative? *Journal of Personality and Social Psychology, 36*, 917–27.

Bryant, F. B. (2003). Savoring Beliefs Inventory (SBI): A scale for measuring beliefs about savoring. *Journal of Mental Health, 12*, 175–96.

Bryant, F. B., Smart, C. M., & King, S. P. (2005). Using the past to enhance the present: Boosting happiness through positive reminiscence. *Journal of Happiness Studies, 6*, 227–60.

Bryant, F. B., & Veroff, J. (2006). *Savoring: A new model of positive experience.* Nahwah, NJ: Erlbaum.

Busseri, M. A., Sadava, S. W., & Decourville, N. (2007). A hybrid model for research on subjective well-being: Examining common- and component-specific sources of variance in life satisfaction, positive affect, and negative affect. *Social Indicators Research, 83*, 413–45.

Cantor, N. (1990). From thought to behavior: "Having" and "doing" in the study of personality and cognition. *American Psychologist, 45*, 735–50.

Cantor, N., & Sanderson, C. A. (1999). Life task participation and well-being: The importance of taking part in daily life. In D. Kahneman, E. Diener, & N. Schwarz (Eds.), *Well-being: The foundations of hedonic psychology* (pp. 230–43). New York: Russell Sage Foundation.

Carver, C. S. (2007). Stress, coping, and health. In H. S. Friedman & R. C. Silver (Eds.), *Foundations of health psychology* (pp. 117–44). New York: Oxford University Press.

Carver, C. S., & Scheier, M. F. (1990). Origins and functions of positive and negative affect: A control-process view. *Psychological Review, 97*, 19–35.

Cash, T. F., Duel, L. A., & Perkins, L. L. (2002). Women's psychosocial outcomes of breast augmentation with silicone gel-filled implants: A 2-year prospective study. *Plastic and Reconstructive Surgery, 109*, 2112–21.

Clore, G. L. (1994). Why emotions are felt. In P. Ekman, & R. Davidson (Eds.), *The nature of emotion: Fundamental questions* (pp. 103–11). New York: Oxford University Press.

Coan, J. A., & Allen, J. J. B. (Eds.) (2007). *Handbook of emotion elicitation and assessment.* Oxford: Oxford University Press.

Coleman, L. M., Jussim, L., & Abraham, J. (1987). Students' reactions to teacher evaluations: The unique impact of negative feedback. *Journal of Applied Social Psychology, 17*, 1051–70.

Compas, B. E., Connor-Smith, J. K., Saltzman, H., Thomsen, A. H., & Wadsworth, M. E. (2001). Coping with stress during childhood and adolescence: Problems, progress, and potential in theory and research. *Psychological Bulletin, 127,* 87–127.

Costa, P. T., McCrae, R. R., & Zonderman, A. B. (1987). Environmental and dispositional influences on well-being: Longitudinal follow-up of an American national sample. *British Journal of Psychology, 78,* 299–306.

Csikszentmihalyi, M. (1990). *Flow: The psychology of optimal experience.* New York: Harper & Row.

Csikszentmihalyi, M., & Larson, R. (1987). Validity and reliability of the experience-sampling method. *Journal of Nervous and Mental Disease, 175,* 526–36.

David, J. P., Green, P. J., Martin, R., & Suls, J. (1997). Differential roles of neuroticism, extraversion, and event desirability for mood in daily life: An integrative model of top-down and bottom-up influences. *Journal of Personality and Social Psychology, 73,* 149–59.

Deci, E. L., & Ryan, R. M. (2000). The "what" and "why" of goal pursuits: Human needs and the self-determination of behavior. *Psychological Inquiry, 4,* 227–68.

Diener, E. (1994). Assessing subjective well-being: Progress and opportunities. *Social Indicators Research, 31,* 103–57.

Diener, E., & Larsen, R. J. (1984). Temporal stability and cross-situational consistency of affective, behavioral, and cognitive responses. *Journal of Personality and Social Psychology, 47,* 871–83.

Diener, E., Lucas, R. E., & Scollon, C. N. (2006). Beyond the hedonic treadmill: Revising the adaptation theory of well-being. *American Psychologist, 61,* 305–14.

Diener, E., Sandvik, E., & Pavot, W. (1991). Happiness is the frequency, not the intensity, of positive versus negative affect. In F. Strack, M. Argyle, & N. Schwarz (Eds.), *Subjective well-being: An interdisciplinary perspective. International series in experimental social psychology* (pp. 119–39). Oxford: Pergamon Press.

Diener, E., Suh, E. M., Lucas, R. E., & Smith, H. L. (1999). Subjective well-being: Three decades of progress. *Psychological Bulletin, 125,* 276–302.

Dunn, E. W., Aknin, L. B., & Norton, M. I. (2008). Spending money on others promotes happiness. *Science, 319,* 1687–8.

Easterlin, R. A. (2005). A puzzle for adaptive theory. *Journal of Economic Behavior and Organization, 56,* 513–21.

Easterlin, R. A. (2006). Life cycle happiness and its sources: Intersections of psychology, economics, and demography. *Journal of Economic Psychology, 27,* 463–82.

Ebstein, R. B., Novick, O., Umansky, R., Priel, B., & Osher, Y. (1996). Dopamine D4 receptor (D4DR) exon III polymorphism associated with the human personality trait of novelty seeking. *Nature Genetics, 12,* 78–80.

Emmons, R. A. (2007). *THANKS! How the new science of gratitude can make you happier.* New York: Houghton Mifflin Company.

Emmons, R. A., & King, L. A. (1988). Conflict among personal strivings: Immediate and long-term implications for psychological and physical well-being. *Journal of Personality and Social Psychology, 54,* 1040–8.

Emmons, R. A., & McCullough, M. E. (2003). Counting blessings versus burdens: An experimental investigation of gratitude and subjective well-being in daily life. *Journal of Personality and Social Psychology, 84,* 377–89.

Frattaroli, J. (2006). Experimental disclosure and its moderators: A meta-analysis. *Psychological Bulletin, 132,* 823–65.

Frederick, S., & Loewenstein, G. (1999). Hedonic adaptation. In D. Kahneman, E. Diener, & N. Schwarz (Eds.), *Well-being:* *The foundations of hedonic psychology* (pp. 302–29). New York: Russell Sage Foundation.

Fredrickson, B. L. (2001). The role of positive emotions in positive psychology: The broaden-and-build theory of positive emotions. *American Psychologist, 56,* 218–26.

Fredrickson, B. L. (2009). *Positivity: Groundbreaking research reveals how to embrace the hidden strength of positive emotions, overcome negativity, and thrive.* New York: Crown Books.

Fredrickson, B. L., & Cohn, M. A. (2008). Positive emotions. In M. Lewis, J. Haviland, & L. F. Barrett (Eds.), *Handbook of emotions* (3rd ed.). New York: Guilford Press.

Fredrickson, B. L., & Levenson, R. W. (1998). Positive emotions speed recovery from the cardiovascular sequelae of negative emotions. *Cognition and Emotion, 12,* 191–220.

Fredrickson, B. L., & Losada, M. F. (2005). Positive affect and the complex dynamics of human flourishing. *American Psychologist, 60,* 678–86.

Fredrickson, B. L., Mancuso, R. A., Branigan, C., & Tugade, M. M. (2000). The undoing effect of positive emotions. *Motivation and Emotion, 24,* 237–58.

Fredrickson, B. L., Tugade, M. M., Waugh, C. E., & Larkin, G. R. (2003). What good are positive emotions in crises? A prospective study of resilience and emotions following the terrorist attacks on the United States in September 11, 2001. *Journal of Personality and Social Psychology, 84,* 365–76.

Frijda, N. H. (1988). The laws of emotion. *American Psychologist, 43,* 349–58.

Frijda, N. H. (1994). Emotions are functional, most of the time. In P. Ekman & R. Davidson (Eds.), *The nature of emotion: Fundamental questions* (pp. 112–22). New York: Oxford University Press.

Frodi, L. M., Lamb, M. E, Leavitt, L. A., & Donovan, W L. (1978). Fathers' and mothers' responses to infants' smiles and cries. *Infant Behavior and Development, 1,* 187–98.

Fujita, F., & Diener, E. (2005). Life satisfaction set point: Stability and change. *Journal of Personality and Social Psychology, 88,* 158–64.

Gable, S. L., Reis, H. T., Asher, E. R., & Impett, E. A. (2004). What do you do when things go right? The intrapersonal and interpersonal benefits of sharing positive events. *Journal of Personality and Social Psychology, 87,* 228–45.

Gerrards-Hesse, A., Spies, K., & Hesse, F. W. (1994). Experimental inductions of emotional states and their effectiveness: A review. *British Journal of Psychology, 85,* 55–78.

Gottman, J. M. (1994). *What predicts divorce? The relationship between marital processes and marital outcomes.* Hillsdale, NJ: Erlbaum.

Gottman, J. M., & Krokoff, L. J. (1989). Marital interaction and satisfaction: A longitudinal view. *Journal of Consulting and Clinical Psychology, 57,* 47–52.

Gottman, J. M., & Silver, N. (1999). *The seven principles for making marriage work.* New York: Three Rivers Press.

Graziano, W. G., Brothen, T., & Berscheid, E. (1980). Attention, attraction, and individual differences in reaction to criticism. *Journal of Personality and Social Psychology, 38,* 193–202.

Hamer, D. H. (1996). The heritability of happiness. *Nature Genetics, 14,* 125–6.

Harker, L., & Keltner, D. (2001). Expressions of positive emotions in women's college yearbook pictures and their relationship to personality and life outcomes across adulthood. *Journal of Personality and Social Psychology, 80,* 112–24.

Headey, B., & Wearing, A. (1989). Personality, life events, and subjective well-being: Toward a dynamic equilibrium model. *Journal of Personality and Social Psychology, 57,* 731–9.

Heath, C., Larrick, R. P., & Wu, G. (1999). Goals as reference points. *Cognitive Psychology, 38,* 79–109.

Helson, H. (1964). Current trends and issues in adaptation-level theory. *American Psychologist, 19,* 26–38.

Hollon, S. D., Haman, K. L., & Brown, L. L. (2002). Cognitive-behavioral treatment of depression. In I. H. Gotlib, & C. L. Hammen (Eds.), *Handbook of depression* (pp. 383–403). New York: The Guilford Press.

Ito, T. A., & Cacioppo, J. T. (2005). Variations on a human universal: Individual differences in positivity offset and negativity bias. *Cognition & Emotion, 19,* 1–26.

Ito, T. A., Larsen, J. T., Smith, N. K., & Cacioppo, J. T. (1998). Negative information weighs more heavily on the brain: The negativity bias in evaluative categorizations. *Journal of Personality and Social Psychology, 75,* 887–90.

Kahneman, D. (1999). Objective happiness. In D. Kahneman, E. Diener, & N. Schwarz (Eds.), *Well-being: The foundations of hedonic psychology* (pp. 3–25). New York: Russell Sage Foundation.

Kahneman, D., Krueger, A. B., Schkade, D., Schwarz, N., & Stone, A. A. (2004). A survey method for characterizing daily life experience: The Day Reconstruction Method. *Science, 306,* 1776–80.

Kahneman, D., & Thaler, R. H. (2006). Anomalies: Utility maximization and experienced utility. *Journal of Economic Perspectives, 20,* 221–34.

Kahneman, D., & Tversky, A. (1979). Prospect theory: An analysis of decision under risk. *Econometrica, 47,* 263–91.

Kahneman, D., & Tversky, A. (1984). Choices, values and frames. *American Psychologist, 39,* 341–50.

Kaiser, R. T., & Ozer, D. J. (1997). Emotional stability and goal-related stress. *Personality and Individual Differences, 22,* 371–9.

Kasser, T. (2002). *The high price of materialism.* Cambridge, MA: MIT Press.

Kasser, T., & Ryan, R. M. (1993). A dark side of the American dream: Correlates of financial success as a central life aspiration. *Journal of Personality and Social Psychology, 65,* 410–22.

Kasser, T., & Ryan, R. M. (1996). Further examining the American dream: Differential correlates of intrinsic and extrinsic goals. *Personality and Social Psychology Bulletin, 22,* 280–7.

Keltner, D., & Bonnano, G. A. (1997). A study of laughter and dissociation: Distinct correlates of laughter and smiling during bereavement *Journal of Personality and Social Psychology, 73,* 687–702.

King, L. A. (2001). The health benefits of writing about life goals. *Personality and Social Psychology Bulletin, 27,* 798–807.

Koo, M., Algoe, S. B., Wilson, T. D., & Gilbert, D. T. (2008). It's a wonderful life: Mentally subtracting positive events improves people's affective states, contrary to their affective forecasts. *Journal of Personality and Social Psychology, 95,* 1217–24.

Koob, G. F., & Le Moal, M. (2001). Drug addiction, dysregulation of reward, and allostasis. *Neuropsychopharmacology, 24,* 97–129.

Lane, E. (2000). *The loss of happiness in market democracies.* New Haven, CT: Yale University Press.

Lawton, M. P., DeVoe, M. R., & Parmelee, P. (1995). Relationship of events and affect in the daily life of an elderly population. *Psychology and Aging, 10,* 469–77.

Layard, R. (2005). *Happiness: Lessons from a new science.* New York: Penguin Press.

Lazarus, R. S. (2000). Toward better research on stress and coping. *American Psychologist, 55,* 665–73.

Leary, M. R., Tambor, E. S., Terdal, S. K., & Downs, D. L. (1995). Self-esteem as an interpersonal monitor: The sociometer hypothesis. *Journal of Personality and Social Psychology, 68,* 518–30.

Leventhal, A. M., Martin, R. L., Seals, R. W., Tapia, E., & Rehm, L. P. (2007). Investigating the dynamics of affect: Psychological mechanisms of affective habituation to pleasurable stimuli. *Motivation and Emotion, 31,* 145–57.

Liberman, V., Boehm, J. K., Lyubomirsky, S., & Ross, L. (in press). Happiness and memory: Affective significance of endowment and contrast. *Emotion.*

Linklater, R. (Producer/Director). (2004). *Before sunset* [Motion Picture]. Burbank, CA: Warner Independent Pictures.

Losada, M. (1999). The complex dynamics of high performance teams. *Mathematical and Computer Modeling, 30,* 179–92.

Lucas, R. E. (2007a). Adaptation and the set point model of subjective well-being. *Current Directions in Psychological Science, 16,* 75–9.

Lucas, R. E. (2007b). Long-term disability has lasting effects on subjective well-being: Evidence from two nationally representative longitudinal studies. *Journal of Personality and Social Psychology, 92,* 717–30.

Lucas, R. (2007c). Personality and subjective well-being. In M. Eid & R. Larsen (Eds.), *The science of subjective well-being.* New York: Guilford Press.

Lucas, R. E. (2005). Time does not heal all wounds: A longitudinal study of reaction and adaptation to divorce. *Psychological Science, 16,* 945–50.

Lucas, R. E., & Clark, A. E. (2006). Do people really adapt to marriage? *Journal of Happiness Studies, 7,* 405–26.

Lucas, R. E., Clark, A. E., Georgellis, Y., & Diener, E. (2003). Reexamining adaptation and the set point model of happiness: Reactions to changes in marital status. *Journal of Personality and Social Psychology, 84,* 527–39.

Lucas, R. E., Clark, A. E., Georgellis, Y., & Diener, E. (2004). Unemployment alters the set point for life satisfaction. *Psychological Science, 15,* 8–13.

Lykken, D. (2000). *Happiness: The nature and nurture of joy and contentment.* New York: St Martin's Press.

Lykken, D., Iacono, W. G., Haroian, K., McGue, M., & Bouchard, T. J., Jr. (1988). Habituation of the skin conductance response to strong stimuli: A twin study. *Psychophysiology, 25,* 4–15.

Lykken, D., & Tellegen, A. (1996). Happiness is a stochastic phenomenon. *Psychological Science, 7,* 186–9.

Lyubomirsky, S. (2008). *The how of happiness: A scientific approach to getting the life you want.* New York: Penguin Press.

Lyubomirsky, S., Dickerhoof, R., Boehm, J. K., & Sheldon, K. M. (2008). *Becoming happier takes both a will and a proper way: Two experimental longitudinal interventions to boost well-being.* Manuscript submitted for publication.

Lyubomirsky, S., King, L. A., & Diener, E. (2005). The benefits of frequent positive affect: Does happiness lead to success? *Psychological Bulletin, 131,* 803–55.

Lyubomirsky, S., Sheldon, K. M., & Schkade, D. (2005). Pursuing happiness: The architecture of sustainable change. *Review of General Psychology, 9,* 111–31.

Lyubomirsky, S., Sousa, L., & Dickerhoof, R. (2006). The costs and benefits of writing, talking, and thinking about life's triumphs and defeats. *Journal of Personality and Social Psychology, 90,* 692–708.

McCullough, M. E., Emmons, R. A., & Tsang, J. (2002). The grateful disposition: A conceptual and empirical topography. *Journal of Personality and Social Psychology, 82,* 112–27.

McGinnis, A. L. (1979). *The friendship factor.* Minneapolis, MN: Augsburg.

McGregor, I., & Little, B. R. (1998). Personal projects, happiness, and meaning: On doing well and being yourself. *Journal of Personality and Social Psychology, 74,* 494–512.

Mischel, W., Ebbesen, E. B., & Zeiss, A. R. (1976). Determinants of selective memory about the self. *Journal of Consulting and Clinical Psychology, 44,* 92–103.

Moll, J., Krueger, F., Zahn, R., Pardini, M., de Oliveira-Souza, R., & Grafman, J. (2006). Human fronto-mesolimbic networks guide decisions about charitable donation. *Proceedings of the National Academy of Sciences, 103,* 15623–8.

Mroczek, D. K., & Spiro, A., III. (2005). Change in life satisfaction during adulthood: Findings from the Veterans Affairs Normative Aging Study. *Journal of Personality and Social Psychology, 88,* 189–202.

Myers, D. G. (2000). The funds, friends, and faith of happy people. *American Psychologist, 55,* 56–67.

Nes, L. S., & Segerstrom, S. C. (2006). Dispositional optimism and coping: A meta-analytic review. *Personality and Social Psychology Review, 10,* 235–51.

Nezlek, J. B., & Gable, S. L. (2001). Depression as a moderator of relationships between positive daily events and day-to-day psychological adjustment. *Personality and Social Psychology Bulletin, 27,* 1692–704.

Niemiec, C. P., Ryan, R. M., & Deci, E. L. (in press). The path taken: Consequences of attaining intrinsic and extrinsic aspirations in post-college life. *Journal of Research in Personality.*

Nolen-Hoeksema, S. (1991). Responses to depression and their effects on the duration of depressive episodes. *Journal of Abnormal Psychology. 100,* 569–82.

Nolen-Hoeksema, S. (2004). *Women who think too much.* New York: Henry Holt.

Nolen-Hoeksema, S., Wisco, B. E., & Lyubomirsky, S. (2008). Rethinking rumination. *Perspectives on Psychological Science, 3,* 400–24.

Oehman, A., Lundqvist, D., & Esteves, F. (2001). The face in the crowd revisited: A threat advantage with schematic stimuli. *Journal of Personality and Social Psychology, 80,* 381–96.

Ohira, H., Winton, W. M., & Oyama, M. (1997). Effects of stimulus valence on recognition memory and endogenous eyeblinks: Further evidence for positive-negative asymmetry. *Personality and Social Psychology Bulletin, 24,* 986–93.

Ong, A. D., Bergeman, C. S., Bisconti, T. L., & Wallace, K. A. (2006). Psychological resilience, positive emotions, and successful adaptation to stress in later life. *Journal of Personality and Social Psychology, 91,* 730–49.

Ortony, A., Clore, G. L., & Collins, A. (1988). *The cognitive structure of emotions.* New York: Cambridge University Press.

Ozer, E., & Weiss, D. S. (2004). Who develops posttraumatic stress disorder? *Current Directions in Psychological Science. 13,* 169–72.

Parducci, A. (1995). *Happiness, pleasure, and judgment: The contextual theory and its applications.* Mahwah, NJ: Erlbaum.

Peeters, G., & Czapinski, J. (1990). Positive-negative asymmetry in evaluations: The distinction between affective and informational negativity effects. In W. Stroebe & M. Hewstone (Eds.),

European review of social psychology (Vol. 1, pp. 33–60). New York: Wiley.

Pennebaker, J. W. (1997). Writing about emotional experiences as a therapeutic process. *Psychological Science, 8,* 162–6.

Pennebaker, J. W., Mayne, T. J., & Francis, M. E. (1997). Linguistic predictors of adaptive bereavement. *Journal of Personality and Social Psychology, 72,* 863–71.

Pennebaker, J. W., & Seagal, J. D. (1999). Forming a story: The health benefits of narrative. *Journal of Clinical Psychology, 55,* 1243–54.

Piliavin, J. A. (2003). Doing well by doing good: Benefits for the benefactor. In C. L. M. Keyes, & J. Haidt (Eds.), *Flourishing: Positive psychology and the life well-lived* (pp. 227–47). Washington, DC: APA.

Porter, S., & Peace, K. A. (2007). The scars of memory: A prospective, longitudinal investigation of the consistency of traumatic and positive emotional memories in adulthood. *Psychological Science, 18,* 435–41.

Pratto, F., & John, O. P. (1991). Automatic vigilance: The attention-grabbing power of negative social information. *Journal of Personality and Social Psychology, 61,* 380–91.

Ratner, R. K., Kahn, B. E., & Kahneman, D. (1999). Choosing less-preferred experiences for the sake of variety. *Journal of Consumer Research, 26,* 1–15.

Reis, H. T., Sheldon, K. M., Ryan, R. M., Gable, S. L., & Roscoe, J. (2000). Daily well-being: The role of autonomy, competence, and relatedness. *Personality and Social Psychology Bulletin, 26,* 419–43.

Rolls, B., Rowe, E., Rolls, E., Kingston, B., Megson, A., & Gunary, R. (1981). Variety in a meal enhances food intake in man. *Physiology and Behavior, 26,* 215–21.

Rozin, P., & Royzman, E. B. (2001). Negativity bias, negativity dominance, and contagion. *Personality and Social Psychology Review, 5,* 296–320.

Sandvik, E., Diener, E., & Seidlitz, L. (1993). Subjective well-being: The convergence and stability of self-report and non-self-report measures. *Journal of Personality, 61,* 317–42.

Scarr, S., & McCartney, K. (1983). How people make their own environments: A theory of genotype→environment effects. *Child Development, 54,* 424–35.

Scheier, M. F., & Carver, C. S. (1993). On the power of positive thinking: The benefits of being optimistic. *Current Directions in Psychological Science, 2,* 26–30.

Scheier, M. F., Weintraub, J. K., & Carver, C. S. (1986). Coping with stress: Divergent strategies of optimists and pessimists. *Journal of Personality and Social Psychology, 51,* 1257–64.

Schueller, S. M. (2006). *Personality fit and positive interventions. Is extraversion important?* Unpublished master's thesis, Department of Psychology, University of Pennsylvania.

Schwarz, N., Kahneman, D., & Xu, J. (in press). Global and episodic reports of hedonic experience. In R. Belli, F. Stafford, & D. Alwin (Eds.), *Using calendar and diary methods in life events research. Thousand Oaks,* CA: Sage.

Scitovsky, T. (1976). *The joyless economy:* The psychology of human satisfaction New York: Oxford University Press.

Skowronski, J. J., & Carlston, D. E. (1989). Negativity and extremity biases in impression formation: A review of explanations. *Psychological Bulletin, 105,* 131–42.

Seligman, M. E. P., Rashid, T., & Parks, A. C. (2006). Positive psychotherapy. *American Psychology, 61,* 774–88.

Seligman, M. E., Steen, T. A., Park, N., & Peterson, C. (2005). Positive psychology progress: Empirical validation of interventions. *American Psychologist, 60,* 410–21.

Shakespeare, W. (1564/1616). *The Oxford Shakespeare: The complete works of William Shakespeare.* London: Oxford University Press.

Sheldon, K. M. (2002). The self-concordance model of healthy goal-striving: When personal goals correctly represent the person. In E. L. Deci & R. M. Ryan (Eds.), *Handbook of self-determination research* (pp. 65–86). Rochester, NY: University of Rochester Press.

Sheldon, K. M., & Elliot, A. J. (1999). Goal striving, need-satisfaction, and longitudinal well-being: The Self-Concordance Model. *Journal of Personality and Social Psychology, 76,* 482–97.

Sheldon, K. M., Elliot, A. J., Kim, Y., & Kasser, T. (2001). What is satisfying about satisfying events? Testing 10 candidate psychological needs. *Journal of Personality and Social Psychology, 80,* 325–39.

Sheldon, K. M., & Lyubomirsky, S. (in press). Change your actions, not your circumstances: An experimental test of the Sustainable Happiness Model. In B. Radcliff & A. K. Dutt (Eds.), *Happiness, economics, and politics.* New York: Edward Elgar.

Sheldon, K. M., & Lyubomirsky, S. (2006a). Achieving sustainable gains in happiness: Change your actions, not your circumstances. *Journal of Happiness Studies, 7,* 55–86.

Sheldon, K. M., & Lyubomirsky, S. (2006b). How to increase and sustain positive emotion: The effects of expressing gratitude and visualizing best possible selves. *Journal of Positive Psychology, 1,* 73–82.

Sheldon, K. M., & Lyubomirsky, S. (2007). Is it possible to become happier? (And, if so, how?). *Social and Personality Psychology Compass, 1,* 129–45.

Sheldon, K. M., & Kasser, T. (2008). Psychological threat and extrinsic goal pursuit. *Motivation and Emotion, 32,* 37–45.

Sheldon, K. M., Ryan, R., & Reis, H. T. (1996). What makes for a good day? Competence and autonomy in the day and in the person. *Personality and Social Psychology Bulletin, 22,* 1270–9.

Skinner, E. A., Edge, K., Altman, J., & Sherwood, H. (2003). Searching for the structure of coping: A review and critique of category systems for classifying ways of coping *Psychological Bulletin, 129,* 216–69.

Smith, N. K., Larsen, J. T., Chartrand, R. L., Cacioppo, J. T., Katafiaz, H. A., & Moran, K. E. (2006). Being bad isn't always good: Affective context moderates the attention bias toward negative information. *Journal of Personality and Social Psychology, 90,* 210–20.

Solomon, R. L. (1980). The opponent-process theory of acquired motivation. *American Psychologist, 35,* 691–712.

Strahilevitz, M., & Loewenstein, G. (1998). The effect of ownership history on the valuation of objects. *Journal of Consumer Research, 25,* 276–89.

Suh, E., Diener, E., & Fujita, F. (1996). Events and subjective well-being: Only recent events matter. *Journal of Personality and Social Psychology, 70,* 1091–102.

Suhara, T., Yasuno, F., Sudo, Y., Yamamoto, M., Inouc, M., Okubo, Y., & Suzuki, K. (2001). Dopamine D2 receptor in the insular cortex and the personality trait of novelty seeking. *NeuroImage, 13,* 891–5.

Taylor, S. E. (1991). Asymmetrical effects of positive and negative events: The mobilization–minimization hypothesis. *Psychological Bulletin, 110,* 67–85.

Taylor, S. E., Lichtman, R. R., & Wood, J. V. (1984). Attributions, beliefs about control, and adjustment to breast cancer. *Journal of Personality and Social Psychology, 46,* 489–502.

Tellegen, A., Lykken, D. T., Bouchard, T. J., Wilcox, K. J., Segal, N. L., & Rich, S. (1988). Personality similarity in twins reared apart and together. *Journal of Personality and Social Psychology, 54,* 1031–9.

Tkach, C., & Lyubomirsky, S. (2007). *Spicing up kindness: The role of variety in the effects of practicing kindness on improvements in mood, happiness, and self-evaluations.* Unpublished manuscript, University of California, Riverside.

Tom, S. M., Fox, C. R., Trepel, C., & Poldrack, R. A. (2007). The neural basis of loss aversion in decision-making under risk. *Science, 315,* 515–8.

Tooby, J., & Cosmides, L. (1990). The past explains the present: Emotional adaptations and the structure of ancestral environments. *Ethology and Sociobiology, 11,* 375–424.

Trivers, R. (1971). The evolution of reciprocal altruism. *Quarterly Review of Biology, 46,* 35–57.

Tversky, A., & Griffin, D. (1991). Endowment and contrast in judgments of well-being. In F. Strack, M. Argyle, & N. Schwarz (Eds.), *Subjective well-being: An interdisciplinary perspective* (pp. 101–18). Elmsford, NY: Pergamon Press.

Urry, H. L., Nitschke, J. B., Dolski, I., Jackson, D. C., Dalton, K. M., Mueller, C. J., et al. (2004). Making a life worth living: Neural correlates of well-being. *Psychological Science, 15,* 367–72.

Van Boven, L. (2005). Experientialism, materialism, and the pursuit of happiness. *Review of General Psychology, 9,* 132–42.

Warr, P., Jackson, P., & Banks, M. H. (1988). Unemployment and mental health: Some British studies. *Journal of Social Issues, 44,* 47–68.

Watkins, P. C., Grimm, D. L., & Kolts, R. (2004). Counting your blessings: Positive memories among grateful persons. *Current Psychology: Developmental, Learning, Personality, Social, 23,* 52–67.

Wegner, D. M. (1994). Ironic processes of mental control. *Psychological Review, 101,* 34–52.

Weinstein, N. D. (1982). Community noise problems: Evidence against adaptation. *Journal of Environmental Psychology, 2,* 87–97.

Williams, D. E., & Thompson, J. K. (1993). Biology and behavior: A set-point hypothesis of psychological functioning. *Behavior Modification, 17,* 43–57.

Wilson, T. D., Centerbar, D. B., Kermer, D. A., & Gilbert, D. T. (2005). The pleasures of uncertainty: Prolonging positive moods in ways people do not anticipate. *Journal of Personality and Social Psychology, 88,* 5–21.

Wilson, T. D., & Gilbert, D. T. (2003). Affective forecasting. *Advances in Experimental Social Psychology, 35,* 345–411.

Wilson, T. D., & Gilbert, D. T. (2005). Affective forecasting: Knowing what to want. *Current Directions in Psychological Science, 14,* 131–4.

Wilson, T. D., & Gilbert, D. T. (2008). Explaining away: A model of affective adaptation. *Perspectives on Psychological Science, 3,* 370–86.

PART 5

Coping Processes and Positive and Negative Outcomes

Meaning, Coping, and Health and Well-Being

Crystal L. Park

Abstract

This chapter first describes theory regarding meaning-making in the context of major life stress from the perspective of an integrative meaning-making model, which distinguishes global and situational meaning, the latter of which comprises appraised meaning, meaning-making, and meanings made. Using this model, the empirical evidence regarding how these aspects of meaning influence health and well-being is critically reviewed. Results suggest that global meaning, appraised meaning, meaning-making, and meanings made have potent influences on psychological and physical well-being. However, current research is methodologically limited, and much remains unknown about meaning-making and adjustment. Suggestions for future research conclude the chapter.

Keywords: stress, coping, global meaning, situational meaning, meaning-making, stress-related growth

Introduction

Meaning plays a central role in human life and well-being; this centrality is apparent in the structure and conduct of daily living, and is particularly salient in the face of existential questions (e.g., Dalai Lama, 2000; Frankl, 1963). Discussions of meaning resonate deeply for many people, and meaning remains a perennially popular topic among the lay public as well as philosophers and psychologists (Baumeister, 1991). For example, in recent years, books such as *The Purpose-Driven Life* (Warren, 2002) have been best-sellers, and Frankl's *Meaning in Life*, originally published in 1946, continues to be widely read (Amazon.com, 2009). Until recently, most scholarly inquiries into issues of meaning have been from philosophical, spiritual, or theoretical perspectives. Psychologists have just begun to apply empirical methods to issues of meaning. Although daunting conceptual and methodological challenges remain, the psychological study of meaning has already produced a deeper understanding of this core aspect of human experience.

One important advance is the development of theories of meaning-making in the context of stress (e.g., Bonanno & Kaltman, 1999; Davis, Wortman, Lehman, & Silver, 2000; Davis, Nolen-Hoeksema, & Larson, 1998; Janoff-Bulman, 1989, 1992; Joseph & Linley, 2005; Neimeyer, 2001, 2002; Lepore & Helgeson, 1998; Taylor, 1983; Thompson & Janigian, 1988; see Park, 2010, for a review). The present chapter draws on an integrated model of meaning-making (Park, 2005, 2010; Park & Folkman, 1997) that extends earlier theories to explicate the ways in which meaning influences the coping process and, through coping, influences psychological and physical health. In this model, two levels of meaning are considered: global and situational. Global meaning refers to an individual's broad beliefs, goals, and sense of purpose, while situational meaning refers to meaning regarding a specific occurrence. Both levels of meaning are involved in coping with stressful experiences, and the extent to which appraised meaning is discrepant with global beliefs and goals creates distress. Consider the appraised meaning of receiving a diagnosis of a particular disease. The appraisal would be based on characteristics of that disease (e.g., time course, severity) (Leventhal, Weinman, Leventhal, & Phillips, 2008) as well as an individual's beliefs in his or her ability to manage the disease and the perceived impact of the disease on his or her future life and lifestyle. The extent to which the illness is perceived as inconsistent with the individual's global beliefs about identity (e.g., I live a healthy lifestyle) and health (living a healthy lifestyle protects people from illness) and global goals (I want to live with robust health and without disability) determines the extent to which the diagnosis is distressing. Distress, in turn, initiates coping. In cases of loss or threat, such as illness, coping often involves *meaning-making*, the reappraising of global meaning as well as the meaning of the situation. The meaning-making process can lead to changes or products, termed *meanings made*, such as revised identity, growth, or reappraised situational or global meaning.

Through their multiple and pervasive roles in coping with stress, global meaning, appraised meaning, meaning-making, and meanings made exert powerful effects on psychological and physical well-being. This chapter first describes the components of the meaning-making model and then critically reviews the evidence regarding how these aspects of meaning-making influence health and well-being. Suggestions for future research on remaining questions about meaning and adjustment to life stress conclude the chapter.

The Meaning-Making Model of Coping With Life Stress

The meaning-making model of coping addresses both global and situational aspects of meaning. Global meaning refers to individuals' general orienting systems (Pargament, 1997). Situational meaning consists of initial appraisals of a particular situation as well as the processes by which global and appraised situational meanings are revised and the outcomes of these processes. The components of this meaning-making model are depicted in Figure 12.1.

Global meaning

Global meaning consists of the structures through which people perceive and understand themselves and their environment, interpret their past, anticipate their future, and direct their behavior. Global meaning systems encompass beliefs, goals, and subjective feelings of purpose or meaning in life (Dittman-Kohli & Westerhof, 2000; Park & Folkman, 1997). Global beliefs (also called "assumptive worlds," "personal theories," or "worldviews"; see Koltko-Rivera, 2004, for a review) are the core schemas through which people interpret their experiences, including beliefs regarding fairness, justice, luck, control, coherence, benevolence, and identity. Global goals are internal representations of ultimate concerns (Emmons, 2005), one's desired long-term processes, events, or outcomes (Austin & Vancouver, 1996). Goals encompass desired future states as well as—and perhaps more importantly in the context of coping—states that one already possesses and desires to maintain (Karoly, 1999; Klinger, 1998). Common global goals include relationships, work, health, wealth, knowledge, and achievement (Emmons, 2003). Subjective feelings of meaning refer to having a sense of "meaningfulness" or purpose in life (Klinger, 1977; Reker & Wong, 1988). This sense of meaningfulness comes from seeing one's life as containing those goals that one values as well as feeling one is making adequate progress towards important future goals (Steger, in press; Wrosch, Scheier, Miller, Schulz, & Carver, 2003; cf. King, Hicks, Krull, & Del Gaiso, 2006).

In ordinary circumstances, global meaning is important to mental and physical health. A fair amount of research has demonstrated links between many aspects of global meaning (beliefs, goals, and sense of meaning) and various indices of physical health and psychological well-being (see Park, 2011, for a review). However, global meaning may be particularly important to psychological and physical well-being in times of high stress. Through its influences on individuals' management of stressful situations, global meaning has a potent impact on their health and emotional well-being. When encountering potentially stressful situations, global meaning informs individuals as they appraise the significance of those situations and their responses to them (Lazarus & Folkman, 1984).

Situational meaning: The meaning of potentially stressful encounters

Upon encountering potentially stressful situations, people appraise them along a variety of dimensions, such as personal relevance, controllability, and likely implications (Lazarus & Folkman, 1984). These appraised meanings of particular events are to some

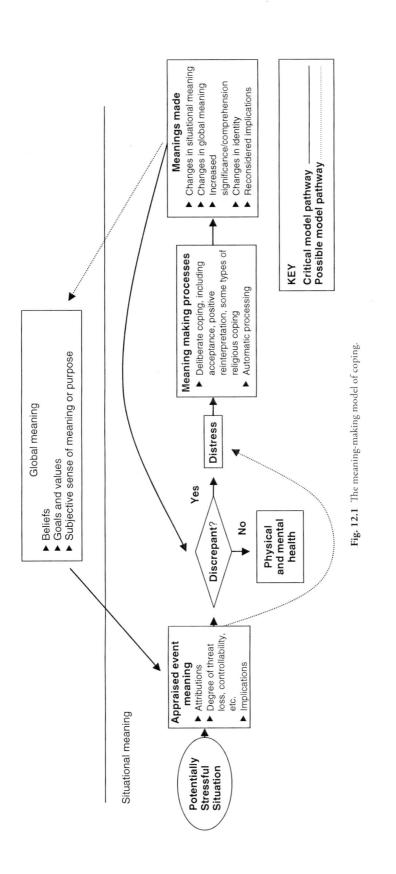

Fig. 12.1 The meaning-making model of coping.

extent determined by the specifics of those situations, but are also greatly informed by individuals' global meaning. For example, some types of global meaning, such as high mastery or control beliefs, may minimize situational stress appraisals (Peacock & Wong, 1996; Weinstein & Quigley, 2006).

Stress as discrepancy between global and situational meaning

The meaning-making model is predicated on the notion that individuals experience stress when they perceive discrepancies between their global meaning (i.e., what they believe and desire) and their appraised meaning of a particular situation (Park & Folkman, 1997). This discrepancy-related distress motivates individuals to somehow resolve their problems and dissipate the resultant negative emotions (Park, 2010). For example, being on the receiving end of a romantic breakup may violate an individual's beliefs in the world (or at least important relationships) as being stable, controllable, predictable, benevolent, and fair. In addition, an individual may experience discrepancies between the breakup and his or her goals of being in a committed relationship, being a good romantic partner, and growing old together. All of these discrepancies would be expected to generate significant distress and prompt the individual's coping efforts (Park, 2005).

Meaning-making coping

Resolving stressful events entails reducing discrepancies between appraised meanings and global meanings (Greenberg, 1995; Janoff-Bulman, 1992; Joseph & Linley, 2005). Discrepancies can be reduced in many ways, and, to this end, people engage in many types of coping (e.g., Manne, Ostroff, Fox, Grana, & Winkel, 2009; Park, Edmondson, Blank, & Fenster, 2008). People may engage in problem-focused coping, taking direct actions to reduce the discrepancy by changing the conditions that create or maintain the problem. Continuing with the breakup example, the individual might try to resurrect the relationship or find another partner, which would resolve at least some of the discrepancies. When encountering stress, individuals can also engage in emotion-focused coping, much of which is targeted at directly alleviating distress, albeit temporarily, by disengaging mentally or behaviorally (e.g., focusing on some distraction). Emotion-focused coping, by definition, does not reduce discrepancies and may be why it is generally associated with distress (Aldwin, 2007).

Stressful situations vary in the extent to which they are amenable to problem-focused coping (e.g., Moos & Holahan, 2007; Park, Armeli, & Tennen, 2004), the type of coping typically considered most adaptive (Aldwin, 2007). In low-control situations such as trauma and loss, meaning-making coping is considered to be particularly relevant and potentially more adaptive because these situations are not amenable to direct repair or problem-solving (Mikulincer & Florian, 1996). In contrast to problem-focused coping, which seeks to directly change the situation, or emotion-focused coping, which aims to alleviate emotional distress, meaning-making refers to approach-oriented intrapsychic efforts to reduce discrepancies between appraised and global meaning. Meaning-focused coping aims to reduce discrepancy by changing either the very meaning of the stressor itself (appraised meaning) or by changing one's global beliefs and goals; either way, the goal of the coping is to improve the fit between the appraised meaning of the stressor and global meaning.

The parameters of what constitutes meaning-making coping are fuzzy. In a study of bereavement, Folkman (1997) identified meaning-making coping as "(a) using positive reappraisal, through which individuals find meaning by interpreting the situation in terms of deeply held values and beliefs; (b) revising goals and planning goal-directed problem-focused coping, which fosters meaning in terms of a sense of purpose and control; and (c) activating spiritual beliefs and experiences, through which individuals find existential meaning" (p. 1216).

However, in addition to these coping strategies explicitly assessed by standard coping inventories, other meaning-making strategies have also been identified. For example, discrepancies between situational and global meaning can be reduced through comparison processes, including making downward social comparisons with less fortunate others or even manufacturing hypothetical normative standards or worse scenarios so that one feels relatively advantaged in comparison (Buunk & Gibbons, 2007; Greenberg, 1995; Taylor, Wood, & Lichtman, 1983; White & Lehman, 2005). The appraised meaning of a situation can be modified by selectively focusing on its positive attributes and identifying benefits or reminding oneself of those benefits (Folkman, 2008; Tennen & Affleck, 2002). Making reattributions such as finding a more acceptable reason for an event's occurrence can also transform the meaning of a situation (Kubany & Manke, 1995; Westphal & Bonanno, 2007).

Meaning-focused coping efforts can also be directed towards goals, such as downgrading one's aspirations or noticing heretofore ignored aspects of alternatives that make them more or less attractive (Brandtstädter, 2002; Folkman, 2008).

Further, coping is usually conceptualized as involving conscious, deliberate effort (Tennen, Affleck, Armeli, & Carney, 2000), but boundaries between deliberate and more automatic types of meaning-making are difficult to distinguish (Folkman & Moskowitz, 2007). Meaning-making has often been theorized to occur below individuals' conscious awareness (e.g., Epstein, 1991; Horowitz, 1992), and constructs such as intrusive thoughts (Horowitz, Wilner, & Alvarez, 1979), which by their nature are unbidden (i.e., conscious but not deliberate), are often considered to be part of meaning-making as well (e.g., Creamer et al., 1992; Lepore & Helgeson, 1998). In addition, even when individuals deliberately employ meaning-making strategies, research has not established whether they are aware of the underlying motive of those strategies as discrepancy reduction. These important theoretical issues also have practical implications in that they limit researchers' ability to directly assess the central constructs of meaning-making. This methodological limitation means that caution is required in interpreting all research conducted to date on meaning-making.

Meanings made

While meaning-making is widely considered essential for adjusting to stressful events (e.g., Gillies & Neimeyer, 2006) and has therefore been the focus of much research, meaning-making *per se* may not be enough. According to the meaning-making model, meaning-making should lead to better adjustment *only to the extent that it enables individuals to make meaning in or through their stressful event* (Park & Folkman, 1997; Roberts, Lepore, & Helgeson, 2005). In other words, meaning-making is helpful to the extent that it produces a satisfactory product (i.e., *meaning made*) (Segerstrom, Stanton, Alden, & Shortridge, 2003).

The outcomes of the meaning-making process involve changes in global or situational meaning. As illustrated in Figure 12.1, individuals may make many different types of meaning through their meaning-making processes. Among the most commonly discussed meanings made are a sense of having "made sense" or found resolution (e.g., Davis et al., 1998), a sense of acceptance (e.g., Pakenham, 2007), causal understanding (e.g., Janoff-Bulman & Frantz, 1997), reconstructed or transformed identity that integrates the stressful experience into one's identity (Gillies & Neimeyer, 2006), reappraised or transformed meaning of the stressor (e.g., Manne et al., 2009), changed global beliefs (e.g., Park, 2005), changed global goals (e.g., Thompson & Janigian, 1988), restoration or changed sense of meaning in life (e.g., Janoff-Bulman & Frantz, 1997), and perceptions of growth or positive life changes, the latter of which is the most commonly assessed meaning made (e.g., Calhoun & Tedeschi, 2006).

Current Review of Literature on Meaning and Adjustment in the Context of Stress

How do these various aspects of meaning influence individuals' health and well-being as they confront stressful encounters? This section reviews the empirical literature regarding links between meaning-making and well-being. As will be seen, research in this area has produced inconsistent results, precluding definitive conclusions. Although much remains to be learned, this area appears to hold great promise for understanding human adaptation to highly stressful experiences.

Global meaning in the context of stressful encounters

All three aspects of global meaning (beliefs, goals, and subjective sense of purpose) can play important roles in individuals' responses to stressful life events. The following sections review the literature to date on these influences in the process of coping with life stress.

GLOBAL BELIEFS IN THE CONTEXT OF STRESSFUL ENCOUNTERS

Certain aspects of global meaning are particularly helpful when individuals face stressors and challenges. In this regard, mastery or control beliefs, the extent to which individuals perceive they have control over the circumstances of their lives, have received much research attention (see Lachman, 2006, for a review). Mastery beliefs can have salutary effects for individuals facing life difficulties. For example, in a sample of community-dwelling elders, a sense of mastery mediated the effects of both earlier- and later-life economic hardships on their current physical and mental health (Pudrovska, Schieman, Pearlin, & Nguyen, 2005), and in a sample of adults with rheumatoid arthritis, mastery predicted lower levels of pain, stress, fatigue, and blood pressure (Younger, Finan, Zautra, Davis, & Reich, 2008). Some physiological pathways through which mastery operates in highly stressful situations have been identified. In a study of Alzheimer's care-givers, mastery moderated the effects of caregiving stress and life events on immune functioning (Mausbach et al., 2006) as well as on antigens implicated in the development of cardiovascular disease (Mausbach et al., 2008).

Other global beliefs are also related to health in stressful times. For example, in one study, higher just world beliefs were related to better physical and psychological recovery following myocardial infarction (Agrawal & Dalal, 1993), and in a sample of mothers whose child was undergoing a bone marrow transplant, higher beliefs in chance were related to better physical health but unrelated to mental health (Rini et al., 2004). In a sample of symptomatic HIV/AIDS patients, beliefs in benevolence and luck were related to less distress and higher mental health-related quality of life, while beliefs in justice were related to higher physical health-related quality of life (Farber et al., 2000).

The effects of global beliefs on health and well-being may be mediated by the types of appraisals they predispose individuals to make when confronting potentially stressful situations. For example, beliefs in control or fairness may allow people to perceive situations as more controllable and challenging and to maintain their views of the world as orderly and coherent, reducing the extent of global meaning disruption (Park, 2010). In addition, positive global beliefs may lead individuals to appraise events as challenges they can successfully meet, thus encouraging them to persist in their coping efforts (Aldwin, 2007; Folkman & Moskowitz, 2007). Surprisingly few studies, however, have traced the pathway from global beliefs through situational meaning to well-being. One experimental study found that participants who had high levels of just world beliefs appraised a laboratory-based stressor as less threatening, which was reflected in lower levels of autonomic reactivity (Blascovich & Tomaka, 1997).

GLOBAL GOALS IN THE CONTEXT OF STRESSFUL ENCOUNTERS

In addition to the powerful role of global beliefs in moderating stress, studies have illustrated how having a strong commitment to core values or goals can buffer stress (Jim, Richardson, Golden-Kreutz, & Andersen, 2006). An extreme example is commitment to a cause that can lead to being subjected to torture. One study found that Turkish political activists had been subjected to relatively more severe torture compared with non-activist prisoners, but showed lower levels of psychopathology and post-traumatic stress disorder symptoms. These authors concluded that having a strong sense of commitment to a cause greater than themselves had helped these torture victims to better endure their ordeal (Basoglu et al., 1997).

SENSE OF MEANING IN LIFE IN THE CONTEXT OF STRESSFUL ENCOUNTERS

The subjective sense of meaning in life is related to many different aspects of well-being, including lower levels of depression and negative affect (e.g., Jim & Andersen, 2007) and higher levels of happiness (e.g., Debats, van der Lubbe, & Wezeman, 1993) and physical well-being (e.g., Scheier et al., 2006). A sense of meaning in life appears to be particularly important in times of major stress or illness, including cancer (Jim & Andersen, 2007; Simonelli et al., 2008), rheumatoid arthritis (Verduin et al., 2008), surgery (Smith & Zautra, 2004), and immigration (Pan, Wong, Chan, & Joubert, 2008).

Stressful encounters as violations of global meaning and adjustment

According to the meaning-making model, distress is created when the meaning assigned to a stressful situation violates global meaning. A positive relationship between the appraisals of events as threats or losses, which essentially *imply* violations of global meaning (i.e., a particular view of the world or a valued goal is being threatened or has been taken away), and distress is well documented (Aldwin, 2007).

Recent research provides more direct evidence regarding the impact of perceived violations of global beliefs on well-being. For example, for a sample of cancer survivors, greater perceptions of their cancer as violating their beliefs in the fairness of the world were related to more subsequent distress (Park et al., 2008), and in a sample of college students dealing with loss, greater perceptions of the loss as violating their global beliefs were related to higher subsequent levels of distress (Park, 2008).

Relative to belief violation, much more research has directly focused on the impact of stressors as violating goals, most of which has been in the context of illness. For example, a study of newly diagnosed gastrointestinal cancer patients found that greater discrepancies between the importance of life values and perceived attainment of them were associated with high levels of anxiety and depression (Nordin, Wasteson, Hoffman, Glimelius, & Sjoden, 2001). A study of chronically ill patients found that greater goal discrepancies (the extent to which patients appraised their goals as not feasible or not important) were associated with more anxiety and depressive symptoms and lower quality of life (Kuijer & De Ridder, 2003), and the extent to which a sample of adults living with HIV perceived HIV as hindering their higher-order goals was related to lower quality of life and higher levels of depressive symptoms (van der Veek, Kraaji, van Koppen, Garnefski, & Joekes, 2007). Additionally, a study of myocardial infarction patients found that the extent to which the myocardial infarction was perceived to violate goals predicted increased depression and lower quality of life 4 months later (Boersma, Maes, & Van Elderen, 2005), and a daily diary study of women with fibromyalgia found that the extent to which they perceived their pain and fatigue as hindering their health and fitness goals was related to subsequent deterioration of positive (but not negative) affect (Affleck et al., 1998).

These results of these studies converge on the notion that highly stressful situations such as serious illness are commonly perceived as violating critically important goals, creating a highly stressful state that is reflected in decrements in physical and emotional well-being. Although sparser, research on the impact of belief violation is also consistent with this notion.

Meaning-making and well-being
Meaning-making coping is widely thought to lead to better adjustment, and many studies have examined the links between meaning-making and a variety of well-being outcomes. Some studies assessed meaning as intrusive thoughts or as reports of "searching for meaning" from stressful encounters. Among these, some have demonstrated that searching for meaning is related to better adjustment. For example, in a cross-sectional study, childhood sexual assault survivors' meaning-making efforts were related to more successful coping and less negative affect (Harvey, Orbuch, Chwalisz, & Garwood, 1991). Favorable findings have also been reported in longitudinal studies, which allow for the examination of the effects of earlier meaning-making on subsequent adjustment. For office workers who had experienced a shooting episode, meaning-making (assessed as intrusive thoughts) was related to subsequent reductions in distress 1 year later (Creamer et al., 1992). A longitudinal study of parents who lost children to sudden infant death syndrome found that while meaning-making related negatively to adjustment cross-sectionally, it was longitudinally related to higher levels of well-being

and lower levels of distress (McIntosh, Silver, & Wortman, 1993). Studies of psychotherapy have also found that meaning-making is related to better adjustment. For example, Hayes and her colleagues (Hayes, Beevers, Feldman, Laurenceau, & Perlman, 2005) found that higher levels of meaning-making (assessed by coded qualitative data) were related to subsequent reductions in depression and increases in perceived growth and self-esteem.

On the other hand, meaning-making coping has also been related to poorer adjustment in many cross-sectional studies. For example, in a study of breast cancer survivors and healthy controls, searching for meaning was correlated with poorer mental functioning and more negative affect; for the cancer survivors, it was also correlated with less positive affect (Tomich & Helgeson, 2002). Such adverse effects have also been reported in longitudinal studies. In a sample of recent widows and widowers, searching for meaning was related to poorer subsequent adjustment (Bonnano, Wortman & Nesse, 2004). Similarly, searching for meaning predicted subsequent increased negative affect 7 months later in breast cancer survivors (Lepore & Kernan, 2009) and poorer mental health and physical health in prostate cancer survivors (Roberts et al., 2005).

These studies explicitly focusing on meaning-making by using measures that ask about attempts to make meaning yield results that are quite varied and discrepant. To further muddy the waters, it should be noted that a broader definition of meaning-making includes a variety of coping strategies (e.g., as suggested by Folkman, 1997), necessitating consideration of the wider literature regarding, for example, effects of the use of coping involving positive reinterpretation, religious coping, emotional social support, acceptance, and emotional processing coping on adjustment. The coping literature is vast and complex (Aldwin, 2007; Skinner, Edge, Altman, & Sherwood, 2003), precluding simple conclusions. It appears that meaning-related strategies are often helpful in adjusting to high-magnitude stressors (e.g., Park, Folkman, & Bostrom, 2001; see Folkman & Moskowitz, 2004, and Aldwin, 2007, for reviews). For example, for a sample of gastrointestinal, colorectal, and lung cancer patients, meaning-focused coping (positive reinterpretation and acceptance) predicted better subsequent emotional and social (but not physical) well-being (Boehmer, Luszczynska, & Schwarzer, 2007). However, a meta-analysis found positive reappraisal to be unrelated to physical well-being and inversely related to psychological well-being (Penley, Tomaka, & Wiebe, 2002).

These mixed findings regarding whether meaning-making is related to better adjustment may be due to the study differences, such as in samples and time frames. Assessment strategies are particularly problematic: The meaning-making literature has been notoriously poor at translating the rich theoretical definitions into operational ones (Park, 2010). In addition, as noted above, it may be that until meaning-making results in some change or product that reduces the discrepancy between appraised and global meaning, meaning-making attempts may be positively related to distress (Bonanno, Papa, Lalande, Zhang, & Noll, 2005). Over time, meaning-making (and concomitant decreases in discrepancies) might more consistently predict better adjustment.

Meanings made and adjustment to stressful life events

An intriguing aspect of the meaning-making model is the notion that meaning-making will be helpful primarily when some adaptive resolution is achieved or meaning made through the process (Davis et al., 2000; Manne et al., 2009). Segerstrom et al. (2003) noted, "the best outcomes are likely to result when people engage in searching that leads to solving, especially when they find positive solutions such as meaning" (p. 212). Thus, the process of meaning-making may be helpful to the extent that it is related to actually *making* meaning, while reports of searching for meaning without successfully finding it may reflect a lack of adequate meaning made (Bower Kemeny, Taylor, & Fahey, 1998).

Many studies have examined the products of meaning-making without explicitly assessing meaning-making, instead implicitly assuming that meaning-making has occurred, often asking participants about the "sense" or "meaning" that they have made or found. Many of these studies have been conducted using cross-sectional correlation designs, limiting their ability to determine temporal order (i.e., does "made meaning" lead to psychological adjustment, or vice versa?). Cross-sectional studies have often reported positive relations between meaning made and adjustment. For example, among bereaved college students, having "made sense" was inversely related to complicated grief (Currier, Holland, & Neimeyer, 2006), and in a community sample of bereaved family members, having found meaning was related to better subsequent adjustment (Davis et al., 1998). However, other studies reported no relation between meaning made and adjustment (e.g., Lepore & Kernan, 2009). For example, for

parents of a child with Asperger syndrome, "having made sense" of their child's disorder was unrelated to their levels of distress, health, or social adjustment (Pakenham, Sofronoff, & Samios, 2004). Having answered the question of "Why me?" has also sometimes (e.g., Affleck et al., 1985) but not always (e.g., Davis & Morgan, 2008) been related to adjustment.

However, as discussed earlier, meaning-making leads to other products in addition to "having made sense," including stress-related growth, changes in identity, and changes in reappraised situational and global meaning. Studies have found that many of these meanings made are positively related to adjustment. To date, the meaning made of stress-related growth has received the vast majority of attention (Park, 2010). Several recent literature reviews provide useful summaries of the research on associations between growth and well-being (Algoe & Stanton, 2008; Bower, Low, Moskowitz, Sepah, & Epel, 2008; Helgeson, Reynolds, & Tomich, 2006; Stanton, Bower, & Low, 2006).

In general, stress-related growth has been positively related to well-being across an array of studies diverse in samples and designs, although not all studies have demonstrated this link. A meta-analysis of growth following a wide range of stressors found that, in the aggregate, growth was associated with less depression and more positive well-being but also with more intrusive and avoidant thoughts about the stressor (Helgeson et al., 2006). However, growth was unrelated to anxiety, global distress, quality of life, and subjective reports of physical health.

Focusing on physical outcomes and potential physiological pathways, Bower et al. (2008) concluded, "Overall, the literature on benefit finding and health supports the hypothesis that individuals who are able to find benefit following stressful experiences show positive changes in various health-related outcomes, including decreases in morbidity and mortality and positive changes in immune and neuroendocrine function" (p. 226). For example, researchers have found that stress-related growth was related to CD4 counts in HIV-positive adolescents (Milam, 2006) and reduced cortisol levels in early-stage breast cancer patients (Cruess et al., 2000). Reviewing longitudinal studies examining growth specifically from chronic illness, Algoe and Stanton (2008) concluded that the effects of growth were stronger and more consistently favorable for physical aspects of adjustment, especially those directly related to the illness (e.g., pain for those with arthritis) than for psychological outcomes (e.g., depressive symptoms).

Although other meanings made have received less attention in the literature, there is some evidence that they are also related to better adjustment. For example, in a sample of people who lost their homes in a fire, a more benign reappraised meaning of their loss was related to less distress (Thompson, 1985). Positive shifts in global meaning are also related to better adjustment (e.g., Rini et al., 2004). In one study, coded narratives of high school students demonstrated that transformations in their understanding of themselves and the world as a result of a life turning point were related to subsequent increases in optimism, generativity, and identity development (McLean & Pratt, 2006). A study of sexual assault survivors found that positive shifts in both situational (i.e., less self-blame for their sexual assaults) and global (i.e., more positive global beliefs) meaning were related to less distress over a 2-year period (Koss & Figueredo, 2004).

In sum, these results are consistent with the meaning-making model of coping, in that having made meaning has often been found to be related to better adjustment to a variety of stressors. However, a true test of this aspect of the model must explicitly address the question of whether meaning-making is associated with adjustment to the extent that meaning is made. This question can only be addressed by studies that examined both meaning-making and meaning made and the relationships *between* meaning-making and meaning made as well as their conjoint relations with adjustment (i.e., mediator or moderator effects).

Studies that have examined the entire linkage of meaning-making→meaning made→adjustment have produced inconsistent results. Meaning-making has generally been linked with distress, but also with meaning made, which has been related to better adjustment. Many of these studies concluded that participants who reported searching for and finding meaning were no better off than those who never searched, but that both groups were better off than those who searched without finding, such as the bereaved who had lost a spouse or child in a motor vehicle accident (Davis et al., 2000). Other studies have even reported that those who never searched for meaning were better adjusted than those who searched, regardless of whether they reported that their search resulted in "meaning made." For example, in a sample of chronic tinnitus sufferers, searching for meaning (asking "Why me?") was related to more distress, even for those who had found an answer to their search (Davis & Morgan, 2008). Several studies suggest that meaning-making is always negative, but its effects can be somewhat mitigated if meaning is found. For example, in a study of bereaved college students, searching for meaning was uniformly related to distress and lower levels of well-being. However, for those students who were searching for meaning but also reported either having "made sense" or experienced growth from their loss, the relationship between searching and distress was somewhat diminished (Michael & Snyder, 2005).

However, numerous other studies have reported that meaning-making resulting in meaning made is indeed related to better adjustment compared with not having searched. Many of these studies have been conducted in the context of bereavement. For example, a study of bereaved HIV-positive men showed that searching for meaning that led to finding positive meaning from bereavement (defined as experiencing a major shift in values, priorities, or perspectives) was related to better physical health (less rapid declines in CD4 T-cell levels and lower rates of AIDS-related mortality) (Bower et al., 1998). However, those who searched and did not find meaning did not differ from those who did not search (Bower et al., 1998). Similarly, a study of bereaved individuals found that those who did not search and those who searched and found meaning experienced less grief than those who searched but did not find meaning; further, those who searched and found meaning were better off than those who had never searched in terms of post-traumatic stress disorder symptoms (Tolstikova et al., 2005).

Evidence for meaning-making leading to meaning made as adaptive has also been shown in other samples. For example, studies have shown that in longer-term cancer survivors, meaning-making was also related to meaning made, which was related to better adjustment cross-sectionally (Fife, 1995) and longitudinally (Park et al., 2008). Similar findings were reported for middle-aged women going through a difficult life experience (Pals, 2006) and for a nationally representative sample of adults following the 9/11 terrorist attacks (Updegraff, Silver, & Holman, 2008).

A review of these findings, central to the question of whether meaning-making efforts are helpful to the extent that they are related to the actual *making* of meaning, provides little clarity. Ample studies, though clearly not all, have demonstrated links between meaning-making (variously defined) and poorer mental and physical adjustment.

Yet very few of these studies have provided evidence regarding whether these reported meaning-making attempts are unhelpful or whether they simply signify a lack of resolution or satisfactory meaning made. The handful of studies that have more explicitly addressed the meaning-making/meaning made/adjustment linkage have produced conflicting results.

Why the discrepant findings? Some of the inconsistency may be due to the different methods, samples, time frames, and statistical techniques used in studying these issues. In addition, different types of meaning-making may be more or less helpful in achieving meaning made. Further, different types of meaning made may differentially help people adapt to highly stressful events. For example, a study of partners of women with breast cancer examined three different types of meaning-making and three different types of meaning made. Results suggested that specific types of meaning-making and meanings made differentially influence their impact on distress (Manne et al., 2009). Only a handful of the study's hypothesized relations of meaning-making and meaning made were supported in their data; among them, searching for meaning was related to increasing cancer-specific distress over time, an effect somewhat attenuated by having found meaning. In addition, for those using emotional expression, positive reappraisal (their [perhaps questionable] proxy for having found a more positive perspective on the cancer) was related to less global distress over time.

Conclusion

This overview of theory and research reveals a complex picture of meaning in the context of coping with stressful life events. The meaning-making model describes a process that, in some form or another, *must* occur (Fillipp, 1999). In other words, in the course of a lifetime, individuals encounter a variety of stressors of magnitudes small and large that are incongruent with their fundamental beliefs about themselves and the world and their goals regarding what they want to occur. They must adjust to these adverse circumstances, and those circumstances that are not amenable to active problem-solving can be resolved only through a transformation of meaning. Theorists have already made a great deal of progress in fleshing out this model and its various components (see Park, 2010, for a review). However, at present, the empirical research examining components of this theoretical model falls far short of giving this model an adequate test.

More sophisticated research is urgently needed to evaluate and refine the meaning-making model as it is currently proposed. In this final section, suggestions are offered for future research directions towards this end.

Future Directions
Improve measurement of meaning-related constructs

Before research on meaning-making can move forward, the methodology requires major improvements. A review of the research makes glaringly obvious the large gap between the rich theoretical constructs of meaning and meaning-making and their actual measurement in extant empirical work. Better measurement approaches to more thoroughly capture constructs relevant to meaning-making are sorely needed to allow the kinds of research from which solid conclusions can be drawn.

Although researchers have developed reasonably good measures of global meaning and appraised situational meaning, there are few measures of discrepancy or violation of global beliefs and goals, which is a core aspect of the meaning-making model. Few studies have examined discrepancies between situational and global meaning (e.g., Boersma, Maes, & Joekes, 2005; Park, 2005, 2008), and in fact, whether individuals can meaningfully report directly on discrepancies between their global and situational meaning remains unknown. Creative approaches to capture discrepancy are needed; these may include daily diaries, narrative coding, and perhaps experimental approaches to assess global meaning violations (e.g., Plaks, Grant, & Dweck, 2005).

Researchers must distinguish between meaning-making and meaning made (e.g., Park et al., 2008; Updegraff et al., 2008) and develop better measures of both. Measures of meaning-making must be solidly based on the theoretical constructs they purport to assess. Is meaning-making deliberate coping? Does meaning-making involve unconscious or automatic processes? According to the meaning-making model, all of these would be aspects of meaning-making, and all should be included in assessment tools designed to assess meaning-making. There are many types of meaning made, and therefore, tools to assess meanings made should assess changes in global and situational meaning, identity change, resolution, and other aspects of made meaning in addition to growth and self-reports of having "made sense," which are the most common current ways of assessing meaning made (Park, 2010).

Improve research designs for investigating meaning-related phenomena

Once conceptual and assessment issues are adequately resolved, studies relying on longitudinal research designs using these measures should be implemented. These studies are necessary to more adequately explore the processes of meaning-making from and adjustment to a variety of highly stressful events. As noted above, much of the extant literature on meaning-making relied on cross-sectional designs, which are woefully inadequate for capturing the dynamic and complex processes that unfold over long periods of time. Multiple assessments are necessary to illuminate important issues such as the timing of these processes, group trajectories, and individual differences. Ideally, prospective studies should be carried out, although the unpredictable nature of highly stressful events makes this an ideal but difficult design to implement.

As researchers design future studies of meaning-making, they must take care to assess the range of meaning-related constructs in order to truly test the meaning-making model. In other words, they should incorporate the multiple constructs depicted in Figure 12.1. This inclusive approach will then allow examination of issues such as whether meaning-making is particularly helpful when meanings are made, whether different types of meaning-making lead to different types of meaning made and are differentially related to adjustment, and so on.

Examine resilience versus vulnerability of global meaning systems

Certain types of global meaning may be less vulnerable to violation at the situational level than other types (Park, 2010). For example, having beliefs that are not overly positive and that acknowledge that negative, random, and unfair events can "happen even to good, careful people" may be protective (p. 277, Thompson & Janigian, 1988). Understanding more about the contents of specific beliefs, as well as the coherence and flexibility of individuals' global meaning (Pöhlmann et al., 2006), will be helpful in understanding the vast individual differences in meaning-making processes and adjustment, and should provide important clues regarding stress-resistance and resilience.

Examine interpersonal aspects of meaning-making

At its most basic level, meaning-making occurs within an individual's mind, and thus that is the level at which it must ultimately be understood.

However, meaning-making can be facilitated (or impeded) by interpersonal interactions. For example, talking with others and getting their perspectives can direct meaning-making (e.g., Clark, 1993). Harvey and his colleagues noted that "not only in personal, private work on one's story, but also in public social interaction, the individual will need to confide part of his or her story to close others over time in order to assimilate different major stressors and losses" (p. 235, Harvey, Carlson, Huff, & Green, 2001). Interpersonal contexts in which interpersonal interaction can influence meaning-making include the family (e.g., Nadeau, 2001; Patterson & Garwick, 1994) and psychotherapy (e.g., Hayes et al., 2007).

Several studies have found that interpersonal contexts that validate the individual and his or her expression of the stressful situation can facilitate meaning-making (e.g., Lepore, Silver, Wortman, & Wayment, 1996). For example, an analysis of a subsample of the parents who lost children to sudden infant death syndrome in the study cited earlier found that early meaning-making was related to subsequent decreased depressive symptoms only for mothers who had unconstrained social relationships; for socially constrained mothers, meaning-making was related to *increased* depressive symptoms (Lepore et al., 1996). While these results suggest the importance of the interpersonal context in which meaning-making may occur, much remains to be learned about social influences on meaning-making.

Design and test meaning-making interventions

Meaning-making plays a central role in the coping and adjustment of most people facing major life stressors. Thus, addressing meaning may be a fruitful approach to clinical interventions aimed at helping people recover from these highly stressful experiences. Many current psychotherapies involve, explicitly or implicitly, meaning-making with an effort towards meaning made (e.g., Hayes et al., 2007). However, to date, only a handful of interventions explicitly targeting issues of meaning-making have been developed and tested in clinical samples. For example, Lee and her colleagues (Lee, Cohen, Edgar, Laizner, & Gagnon, 2006) designed and tested an intervention to promote breast cancer survivors' exploration of existential issues and their cancer experiences through the use of meaning-making coping strategies. Participants receiving the intervention had higher levels of self-esteem, optimism, and self-efficacy than did the control group after controlling for baseline scores, demonstrating the effectiveness of an explicit meaning-making therapy. However, these intervention efforts are in the early stages and much remains to be learned about whether and how meaning-making can be facilitated through interventions and whether this meaning-making is helpful (Chan, Ho, & Chan, 2007).

References

Affleck, G., Tennen, H., & Gershman, K. (1985). Cognitive adaptations to high-risk infants: The search for mastery, meaning, and protection from future harm. *American Journal of Mental Deficiency, 89*, 653–6.

Affleck, G., Tennen, H., Urrows, S., Higgins, P., Abeles, M., Hall, C., et al. (1998). Fibromyalgia and women's pursuit of personal goals: A daily process analysis. *Health Psychology, 17*, 40–7.

Agrawal, M., & Dalal, A. K. (1993). Beliefs about the world and recovery from myocardial infarction. *Journal of Social Psychology, 13*, 385–94.

Aldwin, C. M. (2007). *Stress, coping, and development: An integrative approach.* New York: Guilford.

Algoe, S. B., & Stanton, A. L. (2008). Is benefit-finding good for individuals with chronic illness? In C. L. Park, S. Lechner, A. Stanton, & M. Antoni (Eds.), *Positive life change in the context of medical illness: Can the experience of serious illness lead to transformation* (pp. 173–93). Washington, DC: APA Press.

Amazon.com: http://www.amazon.com/Mans-Search-Meaning-Viktor-Frankl/dp/080701429X/ref=sr_1_1?ie=UTF8&s=books&qid=1241616569&sr=1-1. Accessed May 6, 2009.

Austin, J. T., & Vancouver, J. B. (1996). Goal constructs in psychology: Structure, process, and content. *Psychological Bulletin, 120*, 338–75.

Baumeister, R. F. (1991). *Meanings in life.* New York: Guilford.

Basoglu, M., Mineka, S., Paker, M., Aker, T., Livanou, M., & Gok, S. (1997). Psychological preparedness for trauma as a protective factor in survivors of torture. *Psychological Medicine, 27*, 1421–33.

Boehmer, S., Luszczynska, A., & Schwarzer, R. (2007). Coping and quality of life after tumor surgery: Personal and social resources promote different domains of quality of life. *Anxiety, Stress & Coping, 20*, 61–75.

Boersma, S. N., Maes, S., & Joekes, K. (2005). Goal disturbance in relation to anxiety, depression, and health-related quality of life after myocardial infarction. *Quality of Life Research: An International Journal of Quality of Life Aspects of Treatment, Care and Rehabilitation, 14*, 2265–75.

Boersma, S. N., Maes, S., & van Elderen, T. (2005). Goal disturbance predicts health-related quality of life and depression 4 months after myocardial infarction. *British Journal of Health Psychology, 10*, 615–30.

Bonanno, G. A., & Kaltman, S. (1999). Toward an integrative perspective on bereavement. *Psychological Bulletin, 125*, 760–76.

Bonanno, G. A., Papa, A., Lalande, K., Zhang, N., & Noll, J. G. (2005). Grief processing and deliberate grief avoidance: A prospective comparison of bereaved spouses and parents in the united stated and the People's Republic of China. *Journal of Consulting and Clinical Psychology, 73*, 86–98.

Bonanno, G. A., Wortman, C. B., & Nesse, R. M. (2004). Prospective patterns of resilience and maladjustment during widowhood. *Psychology and Aging, 19*, 260–71.

Bower, J. E., Low, C. A., Moskowitz, J. T., Sepah, S., & Epel, E. (2008). Benefit finding and physical health: positive psychological changes and enhanced allostasis. *Social and Personality Psychology Compass, 2*, 223–44.

Bower, J. E., Kemeny, M. E., Taylor, S. E., & Fahey, J. L. (1998). Cognitive processing, discovery of meaning, CD4 decline, and AIDS-related mortality among bereaved HIV-seropositive men. *Journal of Consulting and Clinical Psychology, 66*, 979–86.

Brandtstädter, J. (2002). Searching for paths to successful development and aging: Integrating developmental and action-theoretical perspectives. In L. Pulkkinen & A. Caspi (Eds.), *Paths to successful development: Personality in the life course* (pp. 380–408). New York: Cambridge University Press.

Buunk, A. P., & Gibbons, F. X. (2007). Social comparison: The end of a theory and the emergence of a field. *Organizational Behavior and Human Decision Processes, 102*, 3–21.

Calhoun, L. G., & Tedeschi, R. G. (Eds.) (2006). *Handbook of posttraumatic growth: Research & practice.* Mahwah, NJ: Erlbaum.

Chan, T. H. Y., Ho, R. T. H., & Chan, C. L. W. (2007). Developing an outcome measurement for meaning-making intervention with Chinese cancer patients. *Psycho-Oncology, 16*, 843–50.

Clark, L. F. (1993). Stress and the cognitive-conversational benefits of social interaction. *Journal of Social and Clinical Psychology, 12*, 25–55.

Creamer, M., Burgess, P., & Pattison, P. (1992). Reaction to trauma: A cognitive processing model. *Journal of Abnormal Psychology, 101*, 452–9.

Cruess, D. G., Antoni, M. H., McGregor, B. A., Kilbourn, K. M., Boyers, A. E., Alferi, S. M., Carver, C. S., & Kumar, M. (2000). Cognitive-behavioral stress management reduces serum cortisol by enhancing benefit finding among women being treated for early stage breast cancer. *Psychosomatic Medicine, 62*, 304–8.

Currier, J., Holland, J., & Neimeyer, R. (2006). Sense-making, grief, and the experience of violent loss: Toward a mediational model. *Death Studies, 30*, 403–28.

Dalai Lama (Gyatso, T.) & Hopkins, J. (Translator) (2000). *The meaning of life: Buddhist perspectives on cause and effect.* Boston: Wisdom Publications.

Davis, C., & Morgan, M. (2008). Finding meaning, perceiving growth, and acceptance of tinnitus. *Rehabilitation Psychology, 53*, 128–38.

Davis, C. G., Nolen-Hoeksema, S., & Larson, J. (1998). Making sense of loss and benefiting from the experience: Two construals of meaning. *Journal of Personality and Social Psychology, 75*, 561–74.

Davis, C., Wortman, C. B., Lehman, D. R., & Silver, R. (2000). Searching for meaning in loss: Are clinical assumptions correct? *Death Studies, 24*, 497–540.

Debats, D. L., van der Lubbe, P. M., & Wezeman, F. R. A. (1993). On the psychometric properties of the Life Regard Index (LRI): A measure of meaningful life. *Personality and Individual Differences, 14*, 337–45.

Dittman-Kohli, F., & Westerhof, G. J. (1999). The personal meaning system in a life-span perspective. In G. T. Reker & K. Chamberlain (Eds.), *Exploring existential meaning: Optimizing human development across the life span* (pp. 107–22). Thousand Oaks, CA: Sage.

Emmons, R. A. (2003). Personal goals, life meaning, and virtue: Wellsprings of a positive life. In C. L. M. Keyes & J. Haidt (Eds.), *Flourishing: Positive psychology and the life well-lived* (pp. 105–28). Washington, DC: American Psychological Association.

Epstein, S. (1991). The self-concept, the traumatic neurosis, and the structure of personality. In D. Ozer, J. N. Healy, & A. J. Stewart (Eds.), *Perspectives in personality* (pp. 63–98). London: Jessica Kingsley.

Farber, E. W., Schwartz, J. A. J., Schaper, P. E., Moonen, D. J., & McDaniel, J. S. (2000). Resilience factors associated with adaptation to HIV disease. *Psychosomatics; 41,* 140–6.

Fife, B. (1995). The measurement of meaning in illness. *Social Science & Medicine, 40,* 1021–8.

Filipp, S. H. (1992). Could it be worse? The diagnosis of cancer as a prototype of traumatic life events. In L. Montada, S. H. Filipp, & M. J. Lerner (Eds.), *Life crises and experiences of loss in adulthood* (pp. 23–56). Englewood Cliffs, NJ: Erlbaum.

Folkman, S. (1997). Positive psychological states and coping with severe stress. *Social Science & Medicine, 45,* 1207–21.

Folkman, S. (2008). The case for positive emotions in the stress process. *Anxiety, Stress & Coping, 21,* 3–14.

Folkman, S., & Moskowitz, J. (2004). Coping: Pitfalls and promise. *Annual Review of Psychology, 55,* 745–74.

Folkman, S., & Moskowitz, J. T. (2007). Positive affect and meaning-focused coping during significant psychological stress. In M. Hewstone et al. (Eds.), *The scope of social psychology: Theory and applications* (pp. 193–208). New York: Psychology Press.

Frankl, V. E. (1963). *Man's search for meaning: An introduction to Logotherapy.* Oxford, England: Washington Square Press.

Gillies, J., & Neimeyer, R. A. (2006). Loss, grief, and the search for significance: Toward a model of meaning reconstruction in bereavement. *Journal of Constructivist Psychology, 19,* 31–65.

Greenberg, M. A. (1995). Cognitive processing of traumas: The role of intrusive thoughts and reappraisals. *Journal of Applied Social Psychology, 25,* 1262–96.

Harvey, J. H., Carlson, H. R., Huff, T. M., & Green, M. A. (2001). Embracing their memory: The construction of accounts of loss and hope. In R. A. Neimeyer (Ed.), *Meaning reconstruction and the experience of loss* (pp. 231–43). Washington, DC: American Psychological Association.

Harvey, J., Orbuch, T., Chwalisz, K., & Garwood, G. (1991). Coping with sexual assault: The roles of account-making and confiding. *Journal of Traumatic Stress, 4,* 515–31.

Hayes, A. M., Beevers, C. G., Feldman, G. C., Laurenceau, J., & Perlman, C. (2005). Avoidance and processing as predictors of symptom change and positive growth in an integrative therapy for depression. *International Journal of Behavioral Medicine, 12,* 111–22.

Hayes, A. M., Laurenceau, J., Feldman, G., Strauss, J. L., & Cardaciotto, L. (2007). Change is not always linear: The study of nonlinear and discontinuous patterns of change in psychotherapy. *Clinical Psychology Review, 27,* 715–23.

Helgeson, V. S., Reynolds, K. A., & Tomich, P. L. (2006). A meta-analytic review of benefit finding and growth. *Journal of Consulting and Clinical Psychology, 74,* 797–816.

Horowitz, M. J. (1992). Person schemas. In M. Horowitz (Ed.), *Person schemas and maladaptive interpersonal patterns* (pp. 13–32) Chicago: University of Chicago Press.

Horowitz, M. J., Wilner, N., & Alvarez, W. (1979). Impact of Event Scale: A measure of subjective stress. *Psychosomatic Medicine, 41,* 209–18.

Janoff-Bulman, R. (1989). Assumptive worlds and the stress of traumatic events: Applications of the schema construct. *Social Cognition, 7,* 113–36.

Janoff-Bulman, R. (1992). *Shattered assumptions: Towards a new psychology of trauma.* New York: Free Press.

Janoff-Bulman, R., & Frantz, C. M. (1997). The impact of trauma on meaning: From meaningless world to meaningful life. In M. J. Power & C. R. Brewin (Eds.), *The transformation of meaning in psychological therapies: Integrating theory and practice* (pp. 91–106). Hoboken, NJ: Wiley.

Jim, H. S., & Andersen, B. L. (2007). Meaning in life mediates the relationship between social and physical functioning and distress in cancer survivors. *British Journal of Health Psychology, 12,* 363–81.

Jim, H. S., Richardson, S. A., Golden-Kreutz, D. M., & Andersen, B. L. (2006). Strategies used in coping with a cancer diagnosis predict meaning in life for survivors. *Health Psychology, 25,* 753–61.

Joseph, S., & Linley, P. A. (2005). Positive adjustment to threatening events: An organismic valuing theory of growth through adversity. *Review of General Psychology, 9,* 262–80.

Karoly, P. (1999). A goal systems-self-regulatory perspective on personality, psychopathology, and change. *Review of General Psychology, 3,* 264–91.

King, L. A., Hicks, J. A., Krull, J. L., & Del Gaiso, A. K. (2006). Positive affect and the experience of meaning in life. *Journal of Personality and Social Psychology, 90,* 179–96.

Klinger, E. (1977). *Meaning & void: Inner experience and the incentives in people's lives.* Minneapolis: University of Minnesota Press.

Klinger, E. (1998). The search for meaning in evolutionary perspective and its clinical implications. In P. T. P. Wong & P. S. Fry (Eds.), *The human quest for meaning: A handbook of psychological research and clinical applications* (pp. 27–50). Mahwah, NJ: Erlbaum.

Koltko-Rivera, M. E. (2004). The psychology of worldviews. *Review of General Psychology, 8,* 3–58.

Koss, M. P., & Figueredo, A. J. (2004). Change in cognitive mediators of rape's impact on psychosocial health across 2 years of recovery. *Journal of Consulting and Clinical Psychology, 72,* 1063–72.

Kubany, E. S., & Manke, F. P. (1995). Cognitive therapy for trauma-related guilt: Conceptual bases and treatment outlines. *Cognitive and Behavioral Practice, 2,* 27–61.

Kuijer, R. G., & de Ridder, D. T. D. (2003). Discrepancy in illness-related goals and quality of life in chronically ill patients: The role of self-efficacy. *Psychology & Health, 18,* 313–30.

Lachman, M. E. (2006). Control: Perceived control over aging-related declines: Adaptive beliefs and behaviors. *Current Directions in Psychological Science, 15,* 282–6.

Lazarus, R. S., & Folkman, S. (1984). *Stress, appraisal, and coping.* New York: Springer.

Lee, V., Cohen, S. R., Edgar, L., Laizner, A. M., & Gagnon, A. J. (2006). Meaning-making intervention during breast or colorectal cancer treatment improves self-esteem, optimism, and self-efficacy. *Social Science & Medicine, 62,* 3133–45.

Lepore, S. J., & Helgeson, V. S. (1998). Social constraints, intrusive thoughts, and mental health after prostate cancer. *Journal of Social and Clinical Psychology, 17,* 89–106.

Lepore, S. J., & Kernan, W. D. (2009). Searching for and making meaning after breast cancer: Prevalence, patterns, and negative affect. *Social Science & Medicine, 68,* 1176–82.

Leventhal, H., Weinman, J., Leventhal, E. A., & Phillips, L. A. (2008). Health psychology: The search for pathways between behavior and health. *Annual Review of Psychology, 59,* 477–505.

Manne, S., Ostroff, J., Fox, K., Grana, G., & Winkel, G. (2009). Cognitive and social processes predicting partner psychological adaptation to early stage breast cancer. *British Journal of Health Psychology, 14,* 49–68.

Mausbach, B. T., Mills, P. J., Patterson, T. L., Aschbacher, K., Dimsdale, J. E., Ancoli-Israel, S., et al. (2007). Stress-related reduction in personal mastery is associated with reduced immune cell β_2-adrenergic receptor sensitivity. *International Psychogeriatrics, 19,* 935–46.

Mausbach, B. T., von Känel, R., Patterson, T. L., Dimsdale, J. E., Depp, C. A., Aschbacher K., et al. (2008). The moderating effect of personal mastery and the relations between stress and plasminogen activator inhibitor-1 (PAI-1) antigen. *Health Psychology, 27,* S172–S179.

McIntosh, D. N., Silver, R. C., & Wortman, C. B. (1993). Religion's role in adjustment to a negative life event: Coping with the loss of a child. *Journal of Personality and Social Psychology, 65,* 812–21.

McLean, K. C., & Pratt, M. W. (2006). Life's little (and big) lessons: Identity statuses and meaning-making in the turning point narratives of emerging adults. *Developmental Psychology, 42,* 714–22.

Michael, S. T., & Snyder, C. R. (2005). Getting unstuck: The roles of hope, finding meaning, and rumination in the adjustment to bereavement among college students. *Death Studies, 29,* 435–58.

Mikulincer, M., & Florian, V. (1996). Coping and adaptation to trauma and loss. In M. Zeidner & N. S. Endler (Eds.), *Handbook of coping: Theory, research, applications* (pp. 554–72). New York: John Wiley & Sons.

Moos, R. H., & Holahan, C. J. (2007). Adaptive tasks and methods of coping with illness and disability. In E. Martz & H. Livneh (Eds.), *Coping with chronic illness and disability: Theoretical, empirical, and clinical aspects* (pp. 107–26). New York: Springer.

Nadeau, J. W. (2001). Family construction of meaning. In R. A. Neimeyer (Ed.), *Meaning reconstruction and the experience of loss* (pp. 95–111). Washington, DC: American Psychological Association.

Neimeyer, R. A. (2001). The language of loss: Grief therapy as a process of meaning reconstruction. In R. A. Neimeyer (Ed.), *Meaning reconstruction and the experience of loss* (pp. 261–92). Washington, DC: American Psychological Association.

Neimeyer, R. A. (2002). Traumatic loss and the reconstruction of meaning. *Journal of Palliative Medicine, 5,* 935–42.

Nordin, K., Wasteson, E., Hoffman, K., Glimelius, B., & Sjoden, P.O. (2001). Discrepancies between attainment and importance of life values and anxiety and depression in gastrointestinal cancer patients and their spouses. *Psycho-Oncology, 10,* 279–89.

Pakenham, K. I. (2007). Making sense of multiple sclerosis. *Rehabilitation Psychology, 52,* 380–9.

Pakenham, K. I., Sofronoff, K., & Samios, C. (2004). Finding meaning in parenting a child with Asperger syndrome: Correlates of sense making and benefit finding. *Research in Developmental Disabilities, 25,* 245–64.

Pals, J. L. (2006). Narrative identity processing of difficult life experiences: Pathways of personality development and positive self-transformation in adulthood. *Journal of Personality, 74,* 1079–110.

Pan, J. Y., Wong, D. F. K., Chan, C. L. W., & Joubert, L. (2008). Meaning of life as a protective factor of positive affect in acculturation: A resilience framework and a cross-cultural comparison. *International Journal of Intercultural Relations, 32,* 505–14.

Pargament, K. I. (1997). *The psychology of religion and coping: Theory, research, practice.* New York: Guilford.

Park, C. L. (2005). Religion and meaning In R. F. Paloutzian & C. L. Park (Eds.), *Handbook of the psychology of religion and spirituality* (pp. 295–314). New York: Guilford.

Park, C. L. (2008). Testing the meaning making model of coping with loss. *Journal of Social and Clinical Psychology, 27,* 970–94.

Park, C. L. (2010). Making sense of the meaning literature: An integrative review of meaning making and its effects on adjustment to stressful life events. *Psychological Bulletin, 136,* 257–301.

Park, C. L. (2011, forthcoming). Meaning, spirituality, and growth: Protective and resilience factors in health and illness. In A. S. Baum, T. A. Revenson, & J. E. Singer (Eds.), *Handbook of health psychology* (2nd ed.).

Park, C. L., Armeli, S., & Tennen, H. (2004). Appraisal-coping goodness of fit: A daily Internet study. *Personality and Social Psychology Bulletin, 30,* 558–69.

Park, C. L., Edmondson, D., Fenster, J. R., & Blank, T. O. (2008). Meaning making and psychological adjustment following cancer: The mediating roles of growth, life meaning, and restored just-world beliefs. *Journal of Consulting and Clinical Psychology, 76,* 863–75.

Park, C. L., & Folkman, S. (1997). Meaning in the context of stress and coping. *Review of General Psychology, 1,* 115–44.

Park, C. L., Folkman, S., & Bostrom, A. (2001). Appraisals of controllability and coping in caregivers and HIV+ men: Testing the goodness-of-fit hypothesis. *Journal of Consulting and Clinical Psychology, 69,* 481–8.

Patterson, J. M., & Garwick, A. W. (1994). Levels of meaning in family stress theory. *Family Process, 33,* 287–304.

Peacock, E. J., & Wong, P. T. P. (1996). Anticipatory stress: The relation of locus of control, optimism, and control appraisals to coping. *Journal of Research in Personality, 30,* 204–22.

Penley, J. A., Tomaka, J., & Wiebe, J. S. (2002). The association of coping to physical and psychological health outcomes: A meta-analytic review. *Journal of Behavioral Medicine, 25,* 551–603.

Plaks, J. E., Grant, H., & Dweck, C. S. (2005). Violations of implicit theories and the sense of prediction and control: Implications for motivated person perception. *Journal of Personality and Social Psychology, 88,* 245–62.

Pöhlmann, K., Gruss, B., & Joraschky, P. (2006). Structural properties of personal meaning systems: A new approach to measuring meaning of life. *Journal of Positive Psychology, 1,* 109–17.

Pudrovska, T., Schieman, S., Pearlin, L. I., & Nguyen, K. (2005). The sense of mastery as a mediator and moderator in the association between economic hardship and health in late life. *Journal of Aging and Health, 17,* 634–60.

Reker, G. T., & Wong, P. T. P. (1988). Aging as an individual process: Toward a theory of personal meaning. In J. E. Birren & V. L. Bengtson (Eds.), *Emergent theories of aging* (pp. 214–46). New York: Springer.

Rini, C., Manne, S., DuHamel, K. N., Austin, J., Ostroff, J., Boulad, F., et al. (2004). Changes in mothers' basic beliefs following a child's bone marrow transplantation: The role of prior trauma and negative life events. *Journal of Traumatic Stress, 17,* 325–33.

Roberts, K. J., Lepore, S. J., & Helgeson, V. S. (2006). Social-cognitive correlates of adjustment to prostate cancer. *Psycho-Oncology, 15,* 183–92.

Segerstrom, S. C., Stanton, A. L., Alden, L. E., & Shortridge, B. E. (2003). Multidimensional structure for repetitive thought: What's on your mind, and how, and how much? *Journal of Personality & Social Psychology, 85,* 909–21.

Simonelli, L. E., Fowler, J., Maxwell, G. L., & Andersen, B. L. (2008). Physical sequelae and depressive symptoms in gynecologic cancer survivors: Meaning in life as a mediator. *Annals of Behavioral Medicine, 35,* 275–84.

Skinner, E. A., Edge, K., Altman, J., & Sherwood, H. (2003). Searching for the structure of coping: A review and critique of category systems for classifying ways of coping. *Psychological Bulletin, 129,* 216–69.

Smith, B. W., & Zautra, A. J. (2004). The role of purpose in life in recovery from knee surgery. *International Journal of Behavioral Medicine, 11,* 197–202.

Stanton, A. L., Bower, J. E., & Low, C. A. (2006). Posttraumatic growth after cancer. In L. G. Calhoun & R. G. Tedeschi (Eds.), *Handbook of posttraumatic growth: Research and practice* (pp. 138–75). Mahwah, NJ: Erlbaum.

Steger, M. F. (in press). The pursuit of meaningfulness in life. In S. J. Lopez (Ed.), *Handbook of positive psychology* (2nd ed.). Oxford, UK: Oxford University Press.

Taylor, S. E. (1983). Adjustment to threatening events: A theory of cognitive adaptation. *American Psychologist, 38,* 1161–71.

Taylor, S. E., Wood, J. V., & Lichtman, R. R. (1983). It could be worse: Selective evaluation as a response to victimization. *Journal of Social Issues, 39,* 19–40.

Tennen, H., Affleck, G., Armeli, S., & Carney, M. (2000). A daily process approach to coping: Linking theory, research, and practice. *American Psychologist, 55,* 626–36.

Tennen, H., & Affleck, G. (2002). Benefit-finding and benefit-reminding. In C. R. Snyder & S. J. Lopez (Eds.), *Handbook of positive psychology* (pp. 584–97). New York: Oxford University Press.

Thompson, S. C. (1985). Finding positive meaning in a stressful event and coping. *Basic and Applied Social Psychology, 6,* 279–95.

Thompson, S., & Janigian, A. (1988). Life schemes: A framework for understanding the search for meaning. *Journal of Social and Clinical Psychology, 7,* 260–80.

Tolstikova, K., Fleming, S., & Chartier, B. (2005). Grief, complicated grief, and trauma: The role of the search for meaning, impaired self-reference, and death anxiety. *Illness, Crisis & Loss, 13,* 293–313.

Tomich, P. L., & Helgeson, V. S. (2002). Five years later: A cross-sectional comparison of breast cancer survivors with healthy women. *Psycho-Oncology, 11,* 154–69.

Updegraff, J. A., Silver, R. C., & Holman, E. A. (2008). Searching for and finding meaning in collective trauma: Results from a national longitudinal study of the 9/11 terrorist attacks. *Journal of Personality and Social Psychology, 95,* 709–22.

Van der Veek, S., Kraaij, V., van Koppen, W., Garnefski, N., & Joekes, K. (2007). Goal disturbance, cognitive coping and psychological distress in HIV-infected persons. *Journal of Health Psychology, 12,* 225–30.

Verduin, P. J. M., de Bock, G. H., Vlieland, T. P. M. V., Peeters, A. J., Verhoef, J. & Otten, W. (2008). Purpose in life in patients with rheumatoid arthritis. Purpose in life in patients with rheumatoid arthritis. *Clinical Rheumatology, 27,* 899–908.

Weinstein, S. E., & Quigley, K. S. (2006). Locus of control predicts appraisals and cardiovascular reactivity to a novel active coping task. *Journal of Personality, 74,* 911–32.

Westphal, M., & Bonanno, G. A. (2007). Posttraumatic growth and resilience to trauma: Different sides of the same coin or different coins? *Applied Psychology: An International Review, 56,* 417–27.

White, K., & Lehman, D. R. (2005). Looking on the bright side: Downward counterfactual thinking in response to negative life events. *Personality and Social Psychology Bulletin, 31,* 1413–24.

Younger, J., Finan, P., Zautra, A. Davis, M., & Reich, J. (2008). Personal mastery predicts pain, stress, fatigue, and blood pressure in adults with rheumatoid arthritis. *Psychology & Health, 23,* 515–35.

Benefit-Finding and Sense-Making in Chronic Illness

Kenneth I. Pakenham

Abstract

In this chapter I will discuss the theoretical origins of benefit-finding and sense-making. In particular, proposals as to how these two meaning-making processes might fit into the stress and coping framework will be examined (Lazarus & Folkman, 1984; Park & Folkman, 1997). Research that has examined the measurement, nature, and role of benefit-finding and sense-making in coping with chronic illness will be reviewed. The interpersonal context of sense-making and benefit-finding will also be considered, particularly the role of shared meaning-making within patient–caregiver dyads. Although the body of research investigating benefit-finding in chronic illness is growing, the role of sense-making has been neglected, as has consideration of the joint role of these two related meaning-making processes. The implications of sense-making and benefit-finding research outcomes for interventions designed to promote health and quality of life in people with chronic illness will be discussed. Finally, future research directions will be delineated.

Keywords: stress, coping, benefit-finding, sense-making, chronic illness

Introduction

Chronic illness can confront an individual with his or her mortality and often forces a range of physical and symbolic losses that oscillate over time and require an ongoing process of adjustment. These losses can disrupt a person's self-definition, life goals, and sense of meaningfulness. According to Frank (1995), "serious illness is a loss of the 'destination and map' that had previously guided the ill person's life" (p. 1). Restoration of meaning is an important part of adjusting to an illness (Taylor, 1983). Two frequently cited meaning-reconstruction processes are benefit-finding and sense-making. Benefit-finding refers to finding benefits in adversity, and sense-making involves the development of explanations for adversity, or making sense of it within existing "assumptive schemas" (Davis, Nolen-Hoeksema, & Larson, 1998; Janoff-Bulman, 1992).

The focus on sense-making and benefit-finding is consistent with the upsurge of positive psychology generally (Seligman & Csikszentmihalyi, 2000) and specifically within the health and rehabilitation psychology areas (Dunn & Dougherty, 2005). There is a growing interest in the application of existential frameworks to coping with illness (Lee & McCormick, 2002), and a call for the conceptualization of adjustment processes to be expanded to include positive outcomes (Folkman & Moskowitz, 2000). In addition, in recent years the stress and coping model has been extended to include meaning-making processes (Park & Folkman, 1997).

In general, although some of the earlier frameworks have conceptualized benefit-finding and sense-making as related meaning-reconstruction processes, there has been vastly more research into benefit-finding than sense-making in the broader literature and in the chronic illness field. This is despite recent calls for researchers to investigate sense-making in people with chronic illnesses and disabilities (e.g., Lee & McCormick, 2002).

With respect to terminology, sense-making has been used interchangeably with "making sense," "comprehensibility," "account-making," and "explaining" the event. Similarly, benefit-finding has been used interchangeably with a variety of terms, including "post-traumatic growth," "stress-related growth," "growth," "adversarial growth," or "perception of positive change." At this stage there is no consensus on terminology for either construct. Throughout this chapter I will use the more commonly used terms *sense-making* and *benefit-finding*, but where appropriate I will use specific terms when referring to literature that has used these terms. An additional point of clarification regarding terminology concerns benefit-finding. Benefit-finding may refer to actual or veridical changes that people have made, or it may refer to perceptions of change. In the main, researchers have used self-report instruments that assess self-perceptions of change. Hence, use of the term *benefit-finding* typically refers to perceptions of change assessed via self-report instruments. This issue will be elaborated in the section on measurement.

Nature of Sense-Making and Benefit-Finding in Illness
Benefit-finding
A wide range of benefits arising from experiencing an illness have been reported by people with many different chronic illnesses, including strengthened relationships, spiritual growth, greater appreciation of life, personal growth, changed life priorities and goals, enhanced health behaviors, and acceptance (Algoe & Stanton, 2009; Helgeson, Reynolds, & Tomich, 2006; Pakenham, 2007b; Stanton, Bower, & Low, 2006; Tennen & Affleck, 2002). It appears that fairly high rates of benefit-finding occur in people with chronic illness. For example, 78% of non-Hodgkin's lymphoma survivors (Bellizzi, Farmer Miller, Arora, & Rowland, 2007) and 83% of breast cancer survivors (Sears, Stanton, & Danoff Burg, 2003) and women living with HIV/AIDS (Siegel & Schrimshaw, 2000) reported at least one positive life change related to their illness, and all but one

of 477 people with MS endorsed one or more benefits related to their illness (Pakenham, 2005a).

Sense-making
Although sense-making has largely been investigated in relation to bereavement, it has emerged as a prominent theme in recent qualitative studies of various illnesses, including prostate cancer (Gray, Fitch, Phillips, Labrecque, & Fergus, 2000), colorectal cancer (Dunn et al., 2006), mixed cancer (Fife, 1994), diabetes (Lang, 1989), dementia (Robinson, Clare, & Evans, 2005), somatization disorders (Baarnhielm, 2005), and multiple sclerosis (MS; Pakenham, 2008b). Although these qualitative studies identified sense-making as an important process, there is a lack of qualitative data that systematically maps out the nature of sense-making in chronic illness. Pakenham (2008b) derived 16 prominent sense-making themes from qualitative data on sense-making in people living with MS. The more frequently reported sense-making themes were causal explanations, acceptance, experienced growth, spiritual/religious explanations, and "wake-up call" for lifestyle change.

Rates of sense-making appear to be somewhat lower than rates of benefit-finding in chronic illness populations. For example, in a sample of 82 women with breast cancer, 56% within 3 months of diagnosis and 58% 18 months later reported that they had been successful in making sense of their illness (Kernan & Lepore, 2009). In a study of 408 persons with MS, 43% indicated that they could make sense of their illness (Pakenham, 2008b). Of the 53% who indicated that they could not make sense of their illness, just over a third (37%) indicated that they anticipated that they would eventually make sense of their illness, and the strength of this anticipation was positively correlated with life satisfaction. Of concern were the 130 participants who did not report sense-making of their illness and who also reported no or low anticipation of eventual sense-making. For such individuals the sense-making process may be prolonged or never resolved adequately, placing them at risk for significant adjustment problems.

Although illnesses vary across a number of dimensions and present unique clusters of adaptive tasks, we know little about whether the nature of sense-making and benefit-finding varies across different illness contexts. There are more data on this issue with respect to benefit-finding, and it would appear that the types of benefits described are relatively consistent across different illnesses.

Theoretical Background

Below I briefly summarize the theoretical frameworks that have specified roles for sense-making and benefit-finding in restoring meaning in the context of adversity. While some theories specify equivalent roles for both (e.g., Gillies & Neimeyer, 2006; Janoff-Bulman, 1992), others propose sense-making as one of many determinants of benefit-finding, with the latter being conceptualized as an outcome (e.g., Tedeschi & Calhoun, 2004), whereas others identify a role for one but not the other (e.g., Antonovsky, 1987).

Assumptive world theory

The roles of both sense-making and benefit-finding in building meaning were first given prominence in the work of Janoff-Bulman and colleagues (see review Janoff-Bulman & Yopyk, 2004). Janoff-Bulman (1992) described how traumatic events and losses can shatter a person's "assumptive world," the network of cognitive schemas that bear on the benevolence and meaningfulness of the world and the worthiness of the self and that provide a sense of order and predictability. To the extent that an event, such as a health threat, undermines these assumptions it causes profound distress. Janoff-Bulman and Yopyk (2004) distinguished between two meaning-making processes that are involved in rebuilding one's assumptive world in the face of significant adversity: "meaning-as-comprehensibility" or sense-making and "meaning-as-significance" or benefit-finding.

The importance of making sense of one's life in a meaningful way in the context of adversity is highlighted by Frankl's (1984) caution to those who are unable to do this, "Woe to him who saw no sense in his life, no aim, no purpose, and therefore no point in carrying on. He was soon lost." (p. 76). According to Janoff-Bulman and Frantz's (1997) theory, making sense of adversity is achieved through developing new worldviews, or via modifying existing assumptive schemas or worldviews. Sense-making is a cognitive processing mechanism that may involve at first automatic and then later volitional reflective ruminating (Janoff-Bulman, 2004) as it serves to rebuild the shattered assumptive world. Gillies and Neimeyer (2006) suggest that sense-making first involves a causal analysis answering the question "why?" But when this is resolved, the individual then turns to other more complex questions, "Why me?" and "Where is the sense in life when such things happen?" Eventually shattered assumptions are rebuilt or

modified and ideally include a balanced view of the world as both controllable and random.

Sense-making is also included in Antonovsky's (1987) meaning concept "sense of coherence." Antonovsky (1987) noted that this component is the core of the sense of coherence concept. Pennebaker's recent work on writing about traumatic events suggests that benefits may arise from this activity because writing or talking about the trauma helps the individual make sense of what he or she suffered (Esterling, L'Abate, Murray, & Pennebaker, 1992).

Benefit-finding involves re-evaluating adverse circumstances positively, thereby mitigating the negative implications, and protecting self-worth (Taylor, 1983). Janoff-Bulman (2004) proposed three explanatory models of benefit-finding. She posited that these are not mutually exclusive and that they are differentially related to the various domains of benefit-finding. Each model contributes to the cognitive processing involved in rebuilding assumptions. The first, "strength through suffering," refers to the process of grappling with the challenges inherent in suffering, and discovering new strengths and possibilities forged through living with a new life reality. The second, "psychological preparedness," refers to changes to the assumptive world associated with successful coping with adversity that better prepare the individual for subsequent trauma. The third model, "existential revaluation," involves an existential struggle that propels a meaning-making process, leading to a fuller awareness of one's existence in the world with respect to a new appreciation of life, relationships, and the unseen.

Another theory that refers to sense-making and benefit-finding is Taylor's (1983) cognitive adaptation theory, which highlights the flexibility of cognitions in three areas: maintaining mastery, self-enhancement, and the search for meaning. The latter is achieved through making causal attributions about the event and understanding the relevance or significance of the event for one's life. This search for meaning incorporates the sense-making process that Janoff-Bulman described. Self-enhancement involves construing personal benefit from the experience and is, therefore, similar to benefit-finding. Mastery involves attempts to gain control over the event and one's life. Taylor proposed that resolving these three tasks rested on illusions that provided a positively oriented slant on objective characteristics of the event.

Gillies and Neimeyer (2006) have also proposed central roles for sense-making and benefit-finding in their model of meaning reconstruction in bereavement. Drawing on Janoff-Bulman's theoretical work, they posited sense-making and benefit-finding as two of three meaning-reconstruction processes in response to significant loss, the other being identity change.

These theoretical frameworks imply that with the disruption of the assumptive world an awakening to the world and self as they are occurs. In the context of this awakening, sense-making concerns cognitive processing and struggle with the meaning of life, whereas benefit-finding concerns the creation of meaning by recognizing a renewed sense of the worth of self, others, and life, leading to new commitments and choices that create new meanings. Janoff-Bulman and Yopyk (2004) suggest that following trauma, people first deal with making sense of the event in the context of their life, and then deal with constructing value and worth in their own lives through finding benefit. They suggest that in the context of trauma, sense-making serves "as a catalyst for the creation of meaning" via benefit-finding.

Post-traumatic growth models

Several theorists have proposed a role for sense-making in the development of post-traumatic growth (PTG). In these models, benefit-finding is the outcome, and sense-making is posited as one of several process variables that lead to benefit-finding. Tedeschi and Calhoun (2004), in their model of PTG, refer to growth from trauma as the reconstruction and reorganization of global beliefs or schematic structures that have guided goals, understanding, decision-making, and meaningfulness following "seismic events" that threaten individuals. They conceptualize sense-making as integral to the cognitive processing of trauma-related information and experiences. Within this framework, sense-making involves revisions of shattered schemas that produce comprehensibility. This process is regarded as an intermediate step to PTG.

More recently, sense-making has been posited as an important meaning-making process in a two-component model of PTG (Zoellner & Maercker, 2006), and in an integrative model of growth through adversity (Joseph & Linley, 2006). For example, Joseph and Linley (2006) suggest that the sense-making or search for meaning process can be triggered not only by a "seismic shattering," but also through a more gradual breakdown of the assumptive world. In the context of chronic illness both processes are likely to occur. While one-off traumatic events eventually cease to define the survivor's world and daily living, chronic illness is ongoing and produces many stressors, such as negative treatment side effects, problematic symptoms, disability, and losses that fluctuate over the course of the illness. A seismic shattering of the assumptive world is likely to occur around crisis points such as receiving a diagnosis. In contrast, a gradual breakdown of the assumptive world is likely to ebb and flow over the long haul of the illness as health deteriorates and disability increases until such point that the individual is able to accommodate the illness experience within his or her assumptive world.

Stress process models

Park and Folkman (1997) extended Lazarus and Folkman's (1984) stress and coping theory to include meaning-making processes, such as benefit-finding, in the context of stressful conditions, and provided a comprehensive theoretical analysis of the role of meaning-making in stress and coping processes. This original framework has been elaborated more recently (Folkman, 2008; Park, 2005; Park, Edmondson, Fenster, & Blank, 2008).

Park and Folkman (1997) distinguished between situational and global meaning. Global meaning refers to the person's enduring fundamental assumptions, beliefs, and valued goals. Situational or appraised meaning of the event includes appraisals of loss, harm, threat, or challenge, and may include causal attributions, evaluation of the degree of discrepancy with global meaning structures, and consideration of coping options. According to this framework, the extent of mismatch between the appraised meaning and global meaning determines the resulting levels of distress. For example, compared to the onset of an illness in an elderly person, diagnosis of an untimely illness in young adulthood (e.g., MS) is more likely to violate beliefs about the fairness of the world, and interfere with unrealized life goals related to areas such as building family and career. The appraised and global meaning mismatch may be changed by altering the appraised meaning of the situation so that it is more consistent with one's global meaning (assimilation; Joseph & Linley, 2005), changing global beliefs and goals to incorporate the stressor (accommodation; Joseph & Linley, 2005), or both, thus facilitating integration of the appraised and global meaning structures and resulting in higher well-being. People who are unable to reduce this mismatch become trapped in a continuing reappraisal cycle where they struggle to reconcile situational meaning with their global beliefs in a brooding ruminative process (Michael & Snyder, 2005).

Meaning-making coping processes that may be used to reduce the mismatch between appraised meaning and global structures include sense-making and benefit-finding. Park and Folkman (1997) suggest that sense-making refers to "the extent to which people have managed to reconcile their appraised (or reappraised) meaning of the event with their global meaning" (p. 129). Sense-making may involve reattributing the illness to more benign causes (e.g., making sense of illness by attributing it to God's will, lifestyle, or behaviors). The role of sense-making is not as well articulated in Park and Folkman's framework as the role of benefit-finding.

Although benefit-finding has been conceptualized as a selective appraisal (Taylor, Wood, & Lichtman, 1983), it is more commonly conceptualized as a coping strategy. Park and Folkman (1997) conceptualize benefit-finding as a cognitive reappraisal coping strategy belonging to the meaning-based category of coping processes. However, Tennen and Affleck (2002) argue that benefit-finding is seldom measured as a coping strategy. They distinguish between benefit-reminding as a coping strategy and benefit-finding as a "belief or conclusion" and claim that it is more often measured as the latter. They regard benefit-reminding as involving effortful cognitions in which the person reminds himself or herself of the possible benefits stemming from a negative event, and is conceptualized as a form of coping that follows the perception of benefits. They showed that benefit-reminding was uniquely associated with positive mood but not decreased negative mood in women with fibromyalgia. Folkman (2008) conceptualizes both benefit-reminding and benefit-finding within the meaning-based coping classification. The distinction between benefit-reminding and benefit-finding has not been adequately explored empirically, and has implications for how each of these constructs is best measured and the timing of measurement in the coping process. As might be expected, several studies show that meaning-based coping strategies such as positive reappraisal coping are related to benefit-finding in people with chronic illness (Pakenham, 2006; Park et al., 2008; Sears et al., 2003).

In the context of an ongoing chronic stressor, benefit-finding can be viewed as both a coping process variable and an outcome (Folkman, 2008; Park & Folkman, 1997; Updegraff, Taylor, Kemney, & Wyatt, 2002). Park et al. (2008) distinguished between meaning-making coping efforts (e.g., positive reframing and reappraisal coping) and the outcomes of this process, meanings made, including benefit-finding as it is typically measured. The distinction between meaning-making efforts and meanings made is in line with Tennen and Affleck's (2002) distinction between benefit-finding conceptualized and measured as a coping strategy and benefit-finding as a belief or conclusion.

Similarly, sense-making may also serve the two purposes of process and outcome in the context of illness, although there has been much less theoretical and empirical research addressing this issue. Sense-making coping processes may include active questioning and reflective rumination directed towards understanding how and why the illness occurred and its relevance to one's life. It may also include seeking information about the illness and "testing out" one's sense-making explanations by sharing them with significant others. Sense-making as an outcome or made meaning refers to the arrived-at or found sense-making explanations that make the person's illness experience comprehensible. Kernan and Lepore (2009) distinguished between these two conceptualizations by assessing both the sense-making process ("How often have you found yourself searching to make sense or meaning of your illness?") and sense-making outcome ("Have you been successful in making sense of your illness?").

Measurement
Sense-making

There is considerable variability in the way sense-making has been operationalized and measured. For example, sense-making has been limited to the assessment of causal attributions, particularly in the chronic illness area, whereas others have assessed sense-making via an interview focusing on responses to the question "Why me?" (Affleck & Tennen, 1993). Davis et al. (1998) interviewed bereaved participants and directly asked them whether they had made sense of their loss and, if so, how. Sense-making is typically measured and conceptualized as a dichotomous variable (present or absent). However, recently I undertook research to develop multi-item scales of sense-making in persons with MS and their caregivers, given the qualitative data that have suggested multiple distinct sense-making themes (Pakenham, 2008b, 2008c). Multi-item sense-making inventories were developed for these patients (Sense-Making Scale [SMS]) (Pakenham, 2007a) and their caregivers (Caregiver Sense-Making

Scale [CSMS]) (Pakenham, 2008a). Items were derived from extensive qualitative data.

Item-level sense-making explanations reflected one or more of the key elements of world assumptions, including viewing self as having control over events (e.g., *I have new life goals because of MS*), perceiving events as predictable and meaningful (e.g., *I got MS for a purpose*), believing that life has purpose (e.g., *MS has helped me find purpose in life*), and regarding self as worthy (e.g., *It is not the MS that is important, it is how I manage it that's important*) (Janoff-Bulman & Frantz, 1997). Some of the sense-making explanations reflected culturally prescribed themes. For example, a conventional religious explanation is "my MS is part of God's plan/will for me." Some sense-making explanations reflected negative illness meanings (e.g., *MS has added nothing to my life*), which may be essential at various points in the process of rebuilding assumptions. Taylor (2000) found that women recently diagnosed with breast cancer reported going through periods of "darkness" and then eventually emerging into "light."

Factor analyses performed on the SMS revealed a 38-item scale with six factors: Redefined Life Purpose, Acceptance, Spiritual Perspective, Luck, Changed Values and Priorities, and Causal Attribution. Factor analyses performed on the CSMS revealed a 57-item scale also with six factors: Catalyst for Change, Acceptance, Spiritual Perspective, Incomprehensible, Relationship Ties, and Causal Attribution. Interestingly, some of the factors in both scales were similar; both had factors reflecting acceptance, causal attribution, spiritual, change, interpersonal, and negatively oriented worldview themes. Regarding the latter, the SMS Luck factor and the CSMS Incomprehensible factor reflected recognition of the randomness of some life events and that not everything can be explained.

Colleagues and I also developed a multi-item scale derived from qualitative data for assessing sense-making in parents of a child with Asperger's syndrome (Samios, Pakenham, & Sofronoff, 2008). This scale yielded some factors that were similar to those identified in the SMS and CSMS, namely spiritual, causal attribution, change, and luck. These themes appear to be core dimensions of sense-making regardless of the context.

All SMS and CSMS factors were psychometrically sound. Internal reliability coefficients were satisfactory and correlations among the subscales were low. Only one SMS factor and two CSMS factors were related to social desirability. Both scales

evidenced adequate convergent validity with Antonovsky's (1987) Sense of Coherence meaningfulness subscale and a dichotomous sense-making variable measured 12 months prior to the measurement of the SMS and CSMS. Regarding criterion validity, the SMS and CSMS factors predicted change in both positive and negative outcomes over a 12-month interval after controlling for the effects of initial adjustment levels, and relevant demographic and illness variables. Furthermore, the factors evidenced differential relations with adjustment dimensions, discussed in more detail below.

The factor structures of the two sense-making inventories suggest seven key sense-making processes for people affected by illness: (1) finding new life purpose that incorporates the illness, (2) contextualizing one's illness in the unseen or spiritual, (3) finding a causal explanation for the illness, (4) revising values, goals, and priorities in view of the illness, (5) appreciating social ties as a source of life meaning and richness, (6) accepting how life includes misfortune such as illness, and (7) acknowledging the randomness of some events and/or that some events cannot be explained. Together, these sense-making dimensions address the key components of the assumptive world, including order, purpose, self, safety, controllability, uncertainty, and impermanence. Further, the seven sense-making processes incorporate the two key characteristics that mark the threat-resistant assumptions or worldviews identified by Thompson and Janigian (1988): that misfortune is not unexpected and that goals are attainable despite negative life events. It would appear that individuals build a network of explanations or a sense-making narrative about their illness that incorporates each of these sense-making processes to varying degrees. The challenge is to build an illness narrative that will make sense, incorporate the new reality, and give value to the experience. In this regard, the sense-making themes may represent "narrative competence," or the ability to tell a coherent story about how individuals relate their illness to their sense of life purpose and meaning.

While the above-mentioned research has provided important foundational steps in multi-item measurement of sense-making in illness, many measurement issues remain unexplored, including temporal stability and validation of the sense-making dimensions on independent samples. In addition, it is not clear whether a more complex sense-making narrative that includes numerous sense-making themes is more adaptive than a simplified narrative that primarily clusters around only one or two sense-making themes. In this regard, narrative assessment strategies might be better placed to capture the potentially complex networks of sense-making explanations. Although these sense-making scales represent meanings made (i.e., "found" sense-making explanations), it is not clear whether they are empirically distinct from sense-making coping strategies or processes. However, using a single item to measure the sense-making search (coping process) and a single item to measure successfully having made sense of cancer (made meaning), Kernan and Lepore's (2009) study of breast cancer patients showed that both measures were unrelated.

Benefit-finding

In general, the measurement of benefit-finding is vastly more developed than that of sense-making. Nevertheless, there are numerous problems with benefit-finding measures, and because these have been comprehensively critiqued by others (e.g., Park & Lechner, 2006; Tennen & Affleck, 2009), I will only briefly discuss these issues with a focus on the illness context.

The most widely used measures of benefit-finding are multi-item self-report scales that assess self-perceptions of positive change. The assessment of only positive changes and not negative changes associated with an illness is problematic for several reasons. First, given that illness can trigger both positive and negative changes, allowing people to report both would provide a more comprehensive account of the illness experience. Second, the use of a unipolar response scale may foster a positive response bias, since respondents may feel obliged to endorse something positive (Tomich & Helgeson, 2004). In response to these criticisms, some benefit-finding scales have been modified to allow respondents to report both positive and negative changes (Armeli, Gunthert, & Cohen, 2001).

DIMENSIONS

There are conflicting findings regarding the dimensional structure of benefit-finding. Factor analytic studies that have examined multi-item benefit-finding measures using community samples have shown these measures to have a single factor (Park, Cohen, & Murch, 1996) and multiple factors (McMillen & Fisher, 1998; Tedeschi & Calhoun, 1996). The dimensional structure of benefit-finding in chronically ill populations has not been clearly delineated, although the research pertaining to this issue is more advanced in the cancer field. Cancer researchers have tended to use the Post-Traumatic Growth

Inventory (PTGI) (Tedeschi & Calhoun, 1996), which has five subscales (e.g., Cordova, Cunningham, Carlson, & Andrykowski, 2001), whereas others have used scales designed for other populations and modified them for cancer patients. For example, the Benefit-Finding Scale (BFS) was adapted from a scale used with parents of disabled children and validated primarily with breast cancer patients (Antoni et al., 2001; Carver & Antoni, 2004; Tomich & Helgeson, 2004). The BFS has undergone several revisions, with the original 17-item scale modified to 22- and 29-item versions. Although factor analyses performed on the BFS suggest that benefit-finding may be represented by multiple dimensions or a single factor, researchers have tended to use the single dimension (e.g., Tomich & Helgeson, 2004). However, Weaver et al. (2008) compared single- and multiple-factor models of the 29-item BFS in prostate and breast cancer patients. They found the six-factor model was a better fit to the data than a single-factor model (Personal Growth, Acceptance, World View, Family Relations, Social Relations, and Health Behaviors).

A difficulty in unraveling the dimensionality of benefit-finding in chronic illness is that researchers have tended to rely on benefit-finding scales that are not context-specific, despite emerging evidence indicating that the nature of benefit-finding may vary with respect to the type of adversity being faced. For example, qualitative studies of people with HIV/AIDS (Siegel & Schrimshaw, 2000) and MS (Pakenham, 2007b) show a wide range of benefit-finding themes, some of which are not reflected in illness-specific benefit-finding scales. Evidence from several studies suggests that the various benefit-finding dimensions in the illness context are differentially related to adjustment outcomes (Pakenham, 2005a; Pakenham & Cox, 2008). For example, a study of people with MS showed that a Family Relations Growth factor emerged as a strong predictor of positive affect, life satisfaction, and dyadic adjustment, whereas Personal Growth predicted only positive affect (Pakenham, 2005a). Delineating the dimensions of benefit-finding for specific populations may have important treatment implications. For example, Bower and Segerstrom (2004) suggest that the success of cognitive-behavioral stress management interventions in promoting benefit-finding in cancer patients may be due to the various treatment components having differential impacts on benefit-finding domains.

To address the need for benefit-finding scales that are sensitive to the illness context, a colleague and I developed the Benefit-Finding in Multiple Sclerosis Scale (BFiMSS) derived from qualitative data obtained from people living with MS (Pakenham & Cox, 2008). Factor analysis of the BFiMSS revealed a seven-factor structure that was stable over a 12-month period. Two of the BFiMSS factors often not included in scales of benefit-finding used in chronic illness populations are the mindfulness and lifestyle gains factors.

VALIDITY

The validity of self-reported benefit-finding is an important yet neglected area of inquiry (Park & Helgeson, 2006). To what extent are the positive changes that people report in adverse circumstances real or to what extent are they imagined? Indeed, Taylor (1983) suggests that when faced with adversity people may create cognitive distortions or illusions that allow them to view themselves and their experience in a more positive light. Studies have neglected examination of the correspondence of scores on a benefit-finding measure and actual real-life change. One view is that perceptions of growth are a phenomenon worth studying and should be taken at face value regardless of whether they are linked with change. Another view is that it is important to establish veridical positive change. Tennen and Affleck (2009) have called for prospective studies that assess both benefit-finding perceptions and veridical growth. It will be important for future research to keep these two types of growth conceptually and operationally distinct (Park, 2009). Ransom, Sheldon, and Jacobsen (2008) in a sample of mixed cancer patients showed that actual change in goal orientation (organic valuing processes) and perceived change in growth-related personal attributes may independently contribute to PTG.

One approach to validating self-reported benefit-finding is by obtaining corroborative data from significant others. The few published studies that have obtained this external validation data show that levels of agreement between benefit-finding scores of respondents and those of significant others vary: .51 for breast cancer patients (Weiss, 2002), .06 to .47 for spinal cord injury patients (McMillen & Cook, 2003), and .23 to .52 for persons with MS across two time points 12 months apart (Pakenham & Cox, 2008). However, this form of external validation has been criticized because of shared method variance, possible discussion between informants and participants (Park, 2009), the tendency for people who have encountered traumatic events to

mobilize people who support their positive change into their network (Tennen & Affleck, 2009), and the fact that not all forms of growth are visible to others.

Regarding convergent validity, Pakenham and Cox (2008) found that six of the seven BFiMSS factors were significantly related to Antonovsky's (1987) Sense of Coherence meaningfulness subscale. Weinrib et al. (2006) also found convergent validity for the PTGI in a study that showed that independent ratings of growth in essays were related to PTGI scores, indicating that endorsement of growth on PTGI could be substantiated by personal accounts.

Using a different approach to testing the validity of self-reported stress-related growth, Frazier and Kaler (2006) found that, compared to a matched comparison group, breast cancer patients did not report more life changes commonly documented by cancer patients (e.g., better relationships or more positive self-images), with the exception of spirituality and use of prayer. In a subsequent study, the authors found that undergraduates who reported that something positive came from a "worst stressor" reported only marginally better well-being in some areas compared to students who reported no positives (Frazier & Kaler, 2006).

SOCIAL DESIRABILITY

Benefit-finding inventories have the potential to be confounded with social desirability response bias, given that many of the benefits included in inventories appear to be very desirable (Tomich & Helgeson, 2004). However, student and community sample scores on the PTGI and stress-related growth inventories have been shown to be unrelated to social desirability (Park et al., 1996; Tedeschi & Calhoun, 1996; Weintraub, Rothrock, Johnsen, & Lutgendorf, 2006). Only one published study has examined relations between benefit-finding and social desirability response bias in the chronic illness field. Pakenham and Cox (2008) found that five of seven BFiMSS factors were weakly correlated with social desirability.

TEMPORAL STABILITY

Another shortcoming of prior benefit-finding research in the chronic illness field is the lack of studies that have examined the temporal stability of benefit-finding. Evers et al. (2001) showed that a six-item benefit-finding scale had a .68 retest coefficient over a 12-month interval, and Pakenham and Cox (2008) found that the seven BFiMSS factors had high retest coefficients ranging from .63 to .76 (also over a 12-month interval). Bower et al. (2005) showed that positive meaning decreased over a mean interval of 2.8 years but did not report retest correlations. Retest reliability coefficients for the PTGI subscales have ranged from .37 to .74 over 2 months (Tedeschi & Calhoun, 1996), and the retest coefficients for the Stress-Related Growth Inventory total score were .81 over 2 weeks and .59 over 6 months (Park et al., 1996). The test–retest correlation for benefit-finding in a sample of breast cancer patients across 5 years was .58 (Carver, Lechner, & Antoni, 2009). Taken together, these results show that people tend to score on perceptions of positive change in the same direction over the short to long term.

Relations Between Sense-Making and Benefit-Finding

Theoretical perspectives suggest that sense-making and benefit-finding are linked processes, although in terms of temporal sequencing most suggest that sense-making precedes benefit-finding. Janolff-Bulman and Frantz (1997) suggest that people first try to make sense of the event and then find some benefit or value in it for their life. For example, with the onset of a serious health problem that poses a threat to one's assumptions about oneself and the world, the person grapples with making sense of the illness through one or more of the seven sense-making processes mentioned earlier. This process leads to a new sense of self-value and worth, and meaningfulness. As the intensity of reflective rumination on the sense-making questions of "Why?" and Why me?" and so forth subsides, the resulting cognitive "space" and emotional leveling then allow for reflections on growth and positive change, such as awakening to previously unrecognized or untested personal strengths.

Only a few studies have examined relations between sense-making and benefit-finding. I conducted correlations between the six SMS factors and the seven BFiMSS factors and found that the SMS factors Redefined Life Purpose, Changed Values and Priorities, and Acceptance were significantly ($p < .01$) correlated with all BFiMSS factors (correlations ranged from .15 to .62). The sense-making factors Spiritual Perspective and Causal Attributions were each weakly related to four of the benefit-finding dimensions (.12 to .40), and Luck was inversely related to two BFiMS dimensions (Spiritual Growth and Life Style Gains). Based on

the proposition that sense-making precedes and paves the way for benefit-finding, this pattern of correlations suggests that finding new life purpose that incorporates the illness, revising life values and goals that account for the illness, and accepting life as it is provide important sense-making pathways to all aspects of benefit-finding. Using spiritual sense-making and causal explanations provides weaker links to only some benefits, and viewing illness as a random event is incompatible with spiritual growth and lifestyle gains.

Findings from other studies also support the link between sense-making and benefit-finding. For example, in a study of parents of children with Asperger's syndrome, colleagues and I (Pakenham, Sofronoff, & Samios, 2004) showed that three indices of sense-making (sense-making present/absent, number of sense-making categories, and anticipated sense-making) were significantly correlated ($p < .01$) with the corresponding benefit-finding variables. Calhoun, Tedeschi, Fulmer, and Harlan (2000) (cited in Tedeschi & Calhoun, 2004) showed that in bereaved parents, attempts to make sense of what happened following the deaths was related to all domains of the PTGI except personal strength.

However, not everyone who finds benefits can also make sense of the adversity, and vice versa. For example, 64% of parents of a child with Asperger's syndrome reported that they were able to both make sense of and find benefit in their situation, while 22% indicated they could do one but not the other (Pakenham et al., 2004). In addition, Davies et al. (1998) found that sense-making and benefit-finding measured as present or absent were unrelated to each other in bereaved persons. Hence, at this stage the empirical data on the extent to which benefit-finding and sense-making are linked are somewhat mixed. It is possible that finding benefits in illness without having made sense of it, or making sense of illness without eventually finding benefits, leads to made meanings that are not robust and lasting. Theories suggest that both processes are necessary for rebuilding a more flexible and realistic assumptive world.

Relations between Benefit-Finding and Sense-Making and Stress and Coping Processes

Although theories incorporate benefit-finding and sense-making as adaptive responses to adversity, they do not clearly articulate the particular characteristics of the person, health difficulty, or coping process that shape these meaning-making processes. There is now a growing body of research providing empirical evidence on the role of benefit-finding relative to other stress and coping processes, although few studies have examined the role of sense-making relative to these. Below I briefly review research in the illness field that has examined relations between benefit-finding and sense-making and the stress and coping predictors, including coping strategies, external coping resources (social support), internal dispositional resources (religious belief and personality), appraisal, and illness characteristics (illness duration and severity).

Coping strategies

In the chronic illness field, coping strategies have been shown to be related to benefit-finding in both cross-sectional (Bellizzi & Blank, 2006; Evers et al., 2001; Urcuyo, Boyers, Carver, & Antoni, 2005) and longitudinal studies (e.g., Luszczynska, Mohamed, & Schwarzer, 2005; Park et al., 2008; Thornton & Perez, 2006). Coping strategies that have been shown to be related to greater benefit-finding include positive reframing/reappraisal (Park et al., 2008; Siegel, Schrimshaw, & Pretter, 2005; Thornton & Perez, 2006; Urcuyo et al., 2005), active coping (Bellizzi & Blank, 2006; Evers et al., 2001; Luszczynska et al., 2005; McMillen & Cook, 2003; Urcuyo et al., 2005), acceptance (Luszczynska et al., 2005; Pakenham, 2006; Urcuyo et al., 2005), seeking social support (McMillen & Cook, 2003; Thornton & Perez, 2006), and religious coping (McMillen & Cook, 2003; Urcuyo et al., 2005). Thus, the coping strategies that would appear to facilitate benefit-finding in the context of chronic illness include active emotional approach and meaning-based coping strategies. These strategies have also been shown to be related to sense-making. For example, reliance on active approach and religious coping strategies and less reliance on behavioral disengagement coping have been shown to be related to sense-making in parents of a child with Asperger's syndrome (Pakenham et al., 2004).

Coping resources
SOCIAL SUPPORT
The pattern of findings regarding associations between social support and benefit-finding in people with chronic illness is a little more complex. Several illness studies have shown an association between greater social support and more benefit-finding cross-sectionally (Littlewood, Vanable, Carey, &

Blair, 2008; McMillen & Cook, 2003) and longitudinally (Luszczynska et al., 2005). However, other studies have shown benefit-finding to be unrelated to social support in cross-sectional (Updegraff et al., 2002), and longitudinal (Abraido-Lanza, Guier, & Colon, 1998; Sears et al., 2003) research designs. Some studies suggest that the association between social support and benefit-finding depends on the aspect of social support that is measured. For example, greater belonging support but not tangible support was related to more benefit-finding in people with spinal cord injury (McMillen & Cook, 2003), social support network but not perceived support was related to greater benefit-finding in people with MS and rheumatoid arthritis (Evers et al., 2001), emotional support but not practical support was related to benefit-finding in women living with HIV/AIDS (Siegel et al., 2005), and a global measure of social support was unrelated to benefit-finding, but talking to others about their cancer was linked to benefit-finding (Cordova et al., 2001). In addition, there is some evidence that social support may be differentially related to various benefit-finding dimensions. For example, greater social support was related to only one benefit-finding dimension, improved family relations, in a longitudinal mixed cancer study (Luszczynska et al., 2005). On balance, the weight of evidence suggests that satisfaction with some types of social support (particularly emotional support) is related to greater benefit-finding, but that this effect may be related to only some dimensions (particularly the interpersonal areas). Greater satisfaction with social support has also been shown to be related to sense-making (Pakenham et al., 2004).

RELIGIOUS BELIEFS
Given that disease often confronts an individual with his or her mortality, one factor that is likely to influence the extent to which people are able to make sense of their illness and derive benefits from their health adversity is their religious or spiritual beliefs. For example, a belief that one's illness is part of God's will or destiny may mitigate the negative impact of the losses and hardship associated with illness, by providing a framework where the health problem is comprehensible in a spiritual or religious sense. In support of this proposal, several studies show that compared to those who do not report religious-spiritual belief, those who do report such belief are more likely to make sense of their adversity, whether it be chronic illness (Pakenham, 2008b),

caring for a chronically ill person (Pakenham, 2008c), or loss of a loved one (Davis et al., 1998). Similarly, religious-spiritual belief has also been shown to be related to higher benefit-finding in people with a chronic illness (Pakenham & Cox, 2009) and caregivers (Pakenham & Cox, 2008).

PERSONALITY ATTRIBUTES
Few studies have examined the association of personality attributes and benefit-finding in chronic illness. Personality dimensions that have been shown to be related to greater benefit-finding include optimism (cross-sectionally [Evers et al., 2001; Updegraff et al., 2002; Urcuyo et al., 2005] and longitudinally [Milam, 2006; Sears et al., 2003; Tallman, Altmaier, & Garcia, 2007]), self-esteem and self-efficacy (Carpenter, Brockopp, & Andrykowski, 1999; Schulz & Mohamed, 2004), hope (Sears et al., 2003), reward responsiveness (Urcuyo et al., 2005), and lower neuroticism and greater extraversion (Evers et al., 2001). However, neuroticism has also been shown to be unrelated to benefit-finding (Lechner et al., 2003). Greater self-efficacy has been shown to be related to sense-making in parents of a child with Asperger's syndrome (Pakenham et al., 2004).

Appraised stressfulness of an illness
In the cancer literature, while most studies have demonstrated an association between higher benefit-finding and greater perceived threat of cancer (Cordova et al., 2001; Lechner et al., 2003; Sears et al., 2003), a few have reported nonsignificant relations (Antoni et al., 2001; Cordova et al., 2001). Consistent with the latter cancer studies, a global appraisal of the stressfulness of MS was found to be unrelated to benefit-finding (Pakenham, 2005a, 2006). There are several difficulties in interpreting findings concerning the association between the appraised stressfulness of illness and benefit-finding, including the wide variations in the operationalization of illness appraisals and the inherent assumption underlying many appraisal measures that illness is a unitary stressor. Regarding the latter, illnesses pose many different adaptive tasks and these ebb and flow over time, such that the extent to which a person perceives an illness as stressful will depend on the particular illness stressors being faced.

Illness and disease characteristics
The illness and disease characteristics most frequently examined in relation to benefit-finding are indicators of disease or illness severity, and illness duration. These two groups of variables will be discussed in turn.

DISEASE AND ILLNESS SEVERITY
The theoretical frameworks reviewed above propose that sense-making and benefit-finding are triggered by seismic health crises; hence, based on this proposition, greater disease or illness severity would be expected to be related to greater sense-making and benefit-finding. However, the reverse of this prediction has been found with respect to sense-making: Lower disability in MS patients has been shown to be related to higher levels of sense-making (Pakenham, 2007a, 2008b). One explanation for this is that illness that is characterized by severe disability may overwhelm worldviews to the point that comprehension of the patient's situation progresses very slowly. In contrast, a diagnosis of MS associated with less disability and minimal life disruption may provide sufficient impetus to trigger sense-making without overwhelming meaning structures, making the illness experience easier to comprehend.

Regarding benefit-finding, consistent with theoretical predictions, several studies show that greater benefit-finding is related to more severe disease indicators, including regional cancer (vs. localized) (Bellizzi & Blank, 2006) and more advanced stage of cancer (Tomich & Helgeson, 2004). However, more studies show benefit-finding to be related to less severe disease indicators, including a relapsing-remitting course of MS (vs. chronic progressive) (Pakenham, 2005a), fewer HIV-related symptoms (Littlewood et al., 2008), and higher motor functioning and lower injury level in persons with spinal cord injury (McMillen & Cook, 2003). In contrast, numerous studies show benefit-finding to be unrelated to disease severity. For example, benefit-finding has been found to be unrelated to cancer stage (Cordova et al., 2001; Rinaldis, Pakenham, & Lynch, 2010; Thornton & Perez, 2006), severity of cancer treatment (Cordova et al., 2001; Lechner et al., 2003; Rinaldis et al., 2010; Thornton & Perez, 2006; Tomich & Helgeson, 2004), disease activity, functional disability, and physical complaints in MS and rheumatoid arthritis (Evers et al., 2001), pain and disability in a mixed chronic illness sample (Abraido-Lanza et al., 1998), *and* HIV/ AIDS disease stage and number of physical symptoms (Siegel et al., 2005), and health status (Updegraff et al., 2002).

There are several possible explanations for the mixed findings. First, stress and coping theory (Lazarus & Folkman, 1984) proposes that the objective characteristics of a stressful event are less potent in shaping outcomes than the person's appraisal of the stressfulness of the event. In the chronic illness field this proposal is supported by empirical data demonstrating that patients' appraisals of their illness-related stressors are much stronger predictors of adjustment outcomes than are illness or disease variables (e.g., Pakenham, 1999). Hence, whether an illness event reaches the seismic levels necessary to trigger meaning-making processes will depend more on an individual's appraisals of the illness than the objective medical characteristics.

Second, disease and illness variables may have differential impacts on the various dimensions of benefit-finding. For example, regional cancer versus localized cancer was associated with only two of the PTGI subscales (Bellizzi & Blank 2006), relapsing-remitting versus chronic progressive course of MS was related only to the personal growth dimension of benefit-finding (Pakenham, 2005a), and the effects of motor functioning and spinal cord injury level varied across benefit-finding domains (McMillen & Cook, 2003).

Third, the relationship between benefit-finding and disease and illness severity may be curvilinear. For example, in a mixed cancer sample, those with stage II disease had significantly higher benefit-finding than those with stage IV or stage 1 cancer (Lechner et al., 2003). The authors proposed that those in early-stage cancer (stage I) had not experienced a serious mortality threat and life disruption; hence, a seismic threshold for triggering benefit-finding had not been reached. In contrast, for those who had experienced very advanced disease (stage IV), particularly a recurrence, this may have triggered such high life stress that cognitive processing and growth were hindered.

Fourth, the relationship between benefit-finding and disease and illness severity may be moderated by other variables. For example, Milam (2006) found that the relationship between PTG and disease status was moderated by dispositional optimism and pessimism; PTG had the greatest impact when these expectancies were low.

Finally, other factors that might explain the mixed findings regarding the association between benefit-finding and disease and illness severity include variations in how disease severity is operationalized, and the possibility that the association varies as a function of illness type.

ILLNESS DURATION

With respect to illness duration, theoretical frameworks reviewed earlier suggest that sense-making is likely to emerge early in the health crisis, followed by benefit-finding. Regarding sense-making, a shorter illness duration was found to be associated with greater sense-making in MS patients (Pakenham, 2008a, 2007b). Although these findings are consistent with the theoretical proposition that sense-making emerges early in the coping process, another interpretation is that sense-making was more likely earlier in the disease progression because neurological deterioration and disability had not progressed markedly, making the illness experience easier to comprehend and fit into existing cognitive schema or worldviews.

Regarding benefit-finding, a longer time since diagnosis has been found to be related to higher benefit-finding in people with cancer (Cordova et al., 2001; Sears et al., 2003), MS (Evers et al., 2001; Pakenham, 2005a), and rheumatoid arthritis (Evers et al., 2001). Greater time since treatment (radiotherapy) completion (mean 10.5 days) was related to higher PTGI scores in breast and prostate cancer patients (Ransom et al., 2008). In one study, MS illness duration was related to only one benefit-finding dimension (personal growth) (Pakenham, 2005a). These findings are consistent with the theoretical proposal that benefit-finding emerges later in the process of coping with illness. However, other studies have found illness duration to be unrelated to benefit-finding in people with cancer (Bellizzi & Blank 2006; Lechner et al., 2003; Park et al., 2008), in people with HIV/AIDS (Littlewood et al., 2008; Siegel et al., 2005), and in mixed chronic illness groups (Abraido-Lanza et al., 1998).

Given the considerable variability among illnesses regarding the extent to which they are characterized by chronic progressive deterioration, fluctuations in symptoms, and marked episodic exacerbations, it is likely that (with at least some illnesses) there may not be a simple linear relationship between illness duration and both sense-making and benefit-finding. In addition, sense-making and benefit-finding are at times likely to occur simultaneously over the course of coping with chronic illness. A further consideration is the fact that, for some diseases, illness duration is confounded by age. For example, in a disease like MS with onset typically in early to mid-adulthood, longer disease duration means progressing through more developmental lifespan stages with the illness.

In summary, the stress and coping variables that appear to be related to higher benefit-finding in the illness context include greater reliance on active emotional approach and meaning-based coping strategies, satisfaction with social support, perceived threat, optimism, and religious-spiritual belief. With respect to sense-making, preliminary findings suggest that the same variables may also be related to making sense of illness. These variables reflect behavioral, dispositional, and interpersonal resources that facilitate the processing of illness-related affect, and cognitions that foster benefit-finding and sense-making. However, the mechanisms by which this cluster of personal resources interrelate to shape meaning-making, or how meaning-making enhances access to these resources, is not clear. Meaning-making may also be related to external formal resources. For example, a colleague and I found that caregivers who accessed respite care reported significantly higher benefit-finding than caregivers who had never used respite care (Jardim & Pakenham, 2010).

NATURE OF THE RELATIONS AMONG STRESS AND COPING PROCESSES AND BOTH SENSE-MAKING AND BENEFIT-FINDING

To shed light on how stress and coping processes are networked with sense-making and benefit-finding, research is needed that employs model-testing approaches that enable examination of the interrelations among these variables simultaneously. In an effort to conduct such research, colleagues and I investigated the role of benefit-finding within a stress and coping model used to explain variations in the quality of life (QOL) of 1,800 survivors of colorectal cancer 5 and 12 months after diagnosis (Rinaldis, Pakenham, & Lynch, in press). We used structural equation modeling to examine the direct and mediational effects among illness appraisals, coping strategies, coping resources (social support and optimism), benefit-finding, and QOL latent variables. We found that increased benefit-finding was associated with reliance on approach coping and higher QOL cross-sectionally. However, increased benefit-finding was also associated with lower threat appraisals and greater social support. Interestingly, the association between higher optimism and more benefit-finding was mediated by appraisal and approach coping. This finding does not support the proposition that benefit-finding is a proxy for optimism; optimism alone had no impact on benefit-finding, but exerted its influence through the other cognitive and behavioral stress and coping

processes. Approach coping also partially mediated the effect of appraised threat on benefit-finding, such that if threat was perceived to be high, approach coping strategies were initiated, thereby increasing benefit-finding.

The patterns of associations among the stress and coping variables and benefit-finding suggest either of two mechanisms or perhaps a combination of the two that foster benefit-finding. The first is consistent with the meaning-making processes proposed in the theoretical frameworks reviewed above, where the diagnosis has been perceived as traumatic, shattering global meaning structures that are consequently rebuilt through cognitive and emotional meaning-based coping. In our study we found that colorectal cancer survivors who reported higher cancer threat were more likely to activate coping strategies involving cognitive and emotional processing that facilitated the perception of benefits. Further, this pattern of coping was more likely when the individuals who perceived high threat, or relied on approach coping, were also more optimistic. The second mechanism is psychological preparedness (Janoff-Bulman, 2004), where the individual perceives the illness as low threat but finds benefits in the situation by reflecting on successful coping with past loss or trauma that led to positive changes. Given that many of the colorectal cancer survivors in this study were older (mean age 65), this pathway to benefit-finding is particularly relevant. Older adults entering the cancer experience may be more likely to draw on wisdom and growth stemming from prior experiences of coping with negative life events (Lerner & Gignac, 1992).

Adjustment and Sense-Making and Benefit-Finding

The theoretical frameworks reviewed above suggest that sense-making and benefit-finding help to restore meaning, which, in turn, facilitates adjustment. The following is a review of the empirical findings concerning the associations between adjustment and both sense-making and benefit-finding, with an emphasis on research that has examined these associations in the illness context.

Benefit-finding

There are several reviews of the research on associations between benefit-finding and adjustment across a range of adverse events (Helgeson et al., 2006; Linley & Joseph, 2004) and specifically within the context of chronic illness (Algoe & Stanton, 2009) and cancer (Stanton et al., 2006). In general, these reviews show that associations between benefit-finding and measures of adjustment are not uniform across outcomes.

There are numerous explanations for the inconsistent relations between benefit-finding and adjustment. First, the relations between benefit-finding and adjustment may be more complex than a simple direct linear link. I briefly discuss the possibility of a curvilinear relationship between benefit-finding and adjustment, and moderators of this relationship, and the potential stress-buffering effects of benefit-finding.

Lechner et al. (2006) found significant curvilinear relations between benefit-finding and adjustment in breast cancer patients. Compared with a group who reported moderate levels of benefit-finding, the groups who reported low and high benefit-finding reported better psychological adjustment. This pattern of findings was replicated by Carver et al. (2009), also using a sample of breast cancer patients. Both studies found that women in the high benefit-finding group had higher optimism and greater reliance on positive reframing and religious coping strategies. The women in the low benefit-finding group did not appear to perceive their cancer as a threat and, therefore, did not experience their illness as a crisis at a magnitude sufficient to trigger benefit-finding. Women who experienced their cancer as a threat and who had greater personal resources, including positive personality attributes and coping strategies, were more likely to report higher benefit-finding. In contrast, women who experienced their cancer as a threat but had fewer personal resources to facilitate positive change reported fewer benefits.

These findings highlight important issues that may explain the inconsistencies in linear relations between benefit-finding and adjustment, particularly the variability in the extent to which people experience their illness as threatening. As mentioned above, illness is not uniformly stressful or threatening for all individuals. Investigation into the curvilinear relations between benefit-finding and adjustment is in the early stages, and both studies above were conducted on breast cancer patients. A colleague and I examined benefit-finding in a sample of 154 thyroid cancer patients. We found no evidence of curvilinear relations between benefit-finding and multiple adjustment outcomes (Costa & Pakenham, submitted manuscript).

The beneficial effects of benefit-finding may depend on the effects of potential moderators. For example, Stanton, Danoff-Burg, and Huggins (2002a) found

evidence of moderator effects of hope. They found that coping with breast cancer using positive reinterpretation was more effective for highly hopeful women. Tomich and Helgeson (2004) showed that disease severity moderated the effects of benefit-finding. They found that for women with more severe breast cancer, benefit-finding 4 months after diagnosis was associated with worse mental functioning 3 months later.

It is also possible that the beneficial effects of benefit-finding are apparent only at high levels of stress. In support of this proposal I found that benefit-finding in the family relations domain buffered the adverse effects of high illness-related stress appraisals on distress in persons with MS (Pakenham, 2005a). The beneficial effects of family relations growth was not evident for those individuals who reported low stress related to their MS. Other studies have also found similar stress-buffering effects of benefit-finding (e.g., McMillen, Smith, & Fisher, 1997).

Another issue concerning the role of benefit-finding in shaping adjustment outcomes is the question of whether benefit-finding is a coping process or an outcome, and as mentioned earlier, to some extent the answer depends on how and when it is measured. In our colorectal cancer survivor study, colleagues and I found evidence supporting the conceptualization of benefit-finding (measured as made meaning) as an interim outcome (Rinaldis et al., in press). For example, benefit-finding had different antecedents and outcomes to a cluster of largely meaning-based coping strategies, and benefit-finding positively influenced QOL outcomes cross-sectionally, which then mediated the effect of benefit-finding on longer-term QOL. Hence, we conceptualized benefit-finding as an interim outcome, representing a consequence of attempts to establish revised priorities and controllability, which restores self-confidence and a sense of mastery that, in turn, leads to better QOL. In this regard, benefit-finding may be the realization or reporting of one's cognitive manipulations, which precedes both actual psychological or behavioral changes and the alleviation of distress (Helgeson et al., 2006).

Park et al.'s (2008) investigation of the meaning-making process and made meaning in a mixed cancer sample also provided support for benefit-finding as an interim outcome. They found that the benefit-finding coping strategy positive reframing (meaning-making) was related to benefit-finding as an outcome (made meaning), which, in turn, was related to better psychological well-being indirectly through life meaningfulness.

Other factors that may account for the lack of consistent findings regarding associations between benefit-finding and adjustment include the measurement problems associated with benefit-finding (reviewed above) and adjustment. Regarding the latter, a wide range of positive and negative adjustment outcomes have been measured. With respect to measures of negative adjustment outcomes, some of those used in prior research have included positive items (e.g., Center for Epidemiologic Studies Depression Scale [CES-D]), and measures of negative feelings have varied considerably as to the domains of affect that have been included (e.g., anxiety, depression, stress). Park (2004) has suggested that benefit-finding may evidence stronger associations with adjustment when the outcomes are more closely tied to the event or illness.

Timing of the assessment of benefit-finding also appears to influence relations between benefit-finding and adjustment. Benefit-finding is more likely to be evident some time after the initial seismic event and following the emergence of sense-making accounts (Janoff-Bulman, 1992). Helgeson et al.'s (2006) meta-analysis showed that there were stronger links between benefit-finding and adjustment when 2 or more years had elapsed since the stressor. Assessing benefit-finding too close to the diagnosis of a serious illness (e.g., within the first year), when the person is still experiencing intense disruption, may gauge benefit-finding before it is fully developed. Tomich and Helgeson (2004) assessed benefit-finding within 9 months of breast cancer diagnosis and found that it had adverse effects. In contrast, our research on colorectal cancer survivors showed that benefit-finding assessed approximately 5 months after diagnosis was related to QOL concurrently and at 12 months after diagnosis (Rinaldis et al., in press). However, the mean age of the women with breast cancer in Tomich and Helgeson's (2004) study was 48, whereas the mean age of the men and women in our colorectal cancer sample was 65. As proposed earlier, given the older age of those in the colorectal sample, these individuals were likely to achieve benefit-finding via the psychological preparedness pathway. Hence, resolution of the initial crisis and sense-making phase may have been quicker for these people, given their lengthy history of surviving negative life events, which is likely to have fostered a speedy processing of cognitions and affect related to their cancer. However, timing of assessment becomes more complex in illnesses that have intermittent episodes of marked progressive deterioration: Each period of increased disability can represent a mini-seismic event that challenges meaning structures.

Another issue is the reporting of positive changes associated with illness relative to negative changes. Failure to distinguish between growth characterized by reports of only positive change and growth that recognizes both positive and negative changes may obscure the relationship between benefit-finding and adjustment. Perceptions of growth that are balanced with an awareness of negative changes as well as positives may be growth that is more strongly predictive of positive adjustment outcomes (Cheng, Wong, & Tsang, 2006). The reporting of only positive change may reflect a cognitive bias (e.g., denial), whereas the reporting of a balance of positive and negative change is likely to be more realistic and adaptive (Taylor, Kemeny, Reed, & Aspinwall, 1991). In support of this proposal, Cheng et al. (2006) found that people affected by severe acute respiratory syndrome (SARS) who gave an exclusive account of benefits had higher levels of defensiveness than those who gave a mixed account and those who gave exclusive accounts of costs. Further, only the perceived impact of benefits given in mixed accounts were related to future accruements in personal and social resources over an 18-month period.

Sense-making

Outside of the chronic illness field, sense-making has been shown to be associated with better adjustment in parents of children with disabilities (e.g., Behr & Murphy, 1993) and high-risk infants (Affleck & Tennen, 1993), and bereaved persons (Davis et al., 1998; Michael & Snyder, 2005). In a prospective study of bereaved persons, Davis et al. (1998) showed that after controlling for pre-loss distress, age at death, religious beliefs, and optimism, sense-making at 6 months after the loss was related to less distress in the first year after the loss.

In contrast to the research above, in a study of 59 parents of a child with Asperger's syndrome, colleagues and I (Pakenham et al., 2004) found that three indices of sense-making (present/absent, number of sense-making categories, and anticipated sense-making) were unrelated to parental adjustment. However, we did find evidence of the stress-buffering effects of sense-making. In other words, parents who reported higher levels of sense-making and stress were more likely to report better adjustment, whereas those who reported lower sense-making and higher stress were more likely to report poorer adjustment.

Few quantitative studies have examined relations between sense-making and adjustment in the chronic illness field. Kernan and Lepore (2009) found that women with breast cancer who engaged in sense-making with a relatively high frequency 11 months after diagnosis reported higher negative affect 18 months later, after controlling for baseline negative affect. Women who engaged in continuous sense-making reported more negative affect than women who reported a relatively low frequency of sense-making or those who reported a resolved sense-making pattern.

I undertook mixed-method cross-sectional research to examine relations between indices of sense-making derived from qualitative data and adjustment in persons with MS (Pakenham, 2008b) and their caregivers (Pakenham, 2008c). In each study the sense-making variable was the number of sense-making categories. Sense-making in persons with MS predicted greater life satisfaction and positive states of mind and lower depression after controlling for illness course, duration and disability, and religious belief. In the caregiver study, after controlling for MS symptoms, relevant caregiver demographics, and religious belief, sense-making predicted greater life satisfaction but was unrelated to positive states of mind and distress.

Most prior research has used dichotomous measures of sense-making or the number of sense-making explanations reported, which do not capture the rich array of sense-making themes. Different sense-making explanations may not evidence uniform associations with adjustment. For example, sense-making explanations that foster a perception of the world as fully unpredictable and uncontrollable are likely to evoke distress, particularly anxiety (Janoff-Bulman & Yopyk, 2004). In contrast, sense-making explanations that afford an individual greater perceived control over aspects of his or her illness, preservation of self-worth, and a balanced and realistic perspective of the randomness and uncontrollability of events may promote greater adjustment. These proposals were in the main supported by the following two studies.

Using a longitudinal design with two assessment points 12 months apart, I examined relations between the MS patient (SMS) and caregiver (CSMS) sense-making multi-item scales (reviewed above) and adjustment in patients (Pakenham, 2007a) and their caregivers (Pakenham, 2008a). In both studies Time 2 sense-making accounted for significant amounts of variance in each of the Time 2 adjustment outcomes after controlling for Time 1 adjustment, and relevant demographic and illness variables. All of the sense-making factors, except Causal Attributions, emerged as significant predictors of one or more adjustment outcomes. In contrast, the Changed Values/Priorities and Luck factors of the SMS and the Catalyst for Change and Incomprehensible factors of the CSMS were related to poorer adjustment. While the association between poorer adjustment and the Luck and Incomprehensible factors is expected, the link between the Changed Values/Priorities and Catalyst for Change factors and poorer adjustment is counterintuitive at first glance. Regarding the latter, both factors reflect a perception of the caregiving situation or illness as a catalyst for change that, in turn, offers new goals and purpose in life. However, the apparent adverse effects of these sense-making processes on adjustment may reflect the tension and difficulties in making changes to various areas of one's life, particularly as some of these changes, although seemingly positive, may be forced and/or not welcomed, and may therefore threaten self-worth, at least in the short term.

In our research on sense-making in parents of a child with Asperger's syndrome (Samios et al., 2008), cross-sectional analyses showed that the six sense-making factors explained significant amounts of variance in parental adjustment. Only the sense-making factor reframing was associated with better adjustment, whereas most of the remaining sense-making factors predicted greater distress.

Consistent with Assumptive World Theory sense-making dimensions that afforded a realistic sense of controllability and predictability in relation to caregiving (Acceptance, Relationship Ties, Spiritual Perspective) or illness (Redefined Life Purpose, Acceptance, Spiritual Perspective) or that preserved self-worth were related to better adjustment, whereas those dimensions that entailed viewing illness (Luck) or caregiving (Incomprehensible) as incomprehensible, fully random, and/or uncontrollable or that did not tend to safeguard self-worth were related to poorer adjustment. The Changed Values and Priorities and Catalyst for Change factors seemed to also fall into the latter category, presumably because of the personal challenges linked to changes forced by illness and caregiving, respectively.

Notably, the Causal Attribution factors of the SMS and the CSMS were unrelated to a measure of meaningfulness and all adjustment outcomes. The causal attribution factor in the parental Asperger's syndrome study was also unrelated to a measure of meaningfulness and was related to higher parental anxiety. Thompson and Janigian (1988) claim that having an attribution for a negative event is not equivalent to finding meaning in the experience, because the attribution may conflict with worldviews and may be formed more by available information (e.g., medical knowledge) than by cognitive structures or meaning-making processes.

The findings reviewed above suggest that sense-making is multidimensional and that the sense-making dimensions are differentially related to adjustment. The fact that some sense-making dimensions are not associated with better adjustment may partially explain why Kernan and Lepore (2009) found some sense-making patterns to be related to higher distress. Findings also highlight the inextricable link between meaning-making and distress. As indicated by the theoretical frameworks reviewed earlier, distress is necessary to propel meaning-making processes. However, distress may also be a consequence or a partner of these processes, particularly when the new meanings emerge from the challenges of a life review (Changed Values and Priorities) or call for change (Catalyst for Change), or when the new meaning includes the realization that some life events cannot be adequately explained (Incomprehensible).

The research reviewed above does not clarify the causal direction between sense-making and adjustment. Just as sense-making may shape adjustment, the reverse may also occur. For example, consistent with the broaden-and-build theory (Fredrickson, 2002), positive states may enable individuals to cognitively process their health trauma and thereby creatively reconstruct their worldviews so as to accommodate illness-related losses and disruptions. It is also important to note that in the studies that examined relations between the sense-making factors and adjustment in MS patients and their caregivers, the amounts of explained variance were relatively small (4% to 9%) in the study of patients and somewhat larger (8% to 17%) in the study of caregivers. However, both studies provided a relatively stringent test of the sense-making model, given that the effects of prior levels of adjustment were controlled for along with numerous pertinent covariates, and that one of the adjustment indices was based on the rating of a partner in the caregiver–patient dyad.

In furthering our understanding of the links between adjustment and both benefit-finding and sense-making, researchers need to examine aspects of psychological functioning that go beyond measures of distress, and limited positive outcomes (Stanton et al., 2006). In particular, the conceptualization of adjustment needs to be broadened to include the more existential or higher-level cognitive and motivational states such as life purpose, sense of fulfillment, self-actualization, spirituality, and wisdom (Calhoun & Tedeschi, 2006; Stanton et al., 2006).

Furthermore, researchers need to examine the relative strength of sense-making and benefit-finding in predicting adjustment to illness. I could find no published research that had examined these associations in the illness field; however, several bereavement studies have addressed this issue. Davis et al. (1998) showed that sense-making at 6 months after the loss was related to less distress in the first year after the loss but not at 13 and 18 months after the loss, whereas benefit-finding was most strongly related to lower distress at 13 and 18 months after the loss. Further, they found evidence indicating that those who made sense of their loss later tended not to experience the decreases in distress that those who made sense earlier reported. On the other hand, the association between benefit-finding and lower distress strengthened over time, whereas the associations between sense-making and distress weakened over time.

In a study of bereaved college students, Michael and Snyder (2005) found that sense-making was more strongly linked to lower bereavement-related rumination than benefit-finding. Furthermore, decreased levels of rumination mediated the beneficial effects of sense-making on well-being. Contrary to the findings by Davis et al. (1998), Michael and Snyder found that benefit-finding was more strongly related to higher well-being in the earlier grieving phase (first year) than in the later phase (after 1 year). For those in the later phase of grieving, benefit-finding was related to higher bereavement rumination. With respect to the latter, in the context of bereavement, continued active benefit-finding in the later stages may represent a more brooding and less purposeful rumination than benefit-finding in the earlier phase. The authors speculated that sense-making is more likely to be a finite process particularly pertinent in the early stages of loss, whereas benefit-finding is more likely to be an ongoing process with different benefits manifesting over time as one searches for how the event has positively influenced one's life.

As mentioned earlier, chronic illness is a multifaceted stressor that is likely to pose various crises or seismic shocks over the long haul of coping with illness. It is not clear how sense-making and benefit-finding might influence each other and link with other coping processes to shape adaptation to the illness. Model-building research that investigates the roles of both sense-making and benefit-finding within the network of coping processes that shape adjustment to illness is necessary.

Interpersonal Aspects of Benefit-Finding and Sense-Making

Theoretically and empirically, most research has examined sense-making and benefit-finding at an individual level. The chronic illness research has largely focused on the person suffering the illness, although recent research has begun to examine sense-making and benefit-finding in caregivers, but this too is on an individual level. However, meaning-making occurs at many levels, including intrapersonal, interpersonal, social, and community levels.

The role of interpersonal and social processing in meaning-making is given prominence in social construction theory. According to this perspective, the social world shapes our meaning structures. Meanings are created through our "ongoing discourse with the social world in which we live" (Gillies & Neimeyer, 2006, p. 58). For example, our social and cultural environments inform our attitudes and beliefs about illness and disability and how to manage illness. In contrast to Park and Fokman's (1997) conceptualization of situational and global meanings, social construction theory regards these meaning structures as fluid and less separable. Meaning-making is regarded as an ongoing process of "storying"—"a way of composing and recomposing one's life through sharable meanings that accumulate into life stories or narratives" (Collie & Long, 2005, p. 846). From this perspective, relationships are important in meaning-making because they allow for deep feelings to be disclosed and the validation of what is revealed (Leitner, Faidley, & Celentana, 2000). Tennen and Affleck (2009) suggest that on the basis of self-verification theory, in the context of a traumatic event people actively draw those into their social network who support their perceived positive self-changes.

In the context of close relationships such as a patient–caregiver dyad, individuals not only tell their own accounts of the illness experience, but they are also likely to tell a joint account of that experience with significant others (Kellas & Trees, 2006). Through collaboratively telling others a story about the illness experience, patient–caregiver dyads together construct meaning about the illness (Kellas & Trees, 2006).

Many of the theories reviewed earlier suggest that sharing one's experience of illness with supportive, noncritical others helps people to make sense of their illness experience and to develop illness narratives that include positive messages. In particular, the role of social processes in meaning-making has been identified in Taylor's (1983) cognitive adaption theory and Tedeschi and Calhoun's (2004) PTG theory. Taylor (1983) found that in a sample of women living with breast cancer, many women engaged in downward social comparison, which she proposed protects self-esteem and leads the way to finding benefits in adversity. Tedeschi and Calhoun (2004) suggest that relationships can facilitate benefit-finding by providing new perspectives and schemas related to growth.

Lepore and Kernan (2009) proposed a social-cognitive processing model of personal growth in the illness context that specified how the social environment can directly facilitate benefit-finding. Drawing on social control and social support theory, they proposed that the social environment could produce increased positive and reduced negative emotional outcomes via buffering the negative effects of stress, providing diversion from one's worries, and reinforcing a sense of belonging and self-worth. However, as reviewed above, the findings regarding the relations between social support and benefit-finding suggest that the link between these constructs is somewhat complex. The extent to which the social environment plays a role in facilitating sense-making and benefit-finding is likely to depend on a range of factors, including the source, type, and timing of support, match between support provided and the recipient's needs, and the quality of the relationship between the support provider and recipient. Support offered by a caregiver can be perceived as intrusive and detracting from one's independence (Pakenham, 1998b), and the sharing of the illness experience between patient and caregiver can be geared towards protecting the other partner from emotional burden (Coyne & Smith, 1991).

Several studies provide findings that support the proposal that meaning-making involves interpersonal processes. Women with breast cancer identified several social and interpersonal factors that were crucial for meaning-making, including confirmation of their experience by significant others, receiving loving support, and solving relationship problems (Jensen, Back-Pettersson, & Segesten, 2000). Fiese and Wamboldt (2003) examined narratives of family experiences related to coping with pediatric chronic illness and found that the construction of meaningful accounts of chronic illness reflected "not only the impact of the illness on family life but the coherent synthesis of family beliefs" (p. 449). Kellas and Trees (2006) used a narrative approach and qualitative data to examine sense-making at the family level with respect to difficult family experiences, some of which included health issues. They found several different forms of family-level sense-making.

Empirical support for the prominence of social processes in shaping sense-making and benefit-finding is evident in the interpersonal themes that have consistently emerged in measures of these constructs within patient and caregiver groups. In addition to facilitating meaning-making, close relationships can themselves become a source of meaning and purpose. For example, the Relationship Ties factor of the CSMS involved an explanation of caregiving and illness that reflected intimacy, reciprocity, duty, rewards, and commitment inherent in the caregiver–care recipient relationship.

Given that the person with illness and the caregiver appear to respond to illness as a social unit (Pakenham, 1998a), both are likely to become engaged in collectively searching for meaning and may become involved in a process of shared sense-making and benefit-finding. However, few studies have examined relations between benefit-finding and sense-making in a person with illness and the same processes in the caregiver. I found that the benefit-finding of MS patients was correlated with the benefit-finding of their caregivers (Pakenham, 2005b). However, there was little evidence indicating that the benefit-finding of one partner influenced the adjustment of the other. The caregiver's benefit-finding was correlated with only one of five care-recipient adjustment outcomes (positive affect), and care-recipient benefit-finding was unrelated to all five caregiver adjustment outcomes.

Samios, Pakenham, and Sofronoff (submitted) examined benefit-finding and sense-making in 81 mother–father dyads who had a child with Asperger's syndrome. Correlations partialling out gender showed that each of the six benefit-finding and six sense-making dimensions in one partner was significantly correlated with that of the other partner, with only one exception.

To examine the effects of each partner's sense-making and benefit-finding on his or her partner's adjustment, Samios et al. (submitted) used the Actor-Partner Interdependence Model (Kenny, Kashy, & Cook, 2006), which takes into account

the non-independence of dyadic data. Results of multi-level modeling showed that a partner's scores on two sense-making dimensions and two benefit-finding dimensions had significant effects on the adjustment of the other partner. With respect to benefit-finding, higher scores on the Positive Effects of the Child dimension in one partner was related to lower depression and higher life satisfaction in the other partner, whereas the New Possibilities dimension was related to less positive affect in partners. Interestingly, the latter association suggests that some types of growth in one partner are not always experienced as a positive by the other partner. Regarding sense-making, higher scores on the Identification with Asperger's syndrome dimension was related to less positive affect in the other partner, whereas Changed Perspective was related to better health in partners. The Identification with Asperger's syndrome factor is likely to be confounded with the presence of Asperger's traits in the parents who endorse it. In such cases the other partner is, therefore, faced with the challenge of dealing with a child and partner who experience Asperger's syndrome-related difficulties.

In summary, theory and preliminary empirical findings support the role of relationships in shaping sense-making and benefit-finding and in serving as a source of made meaning. There are also preliminary data suggesting that the sense-making and benefit-finding in one partner may influence the adjustment of the other and that the various dimensions of these constructs have differential effects not only on one's own adjustment but on that of the partner as well.

Interventions

In general, there are sufficient theoretical and empirical data suggesting that sense-making and benefit-finding processes should be addressed in clinical practice and interventions designed to support people with chronic illness and their caregivers. Findings from research into benefit-finding and sense-making in illness highlight the need for practitioners to facilitate patients' cognitive and emotional processing of the existential implications of their illnesses, and their rebuilding of meaning that integrates their illness experience into global meaning structures.

Sense-making and benefit-finding processes in the context of illness encompass fundamental existential life issues; hence, interventions designed to address the existential crises associated with illness may facilitate sense-making and benefit-finding.

LeMay and Wilson (2007) reviewed eight manualized interventions that explicitly addressed existential themes in the context of life-threatening illness. In general, the interventions targeted "existential distress" experienced in the end-of-life phase of coping with life-threatening illness. The primary outcome variables for the intervention studies were distress and QOL. None of the studies assessed sense-making, benefit-finding, or other related meaning-making processes. However, one intervention explicitly targeted meaning-making without assessing meaning (Kissane et al., 2003; Lee, Cohen, Edgar, Laizner, & Gagnon, 2006a; Lee, Cohen, Edgar, Laizner, & Gagnon, 2006b). The conceptualization of meaning-making was informed by Frankl's (1984) and Janoff-Bulman's (1992) frameworks. Intervention strategies included cognitive-behavioral therapy (CBT) techniques. Results showed that the cancer patients who received the intervention reported higher self-esteem, optimism, and self-efficacy compared to the control group.

Two intervention studies have examined the effects on benefit-finding of a 10-week group CBT stress-management intervention for breast cancer (Antoni et al., 2001) and prostate cancer patients (Penedo et al., 2006). Although the intervention did not target benefit-finding, in both studies the treatment group evidenced more gains in benefit-finding than the control group. Treatment dismantling studies are necessary to identify potent behavior change elements responsible for increased benefit-finding.

Tedeschi and Calhoun (2009) have proposed a "clinician as expert companion" approach to facilitating PTG. Based on their theory of PTG, they suggest that one of the most important intervention tasks is to "guide patients in moving from merely suffering, to suffering meaningfully" (Tedeschi & Calhoun, 2009, p. 216). This involves helping patients to make sense of their illness and to find purpose and meaning in illness experiences. Tedeschi and Calhoun (2009) identify strategies for helping patients negotiate three challenges on the pathway to PTG: managing emotional distress, reconsidering beliefs and life goals, and revising the life narrative. The latter two challenges involve sense-making processes. In this regard, the expert companion "walks alongside" the patient and shares in his or her struggle with difficult life questions and uncertain answers, and the ambiguity of what to believe and how to live.

Given the interpersonal elements to sense-making and benefit-finding, it is important that interventions include strategies that target the social domain, including encouraging social interaction and the sharing of illness experiences, emphasizing the value of relationships, acknowledging illness-related strains on relationships, and promoting awareness of one's own struggle to make sense of the illness situation relative to that of loved ones. Many of the intervention programs reviewed above have used a group format providing opportunities for safe disclosure, support, and exposure to alternative illness perspectives and narratives. Interventions may also address the interpersonal aspects of meaning-making by including both patients and their caregivers in treatment. The benefits of a dyadic treatment approach were made evident in a randomized control trial of a predominantly CBT intervention for people affected by AIDS (Pakenham, Dadds, & Lennon, 2002). Participants were randomly assigned to a patient–caregiver intervention, a caregiver-alone intervention, or a control group. Relative to caregivers and care recipients in the caregiver-alone intervention and control groups, those in the dyadic intervention evidenced greater improvements across social, emotional, relationship, physical health, and target problem outcomes, and these gains were maintained at a 4-month follow-up.

Several studies have demonstrated health gains resulting from written expressive disclosure interventions that focus on writing about the benefits of traumatic events, including illness (King & Miner, 2000; Stanton et al., 2002b). Using a sample of breast cancer patients, Stanton et al. (2002b) found that, compared to a control group (who wrote about their cancer and treatment), women who wrote about either their deepest thoughts and feelings (standard written disclosure condition) or their positive thoughts and feelings (benefit-finding condition) about cancer reported more health benefits.

Fava and colleagues (Fava, Rafanelli, Cazzaro, Conti, & Grandi, 1998a; Fava, Rafanelli, Grandi, Conti, & Belluardo, 1998b) developed a "well-being therapy" that uses CBT approaches to decrease factors that interrupt well-being and to reinforce behaviors that promote well-being in the six areas identified by Ryff (1989): self-acceptance, purpose in life, positive relations with others, personal growth, environmental mastery, and autonomy. In pilot work by Fava et al. (1998a), people with mood and anxiety disorders who received well-being therapy showed gains in personal growth and contentment and a decrease in anxiety symptoms.

An intervention approach that is well suited to facilitating the rebuilding of meaning and that incorporates many of the elements of the interventions mentioned above is Acceptance and Commitment Therapy (ACT). Hayes et al. (2006) define ACT as "a psychological intervention based on modern behavioral psychology, including Relational Frame Theory, that applies mindfulness and acceptance processes, and commitment and behavior change processes to the creation of psychological flexibility" (p. 10). ACT shares common philosophical roots with theoretical frameworks relevant to sense-making and benefit-finding, including constructivism, narrative psychology, social constructivism, and existentialism. ACT promotes acceptance of what cannot be changed (such as an illness), taking responsibility for one's experiences and actions, and drawing on one's fundamental freedom to create a meaningful life through choosing committed action that is in the service of one's life values.

ACT interventions are consistent with Tedeschi and Calhoun's (2009) guidelines for promoting PTG and rebuilding the assumptive world, including the use of metaphors and empathy, acknowledging the paradoxes and ambiguities in life, encouraging direct contact with life as it is rather than as one wants it to be, and managing distress without suppressing it while at the same time acknowledging one's growth in the face of adversity. Noteworthy are the acceptance dimensions that have emerged in measures of benefit-finding, sense-making, and coping strategies in illness and caregiving contexts, which are typically related to better adjustment (Pakenham, 2002, 2006, 2007a, 2008a; Rinaldis et al., 2010).

According to the ACT framework, human language and cognition are learned and contextually controlled and can influence behavior. ACT helps to change the way people view their thoughts and loosen the controls language has over behavior, thereby achieving greater cognitive flexibility. ACT can therefore help to foster more flexible, workable sense-making explanations. In ACT, individuals are cautioned not to hold any beliefs "tightly," including sense-making explanations and perceptions of growth. In addition, ACT includes many of the treatment strategies employed in the intervention programs above, including metaphors, experiential exercises, CBT techniques, and mindfulness. Regarding the latter, mindfulness interventions have become increasingly common in some illness domains (e.g., oncology; Mackenzie, Carlson, & Speca, 2005). The relevance of mindfulness is also evident in the mindfulness dimensions of some benefit-finding scales and the frequently cited reports of people with illness concerning greater appreciation of life and moment-to-moment living. There is now mounting evidence of the efficacy of ACT in treating a range of psychological problems and producing QOL and/or health benefits in people with chronic illnesses (see reviews by Hayes et al., 2006; Powers, Zum Vorde Sive Vording, & Emmelkamp, 2009).

Future Research Directions

This final section summarizes some of the key future research directions and discusses the following: examination of sense-making and benefit-finding within broader theoretical frameworks, issues related to the links between sense-making and benefit-finding and those issues specific to each one, and finally practice implications.

Benefit-finding and sense-making within the broader stress and coping framework

It is now time to place more theoretical and empirical research focus on a broadened examination of the roles of sense-making and benefit-finding within the network of stress and coping processes that shape adaptation to illness. We need to extend our understanding of sense-making and benefit-finding relative to the other coping processes shown to be important in managing illness. In this regard, research using model-testing approaches is required that assesses the range of theoretically relevant variables. Research that has already begun to move in this direction, at least with respect to benefit-finding, suggests that meaning-making is likely to have reciprocal relations with a cluster of personal resources.

Issues related to both sense-making and benefit-finding

Few studies have examined the link between sense-making and benefit-finding. Based on the Janoff-Bulman and Yopyk (2004) proposal that sense-making serves as a catalyst for the creation of meaning via benefit-finding, it is expected that sense-making and benefit-finding would be linked, and that the effects of sense-making on measures of meaningfulness would be mediated by benefit-finding. Alternatively, sense-making may exert an influence on benefit-finding via its effects on other cognitive (e.g., rumination) or emotional (e.g., positive affect) processes. The mechanisms by which benefit-finding and sense-making are linked require further investigation. Preliminary findings suggest three potential pathways between sense-making and benefit-finding. The sense-making processes of finding new life purpose that incorporates the illness, revising life values and goals that account for the illness, and accepting life as it is appear to provide pathways to all aspects of benefit-finding. Spiritual sense-making and causal explanations provide weaker links to only some benefits, and viewing illness as a random event detracts from finding benefits in the spiritual and lifestyle domains.

Researchers need to move away from the simplistic view that all aspects of meaning-making should always be related to less distress. Perhaps this focus reflects society's obsession with ridding ourselves of distress in a desperate search for or attachment to happiness; yet distress is not "bad." Distress is implied as both a trigger and a partner of meaning-making, and recent research suggests that it may also be a consequence of some domains of sense-making and possibly benefit-finding at certain points in the ongoing process of making meaning out of illness. The presence of distress does not mean the absence of positive affect; both may co-occur in the process of coping with illness (Folkman, 1997). Indeed, Janoff-Bulman (2004) suggests that suffering is one of the pathways to growth.

Researchers need to distinguish between benefit-finding and sense-making as meaning-making processes and as made meaning. The former represents those cognitive and behavioral strategies that lead to the latter. Such distinctions need to be reflected in measurement approaches and the timing of assessment in the process of coping with chronic illness.

To better understand the relative sequential unfolding of benefit-finding and sense-making over the course of an illness, longitudinal research designs are required. Longitudinal methodologies should include assessments of benefit-finding, sense-making, and adjustment outcomes at several points from diagnosis to several years later. More regular assessment points may be particularly important in illnesses with episodic courses.

Another question that requires investigation is whether sense-making is necessary for benefit-finding to occur, as the theoretical frameworks suggest. Findings of several studies suggest that both sense-making and benefit-finding may occur independent of each other (e.g., Pakenham et al., 2004). However, it is possible that if one occurs in the absence of the other, "deep" and lasting meaningfulness might not be attained. For example, if benefit-finding occurs in the absence of having made sense of the illness, the benefit-finding may be more reflective of brooding rumination or a denial of the inevitable losses that illness incurs.

There is now considerable evidence indicating that sense-making and benefit-finding are influenced by interpersonal processes and that relationships themselves are a source of meaning. Research that includes data on meaning-making from both patients and their caregivers is necessary. Such research designs should draw on recently developed dyadic data analytic approaches that address problems inherent in dyadic data, such as the non-independence of data. Recent research that has used such approaches provides useful insights into shared meaning-making processes (Samios et al., submitted).

Research is required that examines whether the nature, timing, and sequential unfolding of sense-making and benefit-finding vary across different illness contexts. An important limitation of the body of research that has examined benefit-finding is that much of the research has been conducted on people living with cancer, and many of the cancer studies have been conducted using white middle-class women with breast cancer. There are emerging trends indicating that some of the findings concerning benefit-finding that have come out of the breast cancer studies do not generalize to other cancer samples (e.g., older and predominantly male colorectal cancer survivors; Rinaldis & Pakenham, 2009) or other illness groups. It is important that we do not build a body of knowledge around meaning-making that is limited to one illness or one category of persons within an illness grouping.

Sense-making

Sense-making is in some ways the "poor cousin" to benefit-finding. While benefit-finding has attracted a huge volume of research activity, sense-making has been left in the backdrops, despite many theories of coping with loss and trauma specifying equivalent roles for both constructs. Perhaps the focus on benefit-finding reflects our focus, and that of society's, on the positives (the era of "positive thinking") and our fascination and amazement with how people can grow from suffering. Theory and recent research suggest that sense-making is a potent predictor of adjustment and therefore requires further detailed examination. Because sense-making has been neglected by empirical researchers, there are many gaps in our knowledge with respect to measurement, relations with adjustment, and so forth. Below I elaborate on just a few issues specific to sense-making.

Earlier I proposed a model of sense-making in illness that involved seven processes: finding new life purpose, awakening to the spiritual, finding cause, revising life values and goals, appreciating social ties as a source of meaning, accepting life as it is, and acknowledging the randomness and/or the incomprehensibility of some events. Together these sense-making processes address fundamental life issues of personal vulnerability, relative safety, uncertainty, and impermanence. Further research is required to test and build on this model of sense-making. One interesting avenue of inquiry is whether these sense-making processes arise via different pathways. For example, are these sense-making processes differentially related to the three pathways for developing benefit-finding proposed by Janoff-Bulman (2004)?

Several sense-making measurement issues were discussed earlier. In summary, further research is required to examine the following: the temporal stability and validation of multi-item measures, the superiority of various sense-making measurement approaches (e.g., narrative vs. multi-item scale vs. dichotomous measures), and the development of conceptually distinct measures of sense-making as a process, and sense-making as made meaning. Measurement should also take into account the relative strength of particular sense-making themes within a sense-making narrative.

It may be important for future research to clarify whether some identified sense-making dimensions represent personally derived and chosen meanings, while others reflect adopted socially and culturally prescribed explanations for illness. According to existentialists the former is likely to lead to revised personal values and authentic living, whereas the latter is likely to result in externally defined values that may not be personally valid, blocking unique individual potential (Martin, Campbell, & Henry, 2004).

Benefit-finding

Further research is needed to explore the emerging complex relations between benefit-finding and adjustment, including the curvilinear relations, moderators of this relationship, and the potential stress-buffering effects of benefit-finding. Such relationships may also be relevant to sense-making but have yet to be explored. In addition, keeping in mind the distinction between meaning-making processes and made meaning, researchers need to test the proposal that benefit-finding measured as meaning found represents a cognitive interim outcome that is influenced by stress and coping processes

and that, in turn, results in emotional and functional outcomes.

Two important challenges regarding the measurement and conceptualization of benefit-finding are ensuring that the following pairs of related constructs are operationally distinct: benefit-finding perceptions and veridical growth, and benefit-finding processes and benefit-finding as made meaning.

Interventions

Although a range of psychosocial interventions have been used to assist people with chronic illness and their caregivers, few have examined whether they produce changes in meaning-making processes or made meanings. CBT stress-management intervention studies have demonstrated changes in benefit-finding. However, treatment dismantling studies are needed to isolate the elements of these multicomponent interventions that produce changes in benefit-finding. Experimental intervention studies that examine the mechanisms by which sense-making and benefit-finding change are also required. Finally, the application of ACT to facilitating adjustment to illness is a promising research direction. ACT has theoretical roots and treatment strategies that are consistent with clinical guidelines for promoting PTG and with the theoretical frameworks that account for the roles of sense-making and benefit-finding in adversity.

References

Abraido-Lanza, A. F., Guier, C., & Colon, R. M. (1998). Psychological thriving among Latinas with chronic illness. *Journal of Social Issues, 54*, 405–24.

Affleck, G., & Tennen, H. (1993). Cognitive adaptation to adversity: Insights from parents of medically fragile infants. In A. P. Turnbull, J. M. Patterson, S. K. Behr, D. L. Murphy, J. G. Marquis & M. J. Blue-Banning (Eds.), *Cognitive coping, families, and disability* (pp. 135–50). Baltimore: Paul H. Brookes Publishing Co.

Algoe, S. B., & Stanton, A. L. (2009). Is benefit-finding good for individuals with chronic disease? In C. L. Park, S. C. Lechner, M. H. Antoni & A. L. Stanton (Eds.), *Medical illness and positive life change: Can crisis lead to personal transformation?* (pp. 173–94). Washington, DC: APA.

Antoni, M. H., Lehman, J. M., Klibourn, K. M., Boyers, A. E., Culver, J. L., Alferi, S. M., et al. (2001). Cognitive-behavioral stress management intervention decreases the prevalence of depression and enhances benefit-finding among women under treatment for early-stage breast cancer. *Health Psychology, 20*(1), 20–32.

Antonovsky, A. (1987). *Unraveling the mystery of health.* San Francisco: Jossey-Bass.

Armeli, S., Gunthert, K. C., & Cohen, L. H. (2001). Stressor-appraisals, coping, and post-event outcomes: the dimensionality and antecedents of stress-related growth. *Journal of Social and Clinical Psychology, 20*, 366–95.

Baarnhielm, S. (2005). Making sense of different illness realities: Restructuring of illness meaning among Swedish-born women. *Nordic Journal of Psychiatry, 59*, 350–6.

Behr, S. K., & Murphy, D. L. (1993). Research progress and promise: The role of perceptions in cognitive adaptation to disability. In A. P. Turnbull, J. M. Patterson, S. K. Behr, D. L. Murphy, J. G. Marquis & M. J. Blue-Banning (Eds.), *Cognitive coping, families, and disability* (pp. 151–63). Baltimore: Paul H. Brookes Publishing Co.

Bellizzi, K. M., & Blank, T. O. (2006). Predicting posttraumatic growth in breast cancer survivors. *Health Psychology, 25*(1), 47–56.

Bellizzi, K. M., Farmer Miller, M., Arora, N. K., & Rowland, J. H. (2007). Positive and negative life changes experienced by survivors of non-Hodgkin's lymphoma. *Annals of Behavioral Medicine, 34*(2), 188–99.

Bower, J. E., Meyerowitz, B. E., Desmond, K. A., Bernaards, C. A., Rowland, J. H., & Ganz, P. A. (2005). Perceptions of positive meaning and vulnerability following breast cancer: Predictors and outcomes among long-term breast cancer survivors. *Annals of Behavioral Medicine, 29*(3), 236–45.

Bower, J. E., & Segerstrom, S. C. (2004). Stress management, finding benefit, and immune function: Positive mechanisms for intervention effects on physiology. *Journal of Psychosomatic Research, 56*, 9–11.

Calhoun, L. G., & Tedeschi, R. G. (Eds.). (2006). *Handbook of posttraumatic growth.* New Jersey: Lawrence Erlbaum Associates.

Carpenter, J. S., Brockopp, D. Y., & Andrykowski, M. A. (1999). Self-transformation as a factor in the self-esteem and well-being of breast cancer survivors. *Journal of Advanced Nursing, 29*, 1402–11.

Carver, C. S., & Antoni, M. H. (2004). Finding benefit in breast cancer during the year after diagnosis predicts better adjustment 5 to 8 years after diagnosis. *Health Psychology, 23*(6), 595–8.

Carver, C. S., Lechner, S. C., & Antoni, M. H. (2009). Challenges in studying positive change after adversity: Illustrations from research on breast cancer. In C. L. Park, S. C. Lechner, M. H. Antoni & A. L. Stanton (Eds.), *Medical illness and positive life change: Can crisis lead to personal transformation?* (pp. 51–62). Washington, DC: APA.

Cheng, C., Wong, W.-M., & Tsang, K. W. (2006). Perception of benefits and costs during SARS outbreak: An 18-month prospective study. *Journal of Consulting and Clinical Psychology, 74*(5), 870–9.

Collie, K., & Long, B. C. (2005). Considering "meaning" in the context of breast cancer. *Journal of Health Psychology, 10*(6), 843–53.

Cordova, M. J., Cunningham, L. L. C., Carlson, C. R., & Andrykowski, M. A. (2001). Posttraumatic growth following breast cancer: A controlled comparison study. *Health Psychology, 20*, 176–85.

Costa, R. & Pakenham, K. I. (submitted). *Associations between benefit- finding and adjustment outcomes in thyroid cancer.*

Coyne, J. C., & Smith, D. A. (1991). Couples coping with a myocardial infarction: A contextual perspective on wives' distress. *Journal of Personality and Social Psychology, 61*(3), 404–12.

Davis, C. G., Nolen-Hoeksema, S., & Larson, J. (1998). Making sense of loss and benefiting from the experience: two construals of meaning. *Journal of Personality and Social Psychology, 75*(2), 561–74.

Dunn, D. S., & Dougherty, S. B. (2005). Prospects for a positive psychology of rehabilitation. *Rehabilitation Psychology, 50*(3), 305–11.

Dunn, J., Lynch, B., Rinaldis, M., Pakenham, K. I., McPherson, L., Owen, N., et al. (2006). Dimensions of quality of life and psychosocial variables most salient to colorectal cancer patients. *Psycho-Oncology, 15*, 20–30.

Esterling, B. A., L'Abate, L., Murray, E. J., & Pennebaker, J. W. (1992). Empirical foundations for writing in prevention and psychotherapy: Mental and physical health outcomes. *Clinical Psychology Review, 19*, 280–7.

Evers, A. W. M., Kraaimaat, F. W., Lankveld, W., Jongen, P. J. H., Jacobs, J. W. G., & Bijlsma, J. W. J. (2001). Beyond unfavorable thinking: The Illness Cognition Questionnaire for chronic diseases. *Journal of Consulting and Clinical Psychology, 69*(6), 1026–36.

Fava, G. A., Rafanelli, C., Cazzaro, M., Conti, S., & Grandi, S. (1998a). Well-being therapy. A novel psychotherapeutic approach for residual symptoms of affective disorders. *Psychological Medicine, 28*, 475–80.

Fava, G. A., Rafanelli, C., Grandi, S., Conti, S., & Belluardo, P. (1998b). Prevention of recurrent depression with cognitive behavioral therapy. *Archives of General Psychiatry, 55*, 816–20.

Fiese, B. H., & Wamboldt, F. S. (2003). Coherent accounts of coping with a chronic illness: Convergences and divergences in family measurement using a narrative analysis. *Family Process, 42*(4), 439–51.

Fife, B. L. (1994). The conceptualization of meaning in illness. *Social Science and Medicine, 38*(2), 309–16.

Folkman, S. (1997). Positive psychological states and coping with severe stress. *Social Science and Medicine, 45*(8), 1207–21.

Folkman, S. (2008). The case for positive emotions in the stress process. *Anxiety, Stress, & Coping, 21*(1), 3–14.

Folkman, S., & Moskowitz, J. T. (2000). Positive affect and the other side of coping. *American Psychologist, 55*(6), 647–54.

Frank, A. W. (1995). *The wounded storyteller: Body, illness, and ethics.* London: University of Chicago Press.

Frankl, V. E. (1984). *Man's search for meaning: An introduction to logotherapy* (3rd ed.). New York: Simon & Schuster.

Frazier, P. A., & Kaler, M. E. (2006). Assessing the validity of self-reported stress-related growth. *Journal of Consulting and Clinical Psychology, 74*(5), 859–69.

Fredrickson, B. L. (2002). Positive emotions. In C. R. Snyder & S. J. Lopez (Eds.), *Handbook of positive psychology* (pp. 120–34). New York: Oxford University Press.

Gillies, J., & Neimeyer, R. A. (2006). Loss, grief, and the search for significance: toward a model of meaning reconstruction in bereavement. *Journal of Constructivist Psychology, 19*, 31–65.

Gray, R. E., Fitch, M., Phillips, C., Labrecque, M., & Fergus, K. (2000). Managing the impact of illness: the experiences of men with prostate cancer and their spouses. *Journal of Health Psychology, 5*(4), 531–48.

Hayes, S. C., Luoma, J. B., Bond, F. W., Masuda, A., & Lillis, J. (2006). Acceptance and commitment therapy: Model, processes and outcomes. *Behaviour Research and Therapy, 44*, 1–25.

Helgeson, V. S., Reynolds, K. A., & Tomich, P. L. (2006). A meta-analytic review of benefit-finding and growth. *Journal of Consulting and Clinical Psychology, 74*(5), 797–816.

Janoff-Bulman, R. (1992). *Shattered assumptions: Towards a new psychology of trauma.* New York: Free Press.

Janoff-Bulman, R. (2004). Posttraumatic growth: Three explanatory models. *Psychological Inquiry, 15*(1), 30–4.

Janoff-Bulman, R., & Frantz, C. (1997). The impact of trauma on meaning: from meaningless world to meaningful life. In M. J. Power & C. R. Brewin (Eds.), *The transformation of meaning in psychological therapies: Integrating theory and practice* (pp. 91–106). New York: Wiley.

Janoff-Bulman, R., & Yopyk, D. J. (2004). Random outcomes and valued commitments: Existential dilemmas and the paradox of meaning. In J. Greenberg, S. L. Koole, & T. Pyszczynski (Eds.), *Handbook of experimental existential psychology* (pp. 122–38). New York: Guilford Press.

Jardim, C., & Pakenham, K. I. (2010). Carers of adults with mental illness: A comparison of respite care users and non-users. *Australian Psychologist, 45*(1), 50–58.

Jensen, K. P., Back-Pettersson, S., & Segesten, K. (2000). The meaning of "not giving in": Lived experiences among women with breast cancer. *Cancer Nursing, 23*(1), 6–11.

Joseph, S., & Linley, P. A. (2005). Positive adjustment to threatening events: An organismic valuing theory of growth through adversity. *Review of General Psychology, 9*(3), 262–80.

Joseph, S., & Linley, P. A. (2006). Growth following adversity: theoretical perspectives and implications for clinical practice. *Clinical Psychology Review, 26*, 1041–53.

Kellas, J. K., & Trees, A. R. (2006). Finding meaning in difficult family experiences: Sense-making and interaction processes during joint family storytelling. *Journal of Family Communication, 6*, 49–76.

Kenny, D. A., Kashy, D. A., & Cook, W. L. (2006). *Dyadic data analysis*. New York: Guilford Press.

Kernan, W. D., & Lepore, S. J. (2009). Searching for and making meaning after breast cancer: Prevalence, patterns, and negative affect. *Social Science and Medicine, 68*, 1176–82.

King, L. A., & Miner, K. N. (2000). Writing about the perceived benefits of traumatic events: Implications for physical health. *Personality and Social Psychology Bulletin, 26*(2), 220–30.

Kissane, D. W., Block, S., Smith, G. C., Miach, P., Clarke, D. M., Ikin, J., et al. (2003). Cognitive-existential group psychotherapy for women with primary breast cancer: A randomised controlled trial. *Psycho-Oncology, 12*, 532–46.

Lang, G. C. (1989). "Making sense" about diabetes: Dakota narratives of illness. *Medical Anthropology, 11*(3), 305–27.

Lazarus, R. S., & Folkman, S. (1984). *Stress, appraisal, and coping*. New York: Springer.

Lechner, S. C., Carver, C. S., Antoni, M. H., Weaver, K. E., & Phillips, K. M. (2006). Curvilinear associations between benefit-finding and psychosocial adjustment to breast cancer. *Journal of Consulting and Clinical Psychology, 74*(5), 828–40.

Lechner, S. C., Zakowski, S. G., Antoni, M. H., Greenhawt, M., Block, K., & Block, P. (2003). Do sociodemographic and disease-related variables influence benefit-finding in cancer patients? *Psycho-Oncology, 12*, 491–9.

Lee, V., Cohen, S. R., Edgar, L., Laizner, A., & Gagnon, A. J. (2006a). Meaning-making and psychological adjustment to cancer: Development of an intervention and pilot results. *Oncology Nursing Forum, 33*, 291–302.

Lee, V., Cohen, S. R., Edgar, L., Laizner, A. M., & Gagnon, A. J. (2006b). Meaning-making intervention during breast or colorectal cancer treatment improves self-esteem, optimism, and self-efficacy. *Social Science and Medicine, 62*(12), 3133–45.

Lee, Y., & McCormick, B. P. (2002). Sense-making process in defining health for people with chronic illnesses and disabilities. *Therapeutic Recreation Journal, 36*(3), 235–46.

Leitner, L. M., Faidley, A. J., & Celentana, M. (2000). Diagnosing human meaning-making: An experiential constructivist approach. In R. A. Neimeyer & J. Raskin (Eds.), *Constructions of disorder: Meaning-making frameworks for psychotherapy* (pp. 175–204). Washington, DC: APA.

LeMay, K., & Wilson, K. G. (2007). Treatment of existential distress in life threatening illness: A review of manualized interventions. *Clinical Psychology Review, 28*(3), 472–93.

Lepore, S. J., & Kernan, W. D. (2009). Positive life change and the social context of illness: An expanded social-cognitive processing model. In C. L. Park, S. C. Lechner, M. H. Antoni, & A. L. Stanton (Eds.), *Medical illness and positive life change: Can crisis lead to personal transformation?* (pp. 139–52). Washington, DC: APA.

Lerner, M. J., & Gignac, M. A. M. (1992). Is it coping or is it growth? A cognitive-affective model of contentment in the elderly. In L. Montada, S. Filipp, & M. J. Lerner (Eds.), *Life crises and experiences of loss in adulthood* (pp. 321–37). Hillsdale, NJ: Erlbaum.

Linley, P. A., & Joseph, S. (2004). Positive change following trauma and adversity: A review. *Journal of Traumatic Stress, 17*(1), 11–21.

Littlewood, R. A., Vanable, P. A., Carey, M. P., & Blair, D. C. (2008). The association of benefit-finding to psychosocial and health behavior adaptation among HIV+ men and women. *Journal of Behavioral Medicine, 31*, 145–55.

Luszczynska, A., Mohamed, N. E., & Schwarzer, R. (2005). Self-efficacy and social support predict benefit-finding 12 months after cancer surgery: The mediating role of coping strategies. *Psychology, Health, & Medicine, 10*(4), 365–75.

Mackenzie, M. J., Carlson, L. E., & Speca, M. (2005). Mindfulness-based stress reduction (MBSR) in oncology: Rationale and review. *Evidence-based Integrative Medicine, 2*(3), 139–45.

Martin, L. L., Campbell, W. K., & Henry, C. D. (2004). The roar of awakening: Mortality acknowledgement as a call to authentic living. In J. Greenberg, S. L. Koole, & T. Pyszczynski (Eds.), *Handbook of experimental existential psychology* (pp. 431–48). New York: Guilford Press.

McMillen, J. C., & Cook, C. L. (2003). The positive by-products of spinal cord injury and their correlates. *Rehabilitation Psychology, 48*(2), 77–85.

McMillen, J. C., & Fisher, R. H. (1998). The Perceived Benefit Scales: Measuring perceived positive life changes after negative events. *Social Work Research, 22*(3), 173–86.

McMillen, J. C., Smith, E. M., & Fisher, R. H. (1997). Perceived benefits and mental health after three types of disaster. *Journal of Consulting and Clinical Psychology, 65*, 733–9.

Michael, S. T., & Snyder, C. R. (2005). Getting unstuck: the roles of hope, finding meaning, and rumination in the adjustment to bereavement among college students. *Death Studies, 29*, 435–58.

Milam, J. (2006). Posttraumatic growth and HIV disease progression. *Journal of Consulting and Clinical Psychology, 74*(5), 817–27.

Pakenham, K. I. (1998a). Couple coping and adjustment to multiple sclerosis in care receiver-carer dyads. *Family Relations: Interdisciplinary Journal of Applied Family Studies, 47*(3), 269–77.

Pakenham, K. I. (1998b). Specification of social support behaviours and network dimensions along the HIV continuum for gay men. *Patient Education and Counseling, 34*(2), 147–57.

Pakenham, K. I. (1999). Adjustment to multiple sclerosis: Application of a stress and coping model. *Health Psychology, 18*(4), 383–92.

Pakenham, K. I. (2002). Development of a measure of coping with multiple sclerosis caregiving. *Psychology and Health, 17*(1), 97–118.

Pakenham, K. I. (2005a). Benefit-finding in multiple sclerosis and associations with positive and negative outcomes. *Health Psychology, 24*(2), 123–32.

Pakenham, K. I. (2005b). The positive impact of multiple sclerosis on carers: Associations between carer benefit-finding and positive and negative adjustment domains. *Disability and Rehabilitation, 27*(17), 985–97.

Pakenham, K. I. (2006). Investigation of the coping antecedents to positive outcomes and distress in multiple sclerosis (MS). *Psychology and Health, 21*(3), 633–49.

Pakenham, K. I. (2007a). Making sense of multiple sclerosis. *Rehabilitation Psychology, 52*, 380–9.

Pakenham, K. I. (2007b). The nature of benefit-finding in multiple sclerosis. *Psychology, Health and Medicine, 12*(2), 190–6.

Pakenham, K. I. (2008a). Making sense of caregiving for persons with multiple sclerosis (MS): The dimensional structure of sense-making and relations with positive and negative adjustment. *International Journal of Behavioral Medicine, 15*, 241–52.

Pakenham, K. I. (2008b). Making sense of illness or disability: The nature of sense-making in multiple sclerosis (MS). *Journal of Health Psychology, 13*(1), 93–105.

Pakenham, K. I. (2008c). The nature of sense-making in caregiving for persons with multiple sclerosis (MS). *Disability and Rehabilitation, 30*(17), 1263–73.

Pakenham, K. I., & Cox, S. (2008). Development of the Benefit-finding in Multiple Sclerosis (MS) Caregiving Scale: A longitudinal study of relations between benefit-finding and adjustment. *British Journal of Health Psychology, 13*, 583–602.

Pakenham, K. I., & Cox, S. (2009). The dimensional structure of benefit-finding in multiple sclerosis and relations with positive and negative adjustment: A longitudinal study. *Psychology and Health, 24*(4), 373–93.

Pakenham, K. I., Dadds, M. R., & Lennon, H. V. (2002). The efficacy of a psychosocial intervention for HIV/AIDS caregiving dyads and individual caregivers: A controlled treatment outcome study. *AIDS Care, 14*(6), 731–50.

Pakenham, K. I., Sofronoff, K., & Samios, C. (2004). Finding meaning in parenting a child with Asperger's syndrome: Correlates of sense-making and benefit-finding. *Research in Developmental Disabilities, 25*, 245–64.

Park, C. L. (2004). The notion of stress-related growth: Problems and prospects. *Psychological Inquiry, 15*, 69–76.

Park, C. L. (2005). Religion as a meaning-making framework in coping with life stress. *Journal of Social Issues, 61*(4), 707–29.

Park, C. L. (2009). Overview of theoretical perspectives. In C. L. Park, S. C. Lechner, M. H. Antoni, & A. L. Stanton (Eds.), *Medical illness and positive life change: Can crisis lead to personal transformation?* (pp. 11–30). Washington, DC: APA.

Park, C. L., Cohen, L. H., & Murch, R. L. (1996). Assessment and prediction of stress-related growth. *Journal of Personality, 64*(1), 71–105.

Park, C. L., Edmondson, D., Fenster, J. R., & Blank, T. O. (2008). Meaning making and psychological adjustment following cancer: The mediating roles of growth, life meaning,

and restored just-world beliefs. *Journal of Consulting and Clinical Psychology, 76*(5), 863–75.

Park, C. L., & Folkman, S. (1997). Meaning in the context of stress and coping. *Review of General Psychology, 1*(2), 115–44.

Park, C. L., & Helgeson, V. S. (2006). Introduction to the special section: Growth following highly stressful life events: current status and future directions. *Journal of Consulting and Clinical Psychology, 74*(5), 791–6.

Park, C. L., & Lechner, S. (2006). Measurement issues in assessing growth following stressful life experiences. In L. G. Calhoun & R. G. Tedeschi (Eds.), *Handbook of posttraumatic growth* (pp. 47–67). New Jersey: Lawrence Erlbaum Associates.

Penedo, F. J., Molton, I., Dahn, J. R., Shen, B. J., Kinsinger, D., Traeger, L., et al. (2006). A randomized clinical trial of group-based cognitive-behavioral stress management in localized prostate cancer: Development of stress management skills improves quality of life and benefit-finding. *Annals of Behavioral Medicine, 31*, 261–70.

Powers, M. B., Zum Vorde Sive Vording, M. B., & Emmelkamp, P. M. G. (2009). Acceptance and commitment therapy: A meta-analytic review. *Psychotherapy and Psychosomatics, 78*, 73–80.

Ransom, S., Sheldon, K. M., & Jacobsen, P. B. (2008). Actual change and inaccurate recall contribute to posttraumatic growth following radiotherapy. *Journal of Consulting and Clinical Psychology, 76*(5), 811–9.

Rinaldis, M., Pakenham, K. I., & Lynch, B. (in press). A structural model of the relationships among stress, coping, benefit-finding and quality of life in persons diagnosed with colorectal cancer. *Psychology and Health*.

Rinaldis, M., Pakenham, K. I., & Lynch, B. (2010). Relationships between quality of life and finding benefits in a diagnosis of colorectal cancer. *British Journal of Psychology, 101*, 259–275.

Robinson, L., Clare, L., & Evans, K. (2005). Making sense of dementia and adjusting to loss: psychological reactions to a diagnosis of dementia in couples. *Aging and Mental Health, 9*(4), 337–437.

Ryff, C. D. (1989). Happiness is everything, or is it? Explorations on the meaning of psychological well-being. *Journal of Personality and Social Psychology, 57*, 1069–81.

Samios, C., Pakenham, K. I., & Sofronoff, K. (2008). The nature of sense-making in parenting a child with Asperger's syndrome. *Research in Autism Spectrum Disorders, 2*, 516–32.

Samios, C., Pakenham, K. I., & Sofronoff, K. (submitted). Shared meaning making in couples who have a child with Asperger's syndrome: A dyadic approach to sense-making and benefit-finding.

Schulz, U., & Mohamed, N. E. (2004). Turning the tide: Benefit-finding after cancer surgery. *Social Science and Medicine, 59*, 653–62.

Sears, S. R., Stanton, A. L., & Danoff Burg, S. (2003). The yellow brick road and the emerald city: Benefit-finding, positive reappraisal coping, and posttraumatic growth in women with early-stage breast cancer. *Health Psychology, 22*(5), 487–97.

Seligman, M. E. P., & Csikszentmihalyi, M. (2000). Positive psychology. *American Psychologist, 55*(1).

Siegel, K., & Schrimshaw, E. W. (2000). Perceiving benefits in adversity: Stress-related growth in women living with HIV/AIDS. *Social Science and Medicine, 51*, 1543–54.

Siegel, K., Schrimshaw, E. W., & Pretter, S. (2005). Stress-related growth among women living with HIV/AIDS: Examination of an explanatory model. *Journal of Behavioral Medicine, 28*(5), 403–14.

Stanton, A. L., Bower, J. E., & Low, C. A. (2006). Posttraumatic growth after cancer. In L. G. Calhoun & R. G. Tedeschi (Eds.), *Hanbook of posttraumatic growth* (pp. 138–75). New Jersey: Lawrence Erlbaum Associates.

Stanton, A. L., Danoff-Burg, S., & Huggins, M. E. (2002a). The first year after breast cancer diagnosis: Hope and coping strategies as predictors of adjustment. *Psycho-Oncology, 11*, 93–102.

Stanton, A. L., Danoff Burg, S., Sworowski, L. A., Collins, A. C., Branstetter, A. D., Rodriguez-Hanley, A., et al. (2002b). Randomized, controlled trial of written emotional expression and benefit-finding in breast cancer patients. *Journal of Clinical Oncology, 20*, 4160–8.

Tallman, B. A., Altmaier, E., & Garcia, C. (2007). Finding benefit from cancer. *Journal of Counseling Psychology, 54*(4), 481–7.

Taylor, E. J. (2000). Transformation of tragedy among women surviving breast cancer. *Oncology Nursing Forum, 27*(5), 781–8.

Taylor, S. E. (1983). Adjustment to threatening events: A theory of cognitive adaptation. *American Psychologist, 38*(11), 1161–73.

Taylor, S. E., Kemeny, M. E., Reed, G. M., & Aspinwall, L. G. (1991). Assault on the self: Positive illusions and adjustment to threatening events. In J. Strauss & G. G. R. (Eds.), *The self: Interdisciplinary approaches* (pp. 239–54). New York: Springer-Verlag.

Taylor, S. E., Wood, J. V., & Lichtman, R. R. (1983). It could be worse: Selective evaluation as a response to victimization. *Journal of Social Issues, 39*(2), 19–40.

Tedeschi, R. G., & Calhoun, L. G. (1996). The Posttraumatic Growth Inventory: Measuring the positive legacy of trauma. *Journal of Traumatic Stress, 9*(3), 455–72.

Tedeschi, R. G., & Calhoun, L. G. (2004). Posttraumatic growth: conceptual foundations and empirical evidence. *Psychological Inquiry, 15*(1), 1–18.

Tedeschi, R. G., & Calhoun, L. G. (2009). The clinician as expert companion. In C. L. Park, S. C. Lechner, M. H. Antoni, & A. L. Stanton (Eds.), *Medical illness and positive life change: Can crisis lead to personal transformation?* (pp. 215–36). Washington, DC: APA.

Tennen, H., & Affleck, G. (2002). Benefit-finding and benefit-reminding. In C. R. Snyder & S. J. Lopez (Eds.), *Handbook of positive psychology* (pp. 584–97). London: Oxford University Press.

Tennen, H., & Affleck, G. (2009). Assessing positive life change. In C. L. Park, S. C. Lechner, M. H. Antoni, & A. L. Stanton (Eds.), *Medical illness and positive life change: Can crisis lead to personal transformation?* (pp. 31–50). Washington, DC: APA.

Thompson, S. C., & Janigian, A. S. (1988). Life schemes: a framework for understanding the search for meaning. *Journal of Social and Clinical Psychology, 7*, 260–80.

Thornton, A. A., & Perez, M. A. (2006). Posttraumatic growth in prostate cancer survivors and their partners. *Psycho-Oncology, 15*(4), 285–96.

Tomich, P. L., & Helgeson, V. S. (2004). Is finding something good in the bad always good? Benefit-finding among women with breast cancer. *Health Psychology, 23*(1), 16–23.

Updegraff, J. A., Taylor, S. E., Kemney, M. E., & Wyatt, G. E. (2002). Positive and negative effects of HIV infection in women with low socioeconomic resources. *Personality and Social Psychology Bulletin, 28*, 382–94.

Urcuyo, K. R., Boyers, A. E., Carver, C. S., & Antoni, M. H. (2005). Finding benefit in breast cancer: Relations with personality, coping, and concurrent well-being. *Psychology and Health, 20*(2), 175–92.

Weaver, K. E., Llabre, M. M., Lechner, S. C., Penedo, F., & Antoni, M. H. (2008). Comparing unidimensional and multidimensional models of benefit-finding in breast and prostate cancer. *Quality of Life Research, 17*, 771–81.

Weinrib, A. Z., Rothrock, N. E., Johnsen, E. L., & Lutgendorf, S. K. (2006). The assessment and validity of stress-related growth in a community-based sample. *Journal of Consulting and Clinical Psychology, 74*(5), 851–8.

Weintraub, A. Z., Rothrock, N. E., Johnsen, E. L., & Lutgendorf, S. K. (2006). The assessment and validity of stress-related growth in a community-based sample. *Journal of Consulting and Clinical Psychology, 74*(5), 851–8.

Weiss, T. (2002). Posttraumatic growth in women with breast cancer and their husband: An intersubjective validation study. *Journal of Psychosocial Oncology, 20*(2), 65–80.

Zoellner, T., & Maercker, A. (2006). Posttraumatic growth in clinical psychology - a critical review and introduction of a two-component model. *Clinical Psychology Review, 26*(5), 626–53.

Religion and Coping: The Current State of Knowledge

Kenneth I. Pargament

Abstract

This chapter reviews the current state of knowledge about religion and coping. It begins with a definition and theoretical model of religion, and then addresses several themes that have emerged from this rapidly growing body of study: (1) Religion can be embedded in every part of the coping process; (2) Religion adds a distinctive dimension to the coping process; (3) The role of religion in coping is determined by the availability of religion and perceptions that it offers compelling solutions; (4) Religion can be both helpful and harmful; and (5) Religion can be integrated more fully into the process of treatment. Overall, it has become clear that religion is an integral, rich, and multidimensional part of the coping process, one that should not be overlooked in studies of people experiencing major life stressors. The paper concludes with a discussion of future directions for research in this area of inquiry.

Keywords: religion, spirituality, stress, trauma, coping, struggle, post-traumatic growth, meaning, physical health, mental health

I talk to him all the time. I "keep him up on" what's going on at home and with all of us. I feel the strongest connection at the cemetery. I imagine his spirit in the trees behind his grave. When I begin to talk to him the wind almost always rustles the leaves, which tells me he's there.—Bereaved mother
(Sormanti & August, 1997, p. 464).

The plane was moving more erratically . . . The guy next to me at minus four minutes [before the crash] said, 'We ain't going to make it" . . . I noticed the nun across from me had been praying on her rosary. I remembered I had a cross in my pocket. I pulled it out and held it in my hand for the rest of the ride.—Survivor of Flight 232
("Here I was . . .," 1989, p. 32).

The main support that I receive is my Buddhist practice. That is what has sustained me for the past 25 years. No matter how deep in despair I have become, I've found refuge in Buddhism . . . It helps me find peace and tranquility and love.—Man with HIV/AIDS
(Siegel & Schrimshaw, 2002, p. 94).

God did not protect me either. Why would God not protect a helpless little boy? It was not fair . . . Instead of welcoming and embracing [Jesus] as I want to, I really would like to knock him down. I am mad at him and his Father.—Survivor of clergy sexual abuse
(Anonymous, 1990, p. 119).

Introduction

In times of trial and tribulation, we often find religion. This is not to say that people become religious in a knee-jerk response to stressful situations. The old adage is incorrect; there are at least some atheists in foxholes—but perhaps not too many. The vignettes above are not at all unusual. Empirical studies reveal that many people look to their faith for help in coping with critical life situations. For example, a national survey of Americans shortly after the September 11, 2001, attacks revealed that 90 percent reportedly turned to God for solace and support (Schuster et al., 2001). In a sample of Egyptian patients with cancer, 92 percent voiced their belief that God would help them with their illness (Kesseling et al., 1986). Among some groups, religion is the most common coping resource. Bulman and Wortman (1977) asked a group of people who had been paralyzed how they explained their accidents. The most common response to the question "Why me?" was "God had a reason." Similarly, when asked to identify how they coped with the stresses of caring for their family members with dementia, the most frequent response of Black primary caregivers was prayer or faith in God (Segall & Wykle, 1988-1989).

Given the prominent role of religion in stressful times, it is puzzling that for many years, theorists and researchers largely ignored the role of religion in coping. How do we account for this religious neglect? Perhaps it reflects the fact that psychologists are considerably less religious than the population in the United States (Shafranske, 2001), and as a result underestimate the salience of religion in the lives of many people. Or perhaps it reflects the legacies of central figures in psychology such as Freud and Skinner who viewed religion through jaundiced eyes as a defense mechanism, a form of denial, or a way to avoid the direct confrontation with reality. These stereotypes may still live on, in spite of empirical studies that challenge these over-simplified religious views.

Fortunately, the situation has begun to change. In 1997, I wrote *The Psychology of Religion and Coping: Theory, Research, Practice* in which I articulated a theoretical framework of religion and coping that grew out of the seminal contributions of Lazarus and Folkman (1984). At that time, I was able to identify over 200 empirical studies that addressed the interface among religion, stress, and coping. Since the publication of this book, over 1,000 studies have appeared that deal with religion, stress, and coping.

Thus, the study of religion and coping has grown dramatically over the past decade.

What have we learned? In this paper, I will review the current state of knowledge about religion and coping. As a necessary prelude to this review, I will begin with a definition and theoretical model of religion. I will then address several themes:

- Religion can be embedded in every part of the coping process.
- Religion adds a distinctive dimension to the coping process.
- The role of religion in coping is determined by the availability of religion and perceptions that it offers compelling solutions.
- Religion can be both helpful and harmful in coping.
- Religion can be integrated more fully into the process of treatment.

I will conclude this paper with a discussion of future directions for research in this area of inquiry.

A Definition and Theoretical Model of Religion

Before considering the interface between religion and coping, it is important to consider the meaning of the term "religion." I have defined religion as a search for significance in ways related to the sacred (Pargament, 1997). There are three key terms in this definition: *significance*, *search*, and *sacred*. Below each of these concepts is briefly considered. The meaning of these terms, religion, and the links between religion and coping should become clearer in the remainder of the paper. (see Fig. 14.1)

Significance

Underlying this definition of religion is the assumption that people are more than reactive beings, determined solely by the internal and external forces articulated by Marx, Darwin, and Freud, who, Bennis (1989) once said, would have "our circumstances, present and past, conscious and unconscious, genetic, and learned, make monkeys of us all" (p. 47). People are also goal-oriented, proactive beings, striving to attain something of significance in life. Significance is both objective and subjective in character. It refers to aspects of life or "objects" that hold value and importance to the individual. Virtually any object can take on significance: material, psychological, social, physical, or spiritual. Of course, people generally focus on more than one object of significance in their lives. Thus, it is more accurate to describe significance in terms of a pattern or configuration of goals and values (Karoly, 1993). Significance can also be understood in a subjective manner as a *sense* of value, importance, or worth that accompanies the pursuit and attainment of these ends. It is, in short, what really matters, or, in the words of William James (1902), "the hot place in a man's consciousness" (p. 193).

Search

Significance also has motivational properties; people are drawn to it. More specifically, they are motivated to (a) discover something of significance in their lives, (b) maintain a relationship with it once it has been found, and (c) when necessary transform what they hold significant. We call this process of discovery, conservation, and transformation the search for significance. Religion is intimately involved in this search. In contrast to stereotypical views of religion as a static set of beliefs and practices, religion is a dynamic process, one directed toward the discovery, conservation, and transformation of significance; Pargament, 1997, 2007). Below I provide a brief overview of this process.

People find significance in many aspects of life. The discovery of significance is in part based on socialization. Religious institutions play a particularly key role in teaching what is and is not of primary importance. But the discovery of significance is also based on inner needs and motives. Commenting on the diverse ways people come to understand God, Rizzuto (1979) writes that half of "God's stuffing" comes from "the primary objects the child has 'found' in life. The other half of God's stuffing comes from the child's capacity to 'create' a God according to his needs" (p. 179). Of course, from the perspective of the religiously minded, something is missing here, for those who are most devout experience the discovery of significance as a revelation, something that is given to them rather than created by them.

The search for significance does not end with the process of discovery. Once discovered, people are motivated to nurture and sustain their relationships with whatever they hold significant. It becomes "the place to be." Toward this end, people can take a number of conservational pathways that help them hold on to significance. These include religious pathways, such as the path of knowing (e.g., Bible

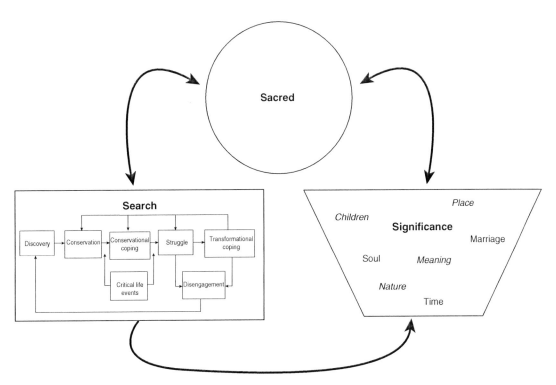

Fig. 14.1 Theoretical model of religion.

study, scriptural interpretation), the path of acting (e.g., ritual, spiritual practice), the path of relating to others (e.g., doing good deeds, proselytizing), and the path of experiencing (e.g., prayer, meditation). In addition, as we will see, people can draw on a variety of religious coping methods that help them conserve significance in stressful times. Conservational pathways are more than a means to an end: they take on a value of their own because they become a stable, overarching orienting system that guides people toward significance.

There are times, though, when people encounter major events that shake or shatter their tried-and-true ways of living. During these times, people become, in essence, disoriented, and struggle to regain their footing. These struggles can be religious as well as psychological, social, or physical. Struggles represent a fork in the road. On one side of the fork, they can lead to transformational forms of coping, often religious in nature, that involve fundamental changes in the character of significance or in the pathways people take in the search for significance. Once it has been transformed, individuals return to the process of conservation in an effort to hold on to and nurture their newly transformed understanding of significance. On the other side of the fork, however, struggles may result in a disengagement from the search for significance. This period of motivational shutdown may be permanent, but more often than not it is temporary: at some later point in life, the individual may experience a rediscovery of significance and engage once again in the processes of conservation and transformation.

Sacred

Religion is not alone in its concern with significance. Almost every social institution, from family and educational systems to governmental and medical institutions, attempts to help people attain significance in their lives. Is there anything special about religion? What sets religion apart from these other institutions is that it brings the sacred to bear in the search for significance. By sacred, I am referring to concepts of God and higher powers (Pargament & Mahoney, 2005). But the sacred is not limited to traditional notions of divinity. As sociologist Emile Durkheim (1915) put it: "By sacred things one must not understand simply those personal beings which are called gods or spirits; a rock, a tree, a pebble, a piece of wood, a house, in a word anything can be sacred" (p. 52). Seemingly secular domains, including marriage, time, self, work, and virtues, can take on sacred character and meaning when they are tied to God or imbued with spiritual qualities, such as transcendence, boundlessness, and ultimacy. Consider, for example, the way one woman perceives loving relationships as sacred:

> The things that make me feel as if I could touch the face of God are times when I am overwhelmed by love and friendship. The last time I went to a family reunion, I was touched by the level of love and caring everyone showed me. There's nothing like the feeling of being loved. I would say that love is the one thing in life that can truly take a person to another level, because the source behind love . . . is God"
>
> (Rosenberg, 2002, p. 8).

Defined in this fashion, the sacred extends the meaning of religion and the psychology of religion as a discipline well beyond a focus on traditional sacred objects.

We say that someone is religious then when he or she involves the sacred in the search for significance. The individual may integrate the sacred in any dimension of this search: in the manner in which significance is defined, in the process of discovery, in the paths the individual takes to conserve significance, in the critical life events the individual encounters and the appraisals of these events, in the struggles the individual experiences, and in the ways significance is transformed. Thus, religion is a complex, multifaceted phenomenon that can evolve in very different ways over the course of the lifespan. In fact, it would not be an exaggeration to say that each individual's religious search for significance is in some ways unique.

In the process of coping, people are also concerned with holding onto, or if necessary, transforming what they find significant in their lives. Nevertheless, it is important to underscore the point that religion is not synonymous with coping. In contrast to the concept of coping, religion is not exclusively focused on periods of stress, but rather has as its overriding concern the place of the sacred in the search for significance in good times and bad. Nevertheless, the sacred is often part and parcel of stressful times, and we find that the most central of religious concerns have a great deal of overlap with issues raised in coping. With this perspective on religion in mind, we turn now to what we have learned about the interface between religion and the coping process.

Religion Can be Embedded in Every Part of the Coping Process

Religion's role is not limited to one aspect of coping. Instead, it can be found in every facet of this process, including the functions of coping; critical life events and the appraisals of these events; coping methods; and the outcomes of coping.

Religion and the functions of coping

Part of the power of religion lies in its ability to serve many purposes for people coping with major life stressors. Consider a few examples. Religion can offer a source of meaning in the face of uncertainty, tragedy, and loss. The effort here, anthropologist Clifford Geertz (1966) wrote, "is not to deny the undeniable—that there are unexplained events, that life hurts, or that rain falls upon the just—but to deny that there are inexplicable events, that life is unendurable, and that justice is a mirage" (pp. 23–4). Similarly, Park and Folkman (1997) assert that religion helps people reconcile the questions of meaning raised by specific stressful situations with their global sense of meaning and purpose in life. There is some evidence that religion can be successful in serving this meaning-making function. For example, Murphy, Johnson, and Lohan (2003) studied 138 parents who had suffered the violent death of an adolescent or young adult child, and tried to identify factors that were associated with the ability to find meaning in these deaths 5 years later. Religion emerged as one of the predictors. Parents who turned to religion for help in coping (e.g., I put my trust in God, I seek God's help) reported that they were able to find greater meaning in their child's death 5 years later.

Durkheim (1915) maintained that religion is first and foremost about community. "The idea of society," he said, "is the soul of religion" (p. 433). In stressful situations, religion can provide people with a sense of belonging, connectedness, and identity. For example, O'Brien (1982) studied dialysis patients and found that those who reported higher levels of faith also indicated more social interaction, less social alienation, and a higher quality of relationships. In a longitudinal study of a community sample in the San Francisco Bay area born in the 1920s, Wink, Dillon, and Larsen (2005) found that greater involvement in religious institutional life buffered the effects of depression associated with poor physical health, even after controlling for general social support. The researchers suggest that religiousness provides people with not only church-based support, but also a strong and historically based sense of identity and values.

Freud (1927/1961) believed that religion was designed to assuage the terror and anxiety that follows from the child's recognition of the parent's inability to master the superior powers of disease, cataclysm, and death. It is not hard to find examples of the comforting function of religion. One analysis of 3,000 Protestant hymns revealed that one third focused on the theme of the return to a loving, protective God; one fourth of the hymns dealt with the comfort and rewards to be experienced in the world to come (Young, 1926). More recently, Hebert, Dang, and Schulz (2007) conducted a longitudinal study of depression and grief among family caregivers to loved ones with dementia. They found that higher religiousness (e.g., prayer, church attendance, faith) among caregivers at baseline predicted lower levels of depression at follow-up.

These examples are merely illustrative. Religion can serve other purposes as well in coping, including impulse control, problem-solving, self-esteem and self-efficacy, bettering the world, and physical health (e.g., Gall & Cornblatt, 2002; Siegel & Schrimshaw, 2002). Important as these psychosocial functions are, they overlook what is, to the religiously minded, the most central religious purpose of all: the spiritual function. "It is the ultimate Thou whom the religious person seeks most of all," Paul Johnson (1959, p. 70) wrote. To put it another way, in the midst of crisis, people are motivated to sustain themselves not only psychologically, socially, and physically, but also spiritually. Here too we find evidence that religion can be quite successful in helping people conserve a relationship with faith itself. For instance, Falsetti, Resick, and Davis (2003) studied trauma survivors and found that those who had experienced more than one trauma reported higher, not lower, levels of religious commitment as assessed by a measure of intrinsic religiousness. More specifically, 70 percent of those who suffered at least one trauma reported no religious change after their experience. Similarly, Cotton et al. (2006) followed HIV patients and reported no significant changes in measures of organized and non-organized religious activity, overall spirituality, positive religious coping, or negative religious coping over 12 to 18 months.

Religion serves one final key function in coping: transformation. When old sources of significance are lost or no longer viable, religion encourages its adherents to "let go" and seek out new sources of value. Though social scientists have generally emphasized the conservational functions of religion, the transformational role of religion should not be underestimated. In this vein, Coe (1916) wrote: "Possibly the chief thing in religion, considered functionally, is the progressive discovery and reorganization of values" (p. 65). Consider this report by a Mormon man who was with his wife when she was killed in a car accident:

> I knew that she was killed. There was a big gash on her wrist, and it wasn't bleeding, and I couldn't get any pulse. And I felt that I could lay my hands on her head and bring her back [a healing practice in the Church of Jesus Christ of Latter-Day Saints]. And a voice spoke to me and said: 'Do you want her back a vegetable! She's fine. She's all right . . . Let her go'
> (Pargament, 1997, p. 234).

The few investigations that have been conducted in this area suggest that religion can be tied to profound change following crises. For example, in one study of female sexual assault victims, those who made use of more religious coping reported a series of positive life changes, including changes in self, relationships, life philosophy or spirituality, and empathy (Frazier et al., 2004).

Religion and events and appraisals

In its efforts to help people find significance in life, religion encourages people to experience some life events and avoid others. For example, members are taught to demarcate and celebrate critical transitional points in life: "holy-days." Because they are replete with religious meaning, these events are not to be confused with their secular counterparts: a ritual circumcision is more than a medical procedure; a wedding within a church is something different than a civil ceremony; a religious funeral is more than the act of depositing a dead body in the earth (Pargament, 1997). On the other hand, religion discourages its members from experiencing other life events, particularly those that represent a threat to the pursuit of the most elevated ends. Thus, members are told to avoid high-risk, immoral behaviors, including drug and alcohol abuse, violence, and sexual promiscuity. And a number of studies have shown that more religious individuals are in fact less likely to engage in these kinds of risky behaviors (e.g., Koenig, McCullough, & Larson, 2001). Thus, religion purposely shapes the topography of events the individual will encounter over the lifespan.

Religious life is also associated with exposure to a variety of undesirable and unanticipated religious-specific life stressors, such as the experience of a church closure, shunning by a church when a member is said to violate church teachings, and clergy sexual abuse. Events of this kind may be particularly stressful because they threaten or damage primary spiritual values. Consider the example of clergy sexual abuse. Sexual abuse perpetrated by a member of the clergy takes on an especially deep and dark significance because it is often appraised as a violation of the sacred (i.e., desecration) on many levels (Pargament, Murray-Swank, & Mahoney, 2008). First, it is a violation of the most sensitive parts of the individual's identity, the soul, or that which makes the person uniquely human. One survivor of clergy sexual abuse put it this way: "This guy had my soul in his hand. It was devastating to know that someone would step out of the powers of spiritual liberty to take over someone else's soul . . . I still have anger about a lot of that and I think more of the anger is about the spiritual loss than anything to do with the sexual abuse" (Fater & Mullaney, 2000, p. 290). Second, clergy sexual abuse can be perceived as a violation of a sacred role and relationship, one that has been set apart from others. Because clergy take formal vows to protect and nurture the spiritual well-being of all of their followers, they are legitimated to enact the role of God. Thus, when a clerical figure violates his or her ordination, responsibility, and privilege as a representative of God in a human relationship, it is as if God himself has committed the violation. Third, it is a violation of a sacred institution that legitimated the cleric, possibly cloaking the acts of the perpetrator, and failing to come to the aide of the survivor. Finally, clergy sexual abuse is a violation of a set of rituals and symbols that were intertwined with the offending clergy and institutions. For example, one woman who had been abused by her minister at the age of 14 described her alienation from the rituals of her church: "I began to have dreams of communion wafers crawling with insects, of pearls oozing mucous, of the pastor blowing up the church just as I was about to serve communion for the first time" (Disch & Avery, 2001, p. 214).

Seemingly secular events can also be appraised in terms of their implications for the individual's sacred values. For example, Pargament, Magyar, Benore, and Mahoney (2005) asked a community sample to report on the most negative life event they had experienced in 2 years. The sample described commonplace major life stressors, including death, illness or injury of a loved one, divorce or separation, job loss, and personal illness. Asked to rate the degree to which they appraised these events as sacred losses and sacred violations, 38 percent of the participants perceived their stressor as a sacred loss and 24 percent perceived their stressor as a sacred violation. Moreover, appraisals of sacred loss and violation were associated with significantly higher levels and differential patterns of emotional distress.

Of course, religion also offers people ways to appraise stressful events in a more benign spiritual context, reducing the threat or damage tied to an event or enhancing the individual's perceived ability to handle the event. Rather than random and senseless, pain and suffering can be appraised as containing a deeper, if elusive, meaning. As one bereaved parent said, "There is a God. And it's an explanation that there's no explanation" (Gilbert, 1989, p. 9). Stressful life events can also be appraised as offering the individual an opportunity to grow spiritually, closer to whatever he or she holds sacred (Gall et al., 2005; Park & Folkman, 1997). One victim of a severe accident who became paraplegic commented: "It's a learning experience; I see God's trying to put me in situations, help me learn about Him and myself and also how I can help other people" (Bulman & Wortman, 1977, p. 358).

Religion and the methods of coping

Efforts to measure coping have generally overlooked the religious dimension. Even when religion has been included in coping instruments, it is usually assessed by only a few items. This approach can offer only a limited view of the ways religion expresses itself in times of crisis. It is important to understand not only *how much* religion is involved in coping, but also *how* religion is involved in coping; specifically, the *who's* (e.g., clergy, congregation members, God), *what's* (e.g., prayer, Bible reading, ritual), *when's* (e.g., acute stressors, chronic stressors), *where's* (e.g., within a congregation, privately), and *why's* (e.g., to find meaning, to gain control) of coping (Pargament, Ano, & Wachholtz, 2005).

In the most comprehensive effort to identify methods of religious coping, Pargament, Koenig, and Perez (2000) developed a measure of 21 religious coping methods (the RCOPE) through interviews, a literature review, and factor analyses (Table 14.1). These methods span a broad spectrum: active, passive, and interactive activities; emotion-focused and problem-focused strategies; and cognitive, behavioral, interpersonal, and spiritual domains. They also address five of the key religious functions: the search for meaning; the search for mastery and control; the search for comfort and closeness to God; the search for interpersonal intimacy and closeness to God; and the search for a life transformation. A brief version of the RCOPE is also available (Pargament, Smith, Koenig, & Perez, 1998).

Questions might be raised why it is important to assess religion at this level of specificity: Why not simply focus on general indicators of religiousness, such as self-rated religiousness or spirituality, frequency of prayer, or frequency of church attendance? Theoretically, there are good reasons to expect that specific religious coping methods will predict the outcomes of stressful life situations more strongly than global religious indicators. We might think of the global indicators (e.g., prayer, Bible study, going to church) as religious television channels and the specific religious coping methods as the potential programming on each channel. Or, to put it another way, we might think of the global religious questions as indicators of a general religious orientation and the religious coping methods as concrete manifestations of this orientation in stressful times. Working collaboratively with God to solve a problem, seeking God's love and care, seeking spiritual support from others, reappraising a situation in a benevolent way, questioning God's power, reappraising the situation as a punishment from God—religious coping methods such as these are directly and functionally related to the situation in hand. In either case, we would expect that these ways of religious coping would have the most immediate and strongest implications for the outcomes of critical events.

In fact, empirical studies have consistently shown that these specific religious coping methods are stronger predictors of stress-related outcomes than global measures of religiousness (see Pargament, 1997, for a review). Other studies indicate that religious coping methods mediate the relationships between general religious variables and outcomes (Nooney & Woodrum, 2002; Roesch & Ano, 2003). For example, working with data from the 1998 General Social Survey, Nooney and Woodrum (2002) found that the relationship between church attendance and depression was mediated through church-based social support. Similarly, the effects of prayer on depression were mediated through religious coping. These studies underscore the importance of attending to the concrete ways people express their faith in response to major life stressors.

Table 14.1 The many methods of religious coping

Religious Methods of Coping to Find Meaning

    Benevolent Religious Reappraisal—redefining the stressor through religion as potentially beneficial

    Punishing God Reappraisal—redefining the stressor as a punishment from God for the individual's sins

    Demonic Reappraisal—redefining the stressor as an act of the Devil

    Reappraisal of God's Powers—redefining God's power to influence the stressful situation

Religious Methods of Coping to Gain Mastery and Control

    Collaborative Religious Coping—seeking control through a partnership with God in problem-solving

    Passive Religious Deferral—passive waiting for God to control the situation

    Active Religious Surrender—active giving up of control to God in coping

    Pleading for Direct Intercession—seeking control indirectly by pleading to God for a miracle or divine intervention

    Self-Directing Religious Coping—seeking control through individual initiative rather than help from God

Religious Methods of Coping to Gain Comfort and Closeness to God

    Seeking Spiritual Support—searching for comfort and reassurance through God's love and care

    Religious Focus—engaging in religious activities to shift focus from the stressor

    Religious Purification—searching for spiritual cleansing through religious actions

    Spiritual Connection—seeking a sense of connectedness with forces that transcend the self

    Spiritual Discontent—expressing confusion and dissatisfaction with God's relationship to the individual in the stressful situation

    Marking Religious Boundaries—clearly demarcating acceptable from unacceptable religious behavior and remaining within religious boundaries

Religious Methods of Coping to Gain Intimacy with Others and Closeness to God

    Seeking Support from Clergy or Church Members—searching for intimacy and reassurance through the life and care of congregation members and clergy

    Religious Helping—attempting to provide spiritual support and comfort to others

    Interpersonal Religious Discontent—expressing confusion and dissatisfaction with the relationship of clergy or church members to the individual in the stressful situation

Religious Methods of Coping to Achieve a Life Transformation

    Seeking Religious Direction—looking to religion for assistance in finding a new direction for living

    Religious Conversion—looking to religion for a radical change in life

    Religious Forgiving—looking to religion for help in shifting from anger, hurt, and fear associated with an offense to peace

Religion and the outcomes of coping

Typically, researchers have focused on the relationships between religious coping and various psychological, social, and physical outcomes. Yet it is important to remember that for many people, the most significant of all outcomes is spiritual in nature. To know God, to grow closer to whatever is held sacred, to become more deeply involved in a spiritual community—these are ultimate goals toward which some strive in difficult times.

A few investigators have begun to measure the changes in religiousness that occur in the process of coping with stressful situations. Many people report growth in their religiousness and spirituality over the course of traumatic events. For example, in the Falsetti et al. (2003) study of people who had experienced multiple traumas, 19 percent stated that they grew more religious after the second trauma; only 8 percent indicated that they had declined in religiousness. In another investigation of adult alcoholics in an outpatient treatment, researchers found significant improvements in spiritual well-being from intake to discharge (Piderman, Schneekloth, Pankratz, Malony, & Altchuler, 2007).

Religious methods of coping have also been linked to desirable religious outcomes in studies of people facing a variety of life stressors (Smith, Pargament, Brant, & Oliver, 2000). For instance, in a 2-year longitudinal study of medically ill elderly patients, greater use of religious methods of coping was predictive of strong increases in feelings of closeness to God, the sense of spirituality, and closeness to one's church (Pargament, Koenig, Tarakeshwar, & Hahn, 2004). These studies make clear that the coping process affects people spiritually as well as psychologically, socially, and physically.

Religion Adds a Distinctive Dimension to Coping

Perhaps because psychologists are, as a group, less religious than the general population, they tend to be particularly skeptical of religious phenomena. Religion is often explained in terms of presumably more basic processes. Beliefs in God, mystical experiences, and religious coping have been interpreted in exclusively physiological terms or as responses to social needs, deep-seated fear and anxiety, or the desire to make sense of the world. Purely reductionistic approaches to religion are problematic. To the extent that religion can be "explained away" by purportedly more basic dimensions, there would be little need to take religion seriously in and of itself (or for a psychology of religion for that matter). Certainly, psychological, social, and physiological explanations provide important insights into the roots of religious experience. Yet, they may not fully account for religious life. There is a difference between explaining religion and explaining religion away (Pargament, 2002). There are some good reasons to propose that religion adds a distinctive dimension to experience and to the coping process more generally.

As noted earlier, religion is by definition unique, for no other human process has as its focus the sacred. Subjectively, many people experience the sacred as the central organizing force of their lives. To live without the sacred becomes almost unimaginable. As Kushner (1989) wrote, "A world without God would be a flat monochromatic world, a world without color or texture, a world in which all days would be the same" (p. 206). Of course, scientists cannot determine whether subjective perceptions of God are in fact real (or unreal). We have no tools to measure God, the truth of Biblical miracles, or the existence of an afterlife.

There is empirical evidence, however, to suggest that religion makes distinctive contributions to the coping process. Some evidence points to the distinc-tive role of religious motivation. Emmons' (1999) research on spiritual motivation and personal strivings is particularly relevant here. In his studies, he asks people to generate their lists of strivings, defined as "what a person is characteristically trying to do" in his or her life. Emmons finds that spiritual strivings or strivings of "ultimate concern" often appear in people's lists of goals. These strivings focus on the transcendent dimension of experience, and most refer to some concept of God or the Divine (e.g., "Discern and follow God's will for my life," "Be aware of the spiritual meaningfulness of my life"; Emmons, 1999, pp. 89-91). Emmons finds a unique role for spiritual motivations. The correlations between spiritual strivings and measures of well-being are stronger than the correlations for other types of strivings. Moreover, these correlations maintain their strength after controlling for intimacy strivings, such as the desire for close, reciprocal relationships. In addition, spiritual strivings are uniquely associated with less conflict in a person's goal system. Emmons asserts that spiritual strivings are "literally at the end of the striving line" and play a critical part in organizing and integrating other goals and strivings (p. 96).

Another body of research has attempted to account for the effects of religion on measures of health and well-being by controlling for a variety of potential psychosocial mediators, but these studies have not been particularly successful. For instance, Ironson, Stuetzle, and Fletcher (2006) studied HIV-positive individuals over a 4-year period. They found that those who reported increases in religiousness/spirituality after diagnosis had significantly greater preservation of CD4 cells. They tested whether these effects could be explained by the pathways of less hopelessness, optimism, secular coping, and social support; none of these explanatory factors accounted for the religion effect. The researchers concluded: "Having ruled out many potential mediators, it is not clear at this point just what is responsible for this relationship and that remains for future study" (pp. S66-S67). Similarly, Ellison and his colleagues conducted a large-scale study of the relationships between religious involvement, psychological distress, and well-being in a probability sample of adults in the Detroit area (Ellison, Boardman, Williams, & Jackson, 2001). The links between the religious variables and the indices of distress and well-being were not mediated by access to social or psychological resources, such as self-esteem, mastery, and social support. Ellison et al. concluded: "The salutary effects of religious involvement cannot be explained away in terms of social or psychological resources, at least insofar as these constructs are conventionally conceptualized and measured . . . Religious groups and traditions may foster distinctive sets of spiritual or psychosocial resources (e.g., distinctive coping styles and practices, doctrines, support patterns) that bolster or undermine health and well-being" (p. 243).

Yet another body of empirical study indicates that religious coping methods are not simply subsets of non-religious forms of coping. Consider a few examples. Gall (2006) studied spiritual coping in 101 adult survivors of childhood sexual abuse. After controlling for abuse descriptors, coping resources of social support, and cognitive appraisals, spiritual coping with a current negative life event continued to predict anxious, angry, and depressed mood. Generally, positive forms of religious coping were tied to better mood, while negative forms of religious coping were tied to greater distress. Tix and Frazier (1998) worked with patients undergoing kidney dialysis and their loved ones. Religious coping predicted life satisfaction 30 months and 12 months after transplantation after controlling for cognitive restructuring, internal control, and social support. They concluded that "religious coping adds a unique component to the prediction of adjustment to stressful life events that cannot be accounted for by other established predictors" (p. 420). Krause (2006) studied a national sample of elders and compared the role of emotional support received from church members with the emotional support received from non-church members as buffers of the effects of financial strain on self-rated health. Church-based emotional support emerged as a buffer, whereas secular support did not. Krause goes on to emphasize the distinctive character of church-based support: It is particularly helpful because it is enacted in a group that shares a spiritual worldview and commitment to God, a common set of sacred beliefs, values, and coping methods, shared religious principles, rituals, and memories, and a support that is "imbued with the mantle of religious authority" (p. S36). Still other studies have shown that religious coping methods predict the outcomes of stressors above and beyond the effects of meaning-oriented secular coping methods in hospice caregivers (Mickley et al., 1998), and control-oriented secular coping methods among loved ones awaiting the outcomes of cardiac surgery in a hospital waiting room (Pargament et al., 1999). One study of German breast cancer patients yielded contrasting results: the effects of religious coping on anxiety and depression were mediated through depressive coping (Zwingmann, Wirtz, Muller, Korber, & Murken, 2006). However, questions arise here about the distinctiveness of the measures of depressive coping and depression and anxiety. Overall, the pattern of these findings indicates that religious coping methods are not redundant with secular methods of coping.

What are the distinctive contributions of religious to coping? A satisfying answer to this question takes us well beyond this chapter. Here, let me reiterate a point I have made elsewhere: religion offers a response to the problem of human insufficiency.

> Try as we might to maximize significance through our own insights and experiences or through those of others, we remain human, finite, and limited. At any time we may be pushed beyond our immediate resources, exposing our basic vulnerability to ourselves and the world. To this most basic of existential crises, religion holds out solutions. The solutions may come in the form of spiritual support when other forms of social support are lacking, explanations when no other explanations seem convincing, a sense of ultimate control through the sacred when life seems out of control, or new objects of significance when old ones are no longer compelling. In any case, religion complements nonreligious coping, with its emphasis on personal control, by offering responses to the limits of personal powers.
> (Pargament, 1997, p. 310).

Consistent with this point of view, empirical studies have shown that religious coping appears to be particularly to helpful to people dealing with more stressful, uncontrollable life events (see Pargament, 1997; Smith, McCullough, & Poll, 2003, for reviews). For example, Maton (1989) studied a group of parents who were recently bereaved (higher stress) and bereaved more than 2 years ago (lower stress). Higher levels of spiritual support were associated with lower levels of depression for both groups, yet spiritual support was related more strongly to less depression and greater self-esteem for the recently bereaved parents. Similarly, in a study of people with HIV/AIDS, Szarflarski et al. (2006) found that the positive effects of religiousness on quality of life were stronger for those who reported lower physical health functioning.

The Role of Religion in Coping is Determined by the Availability of Religion and Perceptions that it Offers Compelling Solutions

It is no accident that a child born in India will likely come to learn many names for God, the Native American infant will learn to see the sacred in the earth, the water, and the sky, and the child born to Christian parents will develop a belief in Jesus as the pathway to everlasting life. Cultural and religious institutional forces make some forms of religious belief, practice, and coping more available to people than others. Thus, although we can find commonalities in religious coping methods across cultures and traditions, we can discover distinctive forms of religious coping as well. Beliefs in karma among Hindus and the impermanence of experience among Buddhists offer novel ways of reframing the meaning of negative life events (Phillips et al., in press; Tarakeshwar, Pargament, & Mahoney, 2003). Similarly, many Swedes derive a sense of spiritual support from nature (Ahmadi, 2006), and the Dutch manifest a religiously "receptive" form of coping that reflects an openness to and trust in the eventual discovery of solutions to problems without specifying a divine agent that makes it possible (Van Uden, Pieper, & Alma, 2004).

At an individual level, religious coping is shaped in part by the person's general orienting system of beliefs, practices, dispositions, and relationships. Not surprisingly, a number of studies have shown that people are more likely to involve religion in coping when religion is a larger part of their orienting system (see Pargament, 1997, for a review). Religious coping methods become more accessible tools for dealing with life problems among those who are more religious (Spencer & McIntosh, 1990). Additional evidence indicates that different kinds of general religious beliefs translate into different kinds of religious coping methods (Belavich & Pargament, 2002; Pargament et al., 1992). For example, working with a sample of family members awaiting the outcome of surgery of a loved one, Belavich and Pargament (2002) found that different forms of attachment to God (i.e., secure, avoidant, anxious/ambivalent) were associated with different types of religious coping and different outcomes in turn.

The role of religion in coping is determined by more than the availability of religion to the individual. One of the consistent findings in the psychology of religion literature is that people tend to draw more deeply on religious resources in times of greatest stress. For example, in a study of fishermen from southern New England, Poggie, Pollnac, and Gersuny (1976) found that religious-like rituals were more common prior to longer, presumably more dangerous fishing trips than shorter ones. Experimental and naturalistic studies have also shown that people are more likely to turn to religion when situations become increasingly threatening and harmful (see Pargament, 1997, for a review). How do we explain these findings? As noted above, more stressful situations are also more likely to reveal the limitations of our ordinary personal and social resources. Pushed closer to the limits of tried-and-true methods of coping, alternatives become more compelling, particularly those that address issues of human insufficiency. Along these lines, one study participant said: "I would feel more like praying in the hour of death because I believe that only prayer can carry you through such a time" (Welford, 1947, p. 317). Philosopher and theologian John E. Smith (1968) put it even more eloquently: "Crisis times . . . direct our thoughts away from the banality of ordinary life to dwell, with awe and proper seriousness, upon the mystery of life itself. . . It is as if the times of crisis were so many openings into the depth of life, into its ground, its purpose, its finite character" (p. 59). In short, the involvement of religion in coping grows out of not only the availability of religion to the individual, but also the degree to which religion is seen to offer compelling solutions to life problems.

Religion can be Both Helpful and Harmful in Coping
Helpful effects

Empirical studies indicate that stereotypical views of religion as merely a passive form of coping or a source of denial are not well founded (see Pargament & Park, 1995). Consider a few examples that challenge the common stereotype that religion promotes denial and passivity in the face of medical illness. Friedman et al. (2006) studied 124 women with breast symptoms and found that in contrast to the religion-as-denial stereotype, those with higher levels of spirituality were less likely to delay seeking a medical consultation for their symptoms. In a study of African American women diagnosed with HIV, Prado et al. (2004) found that women who engaged in more religious behaviors were less likely to rely on avoidant methods of coping, such as denial and suppression. Working with a sample of women dealing with ovarian cancer, Canada et al. (2006)

reported that women who were more involved in religious practices and beliefs made more active attempts to resolve problems associated with their illness. Finally, in a longitudinal study of patients with advanced cancer, patients who reported more positive religious coping were more likely to opt for intensive, life-prolonging end-of-life care in the last week of life (Phelps et al., 2009). These effects remained significant after adjusting for age, race, other coping styles, advance care planning, and terminal illness acknowledgment.

Judging from the research literature, it would be more accurate to say that religion is generally helpful to people coping with major life stressors. According to survey studies of groups dealing with a wide range of critical events (e.g., combat veterans, hospital patients, widows, physically abused spouses, parents of children who are ill), 50 to 85 percent of the samples report that religion was helpful to them in coping (see Pargament, 1997). A meta-analysis of 49 studies revealed significant ties between measures of positive religious coping (e.g., benevolent religious reappraisals, seeking spiritual support and connection) and measures of psychological adjustment (Ano & Vasconcelles, 2005). For instance, religious coping has been associated with greater psychological well-being in studies of women coping with breast cancer (Gall, 2000), informal caregivers (Pearce, 2005), Latinos dealing with arthritis (Abraido-Lanza, Vasquez, & Echeverria, 1998), older adults living in deteriorated neighborhoods (Krause, 1998), church members (Bjorck & Thurman, 2007), and adults in the community under stress (Loewenthal, Macleod, Goldblatt, Lubitsch, & Valentine, 2000).

A methodological note is important here. Cross-sectional studies make it difficult to tease out the effects of two processes that may work in opposite directions—the effects of religious coping on health and well-being, and the mobilizing effects of stressors on religious coping. For example, while religious coping may help to mitigate the effects of a major loss on depression (the direct effects model), higher levels of depression associated with a loss may trigger more religious coping (the religious coping mobilization model). Of course, both models could be operating and, in essence, cancel each other out, in which case we would find a zero correlation between religious coping and depression. To partial out religious coping mobilization effects from the direct effects of religious coping on health, longitudinal studies are needed. In fact, a number of longitudinal studies have been conducted and show that religious coping is predictive of changes in mental health over time (e.g., Ai, Dunke, Peterson, & Bolling, 1998; Alferi, Culver, Carver, Arena, & Antoni, 1999; Krause, 1998; Pargament et al., 2004; Tix & Frazier, 1998).

The majority of the studies cited above focus on the helpful effects of religious coping for measures of psychological health and well-being. However, several studies have also linked religious coping to positive physical health outcomes, particularly among people facing serious medical illnesses. For example, in one study of patients undergoing cardiac surgery, reports of greater strength and comfort from religion were associated with lower 12-month mortality rates (Oxman, Freeman, & Manheimer, 1995). Similarly, Ai, Peterson, Bolling, and Rodgers. (2006) found that more positive religious coping assessed 2 weeks prior to heart surgery was predictive of better physical postoperative functioning, after controlling for depression and other possible confounding variables. In a study of bereaved Japanese elders, Krause, Liang, Shaw, Sugisawa, Kim, et al. (2002) found that those who believed in life after death were less likely to develop hypertension 3 years after the loss than those who did not hold beliefs in an afterlife. Ironson and her colleagues followed a sample of 100 HIV patients over 4 years and found that people who viewed God as loving were considerably more protected against declines in CD4 cell counts (Ironson, Stuetzle, Fletcher, & Ironson, 2006).

Harmful effects

Although religion is generally helpful to people in coping, religion can at times contribute to greater stress and strain. Earlier I noted that major life events can shake or shatter the individual's most fundamental beliefs and values, including religious beliefs and values. When this occurs, the individual is likely to experience a period of religious struggle, a time of tension, question, and conflict centering around spiritual matters. We can distinguish among three types of religious struggle: interpersonal struggles that involve tensions and conflicts with friends, family, clergy, or church around spiritual issues; intrapersonal struggles that embody questions and doubts about matters of faith as well as internal conflicts between higher and lower aspects of oneself; and divine struggles that focus on negative emotions toward God, including anger, anxiety, fear, and feelings of abandonment (Pargament, Ano, & Wachholtz, 2005).

Religious struggles are not unusual. For example, Nielsen (1998) found that 65 percent of an adult sample reported some kind of religious conflict in their lives, often interpersonal in character. In a survey of a national sample of Presbyterians, only 35 percent indicated that they never had any religious doubts (Krause, Ingersoll-Dayton, Ellison, & Wulff, 1999). And surveys reveal that 10 to 50 percent of various samples express negative emotions to God (Exline & Rose, 2005; Fitchett, Rybarczyk, DeMarco, & Nicholas, 1999; Pargament, Koenig, & Perez, 2000).

Religious struggles can be viewed as signs of a religion under stress. At a deeper level, however, religious struggles represent active efforts by the individual to conserve or transform religion itself. This process can be quite painful, as we hear in the words of a 14-year-old Nicaraguan girl:

> Many times I wonder how there can be a God—a loving God and where He is . . . I don't understand why He lets little children in Third World countries die of starvation or diseases that could have been cured if they would have had the right medicines or doctors. I believe in God and I love Him, but sometimes I just don't see the connection between a loving God and a suffering hurting world. Why doesn't He help us—if He truly loves us? It seems like He just doesn't care. Does He?
> (Kooistra, 1990, pp. 91–2).

The relationship between religious struggles and various indicators of psychological distress appears to be robust. Empirical studies, cross-sectional and longitudinal, have linked religious struggles (often measured by negative religious coping subscales from the RCOPE or Brief RCOPE) to poorer psychological functioning (e.g., Ano & Vasconcelles, 2005; Exline, Yali, & Lobel, 1999; McConnell, Pargament, Ellison, & Flannelly, 2006). For example, McConnell et al. (2006) examined the relationships between religious struggles and a battery of measures of psychopathology in a national sample. Higher levels of religious struggles were tied to reports of greater generalized anxiety, phobic anxiety, depression, paranoid ideation, obsessive-compulsiveness, and somatization.

As with studies of positive religious coping, much of the research on religious struggles has focused on psychological criteria of well-being. However, in several studies, religious struggles have also been tied to indicators of poorer physical health status, including declines in independent functional status among medical rehabilitation patients (Fitchett et al., 1999), the development of more addictive behaviors among college students (Caprini-Feagin

& Pargament, 2008), declines in CD4 counts among patients with HIV (Ironson, Stuuezle, Fletcher, & Ironson, 2006; Trevino et al., 2010), elevations in plasma interleukin-6 (a cytokine that has been associated with heart disease) among patients immediately prior to cardiac surgery (Ai, Seymour, Tice, Kronfol, & Bolling, 2009), and even greater risk of mortality among medically ill elderly patients (Pargament, Koenig, Tarakeshwar, & Hahn, 2001). In their longitudinal study of hospitalized elderly patients, Pargament and colleagues (2001) found that religious struggles at baseline were predictive of higher levels of mortality within the next 2 years, even after controlling for selective attrition, demographic factors, and baseline health and mental health. Divine struggles in particular were tied to a 22 to 33 percent greater risk of dying over the 2-year period.

Consistent with research cited earlier on religious coping, attempts to account for the links between religious struggles and measures of health and well-being by controlling for alternate explanations have not been particularly successful. For example, Burke, Evon, Sedway, and Egan (2005) found that religious struggles, particularly those involving God, continued to predict greater depression and anxiety among patients with end-stage lung disease, even after controlling for non-religious coping. In a study of women with panic disorder and other psychological problems, Trenholm, Trend, and Compton (1998) found that intrapsychic religious conflicts continued to predict psychological distress after accounting for conventional predictors of panic (state anxiety, irrational thinking, abnormal illness behavior). Similarly, Pearce, Singer, and Prigerson (2006) studied 162 informal caregivers of terminally ill cancer patients and found that struggles were tied to more burden, poorer quality of life, less satisfaction, and greater likelihood of major depressive and anxiety disorders. The effects were partially but not fully mediated through social support, optimism, and self-efficacy. In an exception to this general pattern of results, Edmondson, Park, Chaudoir, and Wortmann (2008) worked with a sample of patients with end-stage congestive heart failure and found that the relationships between religious struggles and depression were fully mediated by concerns about death. Overall, however, these studies suggest that, as with other dimensions of religiousness, religious struggles may play a distinctive role in the coping process.

Before moving on, it is important to note that a few studies have suggested that religious struggles may be tied to perceptions of growth as well as decline. For instance, Profitt, Calhoun, Tedeshi, and Cann (2004) studied 30 clergypersons and found that higher levels of religious struggle were associated with higher levels of post-traumatic growth. In a study of church members close to the Oklahoma City bombing site, those who reported more religious struggles also manifested higher levels of stress-related growth and symptoms of post-traumatic stress disorder (Pargament, Smith et al., 1998). These findings are provocative: They suggest that religious struggles may represent a fork in the road, one leading to potentially serious declines in physical and mental health, or to potential growth and development. What determines the trajectory of religious struggles and religious coping more generally?

No single key to effective religious coping

There is no single belief, practice, or experience that holds the key to effective religious coping. Certainly we can identify forms of religious coping that are more and less helpful than others. But, as noted earlier, religion (like coping) is a dynamic process that involves many elements interacting and evolving over time. The nature of this process has as much if not more to do with the efficacy of religion in coping than any particular belief or practice (see Folkman, 1992).

A discussion of effective religious coping would take us beyond the focus of this paper (see Pargament, 2007, for a review), but I can offer two illustrative points. First, effective religious coping is discerning. Recall that religious coping methods take many different forms and serve a variety of purposes. The religious methods of coping that are effective in one situation may prove to be ineffective in another. Bickel et al. (1998) illustrated this point in a study of Presbyterian church members. They found that for people under high stress, unlike their low-stress counterparts, a self-directed religious coping style (i.e., coping without God's help) was associated with increases in depression. The opposite pattern emerged with respect to collaborative religious coping (i.e., coping together with God). For people under high stress, in contrast to those under low stress, increases in collaborative religious coping were associated with decreases in depression. Johnson (1959) captures the importance of religious discernment in his comments about prayer:

> Prayer does not work as a substitute for a steel chisel or the wing of an airplane. It does not replace

muscular action in walking or faithful study in meeting an examination. These are not the proper uses of prayer. But prayer may help to calm the nerves when one is using a chisel in bone surgery or bringing an airplane to a landing. Prayer may guide one in choosing a destination to walk toward, and strengthen one's purpose to prepare thoroughly for an examination (pp. 142–3).

Second, effective religious coping is nested in a nurturant social context. The Black church provides one of the best examples of this kind of context. Several studies have shown that African Americans experience particularly high levels of support from their church. For instance, in a study of battered women, Gillum, Sullivan, and Bybee (2006) found that involvement in the church was associated with greater social support for non-White women but not for White women. Similarly, Krause (2003) conducted interviews with a national sample of Black and White older adults and found that those who reported a greater sense of religious meaning (e.g., God has put me in this life for a purpose; God has a reason for everything that happens to me) reported greater life satisfaction, self-esteem, and optimism. These effects were stronger for Black than White elders. Krause suggests that there may be something about the social context of African-American religion that is particularly beneficial. Rooted in the Black church, African Americans may be better equipped to understand the sufferings tied to slavery and racial prejudice and discrimination. Furthermore, the Black church may be especially capable of offering its members spiritual support, religious meaning, and powerful uplifting spiritual emotions that help them withstand life stressors.

Religion can be Integrated More Fully into the Process of Treatment

Building on the body of empirical study that links religious coping with health and well-being, a number of researchers and practitioners have begun to develop and evaluate treatments that draw on religious coping resources or address religious struggles. While this kind of work is still in its early stages of development, the results have been promising (see Pargament, 2007, for review). Below I highlight some of this work.

Wachholtz and Pargament (2008) compared the effects of a spiritually based concentration form of meditation with a secular concentration meditation in a sample of college students suffering from migraine headaches. The students were randomly assigned to one of four groups: those who meditated to a spiritual phrase (e.g., God is peace), those who meditated to an internal secular phrase (e.g., I am happy), or those who meditated to an external secular phrase (e.g., Grass is green). A fourth group of students were taught a progressive relaxation method. The students practiced their technique for a month and were tested before, after, and 1 month after treatment. In comparison to the other three groups, the spiritual mediators reported significantly fewer headaches, less migraine headache pain, reductions in negative mood and anxiety, and greater pain tolerance as measured through a cold pressor task. These findings are intriguing and suggest that the effects of some types of meditation can be enhanced when spiritual resources are integrated more explicitly into the practice.

Richards, Berrett, Hardman, and Eggett (2006) evaluated the relative effectiveness of three treatments for women with eating disorders in an inpatient setting; a spirituality group that read a spiritual workbook and discussed the readings; a cognitive group that read a cognitive-behavioral self-help workbook and then discussed the readings; and an emotional support group that discussed non-spiritually related topics. While all three groups reported positive changes, the spiritual group showed greater improvements in eating attitudes and spiritual well-being, and greater declines in indices of distress and social role conflict.

Tarakeshwar, Pearce, and Sikkema (2005) tested an 8-week spiritual coping group intervention for men and women with HIV. The program focused on helping participants address the spiritual struggles associated with HIV and draw on their religious resources more fully. Participants showed significant reductions in depression and spiritual struggles and significant increases in positive religious coping over the course of the intervention.

Murray-Swank and Pargament (2005) evaluated the effectiveness of an eight-session, spiritually integrated treatment for two female survivors of sexual abuse. The sessions were designed to help the survivors deal with the spiritual struggles that had been triggered by their abuse. An interrupted time-series design tested for changes in religious coping, religious struggles, and religious well-being before, during, and after the intervention. The two clients increased their use of positive religious coping and manifested greater religious well-being during the program.

Gear and colleagues (2008) developed and evaluated a 9-week, manualized, spiritually sensitive group intervention for college students struggling with spiritual issues. The program was designed to help students articulate and normalize their struggles, develop their personal spiritual identity, broaden their coping responses, and engage in psychospiritual self-care. The students demonstrated clinically significant improvements on indices of psychological distress, spiritual struggle, emotional regulation, and congruence between personal behavior and spiritual values. One student described her experience this way: "I'm happy that my spiritual struggle happened because it gave me the chance to reinvent myself and to grow as a person and to question some things. Before I was angry that it was happening. But now I'm happy that it happened. I've had two or three spiritual struggles and I've always come out a better person. So I think they're necessary" (p. 6).

Once again, this area of research is still in its infancy. Perhaps the findings of these studies are idiosyncratic. However, a recent meta-analysis indicates that participants in spiritually integrated treatments showed greater benefits than those in comparative non-spiritual interventions (Smith, Bartz, & Richards, 2007). Thus, efforts to integrate religion in the coping process in treatment appear to be promising.

Future Directions for Research on Religious Coping

Even though research on religious coping has increased dramatically in the past 10 years, questions still outnumber answers. I conclude this paper by noting several of these important questions and directions for future study.

What are the implications of religious coping for other religious traditions? The lion's share of research on religious coping has focused on Christian samples in the United States. Initial steps have been taken to study religious coping among members of other religious traditions, including Muslims (e.g., Abu Raiya et al., 2008; Ai, Peterson, & Huang, 2003), Hindus (Tarakeshwar, Pargament, & Mahoney, 2003), Jews (Rosmarin, Pargament, Krumrei, & Flannelly, in press), and Buddhists (Phillips et al., in press). Interestingly, these studies have identified distinctive forms of religious coping, yet they have also pointed to some commonalities across religious traditions. For example, religious struggles have emerged as predictors of psychological distress for Christians, Muslims, Jews, and Hindus alike.

Nevertheless, these studies are just a beginning: Further research is needed to elaborate on points of similarity and dissimilarity in religious coping and their implications for the health and well-being of members of diverse religious traditions.

What are the implications of religious coping for other social and cultural contexts? Most of the research on religious coping has focused on Western adults facing major medical illnesses or serious life trauma. Little is known about the ways religion expresses itself in coping among people in non-Western cultures. Similarly, little is known about religious coping within other contexts, such as the workplace, school systems, correctional institutions, and families. The few studies that have been conducted have yielded provocative results. For example, working with a sample of 100 adults coping with a recent divorce, Krumrei, Mahoney, and Pargament (in press) found that measures of religious coping and struggles were uniquely tied to adjustment after controlling for the effects of parallel non-religious coping and struggle indices. Similarly, in contrast to the notion that religion doesn't become salient to youngsters until they reach the age of adolescence, two studies found religious coping to be common among children dealing with illness and predictive of their well-being (Benore, Pargament, & Pendleton, 2008; Pendleton, Cavalli, Pargament, & Nasr, 2002).

What forms does religious coping take interpersonally? There is an individualistic bias to the research on religious coping. Yet, as the response to national tragedies such as the Oklahoma City bombing or the September 11 terrorist attacks illustrates, people often respond to crisis by coming together to express their faith through shared prayers and rituals. Religion is expressed communally as well as individually, and the interpersonal nature of religious life may add a distinctive dimension to the coping process. Along these lines, Brelsford and Mahoney (2008) examined the ways parents and their college-age children cope with religious disagreements. Drawing on family systems theory, they defined and measured a relational form of religious coping—"positive religious detriangulation"—in which God becomes an advocate for love and harmony between parent and child rather than taking sides. Higher scores on this measure by parent–child dyads were associated with healthier parent–child relationships. Furthermore, parents and children who talked more about religious and spiritual issues experienced greater satisfaction and intimacy in their relationship. These findings suggest that there may be considerable value to studying religious coping interpersonally as well as individually.

How does religious coping unfold over time? Investigations of religion and coping have tended to rely on "snapshots" of people dealing with stressors taken during one or two points in time. Although this approach has yielded valuable information, it cannot offer a "moving picture" of how religion evolves and changes over the course of the coping process. Toward that end, other methodologies are needed. Narrative studies offer one way of capturing the ebb and flow of religious coping over time (e.g., Ganzevoort, 1998). Diary studies represent another methodological approach. For instance, recognizing the limitations to retrospective reports of coping (e.g., Stone, Greenberg, Kennedy-Moore, & Newman, 1991), Keefe et al. (2001) evaluated the role of daily spiritual experience and daily religious coping among people dealing with the pain associated with rheumatoid arthritis. Participants kept structured daily diaries for 30 consecutive days in which they responded to standardized measures of religious coping, religious coping efficacy, spiritual experiences, pain, mood, and perceived social support. Many of the participants reported spiritual experiences (e.g., feeling touched by the beauty of creation, feeling a desire to be closer to God) on a frequent basis. Moreover, the frequency of daily spiritual experiences was linked with higher levels of daily positive mood, lower levels of daily negative mood, and higher social support.

Finally, does sensitivity to the religious dimension enhance the efficacy of clinical interventions? Building on the established links between religiousness, health, and well-being, psychologists have begun to move from research to practice. As noted above, these initial efforts have yielded promising results, but further research is needed to evaluate the efficacy of spiritually integrated treatments. Particularly needed are controlled clinical trials comparing spiritually integrated treatments with standard treatments, and treatment matching analyses to determine whether the former are especially effective for more religious individuals.

For too long, the religious dimension of coping has been neglected. Fortunately, the picture has changed dramatically in recent years. It has become clear that religion is a potent resource in coping for many people, and a burden for others. In either case, religion is an integral, rich, and multidimensional part of the coping process. Any effort to understand and address the concept of coping that overlooks this distinctive dimension of life will remain incomplete.

References

Abraido-Lanza, A. F., Vasquez, E., & Echeverria, S. E. (2004). En las manos de Dios [in God's Hands]: Religious and other forms of coping among Latinos with arthritis. *Journal of Consulting and Clinical Psychology, 72*, 91–102.

Abu-Raiya, H., Pargament, K. I., Mahoney, A., & Stein, C. (2008). A psychological measure of Islamic religiousness (PMIR): Development and evidence for reliability and validity. *International Journal for the Psychology of Religion, 18*, 291–315.

Ahmadi, F. (2006). *Culture, religion and spirituality in coping: The example of cancer patients in Sweden*. Uppsala, Sweden: Acta Universitatis Upsaliensis.

Ai, A. L., Peterson, C., Bolling, S. F., & Rodgers, W. (2006). Depression, faith-based coping, and short-term postoperative global functioning in adult and older patients undergoing cardiac surgery. *Journal of Psychosomatic Research, 60*, 21–8.

Ai, A. L., Peterson, C., & Huang, B. (2003). The effects of religious-spiritual coping on positive attitudes of adult Muslim refugees from Kosovo and Bosnia. *International Journal for the Psychology of Religion, 13*, 29–47.

Ai, A. L., Peterson, C., Tice, T. N., Bolling, S. F., & Koenig, H. G. (2004). Faith-based and secular pathways to hope and optimism subconstructs in middle-aged and older cardiac patients. *Journal of Health Psychology, 9*, 435–50.

Ai, A. L., Seymour, E. M., Tice, T. N., Kronfol., Z., & Bolling, S. F. (2009). Spiritual struggle related to plasma interleukin-6 prior to cardiac surgery. *Psychology of Religion and Spirituality, 1*, 112–28.

Alferi, S. M., Culver, J. L., Carver, C. S., Arena, P. L., & Antoni, M. H. (1999). Religiosity, religious coping, and distress; A prospective study of Catholic and evangelical Hispanic women in treatment for early-stage breast cancer. *Journal of Health Psychology, 4*, 343–56.

Ano, G. A., & Vasconcelles, E. B. (2005). Religious coping and psychological adjustment to stress: A meta-analysis. *Journal of Clinical Psychology, 61*, 1–20.

Anonymous. (1990). An adult survivor of child abuse speaks up. In S. J. Rosetti (Ed.), *Slayer of the soul: Child sexual abuse and the Catholic church* (pp. 113–22). Mystic, CT: Twenty-Third Publications.

Bade, M. K., & Cook S. W. (2008). Functions of Christian prayer in the coping process. *Journal for the Scientific Study of Religion, 47*, 123–34.

Belavich, T. G., & Pargament, K. I. (2002). The role of attachment in predicting spiritual coping with a loved one in surgery. *Journal of Adult Development, 9*, 13–29.

Bennis, W. (1989). *Why leaders can't lead: The unconscious conspiracy continues*. San Francisco: Jossey-Bass.

Benore, E., Pargament, K.I., & Pendleton, S. (2008). An initial examination of religious coping in children with asthma. *International Journal for the Psychology of Religion, 18*, 267–90.

Bickel, C. O., Ciarrocchi, J., Sheers, N. J., Estadt, B. K., Powell, D. A., & Pargament, K. (1998). Perceived stress, religious coping styles, and depressive affect. *Journal of Psychology and Christianity, 17*, 33–42.

Bjorck, J. P., & Thurman, J. W. (2007). Negative life events, patterns of positive and negative religious coping, and psychological functioning. *Journal for the Scientific Study of Religion, 46*, 159–67.

Bosworth, H. B., Park, K. S., McQuoid, D. R., Hays, J. C., & Steffens, D. C. (2003). The impact of religious practice and religious coping on geriatric depression. *International Journal of Geriatric Psychiatry, 18*, 905–14.

Brelsford, G. M., & Mahoney, A. (2008). Spiritual disclosure between older adolescents and their mothers. *Journal of Family Psychology, 22*, 62–70.

Bulman, R. J., & Wortman, C. B. (1977). Attributions of blame and coping in the "real world": Severe accident victims react to their lot. *Journal of Personality and Social Psychology, 35*, 351–63.

Burker, E. J., Evon, D. M., Sedway, J. A., & Egan, T. (2005). Religious and nonreligious coping in lung transplant candidates: Does adding God to the picture tell us more? *Journal of Behavioral Medicine, 28*, 513–26.

Canada, A. L., Parker, P. A., deMoor, J. S., Basen-Engquist, K., Ramondetta, L. M., & Cohen, L. (2006). Active coping mediates the association between religion/spirituality and quality of life in ovarian cancer. *Gynecologic Oncology, 101*, 102–7.

Caprini-Feagin, C. A., & Pargament, K. I. (2008). *Spiritual struggles as a risk factor for addiction*. Paper presented at American Psychological Society, Chicago.

Coe, G. A. (1916). *The psychology of religion*. Chicago: University of Chicago Press.

Cotton, S., Puchalski, C. M., Sherman, S. N., Mrus, J. M., Peterman, A. H., Feinberg, J., et al. (2006). Spirituality and religion in patients with HIV/AIDS. *Journal of General Internal Medicine, 21*, S5–13.

Disch, E., & Avery, N. (2001). Sex in the consulting room, the examining room, and the sacristy: Survivors of sexual abuse by professionals. *American Journal of Orthopsychiatry, 71*, 204–17.

Durkheim, E. (1915). *The elementary forms of religious life*. New York: Free Press.

Edmondson, D., Park, C. L., Chaudoir, S. R., & Wortmann, J. H. (2008). Death without God: Religious struggle, death concerns, and depression in the terminally ill. *Psychological Science, 19*, 754–8.

Ellison, C. G., Boardman, J. D., Williams, D. R., & Jackson, J. S. (2001). Religious involvement, stress, and mental health: Findings from the 1995 Detroit area study. *Social Forces, 80*, 215–49.

Emmons, R. A. (1999). *The psychology of ultimate concerns: Motivation and spirituality in personality*. New York: Guilford Press.

Exline, J. J., & Rose, E. (2005). Religious and spiritual struggles. In R. F. Paloutzian, & C. L., Park (Eds.), *Handbook of the psychology of religion and spirituality* (pp. 315–30). New York: Guilford Press.

Exline, J. J., Yali, A. M., & Lobel, M. (1999). When God disappoints; Difficulty forgiving God and its role in negative emotion. *Journal of Health Psychology, 4*, 365–80.

Faigin, C. A., & Pargament, K. I. (May, 2008). Filling the spiritual void: Spiritual struggles as a risk factor for addictive behaviors. Paper presented at the American Psychological Society, Chicago.

Falsetti, S. A., Resick, P. A., & Davis, J. L. (2003, August). Changes in religious beliefs following trauma. *Journal of Traumatic Stress, 16*, 391–8.

Fater, K., & Mullaney, J. A. (2000). The lived experience of adult male survivors who allege childhood sexual abuse by clergy. *Issues in Mental Health Nursing, 21*, 281–95.

Fitchett, G., Rybarczyk, B. D., DeMarco, G. A., & Nicholas, J. J. (1999). The role of religion in medical rehabilitation outcomes: A longitudinal study. *Rehabilitation Psychology, 44*, 1–22.

Folkman, S. (1992). Making the case for coping. In B. N. Carpenter (Ed.), *Personal coping: Theory, research, and application* (pp. 31–46). Westport, CT: Prager.

Frazier, P., Tashiro, T., Berman, M., Steger, M., & Long, J. (2004). Correlates of levels and patterns of positive life changes following sexual assault. *Journal of Consulting and Clinical Psychology, 72,* 19–30.

Freud, S. (1927/1961). *The future of an illusion.* New York: Norton.

Friedman, L. C., Kalidas, M., Elledge, R., Dulay, M. F., Romero, C., Chang, J., & Liscum, K. R. (2006). Medical and psychosocial predictors of delay in seeking medical consultation for breast symptoms in women in a pubic sector setting. *Journal of Behavioral Medicine, 29,* 327–34.

Gall, T. L. (2000). Integrating religious resources within a general model of stress and coping: Long-term adjustment to breast cancer. *Journal of Religion and Health, 39,* 167–82.

Gall, T. L. (2006). Spirituality and coping with life stress among adult survivors of childhood sexual abuse. *Child Abuse and Neglect, 30,* 829–44.

Gall, T. L., Charbonneau, C., Clarke, N. H., Grant, K., Joseph, A., & Shouldice, L. (2005). Understanding the nature and role of spirituality in relation to coping and health: A conceptual framework. *Canadian Psychology, 46,* 88–104.

Gall, T. L., & Cornblat, M. W. (2002). Breast cancer survivors give voice: A qualitative analysis of spiritual factors in long-term adjustment. *Psycho-Oncology, 11,* 524–35.

Ganzevoort, R. R. (1998). Religious coping reconsidered, part two: A narrative reformulation. *Journal of Psychology and Theology, 26,* 276–86.

Gear, M. R., Faigin, C. A., Gibbel, M. R., Krumrei, E., Oemig, C., McCarthy, S. K., & Pargament, K. I. (2008, October). The Winding Road: A promising approach to addressing the spiritual struggles of college students. *Spirituality in Higher Education Newsletter, 4,* 1–8.

Geertz, C. (1966). Religion as a cultural system. In M. Banton (Ed.), *Anthropological approaches to the study of religion* (pp. 1–46). London: Tavistock.

Gilbert, K. R. (1989). *Religion as a resource for bereaved parents as they cope with the death of their child.* Paper presented at the meeting of the National Council on Family Relations, New Orleans.

Gillum, T. L., Sullivan, C. M., & Bybee, D. I. (2006, March). The importance of spirituality in the lives of domestic violence survivors. *Violence Against Women, 12,* 240–50.

Hebert, R. S., Dang, Q., & Schulz, R. (2007, April). Religious belief and practices are associated with better mental health in family caregivers of patients with dementia: Findings from the REACH study. *American Journal of Geriatric Psychiatry, 15,* 292–300.

Here I was sitting at the edge of eternity. (1989, August). *Life,* pp. 28–33, 38, 39.

Ironson, G., Stuetzle, R., & Fletcher, M. A. (2006). An increase in religiousness/spirituality occurs after HIV diagnosis and predicts slower disease progression over 4 years in people with HIV. *Journal of General Internal Medicine, 21,* S62–S68.

Ironson, G., Stuezle, R., Fletcher, M. A., & Ironson, D. (2006). *View of God is associated with disease progression in HIV.* Paper presented at the annual meeting of the Society of Behavioral Medicine, March 22–5, San Francisco.

James, W. (1936). *The varieties of religious experience: A study in human nature.* New York: Modern Library. (Original work published 1902).

Johnson, P. E. (1959). *Psychology of religion.* Nashville: Abingdon Press.

Karoly, P. (1993). Goal systems: An organizing framework for clinical assessment and treatment planning. *Psychological Assessment, 5,* 213–80.

Keefe, F. J., Afflect, G., Lefebvre, J., Underwood, L., Caldwell, D. S., Drew, J., Egert, J., Gibson, J., & Pargament, K. I. (2001). Living with rheumatoid arthritis; The role of daily spirituality and daily religious and spiritual coping. *Journal of Pain, 2,* 101–10.

Kesseling, A., Dodd, M. J., Lindsey, A. M., & Strauss, A. L. (1986). Attitudes of patients living in Switzerland about cancer and its treatment. *Cancer Nursing, 9,* 77–85.

Khan, Z. H., & Watson, P. J. (2006). Construction of the Pakistani Religious Coping Practices Scale: Correlations with religious coping, religious orientation, and reactions to stress among Muslim university students. *International Journal for the Psychology of Religion, 16,* 101–12.

Koenig, H. G., McCullough, M. E., & Lasron, D. B. (2001). *Handbook of religion and health.* Oxford, UK: Oxford University Press.

Kooistra, W. P. (1990). *The process of religious doubting in adolescents raised in religious environments.* Unpublished doctoral dissertation. Bowling Green State University.

Krause, N. (1998). Neighborhood deterioration, religious coping, and changes in health during late life. *Gerontologist, 38,* 653–64.

Krause, N. (2003). Religious meaning and subjective well-being in late life. *Journal of Gerontology: Social Sciences, 58B,* S160–S170.

Krause, N. (2006). Exploring the stress-buffering effects of church-based and secular social support on self-rated health in late life. *Journal of Gerontology: Social Sciences, 61B,* S35–S43.

Krause, N., Ingersoll-Dayton, B., Ellison, C. G., & Wulff, K. M. (1999). Aging, religious doubt, and psychological well-being. *Gerontologist, 39,* 525–33.

Krause, N., Liang, J., Shaw, B. A., Sugisawa, H., Kim, H. K., Sugihara, Y. (2002). Religion, death of a loved one, and hypertension among older adults in Japan. *Journal of Gerontology: Social Sciences, 57B,* S96–S107.

Krumrei, E. J., Mahoney, A., & Pargament, K. I. (in press). Divorce and the divine: The role of spirituality in adjustment to divorce. *Journal of Family Psychology.*

Kushner, H. S. (1989). *Who needs God?* New York: Summit Books.

Lazarus, R. S., & Folkman, S. (1984). *Stress, appraisal, and coping.* New York: Springer.

Loewenthal, K. M., Macleod, A. K., Goldblatt, V., Lubitsh, G., & Valentine, J. D. (2000). Comfort and joy? Religion, cognition, and emotion in Protestants and Jews under stress. *Cognition and Emotion, 14,* 355–74.

Maton, K. I. (1989). The stress-buffering role of spiritual support: Cross-sectional and longitudinal investigations. *Journal for the Scientific Study of Religion, 28,* 310–23.

McConnell, K. M., Pargament, K. I., Ellison, C. G., & Flannelly, K. J. (2006). Examining the links between spiritual struggles and symptoms of psychopathology in a national sample. *Journal of Clinical Psychology, 62,* 1469–84.

Mickley, J. R., Pargament, K. I., Brant, C. R., & Hipp, K. M. (1998). God and the search for meaning among hospice caregivers. *Hospice Journal, 13,* 1–17.

Murphy, S. A., Johnson, L. C., & Lohan, J. (2003). Finding meaning in a child's violent death: A five-year prospective analysis of parents' personal narratives and empirical data. *Death Studies, 27,* 381–404.

Murray-Swank, N. A., & Pargament, K. I. (2005). God, where are you? Evaluating a spiritually-integrated intervention for sexual abuse. *Mental Health, Religion, and Culture, 8,* 191–204.

Nielsen, M. E. (1998). An assessment of religious conflicts and their resolutions. *Journal for the Scientific Study of Religion, 37,* 181–90.

Nooney, J., & Woodrum, E. (2002). Religious coping and church-based social support as predictors of mental health outcomes: Testing a conceptual model. *Journal for the Scientific Study of Religion, 4,* 359–68.

O'Brien, M. E. (1982). Religious faith and adjustment to long-term hemodialysis. *Journal of Religion and Health, 21,* 68–80.

Oxman, T. E., Freeman, D. H., & Manheimer, E. D. (1995). Lack of social participation or religious strength and comfort as risk factors for death after cardiac surgery in the elderly. *Psychosomatic Medicine, 57,* 5–15.

Pargament, K. I. (1997). *The psychology of religion and coping: Theory, research, practice.* New York: Guilford Press.

Pargament, K. I. (2002). Is religion nothing but. . .? Explaining religion versus explaining religion away. *Psychological Inquiry, 13,* 239–44.

Pargament, K. I. (2007). *Spiritually integrated psychotherapy: Understanding and addressing the sacred.* New York: Guilford Press.

Pargament, K. I., Ano, G. G., & Wachholtz, A. B. (2005). The religious dimension of coping: Advances in theory, research, and practice. In R. F. Paloutzian & C. L. Park (Eds.), *Handbook of the psychology of religion and spirituality* (pp. 479–95). New York: Guilford Press.

Pargament, K. I., Cole, B., VandeCreek, L., Belavich, T., Brant, C., & Perez, L. (1999). The vigil: Religion and the search for control in the hospital waiting room. *Journal of Health Psychology, 4,* 327–41.

Pargament, K. I., Koenig, H. G., & Perez, L. (2000). The many methods of religious coping: Development and initial validation of the RCOPE. *Journal of Clinical Psychology, 56,* 519–543.

Pargament, K. I., Koenig, H. G., Tarakeshwar, N., & Hahn, J. (2001). Religious struggle as a predictor of mortality among medically ill elderly patients: A two-year longitudinal study. *Archives of Internal Medicine, 161,* 1881–5.

Pargament, K. I., Koenig, H. G., Tarakeshwar, N., & Hahn, J. (2004). Religious coping methods as predictors of psychological, physical, and social outcomes among medically ill elderly patients: A two-year longitudinal study. *Journal of Health Psychology, 9,* 713–30.

Pargament, K. I., & Park, C. L. (1995). Merely a defense? The varieties of religious means and ends. *Journal of Social Issues, 51,* 13–32.

Pargament, K. I., Magyar, G. M., Benore, E., & Mahoney, A. (2005). Sacrilege: A study of sacred loss and desecration and their implications for health and well-being in a community sample. *Journal for the Scientific Study of Religion, 44,* 59–78.

Pargament, K. I., & Mahoney, A. (2005). Sacred matters: Sanctification as a vital topic for the psychology of religion. *International Journal for the Psychology of Religion, 15,* 179–98.

Pargament, K. I., Murray-Swank, N. A., & Mahoney, A. (2008). Problem and solution: The spiritual dimension of clergy

sexual abuse and its impact on survivors. *Journal of Child Sexual Abuse, 17,* 397–420.

Pargament, K. I., Olsen, H., Reilly, B., Falgout, K., Ensing, D., & Van Haitsma, K. (1992). God help me (II): The relationship of religious orientation to religious coping with negative life events. *Journal for the Scientific Study of Religion, 31,* 504–13.

Pargament, K. I., Smith, B. W., Koenig, H. G., & Perez, L. (1998). Patterns of positive and negative religious coping with major life stressors. *Journal for the Scientific Study of Religion, 37,* 710–24.

Park, C. L., & Folkman, S. (1997). Meaning in the context of stress and coping. *Review of General Psychology, 1,* 115–44.

Pearce, M. L., Singer, J. L., & Prigerson, H. G. (2006). Religious coping among caregivers of terminally ill cancer patients: Main effects and psychosocial mediators. *Journal of Health Psychology, 11,* 743–59.

Phelps, A. C., Maciejewski, P. K., Nilsson, M., Balboni, T. A., Wright, A. A., et al. (2009). Religious coping and use of intensive life-prolonging care near death in patients with advanced cancer. *JAMA, 301,* 1140–7.

Pendleton, S. M., Cavalli, K. S., Pargament, K. I., & Nasr, S. Z. (2002). Religious/spiritual coping in childhood cystic fibrosis; A qualitative study. *Pediatrics, 109,* 1–11.

Phillips, R. E. III, Cheng, C. M., Pargament, K. I., Oemig, C., Colvin, S. D., Abarr, A. N., Dunn, M. W., & Reed, A. S. (in press). Spiritual coping in American Buddhists: An exploratory study. *International Journal for the Psychology of Religion.*

Piderman, K. M., Schneekloth, T. D., Pankratz, S., Malony, S. D., & Altchuler, S. I. (2007). Spirituality in alcoholics during treatment. *American Journal of Addictions, 16,* 232–7.

Plante, T. G., & Sherman, A. C. (Eds.), *Faith and health: Psychological perspectives* (pp. 311–38). New York: Guilford Press.

Poggie, J. J. Jr., Pollnac, R., & Gersuny, C. (1976). Risk as a basis for taboos among fishermen in southern New England. *Journal for the Scientific Study of Religion, 15,* 252–67.

Prado, G. Feaster, D. J., Schwartz, S. J., Pratt, I. A., Smith, L., & Szapocznik, J. (2004, September). Religious involvement, coping, social support, and psychological distress in HIV-seropositive African American mothers. *AIDS and Behavior, 8,* 221–35.

Profitt, D. H., Calhoun, L. G., Tedeschi, R. G., & Cann, A. (2003). *Clergy and crisis: Correlates of posttraumatic growth and well-being.* Unpublished manuscript.

Richards, P. S., Berrett, M. E., Hardman, R. K., & Eggert, D. L. (2006). Comparative efficacy of spirituality, cognitive, and emotional support groups for treating eating disorder patients. *Eating Disorders: Journal of Treatment and Prevention, 41,* 401–15.

Rizzuto, A. M. (1979). *The birth of the living God: A psychoanalytic study.* Chicago: University of Chicago Press.

Roesch, S. C., & Ano, G. (2003). Testing an attribution and coping model of stress: Religion as an orienting system. *Journal of Psychology and Christianity, 22,* 197–209.

Rosenberg, R. S. (2002). The religious dimension of life. *America, 187,* 7–9.

Rosmarin, D. H., Pargament, K. I., Krumrei, E. J., & Flannelly, K. J. (in press). Religious coping among Jews: Development and initial validation of the JCOPE. *Journal of Clinical Psychology.*

Schottenbauer, M. A., Klimes-Dougan, B., Rodriguez, B. F., Arnkoff, D. B., Glass, C. R., & Lasalle, V. H. (2006 December). Attachment and affective resolution following a stressful event: General and religious coping as possible mediators. *Mental Health, Religion & Culture*, 9, 448–71.

Schuster, M. A., Stein, B. D., Jaycox, L. H., Collins, R. l., Marshall, G. N., Elliott, M. N. et al. (2001). A national survey of stress reactions after the September 11, 2001, terrorist attacks. *New England Journal of Medicine*, 345, 1507–12.

Segall, M., & Wykkle, M. (1988–1989). The black family's experience with dementia. *Journal of Applied Social Sciences*, 13, 170–91.

Shafranske, E. P. (2001). The religious dimension of patient care within medicine: The role of religious attitudes, beliefs, and personal and professional practices. In T. G. Plante & A. C. Sherman (Eds.), *Faith and health: Psychological perspectives* (pp. 311–38). New York: Guilford Press.

Siegel, K., & Schrimshaw, E. W. (2002). The perceived benefits of religious and spiritual coping among older adults living with HIV/AIDS. *Journal for the Scientific Study of Religion*, 41, 91–102.

Smith, B. W., Pargament, K. I., Brant, C., & Oliver, J. M. (2000). Noah revisited: Religious coping by church members and the impact of the 1993 Midwest flood. *Journal of Community Psychology*, 28, 169–86.

Smith, J. E. (1968). *Experience and God*. New York: Oxford University Press.

Smith, T. B., Bartz, J. D., & Richards, P. S. (2007). Outcomes of religious and spiritual adaptations to psychotherapy: A meta-analytic review. *Psychotherapy Research*, 17, 645–55.

Smith, T. B., McCullough, M. E., & Poll, J. (2003). Religiousness and depression: Evidence for a main effect and the moderating influence of stressful life events. *Psychological Bulletin*, 129, 614–36.

Sormanti, M., & August, J. (1997). Parental bereavement: Spiritual connections with deceased children. *American Journal of Orthopsychiatry*, 67, 460–9.

Spencer, S. J., & McIntosh, D. N. (1990, August). *Extremity and importance in attitude structure: Attitudes as self-schemata*. Paper presented at the meeting of the American Psychological Association, Boston.

Stone, A. A., Greenberg, M. A., Kennedy-Moore, E., & Newman, M. G. (1991). Self-report, situation-specific coping questionnaires: What are they measuring? *Journal of Personality and Social Psychology*, 61, 169–86.

Szaflarski, M., Ritchey, P. N., Leonard, A. C., Mrus, J. M., Peterman, A. H., Ellison, C. G., McCullough, M. E., & Tsevat, J. (2006). Modeling the effects of spirituality/religion on patients' perceptions of living with HIV/AIDS. *Journal of General Internal Medicine*, 31, S28–38.

Tarakeshwar, N., Pargament, K. I., & Mahoney, A. (2003). Initial development of a measure of religious coping among Hindus. *Journal of Community Psychology*, 31, 607–28.

Tarakeshwar, N., Pearce, M. J., & Sikkema, K. J. (2005). Development and implementation of a spiritual coping group intervention for adults living with HIV/AIDS: A pilot study. *Mental Health, Religion, and Culture*, 8, 179–90.

Tix, A. P., & Frazier, P. A. (1998). The use of religious coping during stressful life events: Main effects, moderation, and mediation. *Journal of Consulting and Clinical Psychology*, 66, 411–22.

Trenholm, P., Trent, J., & Compton, W. C. (1998). Negative religious conflict as a predictor of panic disorder. *Journal of Clinical Psychology*, 54, 59–65.

Trevino, K. M., Pargament, K. I., Cotton, S., Leonard, A. C., Hahn, J., et al. (2010). *AIDS and Behavior*, 14, 379–389.

Van Uden, M. H. F., Pieper, J. Z. T., & Alma, H. A. (2004). "Bridge over troubled water": Further results regarding the Receptive Coping Scale. *Journal of Empirical Theology*, 17, 101–14.

Wachholtz, A. B., & Pargament, K. I. (2008). Migraines and meditation: Does spirituality matter? *Journal of Behavioral Medicine*, 31, 351–66.

Welford, A. T. (1947). Is religious behavior dependent upon affect or frustration? *Journal of Abnormal and Social Psychology*, 42, 310–9.

Young, K. (1926). The psychology of hymns. *Journal of Abnormal and Social Psychology*, 20, 391–406.

Zwingmann, C., Wirtz, M., Muller, C., Korber, J., & Murken, S. (2006). Positive and negative religious coping in German breast cancer patients. *Journal of Behavioral Medicine*, 29, 533–47.

Coping, Spirituality, and Health in HIV

Gail Ironson *and* Heidemarie Kremer

Abstract

Although the medical treatment of HIV has improved dramatically since the introduction of effective antiretroviral treatment, people with HIV still face an enormous number of stressors. This chapter reviews the ways of coping that people with HIV use, and the effectiveness of these strategies. It is divided into four primary sections: coping and physical health, coping and psychological health, spiritual coping and physical health, and spiritual coping and mental well-being. There is evidence for the effectiveness of approach coping strategies such as active coping and proactive behavior, maintaining a fighting spirit, and planful problem-solving; for cognitive coping strategies such as positive reappraisal, finding meaning, and optimism; for more enduring personality coping styles, such as extraversion, openness, emotional expression, and altruism; and finally for spirituality. Research findings for the effectiveness of social support are mixed, though it appears to be most helpful as the disease advances. Finally, there is substantial evidence that avoidant coping has a detrimental effect on health and well-being. Clinical recommendations are discussed, including use of the Folkman and Lazarus strategy that matches problem-focused coping with changeable aspects of stressors and emotion-focused coping with unchangeable stressors, and introducing a functional component framework that expands the Folkman and Chesney view (Coping Effectiveness Training [CET]) to include a focus on changeable and unchangeable aspects of the self and the reaction to the stressor in addition to the CET focus on changeable and unchangeable aspects of the stressor alone. In addition, we recommend that emotion-focused coping be broken down into its component parts for clinical purposes: cognitive (reframing, positive outlook), emotion-focused activities to improve mood (relaxation, meditation, exercise), and emotional expression, spirituality, and substance use. Future directions are presented, including preliminary qualitative work from our group. The chapter ends with a summary and clinical suggestions.

Keywords: stress, coping, spirituality, HIV, functional components approach, health, disease progression, psychological well-being

Introduction

Two African American women who shared similar stressors, both diagnosed with HIV in the midrange of the disease, both facing similar struggles with drug addiction, children, jail, and unfaithful partners, have nonetheless had opposite outcomes due to their different ways of coping. Even though Valery (name changed) was diagnosed with HIV at a time when effective antiretroviral therapy was available, she rapidly progressed to AIDS despite treatment. In contrast, Grace (name changed) was diagnosed with HIV long before effective treatment became available, yet she survived, and now, 20 years after her diagnosis, her CD4 cells are in a healthy range (over 1,000 cells/mm³) and her HIV viral load is undetectable. Which coping methods did they use?

Valery stated, "I cannot cope with it. I cannot get close to people because of HIV. I am scared of their reaction. I do not want to be rejected." Valery has limited personal goals, spends most of her time watching TV, and still smokes crack a few times a week. She knows she needs to stop but has been unable to do so. When her CD4 cells dropped into a life-threatening range, it "woke me up" for a few months and she started adhering to her medication. However, the effect did not last. When asked why she does not take her medication, she blames her drug use and the burden of taking care of her children, her grandchildren, and her mother. She feels guilty that she does not keep up with taking her medication because she wants to stay alive for her grandchildren and her mother. She describes herself as "alive, but not living."

Grace, however, feels very vibrant and energetic. Being diagnosed with HIV helped her find new meaning in her life, reconnect with her children, and give love and care not only to her children but also to other people. After hitting rock bottom, Grace grew tired of prostituting herself to support her daily drug use. After ending up homeless on the street with her children, she decided to go to a drug program. She also started praying, befriended a pastor, and found faith in God. "When I got sick [HIV] . . . it saved me from drugs. I never thought that I could go through the day without taking some drugs. It was a whole new way of life; not depending on drugs and depending on God."

With this new outlook on life, and the support from her pastor/friend, she has not only been healthy but also stayed off drugs for almost 20 years and has been consistent with taking her medications. She also participates in programs to feed the homeless and is open with them about her own life and HIV. "Sometimes you have to go through some things and then you can be a help for others going through those same things who don't know which way to go. It's to help somebody else, not just to live on, and to give somebody else an encouraging word to be able to help them."

The above stories illustrate several factors that relate to healthy survival: finding meaning, helping others, connecting with social support, discontinuing drug use, disclosing HIV status, expressing emotion, connecting with one's spirituality, and,

of course, taking antiretroviral therapy (ART). We elaborate below.

From coping with a life-threatening disease to coping with a chronic illness

With the introduction of effective ART in 1996, being diagnosed with HIV has changed from coping with a life-threatening illness to coping with a chronic disease. In industrialized countries, people infected sexually with HIV now experience mortality rates similar to the general population during the first 5 years of their infection (Bhaskaran et al., 2008). For people with HIV taking ART, the mean age at death is estimated to be about 60 years, with 41 percent dying of illnesses not directly attributable to HIV (Braithwaite et al., 2005). For those who have the privilege of having access to ART, mortality largely depends on adherence (Garcia de Olalla et al., 2002). However, the different ways of coping may also contribute importantly to the health and the well-being of people with HIV above and beyond taking medication. We can learn a lot from HIV in terms of coping with both life-threatening as well as chronic diseases. This is not only because there are reliable biological markers of disease progression, such as a decline in CD4 cells or a viral load increase, but also because people with HIV face so many stressors.

STRESSORS OF PEOPLE WITH HIV

Although survival with HIV has increased dramatically with the onset of effective ART, people living with HIV still face multiple stressors. Some of these are common to those with other illnesses and some are unique to HIV. Common stressors are the initial shock of receiving a life-threatening diagnosis, fear of death, the necessity of adhering to treatment, interacting with a complex medical system, and having adequate insurance or access to funding for medical treatment. Unique stressors include the pressure of having a stigmatized illness, incorporating a new identity as someone with a serious illness that is infectious, fear of rejection from friends/family, experiencing symptoms of HIV or side effects of ART, the need to adhere strictly to complex medication regimens, and experiencing the loss of a partner or loved ones. As Barroso (1997) notes, often one needs to renegotiate the friendship group and deal with one's family. For gay men there is the additional stress of disclosing their sexual orientation and often multiple losses of friends/ partners from HIV. People with children also frequently face additional challenges, such as raising children, the consequences of disclosure on their living circumstances and on their children's welfare, and the worry about who will care for their children if their health deteriorates. As the disease progresses, access to medical care becomes even more important, and the additional stress of job loss and financial concerns is present. In a qualitative study of four women with HIV, Mercier, Reidy, and Maheu (1999) point out that uncertainty is an omnipresent stressor. This includes the unknowns of being HIV-positive, such as having the feeling that time and the future are limited; concerns about children and intimate relationships; and difficulties experiencing loss, especially loss of control over one's life. Even with the advent of effective ART, stress has not decreased. Contrary to expectations, compared to a matched sample of HIV-positive women before the ART era (1994–1996), HIV-positive women assessed during the ART era (2000–2003) had more health-related stress, stress from stigma and disclosure, and maladaptive forms of coping (e.g., escape-avoidant coping) (Siegel & Schrimshaw, 2005). Therefore, even in the era of ART the burden of stressors is still quite high, and people with HIV need to find effective ways of coping.

The different ways of coping

Coping is the process by which people try to manage the perceived discrepancy between the demands and resources they appraise in a stressful situation (Lazarus & Folkman, 1984). Aspects of coping that are studied range from strategies generally conceptualized as *approach,* such as active coping, positive cognitive coping (e.g., positive reappraisal coping, finding positive meaning), problem-solving, and seeking emotional and social support, to strategies considered to be *avoidant,* such as denial, distraction, blame, behavioral disengagement, and substance use coping. The diversity of measures and labels used in the study of coping make it a challenge to neatly categorize and summarize (Moskowitz, Hult, Bussolari, & Acree, 2009). While avoidant strategies are generally considered maladaptive and approach strategies are generally thought to be adaptive, this may not always be the case. It is possible that in certain situations, or for certain individuals, avoidance coping may be the most effective coping strategy when it prevents an individual from being overwhelmed to the point where he or she is unable to function. Avoidance may also protect people from focusing on stressors that are not amenable to change. In a meta-analysis

of coping strategies, Suls and Fletcher (1985) found that avoidance was associated with more positive adaptation in the short run (e.g., during the first couple of weeks after the diagnosis), but that more active attention-oriented strategies are better in the long run after this initial period.

Coping strategies can also be grouped into problem-focused and emotion-focused approaches (Lazarus & Folkman, 1984). Problem-focused coping is aimed at reducing the demands of the situation or increasing the resources to deal with it. Emotion-focused coping is aimed at reducing the emotional response to the stressor, generally through either behavioral or cognitive approaches.

The two most widely used measures of coping in HIV studies are Folkman and Lazarus's (1988) Ways of Coping Questionnaire and the COPE of Carver at al. (Carver, 1997; Carver, Scheier, & Weintraub, 1989). The subscales of the Ways of Coping Questionnaire are confrontive, distancing, self-controlling, seeking social support, planful problem-solving, positive reappraisal, self-blame, and escape/avoidance. The COPE subscales comprise 14 types of coping: active coping, planning, denial, behavioral and mental disengagement, seeking emotional and instrumental support, venting of emotions, suppression of competing activities, restraint, turning to religion, substance use, venting, positive reinterpretation and growth, denial, and acceptance. HIV-specific scales have been developed as well, and these cover such additional topics as disclosure/non-disclosure, seeking peer support, seeking information, and managing HIV. A broader discussion of the ways of measuring coping in HIV can be found in Moskowitz et al. (2009). In her meta-analysis, she covered 18 types of coping that were each included in at least two studies in HIV: acceptance, alcohol/drug engagement, behavioral disengagement, confrontive, direct action, distancing, escape/avoidance, maintaining a fighting spirit, hopelessness, planning, positive reappraisal, rumination, seeking social support, self-controlling, self-blame, social isolation, spirituality, and venting. Moskowitz et al. grouped these coping strategies into approach and avoidant types of coping; this method also serves as a starting point for the next section.

Functional Components Approach to Stress and Coping

Based on our literature review and research experience we have conceptualized a functional components approach to stress and coping (Fig. 15.1),

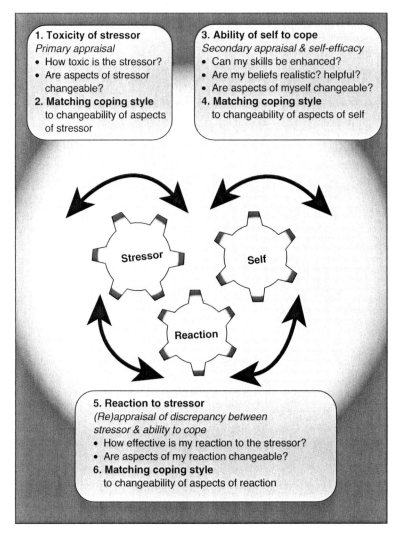

Fig. 15.1 The functional components approach to coping with key clinical questions. The three functional components of coping—the stressor, the self, and the reaction—are represented as cogwheels influencing one another. The arrows show how increases (or decreases) in either the toxicity of the stressor or the appraisal of your ability to cope influence your reaction. Similarly, your reaction can either increase or decrease the toxicity of the stressor and/or your ability to cope.

which addresses three components of the stress and coping paradigm: the **stressor**, the **self**, and the **reaction** of the self to the stressor. This approach extends Folkman et al.'s (1991) Coping Effectiveness Training Approach, which focuses on examining the changeable and unchangeable aspects of the stressor, to include a focus on the changeable and unchangeable aspects of the self and the reaction of the self to the stressor. Consistent with Lazarus and Folkman's (1984) transactional approach, coping is aimed at reducing the discrepancy between the primary appraisal of the toxicity of the stressor and the secondary appraisal of the ability of the self to deal with the stressor. Folkman et al. (1991) suggest

distinguishing changeable from unchangeable aspects of the stressor and matching problem-focused coping with the changeable and emotion-focused coping with the unchangeable aspects of the stressor. Problem-focused coping includes problem-solving, decision-making, interpersonal conflict resolution, information-gathering, advice-seeking, time management, goal-setting, and medication adherence. Emotion-focused coping includes meaning-making, positive reframing, seeing the brighter side of things, using social comparisons, use of humor, relaxation, meditation, religious and spiritual coping, emotional support, and even substance use coping (Folkman et al., 1991).

The functional components approach focuses not only on the changeable and unchangeable aspects of the stressor but also on changeable and unchangeable aspects of the self and the reaction of the self. Furthermore, we suggest that emotion-focused coping be broken down into its component parts: cognitive (reframing, positive outlook), activities to improve mood (relaxation, meditation, exercise), emotional expression, spirituality, and substance use.

As noted, according to the functional components approach, coping with stressors involves three components (stressor, self, and reaction). The functional components are interacting in an iterative and incremental dynamic process of appraisal and matching coping styles. The six steps involved are as follows:

1. Toxicity of stressor (primary appraisal)
2. Matching coping style
3. Ability of self to cope (secondary appraisal)
4. Matching coping style
5. Reaction to stressor (primary reappraisal of changed toxicity of stressor, secondary reappraisal of changed ability to cope, discrepancy between stressor and ability to cope)
6. Matching coping style

Thus, Step 1 in our approach involves primary appraisal of the toxicity of the stressor. This is followed by Step 2, matching coping style by using problem-focused coping for changeable stressors and emotion-focused, cognitive and spiritual coping for unchangeable stressors. Useful clinical questions for these first two steps might be "How toxic is the stressor?" and "Are any aspects of stressor changeable?" Approaches that make the stressful situation less toxic might include changing the stressor directly or by changing one's perception and/or interpretation of the stressor. Problem-solving and direct action (e.g., taking medications, removing oneself from an abusive relationship, getting off drugs) would be examples of a change of the stressor. Examples of using cognitive coping strategies to change the toxicity of the stressor are positive reappraisal and giving meaning to the stressor, reflected in testimonies such as "HIV helped me re-set priorities in my life," "HIV was a wake-up call meant to get me off drugs," "getting HIV led me to start a new agency which gave meaning to my life," and "I have a feeling that I was 'selected' by a higher power for a higher purpose to have HIV."

In Step 3, secondary appraisal evaluates the ability of self to cope. Lazarus and Folkman (1984)

refer to secondary appraisal as "a complex evaluative process that takes into account which coping options are available, the likelihood that a given coping option will accomplish what it is supposed to, and the likelihood that one can apply a particular strategy or set of strategies effectively" (p. 35). The latter expectancy is defined by Bandura as self-efficacy, as the belief in one's ability to exercise control over stressful events (Bandura, 1997, 2001, 2002). Bandura's social cognition theory distinguishes among three modes of agency: personal agency (exercising one's own influence on oneself and one's environment), proxy agency (relying on others to act on one's behest to secure desired outcomes), and community agency (exercised through group action) (Bandura, 2002). None is more central for resilience to taxing stressors than personal agency (Bandura, 1997). However, if one does not feel capable of handling a stressor by oneself, one may extend self-efficacy by seeking help from others, such as believing in the power of God or a higher power, or seeking instrumental or emotional social support from proxy or community agents to deal with the stressor. An example would be a long-term survivor with HIV who managed well by focusing on the aspects of himself that he could change and leaving in the hands of God what he could not change.

Analogous to the primary appraisal of the stressor, secondary appraisal of the self could separate changeable aspects of the self from unchangeable ones. Self-efficacy is changeable by both increasing skills (e.g., becoming an HIV expert) and direct action (e.g., acquiring assertiveness skills or problem-solving to design a pill-taking regimen). When skill levels cannot be changed, the perception of one's ability to handle the stressor may be enhanced by beliefs. The following are several ways that beliefs about the self may be changed:

1. Direct experience
2. Knowing about someone who has successfully coped with a similar situation: This may enhance one's belief in one's ability to handle a difficult situation (social modeling).
3. An authoritative source can help foster a change in a belief, such as the case with one of our participants who was told by a minister that God loved him. As spiritual/religious traditions have emphasized, people may grow spiritually by imitating the life or conduct of spiritual models, whether members of their own family or

community, or the exalted founder or mystic of a world religion (Oman & Thoresen, 2003).

In addition to changing skill levels or beliefs, the ability of the self to cope may be enhanced by proxy—that is, by a belief that God is helping or by finding a supportive empowering person, which in turn could be fostered by having an extraverted personality. Analogous to primary appraisal, matching coping style (Step 4) would involve applying problem-focused coping to the changeable parts of the self and emotion-focused, cognitive, and spiritual coping to the unchangeable parts of the self.

In Step 5, the reaction to the stressor is determined primarily by the discrepancy between the primary reappraisal of the changed toxicity of stressor and the secondary reappraisal of the person's changed ability to cope. Again, there is discernment between changeable and unchangeable aspects of the coping reaction. Uncontrollable aspects of the initial reaction might be the shock or disbelief of getting an HIV diagnosis, or an autonomic response such as increased heart rate, blood pressure, and the like. Furthermore, the genetic predisposition to a physiological reaction to a stressor cannot be changed. In Step 6, matching coping styles again involves using problem-focused coping for changeable aspects of the reaction and emotion-focused, cognitive and spiritual coping for both changeable and unchangeable aspects of the reaction. We suggest that coping efficacy can be further enhanced by asking "What can you change about your reaction to the stressor?" and using not only problem-focused coping but also emotion-focused, cognitive, and spiritual coping strategies to deal with one's reaction. Changeable aspects of one's reaction include the use of distress-reduction techniques such as relaxation exercises, emotion-regulation techniques, exercise, anger management, and emotional expression. Finally, reappraising one's reaction to the stressor may involve accepting one's imperfections in dealing with the stressor and restarting all over again from Step 1, persevering until one has reached one's capacity for stress reduction. Thus, the functional components approach involves a continuous six-step iterative dynamic adjustment of the three components, stressor, self, and reaction.

The functional components approach to stress and coping can be illustrated by using the example of Grace and Valery and their opposing ways of facing HIV. While Grace reduces the toxicity of living with HIV by taking ART consistently, which suppresses viral load and increases her CD4 cells, Valery takes ART inconsistently, jeopardizing her future treatment options and putting herself at risk of developing ART-resistant viral strains. However, Valery woke up temporarily when her CD4 cells dropped to a life-threatening range and started to take ART regularly for a short period. Grace matches problem-focused coping (medication adherence) with changeable aspects of the stressor and emotion-focused coping with the unchangeable reality that HIV cannot be eradicated from her body (Grace perceives that HIV helped her find meaning in life and saved her from drugs), while Valery still sees HIV as a death sentence.

Grace believes in her ability to cope with HIV, while Valery feels unable to do so (lack of self-efficacy). Grace feels very vibrant and energetic "to help somebody else, not just to live on." She wants to be a role model for others going through the same problems she did: hitting rock bottom as a homeless prostitute and drug addict. Grace works in a program to feed the homeless, is open about her HIV infection, and shares her story about how her life changed from depending on drugs to depending on God through the community of a drug program (community agency), her personal prayer and faith (personal agency), and the help of a friend/pastor (proxy agency). In addition, Grace feels supported by her family and reconnected with her children and finds new meaning in HIV by giving love and care to her family. In contrast, Valery blames the burden of taking care for others and her drug use for not being able to adhere to her medications. She feels that she cannot get close to people for fear of rejection due to her HIV. She feels "alive, but not living," lacks the will to live, and has limited personal goals.

Grace changed her reaction to the stressor by reducing the toxicity of the stressor and now feels healthy despite living more than two decades with HIV, and she enhanced her self-efficacy through prayer, faith, and the reciprocal help and care she shares with her loved ones. In contrast, Valery is drowning in a negative spiral of rapidly progressing HIV disease and lack of ability to cope.

According to the functional components approach to stress and coping, which views coping with stress as an iterative dynamic process of primary and secondary appraisal and reappraisal, Valery may get out of this negative spiral by following Grace as a spiritual model.

Coping, Physical Health, and Disease Progression in HIV

For the purposes of this section, the studies are divided into five tables covering different types of coping. The first table covers traditional approach and avoidant strategies generally measured by the major coping scales as noted above by Moskowitz et al. (2009). The second table covers cognitive approaches to coping that are not already included in the first table, and it includes expectancies such as optimism/fatalism, finding meaning, and benefit-finding or post-traumatic growth. The third table summarizes more enduring coping styles related to constructs of personality (e.g., extraversion, openness, conscientiousness), emotional expression, and altruism. The fourth table covers social support; the fifth, spirituality. This division is arbitrary and serves mainly as a way of organizing the data. Our focus is on longitudinal studies and thus is more circumscribed than the Moskowitz et al. (2009) review because we are most interested in the prediction of disease progression, although cross-sectional studies are sometimes noted in the text when they were particularly relevant.

Approach and avoidant coping

Table 15.1 covers the longitudinal studies that examine approach/avoidance coping and their relationship with disease progression in HIV, arranged in order from the oldest to the most recent studies. Only one, the oldest study, a 7-year follow-up Dutch study, which started in 1986, found that avoidance coping predicted slower immunological disease progression (Mulder, de Vroome, van Griensven, Antoni, & Sandfort, 1999). Two studies, one older Norwegian study (Vassend & Eskild, 1998) and the study with the largest sample size (*n* = 414), did not find a relationship between avoidant coping and disease progression (Patterson et al., 1996). However, six studies found that avoidance coping predicted faster progression to AIDS symptoms or mortality (Antoni et al., 1991; Billings, Folkman, Acree, & Moskowitz, 2000; Ironson et al., 1994, 2005b; Leserman et al., 2000; Mulder, Antoni, Duivenvoorden, Kauffmann, & Goodkin, 1995; Solano et al., 2002). One of these studies (Ironson et al., 2005b) was conducted entirely during the era when effective ART was widely available, and findings were maintained even after controlling for both medication prescribed and adherence.

This raises the question of whether avoidance may have been a useful strategy before effective ART became available. Considering all studies, though, especially the more recent ones, there seems to be considerably more support for the notion that avoidant coping predicts faster disease progression. This appears to be true even when taking into account ART and adherence.

Several studies have examined approach-oriented coping strategies. Six of these studies predicted better health (fewer symptoms, slower disease progression, or longer time to AIDS or death) (Ironson et al., 2005a and 2005c; Mulder et al., 1995; Solano et al., 1993; Thornton et al., 2000; Vassend & Eskild, 1998). The specific approach-oriented strategies that predicted better health included maintaining a fighting spirit (Solano et al., 1993), active coping (Mulder et al., 1995), planful problem-solving (Vassend & Eskild, 1998), proactive behavior (Ironson et al., 2005a), acceptance coping (Thornton et al., 2000), and increases in self-efficacy (Ironson et al., 2005c). Only two of these were conducted after effective ART was available (Ironson et al., 2005a, 2005c). However, three other studies showed no relationship between approach-oriented strategies and health (Billings et al., 2000; Mulder et al., 1999; Patterson et al., 1996). None of these studies were conducted in the era of ART. Only one study (Reed, Kemeny, Taylor, Wang, & Visscher, 1994) showed a negative effect: that "realistic acceptance" predicted faster disease progression. However, we believe a perusal of the items used suggests that it measures fatalism rather than "realistic acceptance," as we point out in the next section. Thus, while there is less evidence for protective effects of approach-oriented coping, few studies have been done since 1996, when effective ART became available.

Cognitive coping strategies

The next group of studies (Table 15.2) involves cognitive approaches to coping. We have grouped these into studies involving expectancies (such as optimism or fatalism), studies where finding meaning was measured, and studies where benefit-finding or growth was examined. Cognitive coping strategies such as positive reappraisal and denial have already been covered in the traditional approach/avoidance strategies in Table 15.1 and will not be repeated here. Five studies have examined aspects of optimism as a predictor of disease progression. Most have used dispositional optimism, which is defined as generalized positive expectancies regarding future outcomes. In two of these studies, optimism linearly predicted better health; optimistic outlook was associated with lower mortality in Blomkvist et al. (1994)

Table 15.1 Longitudinal studies of approach/avoidance coping predicting HIV disease progression

Study	Psychological Predictors[1]	Design	Results
Mulder et al., 1999; conducted 1986–93 (Netherlands)	Avoidance, active cognitive & behavioral coping (*Utrecht Coping List*)	*n* = 181 gay men; >200 CD4 cell count, no AIDS symptoms, not using AZT[2]; 7-year follow-up	Only avoidance coping predicted less CD4 decline, CD4↓<200, & syncytium inducing HIV variants; none predicted AIDS symptoms
Vassend et al., 1998; conducted 1988–95 (Norway)	Escape-avoidance, distancing, accepting responsibility, self-controlling, support-seeking, confronting, planful problem-solving, positive reappraisal (*Ways of Coping Scale, WOC*[3], Norwegian version)	*n* = 63 gay men; 97% asymptomatic, 98% not using AZT[2]; mean of 47 months follow-up (range 1–77)	Only planful problem-solving predicted fewer AIDS symptoms
Ironson et al., 1994; conducted 1988–92	Denial increase from before to after notification of HIV+ serostatus (*COPE*[3])	*n* = 23 gay men; asymptomatic; 2-year follow-up	Increased denial predicted AIDS symptoms and mortality
Antoni et al., 1995; conducted 1988–92	Passive (denial, mental & behavioral disengagement) & active (planning, positive reinterpretation/growth, active coping) (*COPE*[3])	*n* = 18 gay men, 82% White; asymptomatic; 1-year follow-up	Only passive coping predicted worse cell-mediated immune response (CD4/CD8 ratio, CD4%, PHA response, CD4CD45RA%)
Reed et al., 1994; conducted 1988–94	Realistic acceptance,[4] community involvement & spiritual growth, active cognitive coping, support & information seeking, self-blame & avoidance (*WOC*[3])	*n* = 74 gay men, 95% White; AIDS diagnosis; 50 months of follow-up	Only low realistic acceptance[4] predicted *higher* mortality after AIDS diagnosis
Patterson et al., 1996; conducted 1989–96	Avoidant & approach coping (*WOC*[3])	*n* = 414 men, 79% White; 77% >200 CD4 cells, 61% asymptomatic; 5-year follow-up	Avoidant & approach coping did not predict disease progression (CD4 decline, AIDS symptoms, mortality)
Billings et al., 2000; conducted 1990–94	Active & social coping, cognitive & behavioral avoidance (*WOC*[5])	*n* = 86 gay male caregivers, 89% White; most using AZT[2], 13 months follow-up	Only behavioral avoidance predicted higher levels of HIV-specific/general symptoms
Leserman et al., 2000; conducted 1990–98	Cumulative denial (*COPE*[3])	*n* = 82 gay men, 79% White; >200 CD4 cells, asymptomatic, no ART[6]; 7.5-year follow-up	Cumulative denial predicted faster progression to AIDS (symptoms/CD4↓<200)
Solano et al., 1993; conducted before 1991 (Italy)	Denial & fighting spirit (*story scores*)	*n* = 100, 74% men; 21% symptomatic; 1-year follow-up	Higher denial & less fighting spirit predicted more symptom progression
Mulder et al., 1995; conducted 1991–93	Active confrontation & optimistic attitude; (*HIV Coping List* [Dutch derivative of *COPE*[3]])	*n* = 51 gay men; no AIDS symptoms; 33% using AZT; 1-year follow-up	Only active confrontation predicted fewer AIDS symptoms

Table 15.1 **Longitudinal studies of approach/avoidance coping predicting HIV disease progression** *(Cont'd)*

Study	Psychological Predictors[1]	Design	Results
Thornton et al., 2000; conducted 1993–96	Acceptance, problem-solving, disengagement, denial, social support, religion *(COPE[3])*	*n* = 143 gay men, 92% White; any disease stage; 30 months of follow-up	Only acceptance coping predicted fewer AIDS symptoms
a) Ironson, O'Cleirigh et al., 2005b; b) Ironson, Balbin et al., 2005a; conducted 1997–2002	a) Baseline & cumulative avoidant coping *(COPE* denial, behavioral disengagement) b) Proactive behavior; *(interviewer ratings)*	*n* = 177, 70% men, 30% White; 150–500 CD4 cells, no AIDS symptoms, 77% using ART[6]; 2-year follow-up	a) Cumulative avoidant coping predicted less CD4 decline & better viral load control, baseline avoidant coping only viral load control; b) proactive behavior only less CD4 decline
Ironson, Weiss et al., 2005c; started 1996	Self-efficacy for AIDS & adherence (post intervention) *(Self-Efficacy Inventory[3])*	*n* = 56 women, 13% White; AIDS stage; 81% using ART[6]; 3 months of follow-up	Increased self-efficacy predicted better viral load control

[1] *measurement in italics*
[2] AZT (azidothymidine) was standard care before effective antiretroviral therapy (ART) in 1996
[3] adapted to HIV/AIDS
[4] "realistic acceptance" construct included items indicating fatalism
[5] adapted to caregiving in gay men
[6] Effective ART became available in 1996

and dispositional optimism with slower disease progression in Ironson et al. (2005a). A third study used positive expectancies as part of a composite (along with positive affect and finding meaning) and found that the composite predicted lower mortality over 5 years (Ickovics et al., 2006). In a recent study of 412 people with HIV by Milam et al. (Milam, Richardson, Marks, Kemper, & McCuthchan, 2004; Milam, 2006), post-traumatic growth and dispositional optimism were examined as predictors. Post-traumatic growth was not associated with disease progression except in Hispanics and those with low optimism, but it was associated with depressive symptoms and alcohol and drug use (Milam, 2006). Dispositional optimism was found to be curvilinear (inverted U-shape) related to the CD4 slope (i.e., moderate optimism predicted the highest CD4 counts). However, Milam et al. (2004) controlled for depression in their analysis, which may have wiped out a linear optimism relationship. Dispositional optimism did not predict viral load in that study, nor did it predict survival in the studies by Reed et al. (1994) and Tomakowsky et al. (Tomakowsky, Lumley, Markowitz, & Frank, 2001). However, Tomakowsky et al. (2001) measured both dispositional optimism and optimistic explanatory style. Against expectations, optimistic explanatory style predicted a *greater* decline in CD4 counts,

while dispositional optimism did not predict the CD4 slope. The authors conclude that health status may be differentially affected through the interaction of optimistic explanatory style with specific types of stressors. Optimistic explanatory style may be considered maladaptive under certain conditions (such as a persistent or uncontrollable stressor like coping with HIV in the pre-ART era), in which realism rather than optimism may be advantageous (Tomakowsky et al., 2001). However, realistic acceptance, perhaps negatively related to an optimistic explanatory style, has to be distinguished from fatalism. Interestingly, fatalism predicted decreased survival time over up to 50 months. Notably, we call this fatalism because this construct included items such as "Prepare myself for the worst," although the authors labeled the construct as "realistic acceptance coping" (Reed et al., 1994) (Table 15.1). Thus, the evidence for optimism is mixed; however, the larger and more recent studies support either a linear or a curvilinear relationship.

Finding meaning has been examined as a predictor of HIV disease progression in only two studies. The first of these was a study of 40 HIV-positive men who had a recent AIDS related loss and were in bereavement (Bower, Kemeny, Taylor, & Fahey, 1998). The discovery of meaning in the loss predicted less loss of CD4 cells and lower mortality over 2 to 3 years. In a

Table 15.2 Longitudinal studies of cognitive approaches to coping (expectancies such as optimism or fatalism, finding meaning, benefit finding or growth predicting HIV disease progression)

Study	Psychological Predictors[1]	Design	Results
Blomkvist et al., 1994; conducted 1985–92, Sweden	Optimistic outlook (*anticipated future activities derived from the Coping Wheel*)	n = 48 hemophiliac men; 1 year after HIV diagnosis; 67% using ART[2]; 7-year follow-up	Optimistic outlook predicted lower mortality, but not physical symptoms
Ironson, Balbin, et al., 2005a; conducted 1997–2002	Dispositional optimism (*Life Orientation Test [LOT, LOT-revised]*)	n = 177, 70% men, 30% White; 150–500 CD4 cells, no AIDS symptoms, 77% using ART; 2-year follow-up	Optimism predicted less CD4 decline & better viral load control
Ickovics et al., 2006; conducted 1993–2000	Psychological resources (finding meaning, positive expectancy, positive affect[3]) (*Psychological Resources Index*)	n = 773 women, 60% African American; no AIDS diagnosis; 5-year follow-up	Psychological resources predicted less HIV-related mortality & CD4 decline
Milam et al., 2004; Milam, 2006; conducted 1999–2001	Dispositional optimism & pessimism (*LOT-R*); post-traumatic growth (PTG) (*PTG Inventory*)	n = 412, 88% male, 40% Latino; 75% using ART[2]; 18–20 months of follow-up	Pessimism predicted higher viral load, optimism curvilinear related to CD4 slope (inverted U); PTG related to low viral load among those low in pessimism
Reed et al., 1994; conducted 1988–94	Dispositional optimism (*LOT*)	n = 74 gay men, 95% White; AIDS diagnosis; 50 months of follow-up	Optimism did not predict survival after AIDS diagnosis
Tomakowsky et al., 2001; conducted 1993–97	Dispositional optimism (*LOT*); optimistic explanatory style (*Expanded Attributional Style Questionnaire*)	n = 47 men, 69% White; no AIDS symptoms, 46% using AZT; 2-year follow-up	Optimistic explanatory style predicted **greater** CD4 decline, dispositional optimism not related to CD4 slope
Bower et al., 1998; started 1987	Cognitive processing & finding meaning from loss (*transcripts of bereavement interviews*)	n = 40 men, 98% White, recent AIDS-related bereavement; 2 to 3 years of follow-up	Only finding meaning from loss predicted less CD4 decline & AIDS-related mortality

[1] *measurement in italics*
[2] After 1996, antiretroviral therapy (ART) consisted of effective combination therapy. Prior to that only less effective monotherapy (e.g., azidothymidine [AZT]) was used.
[3] adapted from Profile of Mood States

larger (n = 773 women) and more recent study noted above (Ickovics et al., 2006), finding meaning was examined as part of a composite of psychological resources also including positive affect and positive expectancy. They found that the composite predicted lower mortality over 5 years. Although meaning looks promising as a predictor of disease progression, results must be viewed as preliminary, given that the first study was small and older, and the second study measured finding meaning as part of a composite.

Coping styles: personality and emotional expression

A third group of studies involves coping factors, which we have labeled coping styles (Table 15.3). These include personality and expression of emotions that are more enduring approaches to coping. Our group examined the five-factor model (i.e., openness, conscientiousness, extraversion, agreeableness, and neuroticism) in a study conducted entirely during the era of ART. Conscientiousness, extraversion, and

Table 15.3   Longitudinal studies of coping styles (more enduring approaches to coping such as personality, expression of emotions, and altruism) predicting HIV disease progression

Study	Psychological Predictors[1]	Design	Results
Ironson, et al., 2008; conducted 1997–2006	Neuroticism, extraversion, openness, agreeableness, conscientiousness	n = 104, 68% men, 37% African American; 150–500 CD4 cells, no AIDS symptoms, 77% using ART[2]; 4-year follow-up	Openness & extraversion predicted less CD4 decline & better viral load control, conscientiousness predicted only better viral load control
O'Cleirigh, et al., 2007; conducted 2002–05	Conscientiousness (*Revised NEO Personality Inventory*)	n = 119, 67% men, 42% African American; 150–500 CD4 cells, no AIDS symptoms, 77% using ART[2]; 1-year follow-up	Conscientiousness predicted less CD4 decline & better viral load control
Thornton et al., 2000; conducted 1993–96	Extraversion, neuroticism, psychoticism (*Eysenk Personality Questionnaire*)	n = 143 gay men, 92% White; any disease stage; 30 months of follow-up	Personality factors did not predict fewer AIDS symptoms
Cole et al., 1996; conducted 1987–88	Concealed homosexual identity (*5-point Likert-type scale*)	n = 80 gay men, 96% White; healthy, CD4% 30–60; 54% using ART[2]; 9-year follow-up	Concealed homosexual identity predicted greater CD4% decline, more AIDS symptoms & mortality
Strachan et al., 2007; conducted 2000–04	Concealed homosexual identity & HIV status (*5-point Likert-type scale*)	n = 373, 88% men, 65% White; 71% using ART[2]; psychiatric comorbidity, 1-year follow-up	Concealed homosexual identity & HIV status predicted greater CD4 decline
Solano et al., 2002; conducted before 2000 (Italy)	Type C (not expressing needs or feelings, presenting pleasant façade) (*Temoshok Coping Vignettes);* hardiness (facing life's events with a sense of challenge, commitment, & personal control) (*Hardiness Scale*)	n = 176, 69% male; asymptomatic, 49% CD4 cells > 500, 51% CD4 cells 200–499, 1-year follow-up	Only type C predicted progression of CDC stage, but only among CDC-A2 (200–499 CD4)
O'Cleirigh et al., 2003; conducted 1997–2001	Emotional processing of traumatic experiences (*essay ratings; cognitive change, self-esteem change, adaptive coping & involvement)* Emotional disclosure (*# of positive & negative emotion words),* finding meaning (*interview ratings*)	n = 97, CD4 cells 100–500, no AIDS symptoms; 1-year follow-up	Emotional processing predicted less CD4 decline and better viral load control; both links were mediated by finding meaning; emotional disclosure did not predict CD4 & viral load slopes
Ironson et al., 2007; conducted 1997–2002	Altruism (care & concern for others (*essay scores*), giving to charities (*questionnaire*), altruism (facet of *Revised NEO Personality Inventory*)	n = 177, 70% men, 30% White; 150–500 CD4 cells, no AIDS symptoms, 77% using ART[2]; 2-year follow-up	Caring (but not concern) for others predicted less CD4 decline & better viral load control, giving to charities & altruism predicted only better viral load control

[1] *measurement in italics*
[2] After 1996, antiretroviral therapy (ART) consisted of effective combination therapy. Prior to that only less effective monotherapy (e.g., azidothymidine [AZT]) was used.

openness were found to predict slower HIV disease progression (G. H. Ironson, O'Cleirigh, Weiss, Schneiderman, & Costa, 2008; O'Cleirigh, Ironson, Weiss, & Costa, 2007). An earlier study using Eysenck's measure of Personality (Thornton et al., 2000) found no relationship between personality and the time to the onset of AIDS-related complex or AIDS in 143 men followed for up to 30 months. Possible reasons for the discrepancy include different measures, constructs, time periods (before vs. after availability of effective ART), and disease stages of participants at study entry.

Several groups have investigated emotional expression and related constructs. We include these because the question of whether it is better coping to express one's emotions or to keep feelings inside when under stress often arises. Cole et al. (Cole, Kemeny, Taylor, Visscher, & Fahey, 1996) found that concealing one's homosexual identity was associated with faster disease progression in HIV. Similarly, in a study of 373 psychiatric outpatients, Strachan et al. (Strachan, Bennett, Russo, & Roy-Byrne, 2007) found that concealment of either HIV status or sexual orientation independently predicted faster CD4 decline over four visits (about one year). Type C personality style, which is defined as a style characterized by emotional inexpression and decreased recognition of needs and feelings, was studied in 185 HIV-positive people who were followed for up to 12 months (Solano et al., 2002). People high on type C did have faster disease progression, but only among those with initial CD4 cells between 200 and 499. In a cross-sectional study (not included in Table 15.3), type C personality was also associated with higher levels of interleukin-6 (Temoshok et al., 2008), a measure that is indicative of inflammation and frailty and that is elevated in aging. Low emotional expression (measured via counting emotional words in essays written about personal traumatic events) was also associated with long survivor status (O'Cleirigh et al., 2003) and remaining asymptomatic even with very low CD4 cell counts (O'Cleirigh, Ironson, Fletcher, & Schneiderman, 2008). Depth processing (scored by rating essays about trauma for cognitive appraisal change, self-esteem enhancement, problem-solving, and involvement) was even more protective of health than emotional expression alone in the two studies just noted on emotional expression, as well as in a longitudinal study by our group (O'Cleirigh et al., 2002). Interestingly, both the Bower et al. (1998) study previously described (in Table 15.2) and our study (O'Cleirigh et al., 2002)

suggest that one way in which depth processing may be related to health is through meaning-making. Finally, it is important to note that while emotional expression/depth processing appears to be beneficial, one must distinguish this from merely venting, which has been associated with a greater increase in HIV-related symptoms in 65 men living with HIV/AIDS (Ashton et al., 2005) (Table 15.4). Summarizing the emotional expression studies, it appears that venting may be detrimental, expressing emotions is protective, depth processing is more protective, and processing toward meaning may be most protective of health in HIV.

Altruism is the final coping style we cover in Table 15.3. We have grouped it into the section on enduring personality styles because being a giving person may be enduring rather than simply situation-specific. Participants in our longitudinal study (Ironson et al., 2005b) who reported taking care of others in written essays about trauma had slower disease progression over 4 years than those who did not report caring for others (Ironson, 2007).

Social support

Because seeking social support can be considered a form of coping, we are including it as a potential predictor of health in HIV. Social support is one of the most researched psychosocial factors. However, the results from longitudinal studies of disease progression are mixed. Eleven longitudinal studies have used social support as a predictor of HIV disease progression. Five of these have found a protective effect of social support and only one study found that social support was associated with faster disease progression. Of the five studies, the one with the longest follow-up (96 gay men followed up to 9 years), Leserman et al. found that more cumulative social support predicted slower time for progression to AIDS (Leserman et al., 1999, 2000, 2002) (the three studies are counted only once since they are within the same cohort). Forty-nine percent of people with low social support had developed AIDS after 7.5 years; in those with high social support, only 24 percent had developed AIDS. The largest of the five studies where social support was related to better health was by Patterson et al. (1996), who followed 414 men over 5 years, examining social network size and emotional and informational support. Large social network size predicted survival, but only among those with AIDS symptoms at baseline. However, for those asymptomatic at baseline, large network size predicted *faster* disease progression, while neither emotional

Table 15.4 Longitudinal studies of social support predicting HIV disease progression

Study	Psychological Predictors[1]	Design	Results
Leserman et al., 1999, 2000, 2002; conducted 1990–2000	Cumulative satisfaction with social support (*Sarason Brief Social Support Questionnaire*)	*n* = 82 gay men, 79% White; >200 CD4 cells, asymptomatic; none using ART[2]; 9-year follow-up	Cumulative satisfaction with social support predicted faster progression to AIDS (symptoms/CD4↓<200)
Patterson et al., 1996; conducted 1989–96	Social network size (*# of social support contacts*); emotional & informational support (*Social Support Questionnaire*)	*n* = 414 men, 79% White; 77% >200 CD4 cells, 61% asymptomatic; 5-year follow-up	Larger social network size and informational support predicted survival, but only among those initially in CDC stage C (AIDS symptoms); larger network size predicted **faster** CDC stage B/C progression among those initially in stage A (asymptomatic); informational support predicted less CDC stage C progression among those in stage B (symptomatic HIV infection) at baseline
Solano et al., 1993; conducted before 1991 (Italy)	Perceived support from the environment (*Social Support Scale*)	*n* = 100, 74% men; all CD4 stages, 21% symptomatic; 1-year follow-up	Perceived social support predicted less symptom progression, but only among those with <400 CD4 cells at baseline
Ashton et al., 2005; conducted 1996–2000	Satisfaction with social support (*UCLA Social Support Inventory*), venting (*Brief COPE*)	*n* = 65 men, 61% men, 69% White; 44% AIDS diagnosis, 81% using ART[2];1-year follow-up	Satisfying social support and less venting predicted fewer HIV-related physical symptoms
Theorell et al., 1995; conducted 1985–90 (Sweden)	Social & emotional support in difficult situations (*Availability of attachment Index of Social Network-Support Questionnaire*)	*n* = 48 hemophiliac men; 1 year after HIV diagnosis; 5-year follow-up	Low social & emotional support predicted CD4 decline, but not physical symptoms & mortality
Miller et al., 1997; conducted 1987–90	Social integration (adapted from *UCLA Social Support Inventory*), loneliness (*UCLA Loneliness Scale*)	*n* = 205 men, 90% White, no AIDS symptoms; 38% using ART[2]; 3-year follow-up	Lower levels of loneliness predicted **greater** CD4% decline, but not AIDS symptoms & mortality. Social integration did not predict CD4%, AIDS & mortality.
Ironson, O'Cleirigh, et al., 2005b; conducted 1997–2002	Social support (*ENRICHED Social Support Instrument*)	*n* = 177, 70% men, 30% White; 150–500 CD4 cells, no AIDS symptoms, 77% using ART[2]; 2-year follow-up	Social support did not predict CD4 & viral load slopes

(Continued)

Table 15.4   Longitudinal studies of social support predicting HIV disease progression   *(Cont'd)*

Study	Psychological Predictors[1]	Design	Results
Solano et al., 2002; conducted before 2000 (Italy)	Perceived availability and acceptance of potential sources of support (*Social Support Scale);* loneliness (*UCLA Loneliness Scale*)	n = 176, 69% male; asymptomatic, 49% CD4 cells >500, 51% CD4 cells 200–499, 1-year follow-up	Perceived social support & loneliness did not predict CDC stage progression, but there was a trend towards lower perceived social support in those with CDC stage progression
Thornton et al., 2000; conducted 1993–96	Perceived available social support (*Interpersonal Support Evaluation List*)	n = 143 gay men, 92% White; any disease stage; 30 months of follow-up	Perceived available social support did not predict fewer AIDS symptoms, but there was a trend towards less CD4↓<200
Perry et al., 1992; conducted 1986–91	Social support (*Interpersonal Support Evaluation List*)	n = 221, 93% men; no AIDS diagnosis, AZT-naïve, 1-year follow-up	Social support did not predict CD4 slope
Eich-Hochli et al., 1997; conducted 1989–92 (Switzerland)	Emotional & practical social support, # of relationships (*Social Network Questionnaire*)	n = 89, 76% men; asymptomatic, CD4 cells >200, 34% using AZT; 2-year follow-up	Social support & network did not predict progression to AIDS

[1] *measurement in italics*

[2] After 1996, antiretroviral therapy (ART) consisted of effective combination therapy. Prior to that only less effective monotherapy (e.g., azidothymidine [AZT]) was used.

nor informational support predicted better health. For participants with symptomatic HIV infection (but without AIDS-defining events) informational support was associated with slower onset of AIDS symptoms. For men in the advanced stages of AIDS, informational support predicted survival, in addition to larger network size. Higher social support also predicted slower disease progression in a study of 100 men and women followed for 1 year, but this relationship was found only for those whose immune systems were more impaired at the start of the study (i.e., those with CD4 counts < 400) (Solano et al., 1993). In a smaller study (65 men and women with HIV), those with higher social support and those with low levels of venting had fewer physical health symptoms (technically less increase in symptoms) at the end of 12 months (Ashton et al., 2005). In an analysis with both venting and social support as potential predictors in the model together, only social support remained a significant predictor of symptoms (Ashton et al., 2005). Finally, Theorell et al. (1995) followed a small sample of 48 men with hemophilia and found that those with low social support at entry had faster declines in CD4 cells over 5 years. Only the Ashton et al. (2005) study was conducted entirely after 1996 when

effective treatment became available, and this study had a short follow-up (12 months).

In contrast, five studies showed no significant longitudinal association of social support with health (two with trends showing higher social support with slower disease progression, two with no trends, and one with a trend in the opposite direction), and one study showed a significant relationship between low social support and slower disease progression (Miller, Kemeny, Taylor, Cole, & Visscher, 1997). The latter, which was the largest study (n = 205 gay men), showed no relationship between loneliness as an indicator of social support and the development of AIDS or mortality. However, contrary to expectations, loneliness at entry was significantly associated with an *increase* in CD4 cells. While this study was conducted before the ART era, another study conducted entirely when effective ART was available (Ironson et al., 2005b) found a similar lack of association between social support and either viral load or CD4 cells, but with a trend for higher social support to predict faster disease progression (CD4 decline). Two studies (n = 176 and 143) showed trends (p <.10) of social support predicting slower disease progression, specifically less CDC stage progression (Solano et al., 2002) and less CD4 decline below 200 (Thornton et al., 2000). Finally, two smaller studies (*n* = 87 and 89) showed no association between social support and disease progression (Eich-Hochli, Niklowitz, Luthy, & Opravil, 1997; Perry, Fishman, Jacobsberg, & Frances, 1992).

Although this literature is quite mixed, there are some important patterns. Both Patterson et al. (1996) and Solano et al. (1993) found a protective effect only among those with more advanced disease. Finally, the Leserman et al. study, which used a cumulative measure of social support and followed men over the longest period of time, found the greatest support for a protective effect of social support (Leserman et al., 1999, 2000, 2002). In conclusion, though the evidence is mixed, social support may be particularly helpful when measured over time and with advanced disease.

Stress-reducing coping activities (nonspecific)

Although often not included in the psychological coping literature, it is important to mention that there are other, non-psychological techniques that people use to cope by diffusing stress. These include, but are not limited to, exercise, relaxation techniques, and massage. A review of these is beyond the scope of this chapter, but all of these have been examined in HIV, and there is some evidence of beneficial effects for both health and well-being. LaPerriere et al. (1994) noted improvements in mood and immune function with exercise. Frequency of practicing relaxation techniques predicted greater survival and less progression to AIDS symptoms at 2-year follow-up (Ironson et al., 1994) and improved immune measures (Antoni et al., 1991). Massage has also been associated with improved immune measures and mood (Ironson et al., 1996). Interestingly, a recent review of exercise studies, although not done in people with HIV, showed that the effect of exercise may be comparable to that of cognitive or group psychotherapy for depression, and similar in percentages of people no longer meeting criteria for depression (60.4 percent) compared to medication (68.8 percent) (Sidhu, Vandana, & Balon, 2009). The recommended prescription includes 30 minutes of moderate to vigorous exercise on all or most days.

Mediators between coping and health behaviors

Potential mediators between coping and health behaviors include optimism, positive states of mind, proactive behavior, and social support. Studies suggest that optimists adopt healthier behaviors such as adhering better to medication (Ironson et al., 2005a; Milam et al., 2004), exercising more (Ironson et al., 2005a), using illicit drugs less (Milam et al., 2004), smoking less (Ironson et al., 2005a; Tomakowsky et al., 2001), exhibiting more adaptive coping and proactive behavior (Ironson et al., 2005a), and using fewer avoidant coping strategies (Cole, 2008; Ironson et al., 2005a). Conversely, optimism has been related to a *higher* incidence of risky sexual behavior in a study examining HIV-negative gay men (Gonzalez et al., 2004). In addition, positive states of mind have been related to better adherence (Taylor et al., 1992). Similarly, social support may play a mediating role by facilitating adherence to medication (Ironson et al., 2002; Kremer, Ironson, Schneiderman, & Hautzinger, 2006). Cacioppo et al. (Cacioppo, Hawkley, & Berntson, 2003) found an association between better social support and receiving better treatment from physicians. Furthermore, Simoni et al. (Simoni, Frick, & Huang, 2006) found that social support was associated with less negative affect and greater spirituality.

Coping and Psychological Well-Being in People with HIV

Studies addressing the association between coping and psychological well-being in people with HIV have encompassed both positive affect, such as happiness, life satisfaction, personal growth, and quality of life, as well as negative affect, such as depression, anxiety, and psychological distress. One of the biggest challenges in comparing the findings across various studies is the diversity of measures and labels used to examine coping as well as psychological well-being. There is an interesting trend in that approach coping and avoidant coping have been examined in particular in relation to physical health, whereas cognitive coping approaches, such as finding meaning, have been examined more often in relation to psychological well-being. Some studies have conceptualized personal growth as a coping strategy, whereas others viewed personal growth as part of psychological well-being and an outcome of successful coping.

We will present a recent meta-analysis to give a broad picture of which coping strategies work best to enhance psychological well-being, look at the few longitudinal studies available, and then go into the details of some cross-sectional studies, including an examination of the role of gender in coping and psychological well-being.

The big picture

A recent meta-analysis of 63 studies (Moskowitz et al., 2009) including a total of 15,490 people with HIV classified coping into two categories: approach coping (i.e., acceptance, confrontive, direct action, fighting spirit, planning, positive reappraisal, seeking social support, self-blame) and avoidance coping (i.e., alcohol/drug disengagement, behavioral disengagement, distancing, escape/avoidance, social isolation). As expected, approach coping was associated with greater well-being and avoidant coping with less well-being; effect sizes ranged between small and medium (Moskowitz et al., 2009). However, some approach coping strategies, such as confrontive coping and self-blame, appear to be inversely associated with psychological well-being. The meta-analysis also examined which of the single coping strategies was most strongly related to well-being. Direct action, which is a combination of active and problem-solving coping, and positive reappraisal were the most effective approach coping strategies, and social isolation had the largest (negative) effect size as an avoidance coping strategy (Moskowitz et al., 2009).

The findings also suggest differences in the effectiveness of coping as a function of gender, time since diagnosis, and the advent of ART. The correlation between approach coping and positive affect was stronger among men, whereas the correlation between avoidance coping and negative affect was stronger among women (Moskowitz et al., 2009). Both approach and avoidance coping became less adaptive with a longer time since diagnosis (Moskowitz et al., 2009). Approach coping appeared to be more effective after the introduction of better ART (Moskowitz et al., 2009).

What works in the long run?

Besides the issue of the different measurements and labels for coping and psychological well-being, the other challenge is that there are very few longitudinal studies examining coping and well-being in people with HIV. We will discuss the findings of longitudinal studies conducted on samples that were diverse with respect to age, sex, and race/ethnicity after the advent of ART.

Patterns of coping responses, their change, and their relationship to emotional well-being were examined in a nationally representative sample (n = 2,864) followed over one year (Fleishman et al., 2003). Four coping patterns were identified: blame-withdrawal coping, distancing, active approach coping, and passive coping (i.e., infrequent use of all three coping strategies). At the one-year follow-up, 46 percent reported the same coping pattern. Those using blame-withdrawal coping had the lowest emotional well-being at baseline and at follow-up, whereas passive coping was associated with higher emotional well-being at both times. The authors conclude that those with a passive coping pattern may not have engaged in coping responses in part because they experienced little emotional distress, whereas blame-withdrawal coping may be a response to more emotional distress (Fleishman et al., 2003). This theory is further supported by two other studies. One study (n = 116), done in our laboratory, found that distress tolerance (i.e., the ability to experience and endure emotional distress) significantly moderated the relationship between major life events in the previous six months and depressive symptoms and substance use coping, indicating that low distress tolerance may present a challenge to effective coping with HIV (O'Cleirigh, Ironson, & Smits, 2007). Another study (n = 85) (Gore-Felton et al., 2006) confirmed that while both "maladaptive" coping (i.e., denial, behavioral disengagement, substance use) and quality of life (i.e., cognitive functioning, health distress) predicted depression at three months, quality of life was the single most important predictor. Thus, there may be a negative spiral of high distress, low distress tolerance, "maladaptive" coping strategies, reduced quality of life, and depressive mood. Conversely, there might also be a positive spiral associated with a high tolerance for adversity, acceptance coping, spiritual striving, and greater psychological well-being. This is suggested by a study with a 6-month follow-up (n = 180) examining the relationship between depression and spiritual striving, defined as the process of consciously trying to grow spiritually and pursuing a meaningful and fulfilling daily life (Perez et al., 2009). The inverse relationship between depression and spiritual striving was partially mediated by acceptance coping, but not by social support (Perez et al., 2009). The construct of acceptance coping includes the ability to recognize the experience of emotional distress, connect it to the situation, and act effectively, while still experiencing discomfort (Perez et al., 2009), which is somewhat related to distress tolerance and active coping.

Thus, one might hypothesize the existence of a negative spiral started by a stressor combined with poor distress tolerance that fosters "maladaptive" coping. This may lead to increased depression and decreased quality of life in the long run. Since there are very few longitudinal studies, and these mostly had short follow-ups, we cannot answer the question of what works in the long run with certainty. Therefore, the next section will focus on what works in the short run and reviews cross-sectional studies examining specific groups in more detail.

Which coping strategies have the strongest influence on psychological well-being?

Several studies in men with advanced HIV/AIDS suggest that positive cognitive coping strategies, in particular positive reappraisal, have a stronger influence on positive well-being than support coping strategies. A study of 203 people with advanced HIV/AIDS (mainly African American men) found that ascribing more positive meaning to the illness was linked to more positive well-being (e.g., happiness, life satisfaction) and less depressed mood, even after controlling for the contributions of social support and problem-focused coping (Farber, Mirsalimi, Williams, & McDaniel, 2003). A Dutch study of 104 gay men showed that positive reappraisal strategies (e.g., attaching a positive meaning to being HIV-positive, thinking about joyful and pleasant issues), focusing on goals, and less use of other blame were related to more personal growth (Kraaij, Garnefski, et al., 2008) and less depression and anxiety (Kraaij, van der Veek, et al., 2008). The finding that positive reappraisal coping was related to higher levels of personal growth was also confirmed in a study of 138 women with HIV, but depressive affect and emotional support explained more variance in personal growth than positive reappraisal coping (Siegel, Schrimshaw, & Pretter, 2005). Interestingly, African American women in that study reported significantly more personal growth than White women did, and the authors discussed a greater salience of spirituality/religiousness among African Americans as a potential explanation (Siegel et al., 2005). The connection between spirituality/religiousness and finding a new meaning in living with HIV will be further discussed in the section on spiritual coping in this chapter.

Notably, another study of 90 predominately minority women found that religious coping was not related with HIV/AIDS-associated quality of life (Weaver et al., 2004). However, even after controlling for demographic and disease-related variables, cognitive coping strategies (e.g., positive reframing, acceptance) were positively related while denial was negatively related with HIV/AIDS-associated quality of life. Since these relationships were both mediated by perceived stress, the authors suggest that use of certain coping strategies may lessen or heighten perceptions of life stressfulness, thereby influencing the quality of life in minority women (Weaver et al., 2004).

Another study of 265 low-income African American mothers found that coping resources and coping responses jointly mediated the relationship between stressors (i.e., daily hassles, difficult life circumstances, major life events) and psychological distress (Burns, Feaster, Mitrani, Ow, & Szapocznik, 2008). Having more stressors was associated with more use of avoidance coping, such as denial, self-distraction, behavioral disengagement, and self-blaming. Of the three coping strategies examined, avoidance coping was the largest single contributor to this meditational effect, particularly among mothers with a history of substance use. Active coping (e.g., positive reframing, planning, taking actions) had a significant meditational effect, whereas use of the available social support did not. Nevertheless, coping resources, such as available social support and perceived control, were associated with more use of active coping. Having feelings of control was associated with less psychological distress beyond the choice of coping responses (Burns et al., 2008). The results of the studies focusing on a single gender raise the question of whether there may be gender differences in coping with HIV. Gender differences in coping are described in more detail in Chapter 4 in this book. As indicated above, there might also be both post-traumatic distress as well as stress-related personal growth.

Can stressors make people with HIV feel better?

The phenomenon of stress-related growth raises the provocative question of whether stressors can make people with HIV feel better. The link between self-efficacy and post-traumatic growth is further supported by a cross-sectional study among hurricane survivors living with HIV by Cieslak et al. (2009), which tested the model of Benight and Bandura (2004). The model postulates that post-traumatic recovery is directly mediated by perceived coping self-efficacy and indirectly by social support (Benight & Bandura, 2004). Among those with intense post-traumatic stress disorder, post-traumatic growth 14 months after the hurricane was associated with coping self-efficacy but not with social support. Self-efficacy influences whether people think pessimistically or optimistically and strengthens resiliency to adversity (Bandura, 2001). It is partly based on self-efficacious beliefs that people act in ways that are self-enhancing or self-hindering (Bandura, 2001).

To enhance self-efficacy, people do not work in social isolation, but rather in coordination with others (proxy and community agency) to secure what they cannot accomplish on their own (Bandura, 2001, 2003). Thus, turning to God/higher power or a successful role model (e.g., someone who is coping well with HIV) as a proxy agent may enhance self-efficacy (Bandura, 2003), paving the way to more effective coping and post-traumatic growth. Thus, current research indicates that enhancing self-efficacy, whether related to HIV or not, may actually enhance psychological well-being.

Spirituality, Health, and Well-Being in People with HIV

Spirituality is defined as a search for a connection with the sacred (Ironson, Kremer, & Ironson, 2006a; Pargament, 2006; Chapter 14 in this book). We purposely chose this definition of spirituality to be broad so that individuals would be able to frame spirituality within their own experience. Spirituality is not limited to religion or belief in a God/higher power, but can also include aspects of life perceived as sacred by the individual (Pargament, 2006). This shares similarities with religiousness; however, spirituality refers to the personal search for this connection, whereas religiousness involves that search within an institutional context (Ironson et al., 2006a). Given the stigma of HIV that is present in some religious institutions, people with HIV sometimes perceive a disconnection with religious institutions but still maintain a sense of their spirituality in coping with their disease (Ironson & Kremer, 2009; Kremer & Ironson, 2009; Kremer, Ironson, & Kaplan, 2009; Pargament et al., 2004). As we discuss below, spirituality and religiousness are important coping resources for people with HIV.

Importance of spirituality/religiousness in people with HIV

A nationally representative sample of 2,266 patients with HIV found that 85 percent reported that spirituality was "somewhat" or "very" important to them, and 65 percent was the comparable figure for religion (Lorenz et al., 2005). This is consistent with another sample of people with HIV, who reported being significantly more spiritual (mean of 6.97 on a scale of 1 to 10) than religious (mean of 4.30) (Ironson et al., 2006a). Groups that are more religious and/or spiritual include women, non-Caucasians, and older patients (Lorenz et al., 2005). African Americans view religion as extremely important, whereas gay men were less religious than African Americans but tend to see themselves as spiritual (Ridge, Williams, Anderson, & Elford, 2008).

Numerous studies have demonstrated that a large proportion of people with HIV use spirituality/religion to cope. In a national survey of people with HIV, 65 percent said they rely on spiritual or religious means when confronting problems. In another study of 450 people with HIV interviewed across four sites (Cotton et al., 2006), 23 percent of participants attended religious services weekly, and 32 percent engaged in prayer or meditation at least daily. Prayer was used as a self-care strategy to combat symptoms of fatigue, nausea, anxiety, and depression by over 50 percent of 448 HIV-positive African American respondents (Coleman et al., 2006) and was rated highly efficacious. Ironson et al. (Ironson, Stuetzle, & Fletcher, 2006c) found that 45 percent of people had increased spirituality/religiousness during the year after their diagnosis (compared to only 13 percent who decreased and 42 percent who remained the same). Similar figures were found by Cotton et al. (Cotton, Tsevat et al., 2006), with 41 percent becoming more spiritual after the diagnosis and 25 percent more religious. Surprisingly, about one third of a volunteer sample of people with HIV had had a profound enough change to be labeled as having had a spiritual transformation (preliminary analysis in Ironson et al., 2006a, complete analysis in Ironson and Kremer 2009). Given the stigma associated with HIV, and non-acceptance of gays in some churches, one of the tasks involved in using spirituality/religiousness to cope is finding an accepting supportive spiritual community. Cotton, Tsevat, et al. (2006) note that 1 in 4 participants felt more alienated by their church after the diagnosis, and 1 in 10 changed their place of worship.

Ways in which spirituality/religiousness can help or hinder coping

Two major ways in which spirituality/religiousness play a part in the management of HIV and its stressors are in influencing decision-making (72 percent) and in coping with problems (65 percent) (Lorenz et al., 2005). First, we will discuss its impact on coping with problems and then its influence on decision-making.

In the face of HIV, people often tap into spiritual resources. Pargament (1997; Pargament et al., 2004) suggests that religion contributes to the coping process by "shaping the character of life events, coping activities, and outcomes of events." Qualitative studies of people with HIV indicate that spirituality/religiousness gives them hope, gives meaning and purpose to life, makes them feel empowered (i.e., having guidance and support from a higher transcendent force), makes some feel more connected (to both a community and God/higher power), can bring a sense of peace, and finally can take them out of the realm of suffering through transcendence (Frankl, 1955, 1963; Ironson et al., 2006a; Ironson et al., 2002; McCormick, Holder, Wetsel, & Cawthon, 2001; Park & Folkman, 1997; Reed, 1987; Tarakeshwar, Khan, & Sikkema, 2006). A qualitative study of interviews of 40 women with HIV in Africa illustrates several of these outcomes (Maman, Cathcart, Burkhardt, Omba, & Behets, 2009): Women used prayer to help overcome the initial shock of diagnosis, turned to clergy to help them prepare for disclosure, conceptualized their infection as a path chosen by God, and turned to their faith for hope. Our research shows that spirituality/religiousness can be empowering: many of our sample (about one third) reported that having a feeling that a higher power is helping them can be instrumental in giving them the fortitude to get off drugs (Ironson et al., 2006a; Kremer & Ironson, 2009).

Spiritual framework, beliefs, and the appraisal process

The use of spiritual/religious cognitive coping strategies may also affect the appraisal process, both of the self (e.g., I can do this with God's help, God's help gives me more strength to deal with the stressor of HIV) and of the stressor (e.g., being chosen by God to get HIV for a special purpose, or as part of a divine plan). The stressor is therefore seen as less toxic and the self is seen as more capable of handling the stressor. Two opposite answers to the question of "Why me?" illustrate the effect of beliefs about HIV and God on behavior. Sarah (name changed) interpreted getting HIV as part of a divine plan. She felt that God was using her to help the HIV community, and her response was to establish a community center to help people with HIV. She said, "Volunteering in the HIV community gave me a sense God was using me" (Ironson et al., 2006a, pp. 246-7). On the other hand, Yvonne (name changed) felt God had cursed her: She was angry with God and with everybody. Because of this she did not disclose her HIV status and continued having unprotected sex (Ironson et al., 2006a, p. 247). Sarah's reframe turned the stressor of HIV into a way to find new meaning in her life, whereas Yvonne's belief made the stressor of HIV more toxic.

The perceived relationship with God has been noted by several authors to be a key factor in dealing with the stressors of living with HIV (Polzer Casarez & Miles, 2008; Tarakeshwar et al., 2006). The transition from a view of God who is punishing and judgmental to one who is loving and benevolent is an example of reframing that has an enormously positive impact on coping. As an example, Carlos (name changed) said, "I was on a downward spiral . . . I was at my worst . . . I felt I was being judged, that I was being punished . . . and the minister basically said, as an individual you don't have to believe in any God that doesn't love you or any God that isn't here to help you . . . When I heard that, [it] changed my God to one that was loving and helpful. It was revolutionary" (Ironson et al., 2006a, p. 249). Carlos noted this as the turning point that gave him the strength to go to Alcoholics Anonymous and become sober.

The belief that God gives one the strength to take action was reflected in other's stories (Ironson et al., 2006a, p. 251). Vanessa (name changed) had hit rock bottom, being HIV-positive and pregnant with her fourth child. Living as a prostitute in the streets and addicted to crack, she wanted to quit using drugs. She said, "Trying program after program, going to jail over and over, I knew there was no other way . . . I was way down in that hole. I didn't have any more options. At that moment, I looked up and told God 'I need you.' On the street, I started praying. 'God help me. I know this is not what you created me for'. I knew that I had to give my life to Christ if I wanted to stay clean." She walked over a mile to the addiction treatment center, noting "God gave me the strength and he gave me the courage to keep walking, and I am so grateful to God . . . from that moment on I believe in God in everything I say and do." Fifteen years later, she is a responsible mother of four and a grandmother, she is still clean, and her HIV infection remains asymptomatic with a CD4 cell count of 675. Vanessa's story reflects several themes that were present in many stories: asking God/higher power for help, surrendering to God/higher power, and perceiving strength from God/higher power.

The extra strength that one can garner for withstanding pain by enlisting the support of a higher power is also illustrated by a study by Wacholtz and Pargament (2005). Although this study was not done in people with HIV, the researchers found that people who meditated using a spiritual word were able to keep their hand in ice water longer than those meditating using a secular word.

Another cognition that could help strengthen one's self-perception is the often-expressed theme of being a vessel of God/higher power, or having a divine spirit within. This is often followed by a statement that the individuals feel they must therefore take care of themselves (e.g., The body is the temple of the soul and you need to keep the body in a condition so that you'll be able to use it; I know I have a higher power within myself that allows me to get up this morning and to be able to take my medication; God uses us to show his divine).

The above beliefs dovetail with a qualitative analysis of 38 African American mothers with HIV (Tarakeshwar et al., 2006). The study revealed two aspects of the perception of God relevant for coping: *God in control* and *God requires participation*. The *God in control* belief may make people feel they do not have to shoulder the entire burden themselves. The *God requires participation* belief was reflected in our examples as well. For example, people need to participate in taking medication. Another example is reflected in a woman who felt she got HIV because she was chosen for a higher purpose. She stated, "God uses us to show his divine. . . . I was chosen to help people see the way they look at the world . . . to learn to love myself, to love other people." This person subsequently started a community organization for people with HIV.

Thus, spiritual/religious beliefs can assist the coping process when they render the appraisal of the stressor to be less toxic and the appraisal of the self to be stronger, or at least to be the recipient of guidance and support.

Practical aspects: spirituality, decision-making, and health behaviors

Lorenz et al. (2005) noted that spirituality or religion was used by 72 percent of a sample of people with HIV when making decisions. In another study of 79 men and women with HIV (Kremer, Ironson, & Porr, 2009), participants believing that health is controlled by God or a higher power were 4.75 times more likely to refuse ART compared to those not sharing this control belief. Participants believing that spirituality helps them to cope with the side effects reported significantly better adherence and fewer symptoms. One of our study participants described eloquently how spirituality helped concretely to cope with the daily challenge of adherence: "Every day God gives me is a gift, so I take my medicines because I need to honor life."

Ironson et al. (2006c) found that an increase in spirituality following HIV diagnosis was associated

with practicing safer sex and consuming less alcohol and fewer cigarettes. Simoni et al. (2006) showed a relationship between greater spirituality and better self-reported medication adherence at three months and higher viral load suppression at six months. Similarly, forgiveness has been associated with better medication adherence and safer sex (Temoshok & Wald, 2006). Our own qualitative study demonstrated the diverse ways in which spirituality affects medication-taking. It may enhance the commitment to adhere to medications: "I strongly believe that not taking medication is a sin." Conversely, it may also lead to the rejection of ART: "I do not have faith in medicine. I put my hands in God." (Kremer et al., 2006). Moreover, spirituality and worldview were considered by 58 percent of participants in their decision to take or not to take ART (Kremer et al., 2006). Furthermore, spirituality/religiosity may facilitate positive reappraisals of stressful situations, which in turn may support positive psychological states (Folkman, 1997).

Spiritual/religious practices are another mechanism for coping and have even been used to cope with side effects of ART (Kremer, Ironson, & Porr, 2009). McCormick et al. (2001) suggests that those practices can be either primarily religious (e.g., worshiping, reading religious materials, practicing forgiveness, connecting to God/higher power) or primarily existential (e.g., meditation, imagery, visualization).

In summary, spiritual coping gives one more options and choices about how to see and deal with stressful situations. Figure 15.2 summarizes the ways that spirituality may help coping, which have been noted in the past three sections.

Spirituality and physical health

Several longitudinal studies have examined the connection between spirituality and physical health in people with HIV (Table 15.5). Fitzpatrick et al. (2007) found that use of spiritual therapies (e.g., prayer, meditation, affirmations, visualizations) was associated with a reduced mortality over one year, but only in people not taking effective ART. Our group found a slower decline in CD4 cell counts and better control of viral load over four years among people with HIV who became more spiritual after their diagnosis (Ironson et al., 2006c). Furthermore, survival over three to five years was 5.35 times more likely for those who had a spiritual transformation (Ironson & Kremer, 2009). In addition, the spiritual belief that "God is merciful" was protective of health over four years, whereas the belief that "God is judgmental and punishing and is going to judge them

1. **May provide hope by fostering a belief in a power greater than oneself**
   - Makes one feel empowered and guided by a transcendent force
   - Provides a source of strength one can rely upon

2. **Can promote more positive appraisals**
   - Appraisal of the stressor to be less toxic: "*Being chosen by God to get HIV as part of a divine plan.*"
   - Appraisal of self to be stronger or as the recipient of guidance & support: "*I can do this with God's help.*"

3. **May enable a feeling of well-being, peace, and safety in the face of major challenges and uncertainties**
   - Helps one feel calm
   - Gives one a sense that everything will be all right

4. **May provide a feeling that one has support and guidance and is not alone**
   - Being connected to a higher power: "*God is with you always.*"
   - Provides for social support through a spiritual/religious community

5. **Potentially engenders a greater respect for one's body**
   - Belief that one's body is "*a gift from God*" may enhance adherence and good health practices, safer sex, and less drug and alcohol use.
   - A belief that the "*body is the temple of the soul*" may enhance the desire to take better care of one's health.

6. **May take one out of the realm of suffering via transcendence**
   - Enhances a transcendent perspective, which takes one out of the immediate stressful situation
   - Allows one to rise above things so one doesn't feel victimized by one's situation

7. **May help one make meaning**
   - Gives meaning and purpose to life
   - Helps one search for the higher good in difficult situations
   - Fosters reframing: "*Maybe this happened for a higher reason/purpose.*"

8. **May activate surrendering to God/higher power**
   - One does not have to shoulder the burden all by him/herself.

In summary, spiritual coping may provide additional options and choices about how to see and deal with stressful situations.

[1]Notably, spirituality may not only help but may also hinder one to cope in the presence of spiritual struggle.

Fig. 15.2 Spirituality: How it may help one to cope.[1]

harshly someday" was associated with faster deterioration of the CD4 cell count and poorer viral load control (Ironson, Stuezle, Fletcher, & Ironson, 2006b). Consistent with this was another recent study relating higher levels of religious struggle to faster disease progression in HIV over 12 to 18 months (Trevino et al., 2010).Thus, depending on the spiritual/religious belief, one's view of God may be either helpful or harmful.

Spirituality and psychological health

In general, higher spirituality/religiousness is related to lower distress and better mental health (Koenig, 2007, 2009). A number of studies have shown that spirituality/religiousness in HIV is also associated with less distress and lower depression.

Simoni and Ortiz (2003) found that 66 percent of 142 HIV-positive Puerto Rican women scored above the conventional threshold for depression. Spirituality was high in this sample, and those higher in spirituality had significantly lower depressive symptoms on the Center for Epidemiologic Studies Depression Scale (CES-D). A multicenter sample of 450 individuals with HIV revealed that 53 percent had depressive symptoms (CES-D >10) (Yi et al., 2006). Lower spiritual well-being was significantly associated with greater depressive symptoms (however, personal religiosity and having a religious affiliation were

Table 15.5   Studies of spirituality predicting HIV disease progression

Study	Psychological Predictors[1]	Design	Results
Fitzpatrick et al., 2007; conducted 1995–99	Use of spiritual therapies (e.g., prayer, meditation, affirmations, visualizations) (*questionnaire*)	*n* = 901, 75% men, 66% White; 47% AIDS symptoms; 1-year follow-up	Use of spiritual therapies predicted lower mortality, but only in those not taking ART[2]
Ironson et al., 2006c; conducted 1997–2004	Increase in spirituality/ religiousness after HIV diagnosis (*INCRS*); positive & negative view of God (*View of God Scale*)	*n* = 100, 64% men, 38% African American; 150–500 CD4 cells, no AIDS symptoms, 79% using ART[2]; 4-year follow-up	Greater INCRS & positive view of God predicted less CD4 decline & better viral load control; negative view of God predicted the opposite
Ironson & Kremer, 2009; conducted 2002–2007	Spiritual transformation (*interview rating*)	*n* = 147, 60% men, 48% African American; any disease stage; 90% using ART[2]; 5-year follow-up	Spiritual transformation predicted less CD4 decline, better viral load control & survival
Trevino et al., 2010; conducted 2002–05	Positive religious coping & spiritual struggle (*Brief RCOPE*)	*n* = 329, 86% men, 53% African American, all HIV/ AIDS stages; 18 months of follow-up	Only spiritual struggle predicted log CD4 decline, but not undetectable viral load

[1] *measurement in italics*
[2] After 1996, antiretroviral therapy (ART) consisted of effective combination therapy. Prior to that only less effective monotherapy (e.g., azidothymidine [AZT]) was used.

not after controlling for other factors). Phillips and Sowell (2000) examined which coping strategies were used to maintain a sense of hope for the future, even in the face of illness, economic stress, and racial stigma, by HIV-positive African American women of reproductive age. Among other results, they found that engagement in spiritual activities was significantly correlated ($r = .40$) with the maintenance of hope. Engaging in spiritual activities also moderated the relationship between HIV-related stressors (functional impairment, work impairment, and HIV-related symptoms) and emotional distress in another sample of HIV-positive women (Sowell et al., 2000).

In another study of 308 African American women recruited from clinics across the Southeast where measures were taken on quality of life, depression, coping, and spirituality, spirituality accounted for a significant proportion of variance in reducing depressive symptoms after accounting for demographic variables and other psychosocial factors (Braxton, Lang, Sales, Wingood, & DiClemente, 2007; Perez et al., 2009). In a cross-sectional study of 279 people with HIV, spirituality/religiousness was significantly associated with lower depression ($r = -.29$) (Ironson et al., 2002). In a smaller sample of 52 HIV-positive men, the Existential Well Being subscale of the Spiritual Well Being scale was sig-

nificantly associated with lower perceived stress, distress, uncertainty, higher quality of life, social support, and use of effective coping strategies (Tuck, McCain, & Elswick, 2001). Another study found the Existential Well Being Scale, which the study's authors interpret as a measure of meaning and purpose, was significantly related to psychological well-being in 117 African American men and women (74 percent were HIV-positive), and did so more than religious well-being (Coleman & Holzemer, 1999).

Adding to evidence on the positive side is a study by Cotton et al. (2006), who interviewed 450 patients with HIV from four clinical sites. Patients who were more spiritual/religious had greater optimism, self-esteem, and life satisfaction and consumed less alcohol. A number of studies support the notion that spirituality can be an instrument to finding meaning and purpose in living with HIV, which can be a bridge to benefit-finding and a better quality of life (Barroso, 1999; Barroso & Powell-Cope, 2000; Fryback & Reinert, 1999; Hall, 1998; Ironson et al., 2002, 2006a; Kremer & Ironson, 2009; Siegel & Schrimshaw, 2000; Tarakeshwar et al., 2006). Turning to spirituality after the HIV diagnosis was associated with perceiving HIV as the most positive turning point in one's life (Kremer, Ironson, & Kaplan, 2009). Finally, in a study of

80 HIV-positive women, Gray and Cason (2002) found that mastery over stress was predicted by social support and holding a spiritual perspective. Thus, spirituality has been associated with both better psychological well-being and a feeling of mastery over stress.

Preliminary research on spiritually oriented interventions in HIV

A few studies have examined translating findings on spirituality and health in HIV into interventions. In addition to studies looking at associations of spiritual practices such as prayer and attending church (Ironson et al., 2006c) various spiritually oriented practices have been tested in the context of randomized trials in HIV. Bormann et al. (2006) compared the efficacy of distress reduction in people with HIV between two groups, a mantram (a spiritually oriented word or phrase) repetition group and an attention control group. The mantram group had significant reductions in trait anger and increases in spiritual faith. Qualitative analysis suggested using a mantram was especially helpful with managing uncontrollable stressors. One mechanism for the reduction in anger was an increase in positive reappraisal coping (Bormann & Carrico, 2009). The authors suggest that use of a mantram may replace anger with responding in a nonjudgmental, more accepting manner. Another intervention tested spiritual growth groups (McCain et al., 2008; Tuck, 2004).These groups facilitated three aspects of personal exploration of spirituality: (1) an experiential component of interconnecting one's spirit with self, others, nature, God, or a higher power; (2) an intellectual component of knowing or apprehending spirituality; and (3) a process of weekly journal entries to facilitate increased awareness of and integration of spirituality into daily life. The spiritual growth group had increased quality of life scores, increases in spiritual perspective, and a decrease in perceived stress from before to after the intervention (Tuck, 2004). Another investigative team pilot tested a spiritual coping group (Tarakeshwar, Pearce, & Sikkema, 2005). Their intervention incorporated Lazarus and Folkman's (1984) stress and coping paradigm and Pargament's (1997) framework of religious coping. It focused on how their spirituality helped (or hindered) coping with HIV. It included both positive aspects of spirituality, such as a secure relationship with God and a larger, benevolent purpose to life, and the spiritual struggles that people face (see Pargament, Koenig, Tarakeshwar, & Hahn, 2004), such as feelings of disconnection from church/religious community and feelings of stigma, guilt, and shame. Pargament et al.'s (2004) Lighting the Way intervention included such themes as body and spirit, control and surrender, letting go of anger, shame and guilt, isolation and intimacy, and hopes and dreams. Thus, good preliminary work has been done to identify themes that could be addressed both in spiritually oriented coping interventions and in interacting with patients.

Limitations

While we were able to restrict our review of the relationship between coping (and spiritual coping) and health to longitudinal studies, because there were fewer longitudinal studies on coping (and spiritual coping) and psychological well-being, our review of that literature included predominantly cross-sectional studies. Some caveats with predominantly cross-sectional research should therefore be kept in mind. We illustrate these points in the context of using spirituality/religiousness to cope. Neither the time course (which comes first, spirituality/religiousness or distress?) nor the direction is clear. While spirituality/religiousness could lead to reduced distress, it is also plausible that when people are distressed they turn to religion to cope. For example, Richards and Folkman (1997) showed that those reporting spiritual phenomena were showing higher levels of depression and anxiety and more physical health symptoms. On the other hand, they also had more adaptive coping and found spirituality/religiousness to be a source of solace and meaning. Longitudinal studies may help to clarify this.

Another caveat of the research on spirituality and psychological well-being, as Koenig (2008) notes, is that measures of spirituality and mental health are often confounded. For example, one widely used scale, the spiritual well-being scale, includes several items that measure psychological well-being. Thus, it is important to know the specifics of the measures in a study when interpreting the results.

With respect to studies on general coping, a limitation of the above studies is that none looked at avoidance in relation to time since diagnosis, and it may be that avoidance is beneficial when the shock of the diagnosis is overwhelming (as long as people get the medical care they need). Although not done in HIV, in a meta-analysis of coping strategies, Suls and Fletcher (1985) found that avoidance was associated with more positive adaptation in the short run (e.g., during the first couple of weeks after the diagnosis), but more active attention-oriented strategies were better in the long run after this initial period. Furthermore, most studies also do not separate out denial from behavioral disengagement. One might hypothesize that denial is not that bad if it protects one from failing to function and get proper medical attention and that behavioral disengagement might be more detrimental.

Summary and Clinical Conclusions

Although HIV has turned into a chronic medically manageable disease, people living with HIV still face a multitude of stressors, whether related to HIV or not. The way people cope with those stressors remains an important determinant of health and psychological well-being, even in the effective ART era. Importantly, there are ways to cope effectively with these stressors. Specifically, evidence indicates that finding meaning, positive reappraisal, and active coping are particularly protective of both physical and psychological health. Even if someone is initially not coping well, coping is amenable to change.

Coping and health

Our knowledge of the relationship between coping and health is based on longitudinal studies with reliable biological markers (CD4 cell count and viral load). There is fairly strong support for the notion that avoidant coping predicts faster disease progression, even when taking ART and adherence into account. Specific approach-oriented strategies that predicted better health before effective ART became available included maintaining a fighting spirit, active coping, planful problem-solving, positive reappraisal, accepting responsibility, and acceptance coping. However, too few studies have been done since 1996, when effective ART became available, thus facilitating more valid conclusions in research. Nevertheless, proactive behavior, optimism, and finding meaning are promising factors in protecting health in HIV above and beyond medication. The evidence on social support is mixed, but it appears to be especially helpful as HIV disease progresses. Finally, it also appears that venting may be detrimental, expressing emotions is protective, depth processing is more protective, and processing toward meaning may be most protective of health in HIV.

Coping and psychological well-being

The present research on coping and psychological well-being has focused mainly on cognitive coping approaches, in particular finding meaning and positive reappraisal. In the broad picture, direct action, which is a combination of active and problem-solving coping, and positive reappraisal were the most effective approach coping strategies associated with psychological well-being. However, we do not know much about what works best in the long run, since these findings are based primarily on cross-sectional studies. There are indications in the current research that stressors can make people with HIV feel even better depending on the perceived self-efficacy. Self-efficacy, the belief in one's ability to control the stressor, may determine whether a person perceives a trauma as a stressor or as chance to grow.

Spiritual coping

Two major ways in which spirituality/religiousness plays a part in the management of HIV and its stressors are in influencing the decision to take medications and in coping with problems. Regarding decision-making about HIV treatment, spirituality may enhance the commitment to adhere to ART, although it may conversely lead to the rejection of ART. With respect to coping with stressors, there are several ways in which spirituality/religiousness can help one cope: meaning-making, appraisal of the stressor to be less toxic, appraisal of the self to be stronger, the feeling that one has support and guidance and is not alone, and elicitation of a calming response with a sense of peace and well-being. A perceived positive relationship with God or a higher power can be a key factor in dealing with the stresses of HIV. In terms of health, research shows that an increase in spirituality after HIV diagnosis, a positive view of God, the occurrence of spiritual transformation, and the absence of a religious struggle may be protective of health.

Suggestions for health care workers

Since it appears that coping predicts health and psychological well-being, health care workers need to engage patients in a discussion about how they are coping with HIV and life stressors and how useful their coping strategies are for them. Health care workers should pay attention to spiritual coping as well, especially since it can be a path to growth as well as a cause of struggle. Potentially helpful strategies include seeing the positive potential of people, keeping communication open by holding a nonjudgmental attitude, and connecting people to appropriate resources. Encouraging coping methods such as positive reframing/reappraisal, problem-solving, active coping, proactive behavior, spiritual coping, fighting spirit, acceptance, finding meaning, emotional expression, and social support (especially when disease progresses) may foster effective coping. Research shows that these coping strategies may preserve the health and psychological well-being of people with HIV.

Health care workers should help guide patients to find their best ways to relax and calm down, including the use of spirituality when appropriate. To assist the patient to find coping mechanisms that work for him or her, barriers to successful coping should also be assessed and addressed.

In addition, coping is a dynamic process. Even patients who are not initially coping well can learn to adapt well in the long run after getting through the initial shock; they may even transform the trauma of being diagnosed with HIV into a path to personal growth. What seems maladaptive today may eventually become a path to a profound spiritual transformation, as in the cases of Grace and Vanessa who hit rock bottom with drugs.

Health care workers can play a key role in enhancing their patients' self-efficacy and strengthening their belief in their personal control. Ways of enhancing self-efficacy include teaching patients skills such as positive reframing and, in accordance with Bandura's social cognition theory, providing patients with positive role models. For example, bringing people like Grace and Valery together—two women who share similar problems but display markedly different coping styles—may pave the way for teaching and learning by modeling. People who have learned to cope well can serve as role models of coping attitudes and skills and can motivate others to do better by showing that their difficulties are surmountable by positive attitudes and perseverance. Another way might be to help patients discern changeable from unchangeable stressors and changeable from unchangeable aspects of the self, and to explore the resources individuals have and the resources they need.

Suggestions from the functional components approach to stress and coping

The functional components approach to stress and coping (see Fig. 15.1) extends the Folkman and Chesney (Folkman et al., 1991) clinical approach to stress and coping (which focuses on examining the changeable and unchangeable aspects of the stressor and matching problem-focused coping strategies with changeable and emotion-focused strategies with unchangeable stressors). The functional components approach adds an emphasis on the self and the reaction of the self to the stressor in addition to a focus on the stressor. This is reflected in a six-step functional system approach to stress and coping and involves asking key clinical questions regarding the appraisal and reappraisal of the toxicity of the stressor, the ability of a person to cope, and the individual's reaction. The clinician helps people work through changeable and unchangeable aspects of the stressor, the self, and reaction by using various coping methods, including problem-solving, emotion-focused, cognitively based, behavioral-based, and spiritually based coping strategies.

Acknowledgements

The authors acknowledge the support of the Templeton Foundation (Grant 14536, Ironson, PI) and the NIMH (NIMH R01MH53791 & R01MH066697, Ironson, PI). The opinions expressed herein are those of the authors and do not necessarily reflect the views of the John Templeton foundation or the NIMH. We are especially grateful for the commitment of the study participants in the longitudinal study, the chief clinical interviewer Annie George, and Project Director Elizabeth Balbin. Finally, we thank our editors (Karen Culver, Dale Ironson, Hod Tamir) and students (Stefanie Altmann, Tony Guerra, Erin Kelly, Andrew Melis, Marietta Suarez) for their critical comments.

References

Alter, G., & Altfeld, M. (2006). NK cell function in HIV-1 infection. *Current Molecular Medicine, 6*(6), 621–9.

Antoni, M. H., Baggett, L., Ironson, G., LaPerriere, A., August, S., Klimas, N., et al. (1991). Cognitive-behavioral stress management intervention buffers distress responses and immunologic changes following notification of HIV-1 seropositivity. *Journal of Consulting and Clinical Psychology, 59*(6), 906-15.

Antoni, M. H., Goldstein, D., Ironson, G., LaPerriere, A., Fletcher, M. A., & Schneiderman, N. (1995). Coping responses to HIV-1 serostatus notification predict concurrent and prospective immunologic status. *Clinical Psychology & Psychotherapy, 2*(4), 234–48.

Ashton, E., Vosvick, M., Chesney, M., Gore-Felton, C., Koopman, C., O'Shea, K., et al. (2005). Social support and maladaptive coping as predictors of the change in physical health symptoms among persons living with HIV/AIDS. *AIDS Patient Care and STDs, 19*(9), 587–98.

Bandura, A. (1997). *Self-efficacy: The exercise of control.* New York: Freeman.

Bandura, A. (2001). Social cognitive theory: An agentic perspective. *Annual Review of Psychology, 52*, 1–26.

Bandura, A. (2002). Special section on factors influencing national development and transformation: Indigenous, psychological, and cultural analysis-social cognitive theory in cultural context. *Applied Psychology, 51*(2), 269–90.

Bandura, A. (2003). On the psychosocial impact and mechanisms of spiritual modeling. *International Journal for the Psychology of Religion, 13*(3), 167–73.

Barroso, J. (1997). Social support and long-term survivors of AIDS. *Western Journal of Nursing Research, 19*(5), 554–82.

Barroso, J. (1999). Long-term nonprogressors with HIV disease. *Nursing Research, 48*(5), 242–9.

Barroso, J., & Powell-Cope, G. M. (2000). Metasynthesis of qualitative research on living with HIV infection. *Qualitative Health Research, 10*(3), 340–53.

Benight, C. C., & Bandura, A. (2004). Social cognitive theory of posttraumatic recovery: The role of perceived self-efficacy. *Behaviour Research and Therapy, 42*(10), 1129–48.

Bhaskaran, K., Hamouda, O., Sannes, M., Boufassa, F., Johnson, A. M., Lambert, P. C., et al. (2008). Changes in the risk of death after HIV seroconversion compared with mortality in the general population. *Journal of the American Medical Association, 300*(1), 51–9.

Billings, D. W., Folkman, S., Acree, M., & Moskowitz, J. T. (2000). Coping and physical health during caregiving: The roles of positive and negative affect. *Journal of Personality and Social Psychology, 79*(1), 131–42.

Blomkvist, V., Theorell, T., Jonsson, H., Schulman, S., Berntorp, E., & Stiegendal, L. (1994). Psychosocial self-prognosis in relation to mortality and morbidity in hemophiliacs with HIV infection. *Psychotherapy and Psychosomatics, 62*(3-4), 185–92.

Bormann, J. E., & Carrico, A. W. (2009). Increases in positive reappraisal coping during a group-based mantram intervention mediate sustained reductions in anger in HIV-positive persons. *International Journal of Behavioral Medicine, 16*(1), 74–80.

Bormann, J. E., Gifford, A. L., Shively, M., Smith, T. L., Redwine, L., Kelly, A., et al. (2006). Effects of spiritual mantram repetition on HIV outcomes: A randomized controlled trial. *Journal of Behavioral Medicine, 29*(4), 359–76.

Bower, J. E., Kemeny, M. E., Taylor, S. E., & Fahey, J. L. (1998). Cognitive processing, discovery of meaning, CD4 decline, and AIDS-related mortality among bereaved HIV-seropositive men. *Journal of Consulting and Clinical Psychology, 66*(6), 979–86.

Braithwaite, R. S., Justice, A. C., Chang, C. C., Fusco, J. S., Raffanti, S. R., Wong, J. B., et al. (2005). Estimating the proportion of patients infected with HIV who will die of comorbid diseases. *American Journal of Medicine, 118*(8), 890–8.

Braxton, N. D., Lang, D. L., M Sales, J., Wingood, G. M., & DiClemente, R. J. (2007). The role of spirituality in sustaining the psychological well-being of HIV-positive black women. *Women & Health, 46*(2-3), 113–29.

Burns, M. J., Feaster, D. J., Mitrani, V. B., Ow, C., & Szapocznik, J. (2008). Stress processes in HIV-positive African American mothers: Moderating effects of drug abuse history. *Anxiety, Stress, and Coping, 21*(1), 95–116.

Cacioppo, J. T., Hawkley, L. C., & Berntson, G. G. (2003). The anatomy of loneliness. *Current Directions in Psychological Science, 12*, 71–4.

Cacioppo, J. T., Hawkley, L. C., & Rickett, E. M. (2005). Sociality, spirituality, and meaning making: Chicago health, aging, and social relations study. *Rev Gen Psychol, 9*, 143–55.

Carver, C. S. (1997). You want to measure coping but your protocol's too long: Consider the brief COPE. *International Journal of Behavioral Medicine, 4*(1), 92–100.

Carver, C. S., Scheier, M. F., & Weintraub, J. K. (1989). Assessing coping strategies: A theoretically based approach. *Journal of Personality and Social Psychology, 56*(2), 267–83.

Cieslak, R., Benight, C., Schmidt, N., Luszczynska, A., Curtin, E., Clark, R. A., et al. (2009). Predicting posttraumatic growth among hurricane Katrina survivors living with HIV: The role of self-efficacy, social support, and PTSD symptoms. *Anxiety, Stress, and Coping*, epub ahead of print Mar 18, 1–14.

Coan, J. A., Schaefer, H. S., & Davidson, R. J. (2006). Lending a hand: Social regulation of the neural response to threat. *Psychological Science: A Journal of the American Psychological Society, 17*(12), 1032–9.

Cole, S. W. (2008). Psychosocial influences on HIV-1 disease progression: Neural, endocrine, and virologic mechanisms. *Psychosomatic Medicine, 70*(5), 562–8.

Cole, S. W., Kemeny, M. E., Taylor, S. E., Visscher, B. R., & Fahey, J. L. (1996). Accelerated course of human immunodeficiency virus infection in gay men who conceal their homosexual identity. *Psychosomatic Medicine, 58*(3), 219–31.

Cole, S. W., Korin, Y. D., Fahey, J. L., & Zack, J. A. (1998). Norepinephrine accelerates HIV replication via protein kinase A-dependent effects on cytokine production. *Journal of Immunology 161*(2), 610–6.

Coleman, C. L., & Holzemer, W. L. (1999). Spirituality, psychological well-being, and HIV symptoms for African Americans living with HIV disease. *Journal of the Association of Nurses in AIDS Care, 10*(1), 42–50.

Coleman, C. L., Holzemer, W. L., Eller, L. S., Corless, I., Reynolds, N., Nokes, K. M., et al. (2006). Gender differences in use of prayer as a self-care strategy for managing symptoms in African Americans living with HIV/AIDS. *Journal of the Association of Nurses in AIDS Care, 17*(4), 16–23.

Cotton, S., Puchalski, C. M., Sherman, S. N., Mrus, J. M., Peterman, A. H., Feinberg, J., et al. (2006). Spirituality and religion in patients with HIV/AIDS. *Journal of General Internal Medicine, 21 Suppl 5*, S5–S13.

Cotton, S., Tsevat, J., Szaflarski, M., Kudel, I., Sherman, S. N., Feinberg, J., et al. (2006). Changes in religiousness and spirituality attributed to HIV/AIDS: Are there sex and race differences? *Journal of General Internal Medicine, 21 Suppl 5*, S14–20.

Eich-Hochli, E., Niklowitz, M. W., Luthy, R., & Opravil, M. (1997). Are immunological markers, social and personal resources, or a complaint-free state predictors of progression among HIV-infected patients? *Acta Psychiatrica Scandinavica, 95*(6), 476–84.

Farber, E. W., Mirsalimi, H., Williams, K. A., & McDaniel, J. S. (2003). Meaning of illness and psychological adjustment to HIV/AIDS. *Psychosomatics, 44*(6), 485–91.

Fitzpatrick, A. L., Standish, L. J., Berger, J., Kim, J. G., Calabrese, C., & Polissar, N. (2007). Survival in HIV-1-positve adults practicing psychological or spiritual activities for one year. *Alternative Therapies in Health and Medicine, 13*(5), 18–24.

Fleishman, J. A., Sherbourne, C. D., Cleary, P. D., Wu, A. W., Crystal, S., & Hays, R. D. (2003). Patterns of coping among persons with HIV infection: Configurations, correlates, and change. *American Journal of Community Psychology, 32*(1-2), 187–204.

Folkman, S. (1997). Positive psychological states and coping with severe stress. *Social Science & Medicine (1982), 45*(8), 1207–21.

Folkman, S., Chesney, M., McKusick, L., Ironson, G., Johnson, D., & Coates, T. (Eds.). (1991). *Translating coping theory into intervention*. New York: Plenum.

Folkman, S., & Lazarus, R. S. (1988). *Ways of coping questionnaire*. Palo Alto, CA: Consulting Psychologists Press.

Frankl, V. (1955). *The doctor and the soul*. New York: Knopf.

Frankl, V. (1963). *Man's search for meaning*. Boston: Beacon.

Fryback, P. B., & Reinert, B. R. (1999). Spirituality and people with potentially fatal diagnoses. *Nursing Forum, 34*(1), 13–22.

Garcia de Olalla, P., Knobel, H., Carmona, A., Guelar, A., Lopez-Colomes, J. L., & Cayla, J. A. (2002). Impact of adherence and highly active antiretroviral therapy on survival in HIV-infected patients. *Journal of Acquired Immune Deficiency Syndromes, 30*(1), 105–10.

Gonzalez, J. S., Penedo, F. J., Antoni, M. H., Duran, R. E., McPherson-Baker, S., Ironson, G., et al. (2004). Social support, positive states of mind, and HIV treatment adherence in men and women living with HIV/AIDS. *Health Psychology, 23*(4), 413–8.

Goodkin, K., Blaney, N. T., Feaster, D., Fletcher, M. A., Baum, M. K., Mantero-Atienza, E., et al. (1992). Active coping style is associated with natural killer cell cytotoxicity in asymptomatic HIV-1 seropositive homosexual men. *Journal of Psychosomatic Research, 36*(7), 635–50.

Gore-Felton, C., Koopman, C., Spiegel, D., Vosvick, M., Brondino, M., & Winningham, A. (2006). Effects of quality of life and coping on depression among adults living with HIV/AIDS. *Journal of Health Psychology, 11*(5), 711–29.

Gray, J., & Cason, C. L. (2002). Mastery over stress among women with HIV/AIDS. *Journal of the Association of Nurses in AIDS Care, 13*(4), 43–51.

Hall, B. A. (1998). Patterns of spirituality in persons with advanced HIV disease. *Research in Nursing & Health, 21*(2), 143–53.

Ickovics, J. R., Milan, S., Boland, R., Schoenbaum, E., Schuman, P., Vlahov, D., et al. (2006). Psychological resources protect health: 5-year survival and immune function among HIV-infected women from four US cities. *AIDS, 20*(14), 1851–60.

Imamichi, T., Conrads, T. P., Zhou, M., Liu, Y., Adelsberger, J. W., Veenstra, T. D., et al. (2005). A transcription inhibitor, actinomycin D, enhances HIV-1 replication through an interleukin-6-dependent pathway. *Journal of Acquired Immune Deficiency Syndromes 40*(4), 388–97.

Ironson, G. (2007). Altruism and health in HIV. In S. G. Post (Ed.), *Altruism and health* (pp. 70–81). New York: Oxford University Press.

Ironson, G., Balbin, E., Solomon, G., Fahey, J., Klimas, N., Schneiderman, N., et al. (2001). Relative preservation of natural killer cell cytotoxicity and number in healthy AIDS patients with low CD4 cell counts. *AIDS, 15*(16), 2065–73.

Ironson, G., Balbin, E., Stieren, E., Detz, K., Fletcher, M. A., Schneiderman, N., et al. (2008). Perceived stress and norepinephrine predict the effectiveness of response to protease inhibitors in HIV. *International Journal of Behavioral Medicine, 15*(3), 221–6.

Ironson, G., Balbin, E., Stuetzle, R., Fletcher, M. A., O'Cleirigh, C., Laurenceau, J. P., et al. (2005a). Dispositional optimism and the mechanisms by which it predicts slower disease progression in HIV: Proactive behavior, avoidant coping, and depression. *International Journal of Behavioral Medicine, 12*(2), 86–97.

Ironson, G., Field, T., Scafidi, F., Hashimoto, M., Kumar, M., Kumar, A., et al. (1996). Massage therapy is associated with enhancement of the immune system's cytotoxic capacity. *International Journal of Neuroscience, 84*(1-4), 205–17.

Ironson, G., Friedman, A., Klimas, N., Antoni, M., Fletcher, M. A., Laperriere, A., et al. (1994). Distress, denial, and low adherence to behavioral interventions predict faster disease progression in gay men infected with human immunodeficiency virus. *International Journal of Behavioral Medicine, 1*(1), 90–105.

Ironson, G., & Kremer, H. (2009). Spiritual transformation, psychological well-being, health, and survival in people with HIV. *International Journal of Psychiatry in Medicine, 32*(3), 263–281.

Ironson, G., Kremer, H., & Ironson, D. (2006a). Spirituality, spiritual experiences, and spiritual transformations in the face of HIV. In J. D. Koss & P. Hefner (Eds.), *Spiritual transformation and healing: Anthropological, theological, neuroscientific, and clinical perspectives* (1st ed., pp. 241–62). Lanham, MD: AltaMira Press.

Ironson, G., Leserman, J., O'Cleirigh, C., & Fordiani, J. (2009). Gender differences: Trauma writing in individuals with PTSD symptoms and HIV [abstract]. *Psychosomatic Medicine*.

Ironson, G., O'Cleirigh, C., Fletcher, M. A., Laurenceau, J. P., Balbin, E., Klimas, N., et al. (2005b). Psychosocial factors predict CD4 and viral load change in men and women with human immunodeficiency virus in the era of highly active antiretroviral treatment. *Psychosomatic Medicine, 67*(6), 1013–21.

Ironson, G., Solomon, G. F., Balbin, E. G., O'Cleirigh, C., George, A., Kumar, M., et al. (2002). The Ironson-Woods Spirituality/Religiousness index is associated with long survival, health behaviors, less distress, and low cortisol in people with HIV/AIDS. *Annals of Behavioral Medicine, 24*(1), 34–48.

Ironson, G., Stuetzle, R., Fletcher, M. A., & Ironson, D. (2006b). View of god is associated with disease progression in HIV. *Annals of Behavioral Medicine, 31 (Suppl.)* S074(abstract).

Ironson, G., Stuetzle, R., & Fletcher, M. A. (2006c). An increase in religiousness/spirituality occurs after HIV diagnosis and predicts slower disease progression over 4 years in people with HIV. *Journal of General Internal Medicine, 21 Suppl 5*, S62–8.

Ironson, G., Weiss, S., Lydston, D., Ishii, M., Jones, D., Asthana, D., et al. (2005c). The impact of improved self-efficacy on HIV viral load and distress in culturally diverse women living with AIDS: The SMART/EST women's project. *AIDS Care, 17*(2), 222–36.

Ironson, G. H., O'Cleirigh, C., Weiss, A., Schneiderman, N., & Costa, P. T., Jr. (2008). Personality and HIV disease progression: Role of NEO-PI-R openness, extraversion, and profiles of engagement. *Psychosomatic Medicine, 70*(2), 245–53.

Koenig, H. G. (2007). Religion and depression in older medical inpatients. *American Journal of Geriatric Psychiatry, 15*(4), 282–91.

Koenig, H. G. (2008). Concerns about measuring "spirituality" in research. *Journal of Nervous and Mental Disease, 196*(5), 349–55.

Koenig, H. G. (2009). Research on religion, spirituality, and mental health: A review. *Canadian Journal of Psychiatry. Revue Canadienne De Psychiatrie, 54*(5), 283–91.

Kraaij, V., Garnefski, N., Schroevers, M. J., van der Veek, S. M., Witlox, R., & Maes, S. (2008). Cognitive coping, goal self-efficacy and personal growth in HIV-infected men who have sex with men. *Patient Education and Counseling, 72*(2), 301–4.

Kraaij, V., van der Veek, S. M., Garnefski, N., Schroevers, M., Witlox, R., & Maes, S. (2008). Coping, goal adjustment, and psychological well-being in HIV-infected men who have sex with men. *AIDS Patient Care and STDs, 22*(5), 395–402.

Kremer, H., & Ironson, G. (2009). Everything changed: Spiritual transformation in people with HIV. *International Journal of Psychiatry in Medicine, 32*(3), 243–63.

Kremer, H., Ironson, G., & Kaplan, L. (2009). The fork in the road: HIV as a potential positive turning point and the role of spirituality. *AIDS Care, 21*(3), 368–77.

Kremer, H., Ironson, G., & Porr, M. (2009). Spiritual and mind-body beliefs as barriers and motivators to HIV-treatment decision-making and medication adherence? A qualitative study. *AIDS Patient Care and STDs, 21*(3), 368–77.

Kremer, H., Ironson, G., Schneiderman, N., & Hautzinger, M. (2006). To take or not to take: Decision-making about anti-retroviral treatment in people living with HIV/AIDS. *AIDS Patient Care and STDs, 20*(5), 335–49.

LaPerriere, A., Ironson, G., Antoni, M. H., Schneiderman, N., Klimas, N., & Fletcher, M. A. (1994). Exercise and psychoneuroimmunology. *Medicine and Science in Sports and Exercise, 26*(2), 182–90.

Lazarus, R. S., & Folkman, S. (1984). *Stress, appraisal, and coping.* New York: Springer.

Leserman, J., Jackson, E. D., Petitto, J. M., Golden, R. N., Silva, S. G., Perkins, D. O., et al. (1999). Progression to AIDS: The effects of stress, depressive symptoms, and social support. *Psychosomatic Medicine, 61*(3), 397–406.

Leserman, J., Petitto, J. M., Golden, R. N., Gaynes, B. N., Gu, H., Perkins, D. O., et al. (2000). Impact of stressful life events, depression, social support, coping, and cortisol on progression to AIDS. *American Journal of Psychiatry, 157*(8), 1221–8.

Leserman, J., Petitto, J. M., Gu, H., Gaynes, B. N., Barroso, J., Golden, R. N., et al. (2002). Progression to AIDS, a clinical AIDS condition and mortality: Psychosocial and physiological predictors. *Psychological Medicine, 32*(6), 1059–73.

Lorenz, K. A., Hays, R. D., Shapiro, M. F., Cleary, P. D., Asch, S. M., & Wenger, N. S. (2005). Religiousness and spirituality among HIV-infected Americans. *Journal of Palliative Medicine, 8*(4), 774–81.

Maman, S., Cathcart, R., Burkhardt, G., Omba, S., & Behets, F. (2009). The role of religion in HIV-positive women's disclosure experiences and coping strategies in Kinshasa, Democratic Republic of Congo. *Social Science & Medicine (1982), 68*(5), 965–70.

McCain, N. L., Gray, D. P., Elswick, R. K., Robins, J. W., Tuck, I., Walter, J. M., et al. (2008). A randomized clinical trial of alternative stress management interventions in persons with HIV infection. *Journal of Consulting and Clinical Psychology, 76*(3), 431–41.

McCormick, D. P., Holder, B., Wetsel, M. A., & Cawthon, T. W. (2001). Spirituality and HIV disease: An integrated perspective. *Journal of the Association of Nurses in AIDS Care, 12*(3), 58–65.

Mercier, L., Reidy, M., & Maheu, C. (1999). Uncertainty and hope in seropositive women. *Canadian Nurse, 95*(10), 40–6.

Milam, J. E., Richardson, J. L., Marks, G., Kemper, C. A., & McCutchan, A. J. (2004). The roles of dispositional optimism and pessimism in HIV disease progression. *Psychology and Health, 19*, 167–81.

Milam, J. (2006). Posttraumatic growth and HIV disease progression. *Journal of Consulting and Clinical Psychology, 74*(5), 817–27.

Miller, G. E., Kemeny, M. E., Taylor, S. E., Cole, S. W., & Visscher, B. R. (1997). Social relationships and immune processes in HIV seropositive gay and bisexual men. *Annals of Behavioral Medicine, 19*(2), 139–51.

Moskowitz, J. T., Hult, J. R., Bussolari, C., & Acree, M. (2009). What works in coping with HIV? A meta-analysis with implications for coping with serious illness. *Psychological Bulletin, 135*(1), 121–41.

Mulder, C. L., Antoni, M. H., Duivenvoorden, H. J., Kauffmann, R. H., & Goodkin, K. (1995). Active confrontational coping predicts decreased clinical progression over a one-year period in HIV-infected homosexual men. *Journal of Psychosomatic Research, 39*(8), 957–65.

Mulder, C. L., de Vroome, E. M., van Griensven, G. J., Antoni, M. H., & Sandfort, T. G. (1999). Avoidance as a predictor of the biological course of HIV infection over a 7-year period in gay men. *Health Psychology, 18*(2), 107–13.

O'Cleirigh, C., Ironson, G., Balbin, E., George, A., Antoni, M., Schneiderman, N., et al. (2002). Emotional processing of trauma predicts HIV disease progression at 1 year follow-up: Finding meaning as mediator of this relationship. *Psychosomatic Medicine, 64*(81), 102 (abstract).

O'Cleirigh, C., Ironson, G., Antoni, M., Fletcher, M. A., McGuffey, L., Balbin, E., et al. (2003). Emotional expression and depth processing of trauma and their relation to long-term survival in patients with HIV/AIDS. *Journal of Psychosomatic Research, 54*(3), 225–35.

O'Cleirigh, C., Ironson, G., Fletcher, M. A., & Schneiderman, N. (2008). Written emotional disclosure and processing of trauma are associated with protected health status and immunity in people living with HIV/AIDS. *British Journal of Health Psychology, 13*(Pt 1), 81–4.

O'Cleirigh, C., Ironson, G., Weiss, A., & Costa, P. T., Jr. (2007). Conscientiousness predicts disease progression (CD4 number and viral load) in people living with HIV. *Health Psychology, 26*(4), 473–80.

O'Cleirigh, C., Ironson, G., & Smits, J. A. (2007). Does distress tolerance moderate the impact of major life events on psychosocial variables and behaviors important in the management of HIV? *Behavior Therapy, 38*(3), 314–23.

Oman, D., & Thoresen, C. E. (2003). Spiritual modeling: A key to spiritual and religious growth? *International Journal for the Psychology of Religion, 13*(3), 149–65.

Pargament, K. (1997). *The psychology of religion and coping: Theory, research, and practice.* New York: Guilford Press.

Pargament, K. (2006). The meaning of spiritual transformation. In J. D. Koss & P. Hefner (Eds.), *Spiritual transformation and healing: Anthropological, theological, neuroscientific, and clinical perspectives* (1st ed., pp. 10–24). Lanham, MD: AltaMira Press.

Pargament, K. I., Koenig, H. G., Tarakeshwar, N., & Hahn, J. (2004). Religious coping methods as predictors of psychological, physical and spiritual outcomes among medically ill elderly patients: A two-year longitudinal study. *Journal of Health Psychology, 9*(6), 713–30.

Pargament, K. I., McCarthy, S., Shah, P., Ano, G., Tarakeshwar, N., Wachholtz, A., et al. (2004). Religion and HIV: A review of the literature and clinical implications. *Southern Medical Journal, 97*(12), 1201–9.

Park, C. L., & Folkman, S. (1997). Meaning in the context of stress and coping. *Review of General Psychology, 1*, 115–44.

Patterson, T. L., Shaw, W. S., Semple, S. J., Cherner, M., McCutchan, J. A., Atkinson, J. H., et al. (1996). Relationship of psychosocial factors to HIV disease progression. *Annals of Behavioral Medicine, 18*, 30–9.

Perez, J. E., Chartier, M., Koopman, C., Vosvick, M., Gore-Felton, C., & Spiegel, D. (2009). Spiritual striving, acceptance coping, and depressive symptoms among adults living with HIV/AIDS. *Journal of Health Psychology, 14*(1), 88–97.

Perry, S., Fishman, B., Jacobsberg, L., & Frances, A. (1992). Relationships over 1 year between lymphocyte subsets and psychosocial variables among adults with infection by human immunodeficiency virus. *Archives of General Psychiatry, 49*(5), 396–401.

Phillips, K. D., & Sowell, R. L. (2000). Hope and coping in HIV-infected African-American women of reproductive age. *Journal of National Black Nurses' Association, 11*(2), 18–24.

Polzer Casarez, R. L., & Miles, M. S. (2008). Spirituality: A cultural strength for African American mothers with HIV. *Clinical Nursing Research, 17*(2), 118–32.

Reed, G. M., Kemeny, M. E., Taylor, S. E., Wang, H. Y., & Visscher, B. R. (1994). Realistic acceptance as a predictor of decreased survival time in gay men with AIDS. *Health Psychology, 13*(4), 299–307.

Reed, P. G. (1987). Spirituality and well-being in terminally ill hospitalized adults. *Research in Nursing & Health, 10*(5), 335–44.

Richards, T. A., & Folkman, S. (1997). Spiritual aspects of loss at the time of a partner's death from AIDS. *Death Studies, 21*(6), 527–52.

Ridge, D., Williams, I., Anderson, J., & Elford, J. (2008). Like a prayer: The role of spirituality and religion for people living with HIV in the UK. *Sociology of Health & Illness, 30*(3), 413–28.

Segerstrom, S. C. (2001). Optimism, goal conflict, and stressor-related immune change. *Journal of Behavioral Medicine, 24*(5), 441–67.

Sidhu, K. S., Vandana, P., & Balon, R. (2009). Exercise prescription: A practical effective therapy for depression. *Current Psychiatry, 8*(6), 39–51.

Siegel, K., & Schrimshaw, E. W. (2000). Perceiving benefits in adversity: Stress-related growth in women living with HIV/AIDS. *Social Science & Medicine (1982), 51*(10), 1543–54.

Siegel, K., & Schrimshaw, E. W. (2005). Stress, appraisal, and coping: A comparison of HIV-infected women in the pre-HAART and HAART eras. *Journal of Psychosomatic Research, 58*(3), 225–33.

Siegel, K., Schrimshaw, E. W., & Pretter, S. (2005). Stress-related growth among women living with HIV/AIDS: Examination of an explanatory model. *Journal of Behavioral Medicine, 28*(5), 403–14.

Simoni, J. M., Frick, P. A., & Huang, B. (2006). A longitudinal evaluation of a social support model of medication adherence among HIV-positive men and women on antiretroviral therapy. *Health Psychology, 25*(1), 74–81.

Simoni, J. M., & Ortiz, M. Z. (2003). Mediational models of spirituality and depressive symptomatology among HIV-positive Puerto Rican women. *Cultural Diversity & Ethnic Minority Psychology, 9*(1), 3–15.

Solano, L., Costa, M., Temoshok, L., Salvati, S., Coda, R., Aiuti, F., et al. (2002). An emotionally inexpressive (type C) coping style influences HIV disease progression at six and twelve month follow-ups. *Psychology and Health, 17*, 641–55.

Solano, L., Costa, M., Salvati, S., Coda, R., Aiuti, F., Mezzaroma, I., et al. (1993). Psychosocial factors and clinical evolution in HIV-1 infection: A longitudinal study. *Journal of Psychosomatic Research, 37*(1), 39–51.

Sowell, R., Moneyham, L., Hennessy, M., Guillory, J., Demi, A., & Seals, B. (2000). Spiritual activities as a resistance resource for women with human immunodeficiency virus. *Nursing Research, 49*(2), 73–82.

Strachan, E. D., Bennett, W., Russo, J., & Roy-Byrne, P. (2007). Disclosure of HIV status and sexual orientation independently predicts increased absolute CD4 cell counts over time for psychiatric patients. *Psychosomatic Medicine, 69*, 74–80.

Suls, J., & Fletcher, B. (1985). The relative efficacy of avoidant and nonavoidant coping strategies: A meta-analysis. *Health Psychology, 4*(3), 249–88.

Tarakeshwar, N., Khan, N., & Sikkema, K. J. (2006). A relationship-based framework of spirituality for individuals with HIV. *AIDS & Behavior, 10*(1), 59–70.

Tarakeshwar, N., Pearce, M. J., & Sikkema, K. J. (2005). Development and implementation of a spiritual coping group intervention for adults living with HIV/AIDS: A pilot study. *Mental Health, Religion and Culture, 8*(3), 179–90.

Taylor, S. E., Kemeny, M. E., Aspinwall, L. G., Schneider, S. G., Rodriguez, R., & Herbert, M. (1992). Optimism, coping, psychological distress, and high-risk sexual behavior among men at risk for acquired immunodeficiency syndrome (AIDS). *Journal of Personality and Social Psychology, 63*(3), 460–73.

Temoshok, L., & Wald, R. (2006). Forgiveness and health implications in persons living with HIV/AIDS. *Annals of Behavioral Medicine 31*, S032.

Temoshok, L. R., Waldstein, S. R., Wald, R. L., Garzino-Demo, A., Synowski, S. J., Sun, L., et al. (2008). Type C coping, alexithymia, and heart rate reactivity are associated independently and differentially with specific immune mechanisms linked to HIV progression. *Brain, Behavior, and Immunity, 22*(5), 781–92.

Theorell, T., Blomkvist, V., Jonsson, H., Schulman, S., Berntorp, E., & Stigendal, L. (1995). Social support and the development of immune function in human immunodeficiency virus infection. *Psychosomatic Medicine, 57*(1), 32–6.

Thornton, S., Troop, M., Burgess, A. P., Button, J., Goodall, R., Flynn, R., et al. (2000). The relationship of psychological variables and disease progression among long-term HIV-infected men. *International Journal of STD & AIDS, 11*(11), 734–42.

Tomakowsky, J., Lumley, M. A., Markowitz, N., & Frank, C. (2001). Optimistic explanatory style and dispositional optimism in HIV-infected men. *Journal of Psychosomatic Research, 51*(4), 577–87.

Trevino, K. M., Pargament, K. I., Cotton, S., Leonard, A. C., Hahn, J., Caprini-Faigin, C. A., et al. (2010). Religious coping and physiological, psychological, social, and spiritual outcomes in patients with HIV/AIDS: Cross-sectional and longitudinal findings. *AIDS and Behavior, 14*(2), 379–89.

Tuck, I. (2004). Development of a spirituality intervention to promote healing. *Journal of Theory Construct and Testing, 8*, 67–71.

Tuck, I., McCain, N. L., & Elswick, R. K., Jr. (2001). Spirituality and psychosocial factors in persons living with HIV. *Journal of Advanced Nursing, 33*(6), 776–83.

Vassend, O., & Eskild, A. (1998). Psychological distress, coping, and disease progression in HIV-positive homosexual men. *Journal of Health Psychology, 3,* 243–57.

Vosvick, M., Martin, L. A., Smith, N. G., & Jenkins, S. R. (2010). Gender differences in HIV-related coping and depression. *AIDS and Behavior. 14*(2), 390–400.

Wachholtz, A. B., & Pargament, K. I. (2005). Is spirituality a critical ingredient of meditation? Comparing the effects of spiritual meditation, secular meditation, and relaxation on spiritual, psychological, cardiac, and pain outcomes. *Journal of Behavioral Medicine, 28*(4), 369–84.

Weaver, K. E., Antoni, M. H., Lechner, S. C., Duran, R. E., Penedo, F., Fernandez, M. I., et al. (2004). Perceived stress mediates the effects of coping on the quality of life of HIV-positive women on highly active antiretroviral therapy. *AIDS and Behavior, 8*(2), 175–83.

Yi, M. S., Mrus, J. M., Wade, T. J., Ho, M. L., Hornung, R. W., Cotton, S., et al. (2006). Religion, spirituality, and depressive symptoms in patients with HIV/AIDS. *Journal of General Internal Medicine, 21 Suppl 5,* S21–7.

Self-Regulation of Unattainable Goals and Pathways to Quality of Life

Carsten Wrosch

Abstract

This chapter addresses how people can adapt when goals are unattainable and protect their psychological well-being and physical health. It is argued that the experience of unattainable goals can elicit emotional distress and contribute to patterns of biological dysregulation and physical health problems. However, individuals can avoid these negative consequences of goal failure if they disengage from unattainable goals, protect their emotional and motivational resources, and engage in other meaningful goals. The literature review includes studies examining (a) specific self-regulation processes in response to an unattainable goal and (b) individual difference in self-regulation tendencies applied across different situations. Studies on specific self-regulation processes show that the use of goal disengagement, self-protective, and goal re-engagement processes is associated with high levels of subjective well-being, and these processes become particularly important in older adulthood when individuals confront increasing developmental constraints on the pursuit of their personal goals. In addition, studies examining general self-regulation tendencies show that goal disengagement capacities can reduce levels of negative emotions and thereby contribute to adaptive biological functioning and good physical health. Goal re-engagement capacities, by contrast, did not predict health-related outcomes but were significantly associated with aspects of subjective well-being. Implications of these findings for adaptive development and future directions are discussed.

Keywords: self-regulation, subjective well-being, physical health, goal disengagement, goal re-engagement, secondary control, lifespan development, age

Whether it's pursuing a career, improving a personal relationship, or watching a new movie, working towards desired goals can contribute to a person's quality of life. This notion is a central premise of theories of self-regulation suggesting that personality processes involved in the pursuit of personal goals play an important role in determining a person's subjective well-being and physical health (Carver & Scheier, 1981, 1998; Emmons, 1986; Heckhausen & Schulz, 1995). From this perspective, goals are important because they are the building blocks that structure people's lives and imbue life with purpose, both in the short run and on a long-term basis (Heckhausen, 1999; Ryff, 1989; Scheier et al., 2006). In very concrete ways, goals motivate adaptive behaviors, direct patterns of life-long development, and contribute to defining a person's identity.

At times, however, goals are beyond reach and cannot be attained. In such situations, individuals are at risk of compromising their quality of life, and they may need to abandon the unattainable goal, protect their emotional and motivational resources, and engage in other meaningful goals (Heckhausen, Wrosch, & Schulz, 2010; Wrosch, Scheier, Carver, & Schulz, 2003). These processes contribute to "giving-up" on a desired goal, which has a bad reputation in Western societies and much of the psychological literature (Bandura, 1997; Seligman, 1975; Taylor & Brown, 1998; Wortman & Brehm, 1975). However, studies reviewed in this chapter suggest that individuals can improve their subjective well-being and maintain their physical health if they engage in these processes and successfully adjust to the experience of unattainable goals.

Unattainable Goals and Quality of Life Across Adulthood

Having a goal that cannot be attained is a common psychological experience. If asked directly about the goals they had to stop pursuing, individuals report that they experienced approximately five valued and unattainable goals over a timespan of 5 years (Bauer, 2004; Wrosch, Scheier, Miller, et al., 2003). Moreover, the majority of unattainable goals typically occurred in central life domains, such as education and work, self-development and personal growth, or finances (Bauer, 2004), suggesting that people confront on average one unattainable goal in a central domain of life each year.

Unattainable goals can be experienced for different reasons and at any point during a person's life. For example, individuals may select goals that are beyond their capacities and, for that reason, will never be attained (e.g., being accepted into a graduate program or being promoted without having the necessary credential or skills), or they encounter critical life events that make it impossible to continue the pursuit of a goal (e.g., after an accident or an economic crisis, a person may not be able to or continue to work or pay back a mortgage). In addition, there are life-course–related changes that, over time, can render unattainable some goals that were realistic and attainable at some point in an individual's life. To this end, research from the area of lifespan development has demonstrated that opportunities and resources for attaining personal goals show sharp declines as people age (Baltes, Cornelius, & Nesselroade, 1979; Brandtstädter, 1990; Heckhausen, 1999; Heckhausen, Wrosch, & Schulz, 2010; Heckhausen & Schulz, 1995; Wrosch & Freund, 2001). For example, age-related biological changes render women unable to bear children after a certain age, and make it difficult to maintain

levels of physical health comparable to those experienced in young adulthood. Societal prescriptions also place normative constraints on the pursuit of developmentally-timed goals related to career and family (Neugarten & Hagestad, 1976). Moreover, given the occurrence of age-related declines in personal resources, older adults may need to focus their time and energy on the pursuit of the most important goals (Baltes & Baltes, 1990), and therefore may be forced to abandon other, more peripheral, goals (Wrosch, Scheier, Miller, et al., 2003). Thus, biological, societal, and personal constraints may make it more likely for older adults to experience constraints on the pursuit of their personal goals.

Unattainable goals, emotional distress, and physical health

Regardless of why a goal can no longer be pursued, having an unattainable goal can create a problem for a person's quality of life because failure to attain a desired outcome that is related to a person's overall sense of identity may trigger high levels of emotional distress. This process is captured by self-regulation theories, which postulate that goal-related processes are organized in feedback loops, in which goals provide important reference values for a person's emotional experiences and behaviors (Carver & Scheier, 1981, 1998). In such a feedback loop, a person's perception of current circumstances is compared to a reference value (i.e., a goal; Carver & Scheier, 1998). If the comparison yields a negative discrepancy between perceived and desired circumstances (e.g., an individual perceives failure or insufficient progress towards a goal), he or she is likely to experience high levels of emotional distress (Carver & Scheier, 1990). In support of this assumption, research based on several different theories has demonstrated that negative affect often emerges in circumstances that involve difficulty with goal pursuits (Carver & Scheier, 1990, 1998; Higgins, 1987; Taylor & Brown, 1988; Watson, Clark, & Tellegen, 1988).

Theories and research further suggest that emotional experiences represent a mechanism that can link challenging encounters with the development of physical disease (e.g., Cohen, 1996; Wrosch, Schulz, & Heckhausen, 2004). Stressful encounters have been shown to dysregulate biological processes in the endocrine, immune, metabolic, and central nervous systems (e.g., cortisol disturbances or excessive inflammation), which increase individuals' vulnerability to the development of physical disease

(Dickerson & Kemeny, 2004; Heim, Ehlert, & Hellhammer, 2000; Lupien, Leon, De Santi, et al., 1998; Miller, Chen, & Zhou, 2007; Miller & Wrosch, 2007; Willerson & Ridker, 2004). Further, the experience of physical problems resulting from goal difficulty can lead to even more problems with goal pursuits as well as subsequent emotional and biological problems. This implies that people who confront unattainable goals are at risk of entering into a downward spiral in which goal failure and psychological and physical health problems reciprocally influence each other and compromise their quality of life (Wrosch, Schulz, & Heckhausen, 2004).

Self-regulation of unattainable goals

To avoid the adverse consequences of goal failure on psychological and physical health, it has been suggested that people need to engage in adaptive self-regulation. Several approaches to adaptive self-regulation postulate that two broad categories of responses are involved in the management of failure in goal pursuits (Carver & Scheier, 1990, 1998; Heckhausen & Schulz, 1995; Kukla, 1972; Wright & Brehm, 1989). One category of responses consists of goal engagement processes, which aim at overcoming difficulty by continuing to make investments of time and effort towards attaining a threatened goal. The second category aims at the exact opposite outcome; that is, abandoning the threatened goal, managing the adverse emotional consequences of failure, and engaging in other meaningful goals.

As depicted in Figure 16.1, the adaptive value of these two categories of responses should depend on a person's opportunities to attain the threatened goal in the future. In particular, goal engagement should facilitate adaptive outcomes when people have favorable opportunities (Heckhausen & Schulz, 1995; Heckhausen, Wrosch, & Schulz, 2010). In such situations, people can overcome goal failure and protect their subjective well-being and physical health if they invest more effort in, strengthen their psychological commitment toward, or find an alternative path to realizing the threatened goal (Bandura, 1997; Folkman, Lazarus, Dunkel-Schetter, DeLongis, & Gruen, 1986; Freund & Baltes, 2002; Heckhausen & Schulz, 1995; Scheier et al., 1989; Taylor & Brown, 1988; Wrosch & Schulz, 2008).

However, if it is not possible to make further progress towards a desired goal because the goal itself is unattainable, a person may be more doubtful about future goal success and engage in self-regulation responses aimed at goal disengagement, self-protection, and the pursuit of other meaningful goals (for appraisals, expectancies, and coping, see Carver & Scheier, 1998; Folkman & Lazarus, 1980; Lazarus & Folkman, 1984). These processes of adaptive goal adjustment keep a person engaged in the pursuit of meaningful and attainable goals (see Fig. 16.1) and can contribute to high levels of subjective well-being and physical health (Miller & Wrosch, 2007; Wrosch, Miller, Scheier, et al., 2007; Wrosch, Scheier, Carver, & Schulz, 2003; Wrosch, Scheier, Miller, Schulz, & Carver, 2003).

Consistent with the previous discussion, there are different specific theories of adaptive self-regulation and coping that show how people can avoid the negative psychological and physical consequences that result from the experience of unattainable goals (Brandtstädter & Renner, 1990; Folkman, 1997;

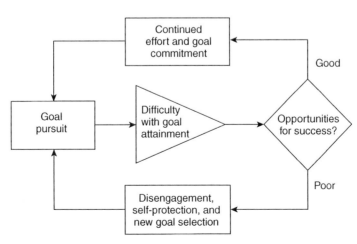

Fig. 16.1 Adaptive self-regulation of difficulty with goal attainment.

Heckhausen & Schulz, 1995; Wrosch, Scheier, Miller, et al., 2003). These theories differ in terms of the terminology that is used to describe adaptive self-regulation processes (e.g., control strategies or coping, Folkman, 1997; Heckhausen & Schulz, 1995). In addition, they examine different levels of aggregation of individuals' self-regulation responses. While some theories focus on how individuals activate specific control strategies or coping tactics in response to an insurmountable stressor (e.g., secondary control or meaning-focused coping; Folkman, 1997; Heckhausen & Schulz, 1995), other theories address the importance of broader individual differences in self-regulation tendencies for successful adjustment to unattainable goals (i.e., accommodation or goal adjustment capacities;Brandtstädter & Renner, 1990; Wrosch, Scheier, Miller, et al., 2003).

A model that conceptualizes how individuals activate specific self-regulation processes to manage the experience of an unattainable goal is the "motivational theory of lifespan development" (Heckhausen, Wrosch, & Schulz, 2010). This approach grew out of the previously developed "lifespan theory of control"(Heckhausen, 1999; Heckhausen & Schulz, 1995; Schulz & Heckhausen, 1996) and considers the importance of control strategies for successful development across the human lifespan. In particular, this theory documents how individuals activate specific types of compensatory secondary control strategies to adjust to age-related increases in constraints on their goal pursuits. Such compensatory secondary control strategies are aimed at changing a person's internal perceptions of goal failure and involve goal disengagement and goal re-engagement processes (e.g., devaluation of an unattainable goal or an increased volitional focus on an alternative goal; Heckhausen, Wrosch, & Fleeson, 2001; Wrosch & Heckhausen, 1999). In addition, compensatory secondary control strategies incorporate self-protective processes, such as positive reappraisals, external attributions of failure, or downward social comparisons (Bauer, Wrosch, & Jobin, 2008; Heckhausen & Brim, 1997; Wrosch & Heckhausen, 2002; Wrosch, Heckhausen, & Lachman, 2000). Compensatory secondary control strategies are used if individuals confront failure in an important life domain and may make it easier for them to accept that a certain goal can no longer be pursued. In addition, these control strategies safeguard individuals' emotional and motivational resources and facilitate engagement in alternative activities (Heckhausen, Wrosch, & Schulz, 2010; Wrosch, Scheier, Carver, & Schulz, 2003).

Conceptually related ideas have been developed by Folkman (1997), who postulated in her elaboration of the cognitive theory of stress and coping (Lazarus & Folkman, 1984) that meaning-based coping processes can contribute to improved levels of positive emotions when individuals confront stressful situations that involve unfavorable resolutions or that cannot be resolved (see also Folkman & Greer, 2000; Folkman & Moskowitz, 2000). Such meaning-based coping tactics include positive reappraisals, relinquishment of unattainable goals, and engagement with new goals. In addition, adaptive meaning-based coping processes can be related to spiritual beliefs, which may help some individuals to adjust to the experience of goal-related constraints (Folkman, 1997).

A theoretical model of goal adjustment that addresses broader individual differences in self-regulation tendencies has been developed by Brandtstädter and colleagues (Brandtstädter, 2006; Brandtstädter & Renner, 1990; Brandtstädter & Rothermund, 2002; Rothermund & Brandtstädter, 2003). Their dual-process theory examines how individuals manage discrepancies between desired and perceived goal progress across the lifespan (Brandtstädter, 2006; Brandtstädter & Renner, 1990; Brandtstädter & Rothermund, 2002; Rothermund & Brandtstädter, 2003). In particular, this theory assumes two modes of goal regulation that are reflected in broader individual tendencies associated with tenaciously pursuing goals (i.e., assimilation) and flexibly adjusting goals (i.e., accommodation). By accommodating to the inability of attaining an important goal through processes of disengagement, reorientation, and acceptance, people may maintain high levels of perceptions of control and subjective well-being (Brandtstädter & Renner, 1990; Brandtstädter & Rothermund, 1994). Further, these accommodation tendencies should become particular important for maintaining high levels of psychological functioning as individuals advance in age by helping them to successfully cope with the growing frequency of uncontrollable events and demands (Brandtstädter & Renner, 1990).

Similar to the previous approach, Wrosch and colleagues have postulated that there exist reliable individual differences in people's general capacities to adjust to unattainable goals across different circumstances (Wrosch, Miller, Scheier, & Brun de Pontet, 2007; Wrosch, Scheier, Miller, et al., 2003). Such individual differences in goal adjustment capacities, in turn, are thought to be functionally associated with individuals' subjective well-being and physical health. Different from Brandtstädter and colleagues' model, however, their model distinguished two separate processes within the domain of goal adjustment: individuals need to (a) disengage from unattainable goals and (b) re-engage in other meaningful goals (Carver & Scheier, 1990; Wrosch, Miller, et al., 2007; Wrosch, Scheier, Carver, & Schulz, 2003; Wrosch, Scheier, Miller, et al., 2003). These two processes are thought to reflect independent self-regulation capacities, and they should therefore be examined as independent constructs in research. In support of this assumption, research has shown that goal disengagement and goal re-engagement capacities are only weakly correlated with each other and can predict different outcomes of subjective well-being and physical health (Bauer, 2004; Kraaij, Garnefski, & Schroevers, 2009; Miller & Wrosch, 2007; Wrosch & Miller, 2009; Wrosch, Miller, et al., 2007).

In addition, Wrosch and colleagues' model identifies specific motivational components involved in goal disengagement and goal re-engagement as well as their adaptive effects (Wrosch, Scheier, Miller, et al., 2003). From their perspective, goal disengagement requires a person to withdraw both *effort* and *commitment* from the pursuit of an unattainable goal. Goal re-engagement, by contrast, involves the *identification of*, *commitment to*, and *pursuit of* alternative goals. Goal disengagement should be primarily adaptive because it prevents a person from experiencing the negative emotional consequences of repeated goal failure(for beneficial consequences of disengagement, see also Carver & Scheier, 1998; Klinger, 1975; Nesse, 2000; Sprangers & Schwartz, 1999). Goal re-engagement, by contrast, should be adaptive particularly because it helps a person to maintain a sense of purpose in life and facilitate positive aspects of emotional well-being. In addition, there are secondary functions of goal adjustment capacities, in which successful goal disengagement can free resources that can be invested in the pursuit of other important goals, and goal re-engagement may reduce some of the negative emotions associated with the inability to make progress towards a desired goal.

Despite the differences in the theoretical approaches to identifying the processes involved in the adjustment to unattainable goals, the different models consist of overlapping ideas and may complement each other. First, they suggest that goal adjustment processes can be conceptualized as specific individual responses to the experience of an unattainable goal, or they can be examined as more general individual tendencies that have important regulatory functions across different circumstances. In this regard, it may be that the outcome of interest determines which theoretical approach is more fruitful. If the outcome involves a specific measure of adaptation (e.g., the emotions that a person experiences with respect to a specific event), models that examine the activation of specific coping or self-regulation responses may be particularly powerful. By contrast, if the outcome involves adaptation across different life domains (e.g., general life satisfaction of global physical health), examining broader tendencies of goal adjustment may show stronger effects on these outcomes (for a discussion of levels of personality processes and outcomes, see Wrosch & Scheier, 2003). Second, the processes defined in the different theoretical models may all play an important role in the adjustment to unattainable goals. Thus, successful goal adjustment may require disengagement from an unattainable goal and re-engagement in other meaningful goals. In addition, self-protective and meaning-based processes may support the goal adjustment process and help individuals to overcome failure by protecting their emotional and motivational resources for future action.

Empirical Evidence

The previous discussion suggests that individuals can protect their quality of life if they successfully adjust to the experience of unattainable goals. In addition, these processes are expected to become particularly important for determining life-long patterns of successful development as people age and experience increasing constraints on the pursuit of their personal goals. The following section reviews the literature examining these propositions empirically. This review is divided in two parts. The first part addresses the effects of specific self-regulation processes on adaptive outcomes. These studies are largely focused on examining outcomes of subjective well-being. The second part addresses the literature on the adaptive consequences of broader individual differences in goal adjustment capacities, and discusses in separate sections studies on predicting both indicators of subjective well-being and physical health.

Specific goal adjustment processes

Over the past decade, different research groups have accumulated empirical evidence suggesting that individual differences in specific reactions to the experience of an unattainable goal can have beneficial effects on an individual's quality of life. Some of these studies were conceptually based on Heckhausen and colleagues' model (Heckhausen & Schulz, 1995; Heckhausen, Wrosch, & Schulz, 2010; Schulz & Heckhausen, 1996). In these studies, the authors assessed goal regulation processes with different methods, including measurements of self-identified goals, goal-related information processing through incidental memory, and self-report scales that were developed to capture specific self-regulation processes. In addition, these studies examined the phenomenon of unattainable goals by conducting age-comparative studies, which assumed that the attainment of certain goals becomes increasingly more difficulty as people age (e.g., having your own children, undoing the consequences of severe life regrets, or establishing a new intimate relationship after divorce; Heckhausen, Wrosch, & Fleeson, 2001; Wrosch & Heckhausen, 1999, 2002).

The findings from this line of research demonstrated consistent evidence across different studies and types of goals. Older, as compared to younger, participants experienced reduced opportunities to attain new intimate relationship goals after a separation (Wrosch & Heckhausen, 1999), to have their own children (Heckhausen, Wrosch, & Fleeson, 2001), or to undo the negative consequences of severe life regrets (Bauer, Wrosch, & Jobin, 2008; Wrosch, Bauer, & Scheier, 2005; Wrosch & Heckhausen, 2002). In addition, the studies showed complementary findings with respect to the use of goal-specific self-regulation processes. For example, older separated adults had disengaged from partnership goals more fully than had younger adults, as reflected in the number of partnership goals they reported and a reduced cognitive reliance on positive versus negative aspects of an intimate relationship (Wrosch & Heckhausen, 1999). In addition, childless women, who had passed the biological clock for childbearing, used compensatory secondary control strategies more frequently than their counterparts who could still have their own children (Heckhausen, Wrosch, & Fleeson, 2001). Finally, older participants were more disengaged from undoing the consequences of their most severe life regrets than younger participants (Wrosch, Bauer, & Scheier, 2005) and activated self-protective downward social comparisons to a greater extent than younger participants if confronted with their regrets (Bauer, Jobin, & Wrosch, 2008).

Of importance, the reported studies also showed that individual differences in self-regulation processes can predict adaptive outcomes, if these processes

were adjusted to the age-related opportunities for goal attainment. To this end, longitudinal data indicated that deactivation of partnership goals predicted improvement of partnership-specific emotional well-being among older separated individuals, but not among their younger counterparts (Wrosch & Heckhausen, 1999). In addition, Heckhausen and colleagues' (2001) study showed that among women who had passed the deadline for having their own children, those who failed to disengage from the goal of having their own children reported particularly high levels of depressive symptomatology. In a similar vein, research on life regrets has documented that being disengaged from undoing the negative consequences of regretted behaviors (Wrosch et al., 2005), using self-protective attributions (i.e., avoiding self-blame, Wrosch & Heckhausen, 2002), and engaging in downward social comparisons (Bauer, Wrosch, & Jobin, 2008) was associated with adaptive outcomes (e.g., reduced regret intensity, low depressive symptoms, or few health problems) among older, but not younger, participants (for beneficial health effects of downward social comparisons in old age, see also Bailis, Chipperfield, & Perry, 2005). Finally, recent experimental work is consistent with these findings by demonstrating that engaging older adults in processes that support goal disengagement (e.g., making self-protective attributions and social comparisons or dwelling on other meaningful goals) can buffer the adverse effect of intense regret on older adults' health problems over time (Wrosch, Bauer, et al., 2007).

Other researchers have begun to examine the adaptive value of specific goal adjustment processes by adjusting Wrosch and colleagues' (2003) model in cross-sectional studies. These studies target populations that confront specific medical problem (e.g., infertility, HIV, cancer; Kraaij et al., 2009; Kraaij, Van der Veek, Garnefski, Schroevers, Witlox, & Maes, 2008; Schroevers, Kraaij, & Garnefski, 2008) and asked participants to report whether they were able to disengage from a specific and important goal that has become unattainable due to the medical problem and to re-engage in other goals. The findings of these studies showed that among middle-aged adults who could not have children because of infertility (Kraaij et al., 2009), disengagement from the goal of having children was associated with lower levels of negative affect, while re-engagement in alternative goals was related to higher levels of positive affect. In addition, a study on cancer patients documented that after controlling for other coping tactics and illness-related and sociodemographic factors, goal re-engagement efforts were independently associated with high levels of positive affect, but not with levels of negative affect. Goal disengagement did not show independent associations with participants' emotional well-being in this study (Schroevers, Kraaij, & Garnefski, 2008). Moreover, goal disengagement and goal re-engagement were associated with lower levels of depressive symptoms in a sample of HIV-positive men, statistically independent of illness characteristics and other coping constructs (Kraaij et al., 2008).

There is also some longitudinal evidence for the beneficial effects of specific goal re-engagement processes. Duke, H. Leventhal, Brownlee, and E. Leventhal (2002) studied older adults, some of whom had to abandon physical activities because of health-related problems. Their study showed that individuals who replaced lost activities with new activities had higher positive affect 1 year after the onset of their illness than those who did not replace their activities.

Another set of studies examined a particularly interesting corollary of disengagement from the pursuit of unattainable goals—that is, the reduction of goal importance (for goal devaluation and disengagement, see Heckhausen, Wrosch, & Schulz, 2010). In this regard, Brandtstädter and Rothermund (1994) showed in a longitudinal study of middle-aged and older adults that participants maintained global perceptions of personal control by reducing the perceived importance of domains with diminished personal control. Similarly, a study examining goal adjustment among couples undergoing infertility treatment found that among individuals for whom treatment was unsuccessful, depressive symptoms were greater if they appraised their child-related goals high in importance and low in attainability (Salmela-Aro & Suikkari, 2008). Convergent findings have been reported in a study of adult women, suggesting that the association between body satisfaction and self-esteem becomes weaker as women advance in age, supposedly because older women tend to accept changes in their bodies to a greater extent (Webster & Tiggemann, 2003).

Studies addressing how individuals cope with disability have also observed adjustments in the importance of threatened goal domains. For example, Weizenkamp and colleagues (2000) reported that spinal cord injury survivors ranked the importance of work and having children lower than the general population. In addition, Tunali and Power (1993) showed that mothers of autistic children downgraded the importance of career success and upgraded the importance of being a good parent (cf. Carver & Scheier, 2000; Sprangers & Schwartz, 1999). In addition, rated importance of being a successful parent was strongly related to life satisfaction among these mothers.

Together, research examining specific self-regulation processes in response to a threatened goal has documented that individuals who have poor opportunities to attain a goal can protect their quality of life if they disengage from the unattainable goal, protect their emotional and motivational resources, and engage in other new goals. In addition, the studies showed that the distribution of opportunities for attaining personal goals undergoes normative age-related declines. In this regard, older, as compared with younger, adults rely to a greater extent on processes involved in the adjustment to unattainable goals. Moreover, there is considerable variability in this process, and individual differences in the activation of goal adjustment processes are functionally associated with older adults' quality of life. Finally, the reviewed studies suggest that certain life events, such as medical illness, can constrain a person's opportunities for goal attainment, independent of age, and therefore may require younger and older individuals to successfully adjust to the experience of unattainable goals.

Goal adjustment capacities

An increasing number of empirical studies have examined the importance of individuals' general goal adjustment capacities for predicting indicators of subjective well-being and physical health. As previously mentioned, these studies are based on the premise that people vary more generally in their capacities to adjust to unattainable goals across different circumstances (Wrosch, Scheier, Miller, et al., 2003). Consequently, they examine whether individuals who are generally better able to abandon unattainable goals and to re-engage in other meaningful activities should experience greater subjective well-being and better physical health than their counterparts who have a more difficult time adjusting to unattainable goals.

To examine these propositions empirically, studies from this line of research typically administer a self-report instrument, the Goal Adjustment Scale (Wrosch, Scheier, Miller, et al., 2003). This instrument contains 10 items that measure how people usually react if they can no longer pursue an important goal. Four items measure a person's capacity to disengage from unattainable goals and six items measure the capacity to re-engage in other new goals. The items on the Goal Adjustment Scale reflect the components of goal disengagement (i.e., withdrawal of effort and commitment) and goal re-engagement (i.e., identification of, commitment to, and pursuit of alternative goals) identified earlier. Both scales have been shown to be internally reliable, to be only weakly correlated with each other, and to predict relevant outcomes (Miller & Wrosch, 2007; Wrosch & Miller, 2009; Wrosch, Miller, et al., 2007; Wrosch, Scheier, Miller, et al., 2003).

PREDICTING SUBJECTIVE WELL-BEING

Several cross-sectional studies examined the influence of goal disengagement and goal re-engagement capacities on indicators of subjective well-being. For example, research among college students has shown that the capacity to disengage from unattainable goals was related to lower levels of perceived stress and intrusive thoughts, and higher levels of self-mastery. In addition, students who were able to re-engage in alternative goals reported lower levels of perceived stress and intrusive thoughts as well as higher levels of purpose in life and self-mastery (Wrosch, Scheier, Miller, et al., 2003). Convergent evidence for an association between goal adjustment capacities and subjective well-being has been reported in a study that compared parents whose children had been diagnosed with cancer and parents of physically healthy children. The study's results showed that goal disengagement and goal re-engagement capacities were independently associated with fewer depressive symptoms, particularly among parents of children with cancer. In fact, among parents of children with cancer, those who were better able to adjust to unattainable goals reported depression scores that were almost as low as the scores of parents of healthy children (Wrosch, Scheier, Miller, et al., 2003).

Other cross-sectional studies suggest that goal disengagement and goal re-engagement capacities can have differential effects on positive versus negative aspects of subjective well-being. For example, and consistent with above-reported findings on goal-specific self-regulation (Kraaij et al., 2009; Schroevers et al., 2008), results from a cross-sectional study of adults showed that goal disengagement capacities were associated with lower levels of negative affect but were unrelated to individual differences in positive affect. Conversely, goal re-engagement capacities predicted high levels of positive affect but were not associated with negative

affect (Bauer, 2004). In addition, O'Connor and Forgan (2007) document a particularly close association between goal re-engagement capacities and purpose for living. Their results from a sample of Scottish students suggest that participants who were better able to identify and pursue new goals reported fewer suicidal thoughts than students who had a more difficult time with goal re-engagement. Goal disengagement capacities were not associated with suicidal thoughts in this study (O'Connor & Forgan, 2007). Moreover, Wrosch and colleagues (2007) showed in a heterogeneous sample of adults that goal disengagement capacities were associated with lower levels of depressive symptoms, while participants' goal re-engagement capacities were unrelated to their depressive symptoms (for effects on other indicators of subjective well-being, see Wrosch, Miller, et al., 2007).

There is also longitudinal evidence suggesting that goal disengagement capacities can be a particularly strong predictor of negative affect. Following a sample of students across the course of one semester, Wrosch and colleagues (2007) demonstrated that high baseline levels of goal disengagement capacities (but not goal re-engagement capacities) predicted fewer increases of emotional distress over time. In addition, results from a 2-year longitudinal study of older adults suggest that participants with poor goal disengagement capacities experienced a large increase in depressive symptoms over time, while depressive symptoms did not increase among older adults with high levels of goal disengagement capacities. Similar to the previous study, goal re-engagement capacities were not related to changes in depressive symptoms (Dunne, Wrosch & Miller, 2010). Consistent with these findings, evidence from a longitudinal study of adolescent girls showed that improvements in goal disengagement capacities (but not in goal re-engagement capacities) over the first year of the study predicted a decline in depressive symptoms during the subsequent 6 months (Wrosch & Miller, 2009).

Finally, research on predicting subjective well-being has shown that goal disengagement and goal re-engagement capacities can produce different types of interaction effects. One pattern of interaction effects suggests that goal re-engagement capacities can buffer the negative effects of inability to disengage on subjective well-being; this has been observed among younger adults. In this regard, different studies conducted by Wrosch and colleagues revealed that among young adults who reported difficulty disengaging from unattainable goals, those with a higher capacity to re-engage reported greater self-mastery, less perceived stress, and better emotional well-being (Wrosch, Scheier, Miller et al., 2003, Study 1 and Study 2; Wrosch, Miller, et al., 2007) than those less able to re-engage. This pattern of results indicates that goal re-engagement may prevent some of the emotional problems associated with failure to disengage from unattainable goals.

Another pattern of interaction effects has been observed among older or vulnerable individuals and indicates that goal re-engagement capacities can become particularly important for maintaining high levels of subjective well-being when individuals tend to disengage from unattainable goals. In this regard, Wrosch and colleagues have shown in two cross-sectional samples of older adults that particularly low levels of subjective well-being were obtained among older adults who disengaged from unattainable goals but had difficulty identifying and engaging in other new goals (Wrosch, Miller, et al., 2007; Wrosch, Scheier, Miller et al., 2003). In a similar vein, a longitudinal study among patients who had a suicidal episode documented that the highest levels of suicidal ideation were found among patients who tended to abandon unattainable goals and had a difficult time engaging in new goals (O'Connor, Fraser, White, MacHale, & Masterton, 2009). This pattern of findings has been explained by the possibility that there are certain contexts that do not provide many potential goals that people could adopt (e.g., because of a reduced availability in old age, or life circumstances that contributed to a suicidal episode; cf. Wrosch, Scheier, Miller et al., 2003). In such circumstances, it may be particularly important to be capable of identifying and pursuing new goals, and for those individuals who cannot identify new goals, it may be even more adaptive to stay committed to unattainable goals than to abandon these goals and have nothing else to pursue in life.

In sum, the reviewed literature has shown that goal disengagement and goal re-engagement capacities are independent constructs that can be associated with high levels of subjective well-being. In addition, the pattern of findings suggests that goal disengagement capacities often show a stronger effect on reduced levels of negative aspects of subjective well-being (e.g., negative affect or depressive symptoms), while goal re-engagement capacities are more closely associated with positive aspects of subjective well-being (e.g., positive affect or purpose in life). These differential effects may be due to the different primary functions of goal disengagement and goal re-engagement capacities. Whereas goal disengagement should prevent the experience of emotional distress associated with repeated goal failure, goal re-engagement is expected to provide purpose for living, and thus may increase positive aspects of a person's subjective well-being. However, the available literature also shows some deviations from this pattern of findings. This may be due to the secondary functions of goal adjustment processes, in which goal disengagement is likely to free resources that facilitate the pursuit of new purposeful goals, and goal re-engagement may reduce some of the distress associated with not being able to make further progress towards an important goal (for a more comprehensive discussion, see Wrosch, Miller, et al., 2007).

PREDICTING PHYSICAL HEALTH

A growing body of research has begun to examine the associations between goal adjustment capacities and indicators of physical health. As discussed earlier, these studies were conducted with the idea that failure to adjust to unattainable goals can have adverse effects on a person's biological functioning (e.g., in the immune or endocrine systems) and physical health. Given that such an association may occur because of the distress derived from failed goal adjustment (e.g., Dickerson & Kemeny, 2004; Heim et al., 2000; Kiecolt-Glaser, McGuire, Robles, & Glaser, 2002; McEwen, 1998; Miller et al., 2007; Segerstrom & Miller, 2004), some of these studies have also explored the mediating role played by emotional well-being in the associations between goal adjustment capacities and physical health.

Evidence in support of an association between goal adjustment capacities and indicators of physical health has been reported in a cross-sectional study of adults. The findings showed that those participants who had difficulty disengaging from unattainable goals reported more physical health problems (e.g., eczema, migraine headaches, constipation) than participants who were able to disengage from unattainable goals. The study, however, did not confirm an association between participants' goal re-engagement capacities and their physical health problems (Wrosch, Miller, et al., 2007). Consistent with these findings, another cross-sectional study of adults confirmed that adaptive goal disengagement capacities (but not goal re-engagement capacities) were associated with a steeper slope of diurnal cortisol secretion. More specifically, the data suggested that adults who had difficulty disengaging from unattainable goals secreted a particularly high volume of cortisol in the day and evening hours, but not the morning hours (Wrosch, Miller, et al., 2007). This implies that goal disengagement capacities are important factors for predicting individuals' biological stress responses during the day, when people typically try to accomplish their goals and may encounter difficulty with goal attainment. Further, to the extent that such flattened diurnal cortisol rhythms can be prognostic of physical disease (Cohen, Janicki-Deverts, & Miller, 2007; Matthews, Schwartz, Cohen, & Seeman, 2006; Sephton, Sapolsky, Kraemer, & Spiegel, 2000; Smyth et al., 1997), the results of this study suggest a mechanism through which poor goal disengagement capacities could predict the physical symptoms reported in other studies.

There are also two longitudinal studies that examined whether goal adjustment capacities can forecast health-related outcomes over time. Results from these studies are of particular importance as they provide some evidence for directional effects. One study examined a group of adolescents and predicted changes in C-reactive protein (CRP), a marker of systemic inflammation, which can be elevated among individuals with high levels of psychological distress (Miller & Blackwell, 2006). The study found that among participants with poor disengagement capacities, levels of CRP increased over approximately 1 year twice as fast as for those with average disengagement capacities. By contrast, levels of CRP did not increase among participants who had an easier time disengaging from unattainable goals. Similar to the previously discussed studies, goal re-engagement capacities were not related to trajectories of systemic inflammation (Miller & Wrosch, 2007). Given that the magnitude and duration of inflammatory responses must be carefully regulated, and excessive inflammation may be a risk factor for diabetes or heart disease (Dandona, Aljada, Chaudhuri, Mohanty, & Garg, 2005; Willerson & Ridker, 2004), this study suggests that adolescents with poor goal disengagement capacities may be at risk of developing serious health problems in the future.

Conceptually consistent results were reported in another longitudinal study that followed a group of college students over the course of one semester (Wrosch, Miller, et al., 2007). The results showed that higher baseline levels of goal disengagement capacities were associated with fewer reported health symptoms and better sleep efficiency at the end of the semester. Similar to the previously reported studies, there was no main effect of goal re-engagement capacities on physical health outcomes, although the findings did suggest evidence of a buffering effect of goal re-engagement, in that goal re-engagement reduced the negative consequences of failure to disengage on participants' cold symptoms.

Finally, some of the reported studies have provided evidence that levels of subjective well-being can mediate the associations between adaptive goal disengagement capacities and physical health outcomes. For example, the previously discussed cross-sectional association between failure in goal disengagement and physical health problems (e.g., eczema, migraine headaches, constipation; Wrosch, Miller, et al., 2007) could be statistically explained by levels of depressive symptoms. Failure in goal disengagement was associated with higher levels of depressive symptoms, and the effect of goal disengagement on physical health outcomes was statistically mediated by participants' depressive symptomatology. In addition, the aforementioned longitudinal study on college students also included measures of emotional well-being. In this regard, the study's findings demonstrated that high levels of goal disengagement capacities were related to fewer increases in emotional distress across the course of the semester, and the effect of goal disengagement on changes in distress over time statistically mediated the associations between goal disengagement and later levels in indicators of physical health (Wrosch, Miller, et al., 2007).

Together, the reported studies document that individual differences in goal disengagement capacities can be associated with physical health outcomes. Difficulty with goal disengagement predicted maladaptive patterns of health-related biological processes (e.g., increased levels of cortisol secretion or systemic inflammation) and was associated with the occurrence of physical health problems (e.g., cold symptoms). Moreover, the findings suggest that the effects of failed goal disengagement on a person's physical health problems can be mediated by the experience of emotional distress. These studies, however, did not show health effects for individuals' goal re-engagement capacities. The absence of an association between goal re-engagement capacities and physical health outcomes may be explained by the previously discussed findings on the emotional consequences of goal adjustment capacities. These results suggested that goal disengagement capacities show strong effects on negative emotional states, while goal re-engagement capacities are mainly associated with positive aspects of subjective well-being. Given that the presence of negative emotions may take a greater toll on a person's physical health than the absence of positive emotions (see Pressman & Cohen, 2005), it is thus not surprising that goal disengagement, but not goal re-engagement, capacities are reliable predictors of physical health. However, the reported findings also showed that goal re-engagement capacities may at times buffer an adverse effect of failed goal disengagement on some physical health problems. This implies that beneficial health effects of goal re-engagement capacities may be more complex and need to be further examined in future research.

Conclusions and Future Directions

This chapter addressed how individuals can adjust to unattainable goals and prevent the adverse effects on their subjective well-being and physical health. Different theories were discussed proposing that effective self-regulation processes can facilitate the adjustment to unattainable goals. These theories conceptualize self-regulation processes either as specific reactions in response to the experience of an unattainable goal or as general individual differences in self-regulation tendencies applied across different circumstances. They further suggest that the adaptive management of unattainable goals requires individuals to disengage from unattainable goals, protect their emotional and motivational resources, and engage in other meaningful goals. These processes are thought to ameliorate the adverse emotional and biological consequences of goal failure and protect individuals' long-term physical health.

The reviewed empirical literature on examining the activation of specific self-regulation processes suggests that goal disengagement, self-protective (e.g., positive reappraisals or attributions), and goal re-engagement processes are associated with high levels of subjective well-being if individuals confront unfavorable opportunities for attaining desired goals. These processes become particularly important as individuals age and enable older adults to successfully cope with declining personal resources and increasing developmental constraints. Moreover, research on examining general goal adjustment capacities suggests that individuals who have difficulty disengaging from unattainable goals experience increased levels of emotional distress, which can contribute to patterns of biological dysregulation and subsequent physical health problems. Goal re-engagement capacities, by contrast, did not predict health-related outcomes but were associated with high levels of positive aspects of subjective well-being.

While the addressed literature has demonstrated that adaptive self-regulation of unattainable goals can benefit individuals' quality of life, several issues need to be addressed in future research. One issue relates to a better understanding of the factors that make it easier for individuals to abandon unattainable goals and to engage in new goals. This is important because it has been suggested that goal attainment processes hold functional primacy in the motivational system that organizes human behavior (Heckhausen, 2000; Heckhausen & Schulz, 1995), which may make disengagement from an unattainable goal difficult or unsuccessful. In fact, although research shows that individuals typically use goal adjustment processes more frequently when they experience constraints on their goal pursuits (Brandtstädter & Renner, 1990; Heckhausen, 1997; Wrosch et al., 2000, 2003, 2005), there is much variability in the success of this process, and little is known about the predictors of successful goal adjustment.

Some of the few studies addressing this research question showed that personality factors, such as dispositional optimism, can predict faster disengagement from unsolvable problems when people have options available (Aspinwall & Richter, 1999). In this regard, it would also be reasonable to assume that certain self-protective control strategies or meaning-based coping tactics, such as positive reappraisals, downward social comparisons, or external attributions, can make it easier to accept that an important life goal can no longer be pursued (Folkman & Greer, 2000; Wrosch, Scheier, Carver, & Schulz, 2003). In addition, there is evidence that negative mood itself can be associated with goal disengagement processes. In a recent longitudinal study of adolescents, Wrosch and Miller (2009) showed that high levels of depressive mood predicted an improvement in participants' goal disengagement capacities over time, and these improved goal disengagement capacities forecasted reduced levels of subsequent depressive mood (for an evolutionary model linking low mood and disengagement, see Nesse, 2000). These findings point to the reciprocal associations between negative emotions and self-regulation, and it would be important to examine whether such effects of depressive mood on improved goal disengagement capacities translate into adulthood and old age. Alternatively, these effects may be specific to adolescent development, as this is a life phase that has been associated with a steep increase in the use of goal adjustment processes and with the frequent adoption of goals that later prove to be unrealizable

(Heckhausen, Wrosch, & Schulz, 2010; Markus & Nurius, 1986; Reynolds, Steward, MacDonald, & Sischo, 2006; Thurber & Weisz, 1997).

In addition, research needs to identify the factors that can contribute to the development of individuals' goal re-engagement processes. It seems likely that these factors are different from the variables that support the development of goal disengagement (Wrosch & Miller, 2009), and they may be associated with processes involved in the attainment of personal goals and the identification and pursuit of new goals (e.g., purpose, optimism, or perceived control; Lachman, 2006; Rasmussen, Wrosch, Scheier, & Carver, 2006; Scheier & Carver, 1985; Scheier et al., 2006). Thus, more comprehensive future studies, involving a variety of predictors, may reveal how people can better adjust to unattainable goals and maintain high levels of subjective well-being and physical health.

Another issue that should be addressed in future research relates to the different functions of self-regulation processes in the association between stressful encounters and physical health outcomes. While the reported research is consistent with the idea that goal adjustment processes can ameliorate the adverse emotional consequences of goal failure and thereby influence adaptive biological functioning and good physical health, recent research from the area of health psychology suggests that personality processes may also moderate the association between biological processes and physical health outcomes. In particular, longitudinal studies have shown that adaptive behaviors and personality functioning (e.g., efficient sleep, low negative affectivity, use of health-related control strategies) can buffer the adverse effects of elevated cortisol level on physical health problems (Wrosch, Miller, Lupien, & Pruessner, 2008; Wrosch, Miller, & Schulz, 2009). This suggests that there are reliable personality–biology interactions in the development of physical health problems, which raises interesting questions about the functions of goal adjustment processes. For example, it would be plausible to assume that goal disengagement and self-protective processes could attenuate the downstream biological consequences of a persistently high cortisol level, and goal re-engagement processes may contribute to new and adaptive behavioral patterns (e.g., seeking medical advice or exercise) that prevent the adverse physical health consequences of dysregulated biological processes. To address these questions, future research should conduct fine-grained longitudinal studies that examine the influence of different self-regulation and biological processes on individuals' physical health outcomes.

The review of the literature also makes it apparent that studies assess general self-regulation tendencies applied across different situations, or examine specific self-regulation behaviors activated in response to an unattainable goal. While both approaches address different and important aspects of self-regulation, there is a lack of research that integrates these approaches. Given that general individual tendencies and specific behaviors may or may not match onto each other (Allport, 1961; Fleeson, 2004; Mischel, 1968), future research is needed that conceptualizes and examines the circumstances under which broader self-regulation tendencies contribute to matching coping or control behaviors and facilitate a person's adjustment to unattainable goals.

Finally, future research should conduct studies that examine the clinical implications of goal adjustment processes. Although clinical scientists and practitioners often focus on techniques that promote individuals' engagement with goals, many of the processes involved in the adjustment of unattainable goals could also be modified through appropriate interventions (cf. Nathan & Gorman, 2007). In this regard, it may be equally important to improve a person's management of unattainable goals, as this could have beneficial consequences for the person's long-term quality of life. In support of this assumption, experimental work that engaged older adults who had life regrets in goal adjustment processes through a writing intervention showed that this intervention prevented the adverse health effects of severe life regrets by ameliorating the experienced intensity of regret (Wrosch, Bauer, Miller, & Lupien, 2007). However, more systematic research is needed to reveal which goal adjustment processes are particularly amendable to interventions, as well as the consequences of effective interventions for subjective well-being and physical health. Future research along these lines can be expected to lead to a more comprehensive understanding of how individuals can adjust to difficult life circumstances and illuminate pathways to subjective well-being and physical health.

Author Note

Preparation of this chapter was supported in part by grants and awards from the Canadian Institutes of Health Research and the Social Science and Humanities Research Council of Canada.

References

Allport, G. W. (1961). *Pattern and growth in personality.* New York: Holt, Rinehart, & Winston.

Aspinwall, L. G., & Richter, L. (1999). Optimism and self-mastery predict more rapid disengagement from unsolvable tasks in the presence of alternatives. *Motivation and Emotion, 23,* 221–45.

Bailis, D. S., Chipperfield, J. G., & Perry, R. P. (2005). Optimistic social comparisons of older adults low in primary control: A prospective analysis of hospitalization and mortality. *Health Psychology, 24,* 393–401.

Baltes, P. B., & Baltes, M. M. (1990). Psychological perspectives on successful aging: The model of selective optimization with compensation. In P. B. Baltes & M. M. Baltes (Eds.), *Successful aging: Perspectives from the behavioral sciences* (pp. 1–34). New York: Cambridge University Press.

Baltes, P. B., Cornelius, S. W., & Nesselroade, J. R. (1979). Cohort effects in developmental psychology. In J. R. Nesselroade & P. B. Baltes (Eds.), *Longitudinal research in the study of behavior and development* (pp. 61–87). New York: Academic Press.

Bandura, A. (1997). *Self-efficacy: The exercise of control.* New York: Freeman.

Bauer, I. (2004). *Unattainable goals across adulthood and old age: Benefits of goal adjustment capacities on well-being.* MA thesis. Concordia University, Montreal, Canada.

Bauer, I., Wrosch, C., & Jobin, J. (2008). I'm better off than most other people: The role of social comparisons for coping with regret in young adulthood and old age. *Psychology and Aging, 23,* 800–11.

Brandtstädter, J. (1990). Entwicklung im Lebenslauf: Ansätze und Probleme der Lebensspannen-Entwicklungspsychologie [Development across the life course: Approaches and problems of life-span psychology]. *Kölner Zeitschrift für Soziologie und Sozialpsychologie, 31,* 322–50.

Brandtstädter, J. (2006). Action perspectives on human development. In R. M. Lerner & W. Damon (Eds.), *Handbook of child psychology* (6th ed.): (Vol 1, Theoretical models of human development, pp. 516–68). Hoboken, NJ: John Wiley & Sons.

Brandtstädter, J., & Renner, G. (1990). Tenacious goal pursuit and flexible goal adjustment: Explication and age-related analysis of assimilative and accommodative strategies of coping. *Psychology and Aging, 5,* 58–67.

Brandtstädter, J., & Rothermund, K. (1994). Self-percepts of control in middle and later adulthood: Buffering losses by rescaling goals. *Psychology and Aging, 9,* 265–73.

Brandtstädter, J., & Rothermund, K. (2002). The life-course dynamics of goal pursuit and goal adjustment: A two process framework. *Developmental Review, 22,* 117–50.

Carver, C. S., & Scheier, M. F. (1981). *Attention and self-regulation: A control-theory approach to human behavior.* New York: Springer Verlag.

Carver, C. S., & Scheier, M. F. (1990). Origins and functions of positive and negative affect: A control-process view. *Psychological Review, 97,* 19–35.

Carver, C. S., & Scheier, M. F. (1998). *On the self-regulation of behavior.* New York: Cambridge University Press.

Carver, C. S., & Scheier, M. F. (2000). Scaling back goals and recalibration of the affect system are aspects of normal adaptive self-regulation: Understanding "Response Shift" phenomena. *Social Science & Medicine, 50,* 1715–22.

Cohen, S. (1996). Psychological stress, immunity, and upper respiratory infections. *Current Direction in Psychological Science, 5,* 86–9.

Cohen, S., Janicki-Deverts, D., & Miller, G. E. (2007). Psychological stress and disease. *Journal of the American Medical Association, 298,* 1685–7.

Dandona, P., Aljada, A., Chaudhuri, A., Mohanty, P., & Garg, R. (2005). Metabolic syndrome: A comprehensive perspective based on interactions between obesity, diabetes, and inflammation. *Circulation, 111,* 1448–54.

Dickerson, S. S., & Kemeny, M. E. (2004). Acute stressors and cortisol responses: A theoretical integration and synthesis of laboratory research. *Psychological Bulletin, 130,* 355–91.

Duke, J., Leventhal, H., Brownlee, S., & Leventhal, E. A. (2002). Giving up and replacing activities in response to illness. *Journal of Gerontology: Psychological Sciences, 57B,* 367–76.

Dunne, E. & Wrosch, C. & Miller, G. E. (2010). Goal disengagement and depressive symptomatology: Reciprocal associations in older adulthood. *Manuscript under review.*

Emmons, R. A. (1986). Personal strivings: An approach to personality and subjective well-being. *Journal of Personality and Social Psychology, 51,* 1058–68.

Fleeson, W. (2004). Moving personality beyond the person-situation debate: The challenge and the opportunity of within-person variability. *Current Directions in Psychological Science, 13,* 83–7.

Folkman, S. (1997). Positive psychological states and coping with severe stress. *Social Science and Medicine, 45,* 1207–21.

Folkman, S., & Greer, S. (2000). Promoting psychological well-being in the face of serious illness: When theory, research, and practice inform each other. *Psycho-Oncology, 9,* 11–9.

Folkman, S., & Lazarus, R. S. (1980). An analysis of coping in a middle-aged community sample. *Journal of Health and Social Behavior, 21,* 219–39.

Folkman, S., Lazarus, R. S., Dunkel-Schetter, C., DeLongis, A., & Gruen, R. J. (1986). Dynamics of a stressful encounter: Cognitive appraisal, coping, and encounter outcome. *Journal of Personality and Social Psychology, 50,* 992–1003.

Folkman, S., & Moskowitz, J. T. (2000). Positive affect and the other side of coping. *American Psychologist, 55,* 647–54.

Freund, A. M., & Baltes, P. B. (2002). Life-management strategies of selection, optimization and compensation: Measurement by self-report and construct validity. *Journal of Personality and Social Psychology, 82,* 642–62.

Heckhausen, J. (1997). Developmental regulation across adulthood: Primary and secondary control of age-related challenges. *Developmental Psychology, 33,* 176–87.

Heckhausen, J. (1999). *Developmental regulation in adulthood.* New York: Cambridge University Press.

Heckhausen, J. (2000). Evolutionary perspectives on motivation. *American Behavioral Scientist, 43,* 1015–29.

Heckhausen, J., & Brim, O. G. (1997). Perceived problems for self and others: Self-protection by social downgrading throughout adulthood. *Psychology and Aging, 12,* 610–9.

Heckhausen, J., & Schulz, R. (1995). A life-span theory of control. *Psychological Review, 102,* 284–304.

Heckhausen, J., Wrosch, C., & Fleeson, W. (2001). Developmental regulation before and after passing a developmental deadline: The sample case of "biological clock" for child-bearing. *Psychology and Aging, 16,* 400–13.

Heckhausen, J., Wrosch, C., & Schulz, R. (2010). A motivational theory of lifespan development. *Psychological Review, 117*, 32–60.

Heim, C., Ehlert, U., & Hellhammer, D. (2000). The potential role of hypocortisolism in the pathophysiology of stress-related bodily disorders. *Psychoneuroendocrinology, 25*, 1–35.

Higgins, E. T. (1987). Self-discrepancy: A theory relating self and affect. *Psychological Review, 94*, 319–40.

Kiecolt-Glaser, J. K., McGuire, L., Robles, T., & Glaser, R. (2002). Emotions, morbidity, and mortality: New perspectives from psychoneuroimmunology. *Annual Review of Psychology, 53*, 83–107.

Klinger, E. (1975). Consequences of commitment to and disengagement from incentives. *Psychological Review, 82*, 1–25.

Kraaij, V., Garnefski, N., & Schroevers, M. J. (2009). Coping, goal adjustments, and positive and negative affect in definitive infertility. *Journal of Health Psychology, 14*, 18–26.

Kraaij, V., Van der Veek, S. M. C., Garnefski, N., Schroevers, M. Witlox, R. & Maes, S. (2008). Coping, goal adjustment, and psychological well-being in HIV-infected men who have sex with men. *AIDS Patient Care and STDs, 22*, 395–402.

Kukla, A. (1972). Foundations of an attributional theory of performance. *Psychological Review, 79*, 454–70.

Lachman, M. E. (2006). Perceived control over aging-related declines: Adaptive beliefs and behaviors. *Current Directions in Psychological Science, 15*, 282–6.

Lazarus, R. S., & Folkman, S. (1984). *Stress, appraisal, and coping*. New York: Springer.

Lupien, S. J., de Leon, M., De Santi, S., Convit, A., et al. (1998). Cortisol levels during human aging predict hippocampal atrophy and memory deficits. *Nature Neuroscience, 1*, 69–73.

Markus, H., & Nurius, P. (1986). Possible selves. *American Psychologist, 41*, 954–69.

Matthews, K.M., Schwartz, J., Cohen, S., & Seeman, T. (2006). Diurnal cortisol decline is related to coronary calcification: CARDIA study. *Psychosomatic Medicine, 68*, 657–61.

McEwen, B. S. (1998). Protective and damaging effects of stress mediators. *New England Journal of Medicine, 338*, 171–9.

Miller, G. E., & Blackwell, E. (2006). Turn up the heat: Inflammation as a mechanism linking chronic stress, depression, and heart disease. *Current Directions in Psychological Science, 15*, 269–72.

Miller, G. E., Chen, E., & Zhou, E. S. (2007). If it goes up, must it come down? Chronic stress and the hypothalamic-pituitary-adrenocortical axis in humans. *Psychological Bulletin, 133*, 25–45.

Miller, G. E., & Wrosch, C. (2007). You've gotta know when to fold 'em: Goal disengagement and systemic inflammation in adolescence. *Psychological Science, 18*, 773–7.

Mischel, W. (1968). *Personality and assessment*. New York: Wiley.

Nathan, P., & Gorman J. (2007). *A guide to treatments that work*. New York: Oxford University Press.

Nesse, R. M. (2000). Is depression an adaptation? *Archives of General Psychiatry, 57*, 14–20.

Neugarten, B.L., & Hagestad, G.O. (1976). Age and the life course. In R. Binstock & E. Shanas (Eds.), *Handbook of aging and social sciences*. New York: Van Nostrand Reinhold.

O'Connor, R. C., Fraser, L., Whyte, M.-C., MacHale, S., & Masterton, G. (2009). Self-regulation of unattainable goals in suicide attempters: The relationship between goal disengagement, goal reengagement and suicidal ideation. *Behaviour Research and Therapy, 47*, 164–9.

O'Connor, R. C., & Forgan, G. (2007). Suicidal thinking and perfectionism: The role of goal adjustment and behavioral inhibition/activation systems. *Journal of Rational-Emotive & Cognitive-Behavior Therapy, 25*, 321–41.

Pressman, S. D., & Cohen, S. (2005). Does positive affect influence health? *Psychological Bulletin, 131*, 925–71.

Rasmussen, H. N., Wrosch, C., Scheier, M. F., & Carver, C. S. (2006). Self-regulation processes and health: The importance of optimism and goal adjustment. *Journal of Personality, 74*, 1721–47.

Reynolds, J., Steward, M., Macdonald, R., & Sischo, L. (2006). Have adolescents become too ambitious? High school seniors' educational and occupational plans, 1976 to 2000. *Social Problems, 53*, 186–206.

Ryff, C. D. (1989). Happiness is everything, or is it? Explorations on the meaning of psychological well-being. *Journal of Personality and Social Psychology, 57*, 1069–81.

Rothermund, K., & Brandtstädter, J. (2003). Coping with deficits and losses in later life: From compensatory action to accommodation. *Psychology and Aging, 18*, 896–905.

Salmela-Aro, K., & Suikkari, A-M. (2008). Letting go of your dreams: adjustment of child-related goal appraisals and depressive symptoms during infertility treatment. *Journal of Research in Personality, 42*, 988–1003.

Scheier, M. F., & Carver, C. S. (1985). Optimism, coping, and health: Assessment and implications of generalized outcome expectancies. *Health Psychology, 4*, 219–47.

Scheier, M. F., & Carver, C. S. (2001). Adapting to cancer: The importance of hope and purpose. In A. Baum & B. L. Andersen (Eds.), *Psychosocial interventions for cancer* (pp. 15–36). Washington, DC: American Psychological Association.

Scheier, M. F., Magovern, G. J., Abbott, R. A., Matthews, K. A., Owens, J. F., Craig Lefebvre, R., & Carver, C.S. (1989). Dispositional optimism and recovery from coronary artery bypass surgery: The beneficial effects on physical and psychological well-being. *Journal of Personality and Social Psychology, 57*, 1024–40.

Scheier, M. F., Wrosch, C., Baum, A., Cohen, S., Martire, L. M., Matthews, K. A., et al. (2006). The Life Engagement Test: Assessing purpose in life. *Journal of Behavioral Medicine, 29*, 291–8.

Schroevers, M., Kraaij, V., & Garnefski, N. (2008). How do cancer patients manage unattainable personal goals and regulate their emotions? *British Journal of Health Psychology, 13*, 551–62.

Schulz, R., & Heckhausen, J. (1996). A life span model of successful aging. *American Psychologist, 51*, 702–14.

Segerstrom, S. C., & Miller, G. E. (2004). Stress and the human immune system:A meta-analytic review of 30 years of inquiry. *Psychological Bulletin, 130*, 601–30.

Seligman, M. E. P. (1975). *Helplessness*. San Francisco: Freeman.

Sephton, S. E., Sapolsky, R. M., Kraemer, H. C., & Spiegel, D. (2000). Diurnal cortisol rhythm as a predictor of breast cancer survival. *Journal of the National Cancer Institute, 92*, 994–1000.

Smyth, J. M., Ockenfels, M. C., Gorin, A. A., Catley, D., et al. (1997). Individual differences in the diurnal cycle of cortisol. *Psychoneuroendocrinology, 22*, 89–105.

Sprangers, M. A. G., & Schwartz, C. E. (1999). Integrating response shift into health-related quality of life research: A theoretical model. *Social Science & Medicine, 48*, 1507–15.

Taylor, S. E., & Brown, J. D. (1988). Illusion and well-being: A social psychological perspective on mental health. *Psychological Bulletin, 103*, 193–210.

Thurber, C. A., & Weisz, J. R. (1997). "You can try or you can just give up": The impact of perceived control and coping style on childhood homesickness. *Developmental Psychology, 33*, 508–17.

Tunali, B., & Power, T. G. (1993). Creating satisfaction: A psychological perspective on stress and coping in families of handicapped children. *Journal of Child Psychology and Psychiatry and Allied Disciplines, 34*, 945–57.

Watson, D., Clark, L. A., & Tellegen, A. (1988). Development and validation of brief measures of positive and negative affect: The PANAS Scales. *Journal of Personality and Social Psychology, 54*, 1063–70.

Webster, J.,& Tiggemann, M. (2003). The relationship between women's body satisfaction and self-image across the life span: The role of cognitive control. *Journal of Genetic Psychology, 164*, 241–52.

Weitzenkamp, D. A., Gerhart, K. A., Charlifue, S. W., Whiteneck, G. G., Glass, C. A., & Kennedy, P. (2000). Ranking the criteria for assessing quality of life after disability: Evidence for priority shifting among long-term spinal cord injury survivors. *British Journal of Health Psychology, 5*, 57–69.

Willerson, J. T.,& Ridker, P. M. (2004). Inflammation as a cardiovascular risk factor. *Circulation, 109*, 2–10.

Wortman, C. B., & Brehm, J. W. (1975). Responses to uncontrollable outcomes: An integration of reactance theory and the learned helplessness model. In L. Berkowitz (Ed.), *Advances in experimental socialpsychology* (Vol. 8, pp. 277–336). New York: Academic Press.

Wright, R. A., & Brehm, J. W. (1989). Energization and goal attractiveness. In L. A. Pervin (Ed.), *Goal concepts in personality and social psychology* (pp. 169–210). Hillsdale, NJ: Erlbaum.

Wrosch, C., Bauer, I., Miller, G. E., & Lupien, S. (2007). Regret intensity, diurnal cortisol secretion, and physical health in older individuals: Evidence for directional effects and protective factors. *Psychology and Aging, 22*, 319–30.

Wrosch, C., Bauer, I., & Scheier, M. F. (2005). Regret and quality of life across the adult life span: The influence of disengagement and available future goals. *Psychology and Aging, 20*, 657–70.

Wrosch, C., Dunne, E., Scheier, M. F., & Schulz, R. (2006). Self-regulation of common age-related challenges: Benefits for older adults' psychological and physical health. *Journal of Behavioral Medicine, 29*, 299–306.

Wrosch, C., & Freund, A. M. (2001). Self-regulation of normative and non-normative developmental challenges. *Human Development, 44*, 264–83.

Wrosch, C., & Heckhausen, J. (1999). Control processes before and after passing a developmental deadline: Activation and deactivation of intimate relationship goals. *Journal of Personality and Social Psychology, 77*, 415–27.

Wrosch, C., & Heckhausen, J. (2002). Perceived control of life regrets: Good for young and bad for old adults. *Psychology and Aging, 17*, 340–50.

Wrosch, C., Heckhausen, J., & Lachman, M. E. (2000). Primary and secondary control strategies for managing health and financial stress across adulthood. *Psychology and Aging, 15*, 387–99.

Wrosch, C., & Miller, G. E. (2009). Depressive symptoms can be useful: Self-regulatory and emotional benefits of dysphoric mood in adolescence. *Journal of Personality and Social Psychology, 96*, 1181–90.

Wrosch, C., Miller, G. E., Lupien, S., & Pruessner, J. C. (2008). Diurnal cortisol secretion and 2-year changes in older adults' acute physical symptoms: The moderating roles of negative affect and sleep. *Health Psychology, 27*, 685–93.

Wrosch, C., Miller, G. E., Scheier, M. F., & Brun de Pontet, S. (2007). Giving up on unattainable goals: Benefits for health? *Personality and Social Psychology Bulletin, 33*, 251–65.

Wrosch, C., Miller, G. E., & Schulz, R. (2009). Cortisol secretion and functional disabilities in old age: The importance of using adaptive control strategies. *Psychosomatic Medicine, 71*, 996–1003.

Wrosch, C., & Scheier, M. F. (2003). Personality and quality of life: The importance of optimism and goal adjustment. *Quality of Life Research, 12*, 59–72.

Wrosch, C, Scheier, M. F., Carver, C. S., & Schulz, R. (2003). The importance of goal disengagement in adaptive self-regulation: When giving up is beneficial. *Self and Identity, 2*, 1–20.

Wrosch, C., Scheier, M. F., Miller, G. E., Schulz, R., & Carver, C. S. (2003). Adaptive self-regulation of unattainable goals: Goal disengagement, goal reengagement, and subjective well-being. *Personality and Social Psychology Bulletin, 29*, 1494–508.

Wrosch, C., & Schulz, R. (2008). Health engagement control strategies and 2-year changes in older adults' physical health. *Psychological Science, 19*, 536–40.

Wrosch, C., Schulz, R., & Heckhausen, J. (2004). Health stresses and depressive symptomatology in the elderly. A control-process approach. *Current Directions in Psychological Science, 13*, 17–20.

Future-Oriented Thinking, Proactive Coping, and the Management of Potential Threats to Health and Well-Being

Lisa G. Aspinwall

Abstract

Proactive coping is the process of anticipating potential stressors and acting in advance either to prevent them or to mute their impact (Aspinwall & Taylor, 1997). This chapter reviews diverse approaches to defining and studying proactivity and highlights applications of the proactive coping concept to the domains of aging, stigma and discrimination, organizational behavior, and health, including genetic testing, health promotion, medical decision-making, and the management of chronic illness. Recent process-oriented interventions demonstrate that proactive approaches to managing health and aging can be taught, with sustained gains in both proactive competence and health outcomes. Continued integration of efforts to understand and improve proactive coping with insights into the social-cognitive processes underlying future-oriented thinking more generally will serve to further inform our understanding of the personal and social resources, individual differences, and component processes that underlie successful proactivity, as will increased attention to the affective and transactional qualities of proactive coping.

Keywords: proactive coping, prevention, future-oriented thinking, self-regulation, aging, discrimination, genetic testing, chronic illness, individual differences, worry

Introduction

Whether we are considering how health, investment, interpersonal, or environmental choices made now will affect us in the years to come, or how current events (a positive genetic test result, an economic recession, a racially prejudiced employer, climate change) will influence our future options and outcomes, our views of the future play a major role in mental life, as we *think through, prepare for, and potentially act to alter* what we believe to be in store for ourselves and our loved ones.

The process of *proactive coping* involves anticipating and/or detecting potential stressors and acting in advance either to prevent them altogether

or to mute their impact (Aspinwall & Taylor, 1997; Aspinwall, 1997a, 2001, 2005). As such, proactive coping blends activities typically considered to be *coping* (activities undertaken to master, reduce, or tolerate environmental or intrapsychic demands perceived as representing potential threat, existing harm, or loss; Folkman & Lazarus, 1985; Lazarus & Folkman, 1984) with those considered to be *self-regulation* (the processes through which people control, direct, and correct their own actions as they move toward or away from various goals; Aspinwall, 2001; Carver & Scheier, 1998; Fiske & Taylor, 1991). Proactive coping combines these two processes by examining people's emotions, thoughts, and behaviors as they anticipate and address potential sources of adversity that might interfere with the pursuit of their goals (Aspinwall & Taylor, 1997).

It is important from the outset to distinguish proactive coping from other forms of coping in advance, such as anticipatory coping. The cardinal property of proactive coping is the possibility of altering one's outcomes by responding to a potential stressor prior to or early in its development, whereas anticipatory coping refers to efforts to brace oneself for the expected consequences of a known and imminent stressor (Aspinwall, Sechrist, & Jones, 2005; Aspinwall & Taylor, 1997; McGrath & Beehr, 1990; Shepperd, Ouellette, & Fernandez, 1996). Accordingly, a central tenet of the proactive coping model is the notion that many (but by no means all) potential stressors related to health, work, social life, and aging allow for preparatory thoughts and actions that may either prevent anticipated negative events or serve to reduce their magnitude and impact (Aspinwall & Taylor, 1997; see also Kahana & Kahana, 1996, 2003).

Chapter Overview

In this chapter, we will review the original Aspinwall and Taylor (1997) proactive coping formulation, distinguish it from related approaches, and consider recent extensions of it, including successful interventions that have been derived from the model. We will review research contributions in new domains of application for the proactivity concept, such as the management of stigma and discrimination, predictive genetic testing for familial disease, health promotion, and the management of chronic illness. Throughout the review, we will also consider what is known about individual differences and situational moderators of proactivity—that is, who undertakes proactive coping efforts, and what determines whether such efforts will be successful? Our discussion of these issues will examine the diverse approaches to defining and measuring proactivity that characterize current research, as well as an emerging literature on the sociodemographics of proactivity. We will also consider whether and in what ways the potential for proactive coping may differ across different situations (for example, educational and occupational stressors vs. those related to health and aging, Aspinwall, 2005; or interpersonal stressors vs. other stressors; cf. Sansone & Berg, 1993; Mallett & Swim, 2005; Ouwehand, de Ridder, & Bensing, 2006).

Finally, because proactive coping inherently involves the consideration of future outcomes, proactive coping may bring to bear a different set of skills and processes involved in trying to understand, predict, and alter various future possibilities than the more reactive kinds of coping efforts that are more typically studied. For this reason, this chapter will also examine recent developments in the study of future-oriented thinking that may have important implications for understanding whether, how, and with what success proactive coping efforts may be undertaken, as well as the kinds of goals that people seek to manage proactively. Our review will highlight specific interventions designed to promote proactive management of health threats that have profitably drawn on these evolving insights into the processes that link different kinds of future-oriented thinking to human action.

Conceptual Approaches to Understanding the Proactive Management of Threats to Health and Well-Being
Defining proactivity

In this section, we will review diverse approaches to defining and studying proactivity in different domains. As we will see, although these frameworks share a common concern with people's active efforts to understand and shape the situations they face, their definitions of proactivity differ in the nature and timing of the behaviors described, as well as in their fundamental goal (e.g., develop or preserve resources, offset incipient problems, create new opportunities). Some authors use the terms *proactive coping* (Aspinwall & Taylor, 1997) or *proactive adaptations* (Kahana & Kahana, 1996) to refer to efforts undertaken in advance to develop or preserve resources useful in coping with subsequent problems. Efforts to identify, understand, and address problems early in their development would still be termed proactive coping in the process model developed by Aspinwall and Taylor but would be termed *corrective adaptations* in the Kahana and Kahana framework. Other authors use the terms *proactivity* or *proactive coping* to refer primarily to the creation of new opportunities, including self-imposed goals and challenges (Crant, 2000; Schwarzer & Knoll, 2003), and refer to efforts to offset potential problems as *preventive coping* (Greenglass, 2002; Greenglass, Schwarzer, & Tauber, 1999; Schwarzer, 2000). Others use related terms such as *personal initiative* to describe efforts both to overcome problems and to develop new opportunities (Frese, Kring, Soose, & Zempel, 1996).

An intriguingly parsimonious alternative definition was recently proposed by Grant and Ashford (2008), who suggested that proactive behaviors are not necessarily a different set of behaviors, but instead are any behavior undertaken *in advance* of a stressful situation—that is, what makes a behavior proactive is its timing rather than its specific form. For example, one may seek feedback proactively or not, and one may build social networks proactively or not. This broad and appealing definition has the potential to expand the study of proactivity by directing researchers' attention to a wide variety of behaviors that may be enacted in advance. However, by suggesting that the component activities of proactive coping are the same as those involved in more reactive ways of managing situations, this definition of proactivity risks underemphasizing some of the forward-looking processes involved in anticipating potential stressors, running them forward in time to see how they might develop, and considering alternative ways to address them (Aspinwall & Taylor, 1997). Further, research on future-oriented thinking indicates that multiple aspects of the way we consider relatively distant-future events and outcomes differ considerably from how we consider present or near-future events and outcomes (see, e.g., Trope & Liberman, 2003; Liberman & Trope, 2008). Thus, a complete account of the activities and skills involved in proactive coping is likely to involve some unique aspects that may not be present in responding to current stressors or opportunities.

Proactive coping as prevention-focused versus promotion-focused coping

The distinction between prevention-oriented and promotion-oriented forms of self-regulation (Higgins, 1997) is just beginning to be applied to the proactive coping literature (see Grant & Ashford, 2008, and Swim & Thomas, 2006, for discussion). This work distinguishes between the motivational and emotional antecedents and consequences of efforts to prevent negative outcomes and efforts to attain positive outcomes. This distinction applies well to frameworks that distinguish between preventive and proactive coping by defining *preventive coping* as efforts to prepare for uncertain events in the long run (as by building general resistance resources that would minimize the impact of potential future events) and *proactive coping* as efforts to build resources that facilitate promotion-oriented goals and personal growth (Greenglass, 2002; Greenglass, Schwarzer, & Tauber, 1999; Schwarzer, 2000;

Schwarzer & Knoll, 2003). In contrast, the Aspinwall and Taylor and Kahana and Kahana formulations, with their emphasis on either preventing problems or reducing their impact, may be more clearly conceptualized as prevention-focused coping. However, as the present review will discuss, it may not be the case that proactive coping is inherently or always prevention-oriented, even with our current focus on the advance detection and management of potential problems. For example, in their discussion of multiple goals that people may adopt in managing anticipated discrimination, Swim and Thomas (2006) point out that someone may approach such a situation with prevention-oriented goals, such as avoidance, prevention of harm to the self, and efforts not to confirm a stereotype, or with promotion-oriented goals, such as demonstrating competence, validating the self, and/or educating a perpetrator (see also Umaña-Taylor, Vargas-Chanes, Garcia, & Gonzales-Backen, 2008). As this example illustrates, proactive coping can serve to meet multiple goals in different situations and may thus resist neat classification as always or inherently prevention-oriented.

That said, there may be some important advantages to conceptualizing proactive coping as prevention-oriented, not least of which is the idea that in this perspective people are more clearly *coping* with potential harm, threat, or loss. Working toward an innovation, improved opportunity, or new accomplishment does not necessarily carry with it the idea that one is managing a potential threat and thus may not invoke twin needs to manage both potential problems and the emotions generated by their consideration. Because our approach to proactivity involves acting in advance to avert or reduce unfavorable outcomes, we believe it is more closely allied to the topics typically considered in the stress and coping literature than are the more promotion-oriented approaches to proactivity.

Expanding the study of proactivity beyond the achievement setting

There are some other important differences between the achievement-oriented settings and goals typically considered in the educational and occupational domains and the potential stressors encountered in other life domains, such as health, aging, and close relationships, that are likely important to understanding proactive coping (see Aspinwall, 2005, for discussion). Specifically, the organizational settings in which such promotion-oriented concepts as personal initiative and proactive personality are studied share common features with many other achievement situations, in that people are free to set goals that they are likely to meet if they acquire realistic information about them and apply sufficient effort (see, e.g., Sohl & Moyer, 2009). Such settings also typically afford opportunities to change and improve one's situation and even to create entirely new situations. In contrast, potential stressors related to stigma and discrimination, preparation for natural or technological disasters, genetic risk for disease, physical disability, chronic illness, and aging are not as amenable to change through personal effort and explicitly involve the consideration of likely, and even inevitable, harm and loss (Aspinwall, 1997b, 2005; Aspinwall et al., 2005).

Of course, the point of this discussion is not to say that one could not take a promotion-oriented approach to the challenges of health and aging (see, e.g., Fiksenbaum, Greenglass, & Eaton, 2006; Greenglass, Marques, deRidder, & Behl, 2005) or to argue that educational and workplace settings are stress-free, but instead to highlight the idea that proactive approaches to stressors in such domains as health and aging necessarily involve the consideration and management of potential harm and loss in ways that many occupational and educational situations do not. Put differently, preparing for aging is inherently different from preparing for an exam or earning a degree, not only in the activities involved, but also in the constraints placed on what one can achieve or sustain. Thus, although people may act in advance to pursue promotion-oriented goals or may construe potentially stressful developmental transitions in promotion-oriented terms, the present review will focus on proactive efforts taken to anticipate and ward off potential threats to health and well-being, and thus will focus on future-oriented thoughts, emotions, and behaviors directed toward situations that are often both undesirable and beyond one's complete control, but that may be proactively understood, prepared for, and managed nonetheless.

The Aspinwall and Taylor (1997) proactive coping model

The original Aspinwall and Taylor (1997) proactive coping model specified five interrelated steps involved in efforts to detect and respond to potential stressors. As shown in Figure 17.1, the first step, *resource accumulation*, refers to efforts to build general resources and skills in advance of any specific anticipated stressor. Such resources may involve

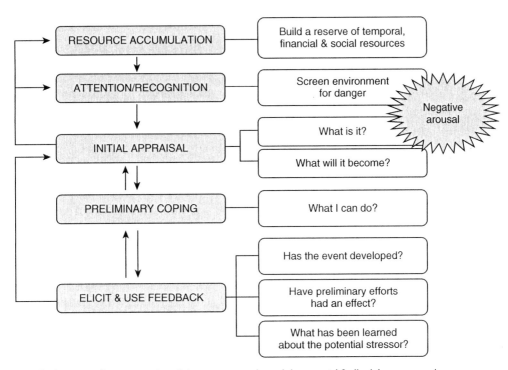

Fig. 17.1 The five stages of proactive coping, their component tasks, and the potential feedback loops among them.
(Figure adapted with permission, © American Psychological Association and L. G. Aspinwall and S. E. Taylor [1997])

personal resources, such as time, money, and energy; social resources, such as information and social support; and skills, such as those involved in planning and organization (cf. Hobfoll, 1989, and Chapter 7 in the present volume). The next step, *attention to and recognition of potential stressors*, involves screening the environment and/or reflecting on one's prospects in order to detect potential or incipient stressors. After a potential stressor has been detected, an *initial appraisal* step involves preliminary assessments of what a potential situation is and what it may become, as well as whether it should be monitored as a potential threat. Next, *preliminary coping efforts* are activities undertaken either to prevent or minimize a recognized or suspected stressor. The last step involves the *elicitation and use of feedback* about both the nature and development of a potential stressor and the effects of one's preliminary efforts on it. This feedback may be used to revise one's appraisals of the potential stressor and to modify one's strategies for addressing it.

Three aspects of the model merit attention with respect to the present review. The first is that the proactive coping model and its component activities are explicitly *forward-looking*. Key tasks of proactive coping involve detecting potential stressors and simulating multiple future forms they may take. Accordingly, multiple social-cognitive skills and processes involved in future-oriented thinking are explicitly part of the model (Aspinwall, 2005; Aspinwall & Taylor, 1997). The second is that the model, in the spirit of the original stress and coping formulation, is *transactional* (Lazarus & Folkman, 1984; Lazarus, 1990). As shown in Figure 17.1, the multiple feedback loops in the model represent the recursive nature of this process as people respond to incipient stressful situations that unfold and change over time and vary their appraisals and efforts accordingly. Because potential or incipient stressors are by definition not fully developed, key challenges of proactive coping involve regulating one's attention to a potential stressor and accumulating both general and specific resources to address it as a function of one's initial appraisals of its nature and potential. Further, preliminary coping efforts—specifically, active preliminary coping efforts—are thought to play a role in eliciting information about the nature of the stressor in ways that may influence its management. A central prediction of the proactive coping model is that active forms of information-seeking and problem-solving are more likely to yield information about a potential stressor than are more avoidant forms of coping (see also Aspinwall, 2001; Aspinwall, Richter, & Hoffman, 2001).

A third key element of the model, represented by the *negative arousal* starburst in Figure 17.1, is the presence of negative emotions that may occur as one detects a potential threat to health and well-being. As suggested earlier, what makes proactive coping different from other kinds of promotion-oriented planning and self-regulatory activity is the active consideration of potential negative outcomes that are serious and enduring. Although a central prediction of the proactive coping model is that potential stressors are likely to create fewer negative emotions and other demands than more fully developed stressors, consideration of potential stressors (e.g., Will I lose my job? Will my instructor discriminate against me? Is it time for a cancer screening? Where will I live when I am unable to care for myself? Is there still time to prevent climate change?) may evoke negative thoughts and feelings, such as alarm or worry. Understanding how such thoughts and feelings influence subsequent stages of the model, such as initial appraisals, preliminary coping efforts, and the use of feedback, is an important and relatively understudied research question. Such thoughts may keep an issue at the fore of one's attention and thus potentiate efforts to prepare for or reduce the threat (Aspinwall et al., 2005; Magnan, Köblitz, Zielke, & McCaul, 2009; McCaul & Mullens, 2003; Norem & Cantor, 1986; Ouwehand, 2005; see also Thoolen, de Ridder, Bensing, Gorter, & Rutten, 2008a). Alternately, negative thoughts and feelings may prioritize emotion-management concerns and thereby divert attention and other resources away from responding to the incipient problem itself (see, e.g., Leith & Baumeister, 1996). Some negative states also have the potential to narrow attention in ways that may compromise both the accuracy of initial appraisals and responsiveness to subsequent feedback about them (see Aspinwall & Taylor, 1997, for review). As these examples illustrate, the recognition that thoughts and feelings about potential stressors in important life domains—our worries, hopes, and fears—are unlikely to be neutral or pallid suggests the necessity of understanding the nature and impact of such thoughts and feelings on different stages of the proactive coping process.

Potential advantages and disadvantages of proactive coping

Consistent with our original title ("A stitch in time saves nine"), the primary advantages of proactive coping likely involve the more modest resource costs of addressing problems earlier in their course and the corresponding reduction in exposure to stress. To the extent that such efforts are successful, the traditional order of the stress and coping process may be reversed: proactive coping may serve to keep chronic stress under control by building resources in advance, by preserving resources through effective early management of potential problems, and by reducing an individual's total stress exposure. Further, we noted that proactive efforts to manage potential or emerging stressors may offer greater coping options and a more favorable ratio of resources to demands at the proactive stage than at later stages, either because resources have not yet been depleted or because the problem has not yet assumed its final form (Aspinwall & Taylor, 1997).

We also identified some potential disadvantages of efforts to address problems prior to or early in their development. The first of these is that a potential stressor to which one may have devoted considerable attention and other resources may not materialize, in which case one has wasted one's efforts. Such costs may, however, be at least partially offset by increased knowledge about the potential stressor and/or the state of one's general resources. For example, a person who prepares for a hurricane that does not ultimately land in her region now has a disaster kit, materials to protect her windows, and information about hurricane safety. A second potential disadvantage is that if one begins coping with a problem prior to having complete information about it, one may "jump the gun" and cope in ineffective ways that may exacerbate the problem.

Third, proactive efforts undertaken without good information about the nature of the problem and the accompanying skills involved in evaluating solutions to problems and responding to feedback can actually backfire. For example, if a tendency to engage in proactive efforts is not moderated by the likelihood of potential problems, proactivity may lead to the excessive devotion of effort to acquiring information about relatively unlikely problems (Newby-Clark, 2004). Poor skill in judging situations may also lead to proactive efforts that backfire. In a cross-sectional study, Chan (2006) found that situational judgment effectiveness, assessed via a test of responses to hypothetical workplace problems, sharply moderated the link between proactive personality and workplace success. Proactivity was linked to better workplace outcomes for employees with high scores on the situational judgment test, but to lower job satisfaction and social integration at work and lower performance ratings from supervisors among employees with low scores on the test.

Finally, proactivity may also have some important social costs. The workplace proactivity literature suggests that proactive efforts to obtain information or to exert influence in the workplace can backfire if they are perceived as stemming from image concerns, as overly frequent, or as insufficiently responsive to feedback. In such cases, proactive efforts may create an impression of the actor as insecure or incompetent (for reviews, see Ashford, Blatt, & VandeWalle, 2003; Grant & Ashford, 2008).

Evidence of Proactive Coping in Different Domains

At the time the proactive coping model was developed, there were few empirical approaches to documenting proactivity or to understanding the specific situations in which it was more or less likely to be enacted (see workplace proactivity studies by Ashford & Black, 1996; Ashford & Cummings, 1983, 1985; and Morrison, 1993a,b; and Sansone & Berg's 1993 study of everyday problem-solving for notable exceptions). Fortunately, there is now a great deal more research evidence available to document proactive coping and the specific forms it may take in different domains. Also, the advent of controlled interventions based on the proactive coping model allows for an understanding of the specific components of proactive coping that may produce benefits, as well as an understanding of the nature and duration of such benefits. Finally, the research base for understanding proactive coping has been expanded not only by considering proactivity in multiple life domains, but also by applying a diverse array of research methods, such as daily diary studies (Mallett & Swim, 2005, 2009), laboratory studies (Mallett & Swim, 2005; Newby-Clark, 2004), and vignette studies (Chan, 2006; Ouwehand, de Ridder & Bensing, 2006), to an increasingly diverse set of respondents. In the following sections, we will review this new evidence concerning the prevalence, nature, and adaptiveness of proactive coping in different domains.

Proactive coping with stigma and discrimination

Frequent, even daily experiences with stigma and discrimination have been linked to a variety of negative mental and physical health outcomes

(Clark, Anderson, Clark, & Williams, 1999; Huebner, Rebchook, & Kegeles, 2004; Meyer, 2003; Pascoe & Smart Richman, 2009; Sellers & Shelton, 2003). In line with an increasing emphasis in the field of social psychology on understanding the experiences of the targets of stereotyping, prejudice, and discrimination (Miller & Major, 2000; Swim & Stangor, 1998; Swim & Thomas, 2006), researchers have increasingly turned their attention to proactive approaches that members of stigmatized groups may take in order to anticipate, detect, and respond to such treatment. Evidence from laboratory experiments and daily diary studies documents the multifaceted efforts of racial and ethnic minorities and members of other stigmatized groups, such as overweight individuals, to be alert to signs that they are being judged negatively and to act to counter such efforts. Such activities may involve highly active primary-control-oriented strategies designed to influence a prejudiced person's impressions through greater preparation (Mallett & Swim, 2005; Miller & Myers, 1998), more careful dress, the use of humor and other social skills, greater attention to or engagement with interaction partners (Frable, Blackstone, & Scherbaum, 1990; Shelton, Richeson, & Salvatore, 2005), or direct confrontation or discussion (Kaiser & Miller, 2004; Umaña-Taylor et al., 2008). Alternatively, potentially stigmatized individuals may avoid potentially prejudiced people or situations or mentally disengage from goal pursuit (see Mallett & Swim, 2009; Swim & Thomas, 2006, for reviews). At the extreme end, efforts to avoid stigma and discrimination may involve complex and demanding forms of concealment (e.g., being closeted, "passing"), which have been shown to exact a toll on mental and physical health (Cole, Kemeny, Taylor, Visscher, & Fahey, 1996; Pachankis, 2007).

In the following section, we will review evidence for proactive coping with stigma and discrimination, including striking evidence that proactive strategies may either reduce or eliminate negative consequences before or during a potentially stressful event. In an intriguing experimental demonstration of this phenomenon, Miller, Rothblum, Felicio, and Brand (1995) found that when overweight middle-aged women believed that an interaction partner could see them on a TV monitor during the course of a telephone conversation, they were able to compensate somehow and did not receive lower evaluations of social skill than normal-weight women; however, when overweight women thought that observers could not see them, they apparently did not engage in compensatory behavior and received lower ratings. These intriguing initial findings suggested that stigmatized participants were aware in advance that they would be judged negatively and were able to alter their behavior in order to counter discriminatory evaluations. However, objective ratings of audiotapes and videotapes of the interactions for both conversational content and nonverbal behavior did not reveal what it was that obese participants who thought they were visible to their interaction partners did differently or what obese participants who thought they were not visible neglected to do.

In an Internet-era twist on this study, Mallett and Swim (2005) used a video-dating manipulation to create a high-impact laboratory experiment to examine behavioral and interpersonal outcomes of overweight women's efforts to manage potential discrimination based on body size. Women who perceived themselves to be overweight were asked to prepare a videotaped interview for an online dating profile to be shown to an attractive potential dating partner. Importantly, each participant was led to believe that the potential partner had received a full-length digital photo of her at the beginning of the session. Participants completed measures of primary and secondary appraisals of the impending interview session (e.g., "I am afraid that my interaction partner will not like me," "I think I will be able to convey the type of person that I really am in my introduction") and then were videotaped as they prepared for the interview. These preparation sessions were coded for time spent reviewing information about how to create a speech, planning one's introduction, grooming, and doing off-task activities, such as reading magazines or playing games on one's cell phone. Participants then created videotaped introductions to be used for the study of online dating and ostensibly shown to the attractive male partner.

The results indicated that perceived weight (but not actual BMI) was associated with greater primary appraisals of potential harm and lower secondary appraisals of ability to manage potential harm. However, women who perceived themselves to be more heavy spent significantly more time preparing their videotaped introductions, and these efforts were clearly successful: Objective ratings of the taped performances indicated that greater preparations resulted in higher subsequent ratings of intelligence, competence, and likability. Thus, women who were most concerned about being judged unfavorably "upped their game" and succeeded in establishing themselves as intelligent, competent, and likable. These experimental studies suggest that when the potential for discrimination is made salient, people who are frequent targets of discrimination may compensate in advance and successfully influence how they are judged.

In an intriguing program of research, Mallett and Swim (2005; 2009) have used daily diary methodology to examine everyday situations in which stigmatized people anticipate discrimination and act either to prevent or avoid it or to respond to it early in the course of an unfolding interaction. In their first such study, Mallett and Swim (2005) examined overweight women's efforts to prevent discriminatory versus nondiscriminatory interpersonal hassles. Sixty-two female participants (a mix of college students and adult community members) used daily diaries for seven days to document their efforts either to prevent such hassles or to respond to them early in their course. Participants were asked specifically to focus only on stressors that involved other people in some way. Discriminatory hassles were predicted to produce (1) higher primary appraisals of harm than nondiscriminatory hassles, as discriminatory treatment based on a core component of one's identity indicates that one is socially devalued, and (2) lower secondary appraisals of resources, as discrimination is difficult to deter. Specific ways of coping with either anticipated or unfolding interactions were derived from the proactive coping model (Aspinwall & Taylor, 1997) and work on how stigmatized individuals manage self-presentation (Miller & Myers, 1998) and devote increased attention to their interaction partners (Frable et al., 1990). Study outcomes included intrapersonal costs and benefits of such efforts.

In total, participants reported 269 discriminatory and 236 nondiscriminatory hassles, with the vast majority of hassles being identified as potentially stressful during, rather than before, the actual interaction. Secondary control coping efforts, such as those involving monitoring one's thoughts, regulating one's emotions, and maintaining self-control when in a stressful situation, were reported in upwards of 92 percent of the situations and were reported more frequently than various primary control strategies directed toward monitoring and altering the situation, which were reportedly used from 54 percent to 86 percent of the time. Specific primary control strategies included emphasizing one's intelligence and other positive attributes, paying extra attention to grooming and clothing, and using humor to counter derogatory remarks and other forms of disrespect. As predicted, discriminatory stressors were perceived as more harmful than nondiscriminatory stressors, and participants perceived fewer resources for coping with them. The results also indicated that discriminatory stressors prompted higher levels of both primary and secondary control-oriented coping than nondiscriminatory ones. Importantly, as was the case with the video-dating study, greater reports of primary control-oriented coping predicted greater self-rated success at preventing negative outcomes.

These data reveal important information about the frequency with which stigmatized individuals must manage discriminatory hassles (more than four times per week on average) and also the specific appraisals and coping efforts employed to manage not only the unfolding situation, but also its impact on their emotions and self-worth. Mallett and Swim (2009) have recently extended this work to examine how African Americans living in a predominantly white rural community cope with anticipated discrimination on a daily basis. They predicted that African Americans may have more experience dealing with discrimination because their minority status is conferred at birth, whereas overweight may be acquired at different times in life. Respondents were 77 African Americans, mostly women college students, ages 18 to 33, who lived in a rural college town in the Mid-Atlantic United States. Participants first completed a retrospective account of their typical use of proactive coping with discrimination and then completed daily diary studies for the next seven days. In both assessments, participants were asked about the degree to which they practiced a variety of proactive strategies in response to potential discrimination based on race/ethnicity.

The results revealed considerable reported practice of proactive coping with racism, with 83 percent of respondents indicating that they did things to cope with racism before it happened or while it was happening. A factor analysis revealed evidence for three distinct sets of strategies for proactive coping with racism: *self-focused efforts* to attend to one's own thoughts, emotions, behavior, and performance, and to maintain self-control; *situation-focused efforts* to pay attention to the unfolding interaction and monitor its potential for discrimination, including monitoring nonverbal responses, such as an interaction partner's eye contact or body position, and less frequently, to alter the situation by trying to educate a prejudiced person about African Americans as a group; and *physical avoidance* of, or early departure from, situations that might involve racism in order to minimize stress. In both the retrospective and daily reports, self-focused coping strategies were endorsed to a greater extent than both situation-focused strategies and physical avoidance. Consistent with the authors' findings regarding weight-based discrimination, participants' primary appraisals of harm, loss, and threat predicted greater reports of all three kinds of proactive coping with racism; secondary appraisals, however, were unrelated to reports of proactive coping.

There were also some interesting differences between the retrospective and daily diary reports that have implications for the interpretation of retrospective self-report measures of proactive coping. Specifically, the diary reports showed significantly greater reports of avoidance and self-focused forms of coping and significantly lower reports of situation-focused proactive coping than participants reported in their retrospective accounts of how they typically handled racial discrimination. It is important to note that the retrospective assessment did not cover the same time period as the daily diary reports and thus cannot be interpreted as a direct comparison of these different methods of reporting on the same events. The authors suggest that several factors may lead people to remember using situation-focused coping more than they actually do— the pressure of the immediate situation and potential costs of confronting racism are high (see also Swim & Thomas, 2006), and although many people report that they would confront a perpetrator in situations involving racism or sexism, few do when actually faced with the situation (see, e.g., Kawakami, Dunn, Karmali, & Dovidio, 2009). The authors also suggest that the events that people considered when they completed the retrospective coping assessment might have been more firmly categorized as blatantly discriminatory, while the events reported in the daily assessments could have been more ambiguous or subtle in nature. Finally, the greater reports of self-focused proactive coping in the daily diaries compared to the general retrospective accounts suggest that actions such as trying to educate a racist and alter his or her view of oneself and one's group may be more salient and more easily remembered over time than either subtle behaviors or non-actions, such as increases in self-focused attention or behavioral avoidance. This last possibility highlights the importance of using daily diaries and other approaches to measuring proactivity as it happens in order to capture cases in which proactive coping may be represented by subtle forms of behavior, including inaction.

Work in the area of discrimination and stigma is unique in its focus on both intra- and interpersonal outcomes of proactivity, its use of controlled laboratory paradigms to examine specific behaviors undertaken proactively to address potential discrimination, its attention to the differences between responses to discriminatory versus nondiscriminatory stressors, and its careful documentation of some of the attentional and performance costs (and benefits) of the extra vigilance required by such situations (see Mallett & Swim, 2009, for review). This work also highlights some of the additional demands created by stressors that are interpersonal in nature—efforts to focus on one's own behavior and to maintain control in order not to exacerbate the situation and to closely monitor the verbal and nonverbal behavior of an interaction partner are complex and involving tasks that are typically not present, or at least not to the same degree, in other coping settings. That one can act to influence, but most surely cannot completely control, or sometimes even predict, the behavior of others adds an extra level of complexity to the challenge of proactive coping with interpersonal stressors (cf. Sansone & Berg, 1993).

The study of proactive coping with discrimination also highlights the multiple goals targets may adopt in responding to actions that are potentially racist, sexist, or homophobic. Swim and Thomas (2006; see also Hyers, 2007; Umaña-Taylor et al., 2008) outlined the multiple different personal and social goals people may adopt in responding to discrimination and suggest that the effectiveness of proactive efforts must be evaluated in light of the particular goal selected. For example, a person's efforts to confront racism directly could be labeled as unsuccessful if the goal was to alter the perpetrator's opinions, but successful if the goal of confrontation was to provide self-validation or stand up for oneself. Alternatively, avoidance and concealment can prevent discrimination and rejection and thus be seen as successful strategies in some respects, but they may create other problems, such as a perceived lack of authenticity and long-term negative health effects (see also Pachankis, 2007). As a third example, a stigmatized person may decide to focus on the task at hand rather than calling out another person's prejudice, in order that an incipient stressor not threaten primary goals involving task completion. People may also decline to respond to discrimination in order to preserve energy or avoid conflict (Hyers, 2007). In such cases, the goal of not allowing discrimination to interfere with one's performance or to escalate a conflict has been pro-actively managed, but the discriminatory behavior has been left unaddressed. These examples highlight some of the complex choices faced by stigmatized people as they consider the proactive management of discrimination and provide insight into the wide range of personal and social goals such efforts may serve. These examples also illustrate the impor-tance of understanding the particular goals with which people are coping in understanding the coping strategies they select and evaluating the success of their efforts (see Aspinwall, 2001, for discussion).

To fully appreciate whether a particular person is coping proactively, we need to know what the person is trying to prevent or to attain, and whether proactive coping in the service of a particular goal involves action or inaction. Understanding these motives is easier in experimentally constructed and circumscribed situations that call for particular performance or interpersonal outcomes, such as being judged as more likable on the basis of one's Internet dating profile. To date, the results of exper-imental studies of proactive approaches to antici-pated discrimination suggest that people can successfully alter others' views of them in ways that are measurable by objective observers. At the same time, however, the results of the daily diary studies also provide strong evidence that efforts to manage the impact of discriminatory situations on the self are reported in nearly all such instances. Thus, even though a variety of primary control options are typ-ically available, a major goal in responding proac-tively to discrimination appears to be limiting damage to the self as the interaction unfolds.

Proactive coping with threats to health
Proactive coping to manage threats to health can take many forms. In the absence of specific health concerns, people may seek to promote their general health and fitness in order to ward off disease and to be better able to handle specific challenges should they arise. People who anticipate they are at risk for disease may undertake efforts to improve diet and exercise, to educate themselves about the disease, to modify specific risk factors, and to seek early detection and other forms of risk screening, such as predictive genetic testing, and people who are diag-nosed with disease may take a proactive approach to

slowing its development and/or reducing its com-plications. Although there are large literatures on the psychological determinants of preventive health and screening behaviors (see, e.g., Miller, Bowen, Croyle, & Rowland, 2009), very little of it has used a proactive coping framework to examine the spe-cific resources, appraisals, and coping efforts that may underlie such actions (see McCaul & Mullens, 2003, for an exception). In the following sections, we will examine how the proactive coping concept might apply to multiple efforts to prevent serious illness or to detect it early in its course, with a spe-cial emphasis on proactive management of familial disease risk through predictive genetic testing. We will also review recent applications of the proactive coping concept to interventions in the areas of health promotion and self-management of chronic illness. Finally, we will examine advance medical directives as a critically important form of proactive coping that presents unique challenges to the pre-diction and management of future negative out-comes (Ditto, Hawkins, & Pizarro, 2005).

PROACTIVITY AND THE PREVENTION AND EARLY DETECTION OF SERIOUS FAMILIAL DISEASE
An important context in which to understand proactivity in the context of disease risk manage-ment is familial disease, notably familial cancer, but also such conditions as heart disease, diabetes, Alzheimer's, osteoarthritis, and other illnesses with a strong known or suspected heritable component. Activities undertaken in advance of the develop-ment of disease may include efforts to build per-sonal resources by improving or maintaining one's general health status, to build social resources by maintaining support, to build financial resources in anticipation of long-term care needs, and to update one's appraisals of one's risk for disease by monitor-ing the medical literature and other sources for new information about the condition and its treatment. More specific forms of proactivity may involve avoiding specific behaviors known to be linked to the development of specific diseases (e.g., fat con-sumption for heart disease) and increasing one's practice of behaviors known or suspected to prevent or forestall disease (e.g., exercise). Other prepara-tory activities, such as the acquisition of life, dis-ability, and long-term care insurance, are probably also common among people with a strong family history of disease, but are understudied from this perspective.

Predictive genetic testing and the proactive management of familial cancer risk

The advent of personalized medicine suggests that people will have the opportunity to receive more information than ever before about their vulnerability to a variety of disorders and to receive it earlier, prior to development of disease, when early detection and potentially also prevention are still possible. Such developments represent important opportunities for studying the proactive management of risk for serious disease. For some genetically linked diseases, it is possible to take early actions, such as prophylactic surgery for ovarian or breast cancer (Botkin, Smith, Croyle, Baty, Wylie, Dutson, et al., 2003), that will virtually eliminate the risk of disease, and for many diseases, such as hereditary cancer, accelerated screening is vital to early detection efforts and corresponding treatment outcomes. As new information about the interactions among genetic vulnerability, personal behavior, and environmental exposure becomes available, there will be an increasing number of genetically linked disorders for which it is possible to alter one's behavior or environmental exposure in ways that may reduce disease risk.

Our own recent research has examined the potential of predictive genetic test results to spur proactive efforts to manage familial melanoma risk (Aspinwall, Leaf, Dola, Kohlmann, & Leachman, 2008; Aspinwall, Leaf, Kohlmann, Dola, & Leachman, 2009; Leaf, Aspinwall, & Leachman, 2010). Malignant melanoma is an aggressive and lethal form of skin cancer, with only a 15 percent survival rate at 5 years for metastatic disease (American Cancer Society, 2008). Because early detection radically improves treatment outcomes, members of high-risk families are counseled to conduct monthly skin self-examinations and to obtain annual professional total body skin examinations. Further, evidence suggests that avoidance of UV exposure may reduce familial melanoma risk. Of all melanomas, 5 to 10 percent have a familial clustering, and 20 to 40 percent of these are associated with a pathogenic mutation in *CDKN2A/p16* (Bishop, Demenais, Goldstein, Bergman, Bergman, Bishop, et al., 2002; Florell, Boucher, Garibotti, Kerber, Mineau, Wiggins, et al., 2005; Goldstein, Chan, Harland, Hayward, Demenais, Bishop, et al., 2007). A mutation in *CDKN2A,* a tumor suppressor that regulates cell cycle and senescence, confers an approximate lifetime risk of 76 percent to people residing in the United States (Bishop et al., 2002); however, geographic variation in this risk suggests that differences in UV exposure might account for different penetrance rates in different countries, from a low of 58 percent in Europe to a high of 91 percent in sunny Australia. Thus, members of melanoma-prone families are counseled to reduce UV exposure through the use of sunscreen and protective clothing or the avoidance of UV exposure.

The impact of cancer genetic test reporting and counseling on proactive risk-reducing lifestyle modifications for hereditary cancers, such as photoprotection to reduce familial melanoma risk, is just beginning to be assessed, primarily because there are no known behaviors analogous to photoprotection that would substantially reduce the risks of the other hereditary cancers for which predictive genetic tests are currently available (e.g., colon and breast cancer; see Aspinwall et al., 2009, for discussion). Thus, as we began our work, it was unknown whether a positive genetic test result, paired with appropriate counseling about photoprotection and early detection, would promote relevant prevention behaviors. Further, scenario or analog studies of how people think about genetic risks suggest that information that a disease has a genetic origin often undermines interest in information about prevention (Senior, Marteau, & Weinman, 2000; see Marteau & Weinman, 2006, for review and discussion).

We began by examining photoprotection and screening behaviors at baseline, prior to genetic test reporting and counseling, among 62 members of melanoma-prone families with a known *CDKN2A/p16* mutation (Aspinwall et al., 2008; Aspinwall et al., 2009). One might imagine that the knowledge that one is a member of a melanoma-prone family, as well as the experience of seeing multiple family members grapple with this aggressive disease, might promote efforts to reduce this risk through prevention and early detection. However, as has been reported in other studies of melanoma-prone families, unaffected participants (those without a personal history of melanoma) reported much lower compliance with prevention and screening recommendations overall than members of the same families who had been diagnosed with the disease. Of particular interest, unaffected family members fell into two quite different groups. Among one third of the unaffected participants, baseline reports of skin self-examinations were exceptionally high and far in excess of medical recommendations, whereas two thirds of unaffected family members reported conducting skin self-examinations far less frequently than recommended. Thus, these findings indicate that although a healthy subset of unaffected members of these melanoma-prone families were actively engaged (arguably overactively so, as frequent examination of one's skin may interfere with the detection of interval changes in specific lesions) in screening behaviors, nearly two thirds were substantially undercompliant with these critical recommendations. Similar results were obtained for reports of professional total body skin examinations in the past 5 years, with participants with a history of melanoma reporting much greater compliance than family members without such a history. Finally, an analysis of the routine daily implementation of the three most frequently recommended photoprotection measures (i.e., sunscreen, protective clothing, UV avoidance) indicated the presence of a large subset (28 percent) of respondents from these high-risk families who had not implemented any of the three recommendations on a regular basis.

We next examined the impact of genetic test reporting on the screening and photoprotection behaviors of participants without a history of melanoma who received positive *CDKN2A* test results. These results were encouraging: such participants showed increases in both the frequency and thoroughness of skin self-examinations and reported greater intentions to obtain professional total body skin examinations in the next year (Aspinwall et al., 2008). They also showed significantly greater intentions to practice photoprotection and marginal gains in such practice at 1 month, with more than one third of participants reporting the adoption of a new prevention behavior or the improvement of an existing one (Aspinwall et al., 2009). A 2-year follow-up revealed that unaffected participants who received positive genetic test results reported significant improvements in the use of protective clothing and reported sustaining fewer sunburns in the past 6 months (Aspinwall, Taber, & Leachman, 2010). These participants also reported sustained improvements in the thoroughness of skin self-examinations and compliance with recommendations regarding professional total body skin examinations that approximated the levels of adherence reported by melanoma patients. By demonstrating that genetic test reporting and counseling can improve prevention and early detection behaviors toward the levels practiced by family members with a personal history of the disease, these findings suggest that one of the major goals of personalized medicine—to alert and motivate healthy asymptomatic people in advance to undertake critical prevention and early detection efforts prior to the development of disease—has been met in this case.

As more diseases are identified for which personal behavior and/or environmental exposure interact with genetic vulnerability, understanding how people conceptualize the necessity and effectiveness of their own proactive actions to detect and manage such diseases will become even more important. Further, as genetic testing is extended to minor children of cancer-prone families, issues involved in the proactive management of disease risk will come to the fore. Critically, such efforts will involve not only accelerated screening, but also risk-reduction efforts with the goal of disease prevention. Here, too, familial melanoma may provide an important model for understanding such efforts, as childhood and adolescent sun exposure is suspected to play an important role in the development of melanoma. For example, parents of children with *CDKN2A* mutations will likely consider such proactive adaptations as choosing indoor hobbies and pursuits for their children (e.g., music lessons, indoor swimming, hockey, gymnastics) instead of outdoor ones for which sustained UV exposure would be chronically high (e.g., soccer or baseball, outdoor swimming). Thus far, our surveys of parents in these high-risk melanoma-prone families suggest that most parents desire such testing for their minor children, although concerns about unduly alarming children were expressed by some parents (Taber, Aspinwall, Kohlmann, Dow, & Leachman, in press). Understanding how parents balance the potential costs and benefits of proactive knowledge of their children's disease risk and decide when and how to share this information with children who carry a pathogenic mutation represent important areas for future research.

Another aspect of this research program involves efforts to identify individual differences in the management of familial cancer risk and in responses to genetic test reporting and counseling that may prove important to efforts to personalize personalized medicine—that is, to tailor health-risk communications and medical management recommendations not only on the basis of genetic risks, but also on the basis of individual differences in future-oriented thinking, psychological distress, health cognitions, and other factors. Thus far, our preliminary findings suggest that optimism predicts better baseline adherence to monthly skin self-examinations among patients with a history of melanoma, whereas low optimism or high anxiety coupled with a personal history of melanoma predicts potentially counterproductive overscreening (Aspinwall, Taber, & Leachman, 2010). As noted earlier, overscreening (for example, conducting skin self-examinations daily rather than monthly) is thought to interfere with one's ability to detect problematic skin changes. We are currently investigating the possibility that such frequent self-examinations may be a strategy undertaken by high-risk patients to reduce worry by verifying that they have not developed a new cancer. An important question for future research that follows from these findings regarding the proactive management of familial disease risk is whether the benefits of such heightened vigilance to the development of cancer outweigh the potential costs.

PROACTIVITY AND THE MANAGEMENT OF CHRONIC ILLNESS

As noted above, although there is a voluminous literature on coping with chronic illness (see multiple chapters, this volume), a primary focus of research in this area concerns adaptation or adjustment to illness, with relatively little research on the proactive efforts individuals may take to slow disease progression or reduce the impact of chronic illness once they have been diagnosed. An impressive intervention to improve the proactive management of diabetes in older adults conducted by Thoolen and colleagues (Thoolen, de Ridder, Bensing, Gorter, & Rutten, 2008b, 2009; Thoolen, de Ridder, Bensing, Maas, Griffin, Gorter, & Rutten, 2007) suggests that this may be a rich area for research and application.

Interventions to promote proactive self-management of chronic illness

The management of chronic illness presents many challenges, especially for diseases like diabetes for which one's health status must be continually monitored and for which inconsistent or poor management has dire health consequences. To benefit maximally from early detection, people must learn to monitor and manage their disease in the absence of symptoms or in the presence of relatively few symptoms that might prompt management efforts. In their studies of screen-detected adult diabetes patients, Thoolen (2007) suggested that the majority of patients recognize the need for self-management in such situations, but often fail to take into account the multiple barriers and situational factors that could undermine their efforts. A group-based intervention by Thoolen and colleagues ("Beyond Good Intentions," Thoolen, 2007; see also Thoolen et al., 2007, 2008b, 2009) tested whether teaching older patients with screen-detected type II diabetes to think about their diabetes self-management goals, anticipate potential threats to their goals, and plan and evaluate their progress accordingly would improve diabetes self-management.

Participants were 180 adults ages 50 to 70 recruited from the Dutch arm of the ADDITION study of the intensive treatment of people with screen-detected type II diabetes in primary care. Participants had been diagnosed 3 to 33 months prior to participation during a population screening. Participants were randomized to either a 12-week proactive self-management intervention or to a control group that received only a brochure on diabetes self-management. Follow-up data were obtained at 3 and 12 months, with medical outcomes at 12 months taken from patients' medical records.

The intervention consisted of four 2-hour group sessions and two 1-hour individual sessions facilitated by a registered nurse. In an initial individual session, patients discussed their knowledge and attitudes with regard to diabetes management, their diabetic history, and their present self-management practices. Initial discussion of areas the patient might like to work on and how the group could help achieve such changes took place during this first session. The next three group sessions covered such topics as physical activity, dieting, medication, and monitoring of the disease. In the fourth session, patients were given the opportunity to work on a personally relevant goal with respect to diabetes self-care. In group sessions designed to promote proactive coping competencies, such as the anticipation of potential stressors, goal-setting, planning, problem-solving, and evaluation, participants wrote their own individual action plans to attain a goal and discussed them with the group. Group members were asked to judge the quality of the goals in terms of concreteness and attainability, to help each other to recognize additional conditions and barriers to be addressed, and to use mental simulation techniques to generate alternative strategies for solving problems in specific situations. Following these sessions, patients were asked to write down their final plans in the form of implementation intentions that specified what they were going to do, how, where, when, and with whom. Patients were then asked to indicate how they were going to evaluate their progress. Finally, participants were given a homework assignment in which they were asked to act on their plan and keep a written daily record of goal attainment.

At 3 months, the proportion of participants who indicated that they had worked on a diabetes management-related goal in the past month rose from 82 percent to 100 percent in the intervention group but remained at 78 to 81 percent in the control group. Further, significant improvements in proactive coping skills (as assessed by a 17-item Proactive Diabetes Management Inventory containing items concerning multiple aspects of anticipating goals and barriers to their attainment, monitoring one's progress, and responding to feedback), self-rated goal attainment, and diabetes management self-efficacy were obtained for the intervention group but not for the control group. At 3 months, 80 percent of intervention patients said that they were planning to continue using the five-step proactive self-management plan in the future, and 85 percent indicated that they would advise other patients to take the course.

At 12 months, the numerous gains reported by the proactive coping intervention group were sustained over time. Specifically, intervention participants reported sustained improvements in intentions with respect to diet and exercise, general self-efficacy, proactive competence, proactive behavior, and goal attainment. Further, patients in the intervention group reported significant positive changes on all self-care measures (general self-care, exercise, diet, fat consumption), except for medication adherence, which was already high at baseline. The authors noted that the magnitude of the reported changes in diet and exercise could be considered clinically relevant—for example, the intervention group reported one additional day of exercise per week. Consistent with this change in self-care behavior, intervention patients lost weight at 12 months, compared to controls, who reported an increase in BMI. Further, the intervention was effective in reducing systolic blood pressure, with especially good results found in patients receiving both intensive medical treatment and the proactive self-management intervention (Thoolen et al., 2007). Interestingly, however, the sustained weight loss in the proactive coping intervention group did not depend on assignment to intensive medical treatment or control in the parent study. Thus, the results of this intervention to promote proactive management of diabetes suggest that important health gains were maintained 1 year later and, critically, that behavioral changes were maintained after contact with health professionals had been withdrawn.

It is important to note that these encouraging results were obtained in a sample in which both diabetes-management intentions and self-efficacy were high at baseline, as was medication adherence, making adherence to diet and exercise goals the critical targets for early diabetes self-management efforts. Of particular interest, proactive coping competencies attained at the end of the intervention predicted improved long-term self-management at 12 months, controlling for baseline self-management, exercise, and dietary habits; baseline intentions, however, did not predict any of the self-management outcomes at 12 months (Thoolen et al., 2009). The authors suggested that baseline self-efficacy and initial intentions may play a role in the initiation of behavior change but do not appear to predict the maintenance of behavior change, whereas proactive preparations to anticipate and manage barriers to self-management appeared to be successful in maintaining new behaviors.

In discussing the mechanisms through which the intervention achieved such results, Thoolen (2007) suggested that the proactive coping intervention may be effective because it helps patients translate an abstract long-term concern about the health impact of diabetes into more concrete challenges patients can deal with in the present. Further, Thoolen (2007, p. 101) noted, "Proactive coping, with its focus on anticipation, planning and continued evaluation of self management activities, may help patients to become more aware of threats to their self management and act accordingly before such threats can undermine their behaviors." In particular, Thoolen (2007) suggested that thinking about goals in advance may help patients to become aware of other competing goals, habits, and activities that may undermine their motivation; to recognize their limited resources; to set concrete, achievable goals; and to recognize an array of potential threats and to plan alternative strategies to deal with problem situations as they arise (cf. Marlatt & Gordon, 1985). Finally, the intervention's emphasis on the evaluation and continued monitoring of one's goal progress might not only help patients evaluate the success of their activities to deal with potential threats, but may also help patients to detect the emergence of new threats to diabetes management.

PROACTIVE APPROACHES TO HEALTH-PROMOTION INTERVENTIONS

Similar encouraging gains in the area of health promotion have recently been obtained by Stadler, Oettingen, and Gollwitzer (2009) in a self-regulatory intervention that paired two important advances in the study of future-oriented thinking, *mental contrasting*

(Oettingen, Pak, & Schnetter, 2001; Oettingen, Mayer, Thorpe, Hanetzke, & Lorenz, 2005) and *implementation intentions* (Gollwitzer, 1999; see Gollwitzer & Sheeran, 2006, for review). Mental contrasting is a technique in which a desired future outcome is jointly considered with present impediments to attaining that outcome in ways that promote goal commitment, while implementation intentions refer to specific plans regarding the nature and timing of goal-related efforts. The goal of the intervention was to use such techniques to promote physical activity in a large sample of middle-aged women in metropolitan Germany. The intervention took place in a single session. Intervention participants were asked to articulate their most important current wish regarding physical activity (e.g., going for a brisk walk during one's lunch break or using a stationary bike at home three times per week), the most positive outcome of realizing this wish, and the most important obstacle to obtaining this wish. Importantly, they were asked to articulate the events and experiences they associated both with the positive outcome and with the critical obstacle to its attainment. Next, participants were asked to form three specific implementation intentions: plans to overcome or circumvent specific obstacles when they occur, specific opportunities to prevent the obstacle from occurring, and specific opportunities to act on the chosen wish. These latter parts of the intervention are a close match to the proactive coping concept in that participants are asked to form intentions not just with respect to how they will respond to the obstacle, but also to identify obstacles in advance and to form specific implementation intentions to actively prevent their occurrence.

As with the diabetes self-management intervention (Thoolen, 2007), specific training in the process of articulating obstacles to goal attainment and developing specific plans to prevent, overcome, or circumvent such obstacles proved to be successful: a 4-month follow-up indicated that intervention participants reported a sustained increase of more than 60 minutes per week of physical activity, compared to an increase of 15 minutes per week for an information-only control group. Given the extraordinary health costs of obesity and the difficulty of sustained weight loss, interventions to prevent the typical annual weight gain among middle-aged participants through modifications to diet and exercise will likely assume critical importance in the health-promotion literature. Efforts to assist people in managing proactive approaches to weight gain, especially when they are informed by contemporary social cognition research on future-oriented thinking, as was the case in the present intervention, have great potential to elucidate and promote proactive efforts to maintain health. Importantly, these efforts both complement and extend prior approaches, such as Marlatt and Gordon's (1985) seminal work on relapse prevention, by using specific techniques, such as mental simulation and mental contrasting, to promote the joint consideration of future goals and current impediments to their attainment and also to prompt proactive efforts not only to recognize, but also to proactively manage some of the situational and motivational factors that create barriers to goal attainment.

PROACTIVE COPING AND MEDICAL DECISION-MAKING

Finally, a particularly interesting and important area in which to examine proactivity and future-oriented thinking with respect to future health and well-being concerns the establishment of advance medical directives. Thus far, we have considered proactive coping situations in which people are free to change their appraisals and modify their efforts as their situation changes. However, advance medical directives specifically require a person to enter a binding contract regarding his or her preferences for medical care in the event he or she becomes either temporarily or permanently incapacitated. In this case, people must not only anticipate potential negative future outcomes and respond to them, but must state binding preferences for future outcomes they have likely never experienced. In a fascinating line of research, Ditto et al. (2005) examined multiple ways in which our future psychological state and corresponding preferences may be quite different from the present state and preferences we use to make advance medical decisions, and questioned the assumption that people can accurately predict their preferences in such different future circumstances. For example, Ditto et al. noted that preferences for different physical states may be altered by pain, disability, fatigue, and experience with these states; and further, that such preferences may be context-dependent in other ways that render them relatively unstable. As a result, determining which set of preferences (the preferences a person expressed when well, the preferences he expresses when critically ill, or the preferences expressed by others on his behalf when he is unable to offer his own) is more "true" and should be binding involves multiple serious ethical and legal considerations.

In general, the notion that one's goals change with one's changing circumstances and increased information about them is quite compatible with transactional approaches to stress and coping; however, advance medical directives and other binding contracts highlight the importance of understanding the limits of, and specific influences on, people's ability to predict what they might want at some future time under very different conditions. Such concerns are likely to play a role in proactive efforts to provide for long-term care, assisted living, and other disability- and aging-related preparations, and suggest further that proactive decisions in other domains in which one's mental and physical health and accompanying preferences are likely to change may be subject to similar complexities.

Proactivity in aging

The last major domain we will review, proactivity in aging, is poised for significant advances. There are well-developed conceptual models that delineate proactive efforts to avert stressors and to build or preserve personal and social resources (Kahana & Kahana, 1996, 2003; Kahana, Kahana, & Kercher, 2003; see also Ouwehand, de Ridder, & Bensing, 2007), research findings linking future orientation and planning, respectively, to older adults' maintenance of exercise behavior (Kahana, Kahana, & Zhang, 2005) and life satisfaction (Prenda & Lachman, 2001), and new interventions to promote goal-setting and goal-attainment competencies among middle-aged and older adults (Bode, de Ridder, Kuijer, & Bensing, 2007; see also Bode & de Ridder, 2007; Bode, de Ridder, & Bensing, 2006). At the same time, however, there are many unanswered questions in the current literature that concern mechanisms underlying the relation between measures of future-oriented thinking and later-life outcomes, as well as the nature of specific efforts that may be strategically undertaken to avoid or minimize particular aging-related stressors.

CONCEPTUAL APPROACHES TO PROACTIVITY IN AGING

The well-developed model of preventive and corrective forms of proactivity in aging (PCP model; Kahana & Kahana, 1996, 2003) explicitly considers proactive efforts both to prevent aging-related losses and to preserve or increase resources for future use. In this model, *preventive adaptations* are undertaken to avert stressors and to build personal and social resources, while *corrective adaptations* are activated by stressors and can be facilitated by existing internal and external resources. Three major kinds of preventive adaptations have been hypothesized among retired adults: exercising to forestall age-related disability, planning ahead, and helping others in order to shore up social resources for the future (Kahana, et al., 2003; see also Midlarsky & Kahana, 2007). Further, these different proactive adaptations are predicted to be influenced by both internal (e.g., future orientation, coping dispositions) and external (e.g., financial, social support, access to health care) resources. In a review of theoretical approaches to successful aging, Ouwehand et al. (2007) similarly proposed that proactive coping aimed at preventing potential threats may confer multiple benefits, especially as older people face documented declines in resources. Drawing on both the proactive coping (Aspinwall & Taylor, 2007) and selective optimization with compensation (Baltes & Baltes, 1990) models, Ouwehand et al. suggested that proactive coping may result in prolonged availability of resources to use in optimization and compensation processes to manage actual losses and may also delay disengagement from important goals.

EVIDENCE REGARDING FUTURE-ORIENTED THINKING AND OUTCOMES IN AGING

Most empirical evidence for the Kahana and Kahana PCP model has been drawn from the authors' large-scale prospective longitudinal study of 1,000 retirees (minimum age, 72; Kahana, Lawrence, Kahana, Kercher, Wisniewski, Stoller, et al., 2002). To date, it has been demonstrated that one of the hypothesized preventive adaptations, self-reported frequency of exercise, predicted fewer instrumental limitations in activities of daily living, decreased mortality risk, increased positive affect, and greater reports of meaning in life over an 8-year period, controlling for initial basic limitations in activities of daily living (Kahana et al., 2002). Of particular interest, even though both physical and mental health outcomes declined over time in this sample of old-old individuals, the rate of decline was slower among adults who reported greater exercise. Thus, these findings represent an important instance in which the proactive maintenance of exercise served to diminish rather than completely prevent adverse outcomes. Additional findings have linked self-reported frequency of thinking about the future to slower declines in exercise frequency over a 4-year period (Kahana, Kahana, & Zhang, 2005). Although these findings suggest that thinking about the future and maintaining exercise behavior may be related to proactive efforts to manage age-related threats to health, the mechanisms through which frequent thoughts about the future are related to proactive adaptations are unspecified, and it is unclear whether respondents had maintained their level of exercise with the specific goal of preserving health rather than enjoyment, habit, social engagement, or other reasons.

A few other studies link thoughts about the future to good later-life outcomes but are similarly inconclusive with respect to the mechanism(s) involved. For example, Kahana, Kahana, and Kelly-Moore (2005) reported that planning for the future at baseline was a significant predictor of greater engagement in valued activities 5 years later. Of particular interest, the future-planning item asked about future plans such as taking a trip, making a major purchase, or starting a new project, not plans for managing disability, illness, or social loss. Thus, these findings make it difficult to distinguish the effects of planning in general or plans to continue valued activities from the effects of plans to prevent specific negative effects of aging. Similarly, in a cross-sectional study with a very large sample of adults ages 25 to 75, Prenda and Lachman (2001) found that reported preference for planning for the future declined with age, but was especially predictive of greater life satisfaction among older adults between 60 and 75 years old. The planning items used in this study were general rather than domain-specific, so it was not possible to determine from these data whether there are specific domains for which planning is especially predictive of life satisfaction or whether it is the practice of planning in general that may confer benefits.

KEY CONCEPTUAL QUESTIONS FOR THE STUDY OF PROACTIVITY IN AGING

Although there is accumulating evidence that planning and future-oriented thinking are associated with good outcomes in aging, it is not yet clear whether these outcomes have resulted from deliberate proactive coping efforts or how these specific forms of future-oriented thinking may be related to proactive efforts to preserve resources and prevent or slow specific forms of age-related decline. Accordingly, key conceptual questions for research on proactivity in aging would be to better understand (1) older adults' appraisals and expectations that may prompt proactive coping efforts with specific age-related stressors, including declines in resources, and (2) how future orientation and planning are related to preventive forms of proactivity in aging.

Understanding specific age-related stressors that may be proactively managed

To date, interventions have used the proactive coping model to teach general goal-setting and goal-attainment skills and to guide middle-aged and older adults through the process of articulating future goals and working to achieve them ("In anticipation of the golden years"; Bode et al., 2007; see also Bode & de Ridder, 2007; Bode et al., 2006). Although this intervention met its stated goal of creating gains in goal-setting and goal-attainment competencies, the specific instructions given to participants about how to select a personal future goal may have limited its applicability to understanding proactive coping to prevent or minimize future stressors. Specifically, participants were asked in an initial homework assignment to anticipate topics about which they would have regrets after 5 years if they did not work on them now and then to select from this list one personal future goal based on its relevance to the aging process and its personal importance. As a result, participants selected a wide variety of goals, only some of which seemed to involve the identification and management of aging-related stressors. Specifically, participants identified goals related to hobbies and sports (26.2 percent); practical goals inside and outside the house that were important to tackle while one was physically well enough to do them (21.3 percent); time management (19.7 percent); preparatory activities including searching for information on euthanasia, reviewing one's last will, or acquiring information about early retirement (13.1 percent); and goals involving social contacts (11.5 percent). To the extent that the instructions pulled for the selection of goals best completed while relatively young, they likely elicited a different set of goals from the specific stressors such respondents might seek to proactively manage in later life. For example, a household project undertaken to make one's home safer and more comfortable for aging residents may be fundamentally different from a project undertaken to beautify one's home. As result, it is difficult to determine whether the intervention promoted specific proactive coping efforts to prevent or minimize potential stressors or more general forms of goal-directed problem-solving.

Applications of the goal-setting and goal-attainment intervention that focus more narrowly on coping with age-related stressors are likely to provide insight into the specific stressors people expect to face in aging and corresponding efforts undertaken to prevent, forestall, or minimize them. It will be important in future studies of this kind to ask participants to specifically anticipate potential sources of aging-related stress in order to be sure that proactive coping is being studied. Indeed, such an approach has been taken in related vignette studies of proactive coping with financial, social, and health-related losses in aging (Ouwehand et al., 2006).

Understanding how future-oriented thinking and planning are related to proactive coping with age-related stressors

Much remains unclear about the relationship of future orientation and planning preferences to later-life outcomes. First, it remains to be determined whether the specific plans and other thoughts about the future linked to good outcomes are related to the anticipation and management of potential stressors, or whether thoughts about the future are beneficial in other ways. For example, older respondents may conceptualize the trips and projects they are planning as activities that would keep them vital and engaged. It is also possible that frequent thoughts about the future may direct one's attention to potential stressors and ways to manage them. Alternatively, the benefits of planning for the future may derive from having something to look forward to, and simply having future goals, projects, and plans may have independent effects on mental and physical health, apart from a desire to take better care of oneself and preserve personal and social resources in order to achieve these plans. As a fourth possibility, the propensity to plan may either reflect or be reciprocally related to a greater sense of perceived control over outcomes in valued life domains (Prenda & Lachman, 2001). As we will review in the next section, such questions of mechanism are by no means unique to the study of proactivity in aging, but they are essential to advancing our understanding of whether and how specific kinds of future-oriented thinking may be related to efforts to preserve resources and address potential stressors early in their course.

Who is Proactive? Individual Differences in Proactivity

Thus far, efforts to find consistent predictors of proactivity in different domains have met with limited success, partly because of the diversity of definitions involved, the multiple component skills included in various measures of proactivity, and the multiple goals people may adopt in responding proactively to different situations. Results concerning the relation of particular individual differences to the enactment and the success of proactive coping efforts may also depend on which part of the process one is studying. As Aspinwall and Taylor (1997) predicted, some individual differences may promote some of the component activities of proactive coping, such as vigilance to potential stressors, but interfere with successful enactment of the other steps, such as active efforts to acquire information about them. Further, other factors may moderate the relationship of proactivity to outcomes, making main effect relationships difficult to detect (Chan, 2006). Finally, there is little systematic study of the particular aspects of potential stressors that would require different proactive coping skills.

Although a comprehensive review is beyond the scope of this chapter, we will identify multiple approaches to defining individual differences in proactive coping and note some of their strengths and limitations. Efforts to identify the individual differences involved in whether proactive efforts are undertaken and are ultimately successful may be classified in several different ways: (a) individual differences in proactive coping style and preferences for planning, (b) the multiple skills required for the successful proactive detection and management of potential stressors, (c) temporal orientation, time perspective, and other forms of future-oriented thinking, (d) the content of future-oriented thinking (e.g., optimism, hope, fatalism), (e) the experience of negative affect or chronic concern with negative events and information (e.g., neuroticism, anxiety, defensive pessimism, worry), and (f) socioeconomic and personal resources, such as income, education, and health status. Also, an important recent contribution to this literature has been the detailed consideration of who enrolls in and who benefits from interventions to promote proactive coping.

Individual differences in proactive coping style and preference for planning

Several individual difference measures have been specifically developed to capture proactivity as a stable preference or style (e.g., Bateman & Crant's Proactive Personality Scale [1993]; see Crant, 2000, for review; and Greenglass et al.'s Proactive Coping Inventory [1999]). The Proactive Coping Inventory uses seven subscales to assess different preferences and skills involved in proactivity. For example, the *proactive coping* subscale includes not only such general self-descriptors as whether one is a "take charge" person, but also multiple concepts from the goal-setting and persistence literatures, such as whether one visualizes one's dreams and tries to achieve them, tries to pinpoint what is necessary for success, and works around obstacles. The *preventive coping* subscale assesses efforts to preserve resources, both in general ("I plan for future eventualities," "I like to save for a rainy day") and for specific situations (financial resources in aging, job skills to protect against unemployment, disaster preparation), while the *reflective coping* subscale captures many of the component activities of the proactive coping model, such as thinking about realistic alternatives to a problem, going through different scenarios in order to prepare oneself for different outcomes, and other activities undertaken to generate multiple solutions to problems. A strength of this approach is that the inventory as a whole captures multiple self-regulatory tasks involved in both promotion-oriented and prevention-oriented forms of proactive coping, but a limitation is that some of the multi-faceted subscales do not allow the determination of whether it is a preference for advance action or the possession of specific self-regulatory skills that confers benefit, or whether both are operating jointly. Further, although it follows clearly from the Greenglass et al. (1999) definition of proactivity as seeking new opportunities and promoting personal growth, the separation of preventive and reflective preferences, skills, and behaviors from the proactive coping subscale implies that such skills and behaviors are somehow less implicated in proactivity, as opposed to being central concepts. Consistent with this point, recent factor-analytic studies suggest that the proactive coping, preventive coping, reflective coping, and strategic coping subscales are highly intercorrelated and may be more parsimoniously represented as a single factor (Roesch, Aldridge, Huff, Langner, Villodas, & Bradshaw, 2009). Finally, most published studies appear to have used only the proactive coping subscale from the inventory, making it difficult to determine the contribution of the other activities thought to represent proactive and preventive coping more generally.

Other approaches assess general preferences for planning and relate these to life satisfaction (e.g., Prenda & Lachman, 2001). As reviewed earlier, this approach suggests that planning is an important correlate of both perceived control and life satisfaction in aging, but it does not provide insight into the specific activities potentiated by planning preferences that may confer benefit or the specific domains in which planning may be most important. Thus, a challenge for research on individual differences in the preference for proactivity and planning is to determine how, specifically, such preferences influence the various component activities involved in proactive coping and also to examine whether such preferences alone are sufficient to promote effective forms of proactivity. Chan's (2006) study of workplace proactivity indicates clearly that a preference for proactivity can backfire if it is not accompanied by competence in judging workplace situations. Put differently, a take-charge orientation is beneficial only if one addresses the right problems in a constructive manner; otherwise, one risks being a bull in a china shop. These findings suggest that a preference for proactivity is not all that is required for success and that further study of how people decide when to be proactive and what to be proactive about will shed light on successful versus unsuccessful forms of proactivity.

An additional challenge for the study of individual differences in proactive coping style is to distinguish such preferences or styles from some of the specific competencies involved, an approach recently undertaken by Bode et al. (2007) in their studies of interventions to improve goal-setting and goal-attainment skills in middle-aged and older adults. Ironically, their vignette studies suggest that proactive style did not predict proactive responses to potential problems, but future temporal orientation, to be discussed in the next section, did (Ouwehand et al., 2006). Further, there was appreciable within-subjects variation in responses to the different vignettes. These findings suggest that increased attention to situational determinants of proactive coping might be useful in understanding when and why particular individual differences are related to proactive efforts.

Individual differences in future orientation and time perspective

Other approaches to predicting proactive behaviors consider the nature of future-oriented thinking itself as a critical determinant of future-oriented behaviors in achievement, health, and other settings. Though these approaches have similar names, they vary in the specific elements of future-oriented thinking considered. Such concepts as *future orientation* and *temporal orientation* refer to multiple aspects of people's thinking about and acting on the future and may include the content of future orientation (e.g., specific expectations, hopes, goals, fears), how far into the future such thoughts are projected, and beliefs about factors that influence the future (Jones, 1988; Lasane & O'Donnell, 2005;

Nurmi, 2005; see also Aspinwall, 2005). Other measures assess stable individual differences in the proportion of cognitive activity devoted to past, present, and future outcomes (*time perspective*, Zimbardo & Boyd, 1999; see Boyd & Zimbardo, 2005, for a review) or the value placed on future versus current outcomes (*consideration of future consequences*, Strathman, Gleicher, Boninger, & Edwards, 1994; Joireman, Strathman, & Balliet, 2006).

Measures of future orientation, variously defined, show an intriguing positive relationship to health behaviors that require planning and/or delay of gratification, such as safer sexual behavior (Rothspan & Read, 1996; see also Boyd & Zimbardo, 2005), and they are also reliable predictors of decreased substance use in adolescents (Wills, Sandy, & Yaeger, 2001). At the other end of the lifespan, a future temporal orientation was found to be the only significant individual difference predictor of reported proactive coping with potential financial, health, and social stressors in Ouwehand et al.'s (2006) vignette study among middle-aged and older adults; neither proactive coping style nor generalized self-efficacy predicted proactive responses to the vignettes. Similarly, as noted earlier, the frequency with which older adults reported thinking about the future predicted slower declines in exercise frequency over a 4-year period (Kahana, Kahana, & Zhang, 2005). These results suggest that there may be something unique and important about future temporal orientation that links it to active, problem-solving forms of coping; however, it is also important to consider the alternative possibility that there is something detrimental about either hedonistic or fatalistic forms of present orientation that may interfere with effective forms of coping (see, e.g., Wills et al., 2001). The ability to disentangle such effects depends on the assessment of multiple, theoretically distinct sets of beliefs regarding time perspective (see, e.g., Boyd & Zimbardo 2005) rather than single items or other limited measures that treat time perspective or temporal orientation as unitary concepts.

This discussion highlights the importance of understanding how distinct forms of present- and future-oriented thinking are linked to specific efforts to preserve resources, appraise potential stressors, and act to manage them. As Holman and Silver (2005) note, many studies linking future orientation to mental and physical health do not consider the content of those future-oriented thoughts, such as whether a positive or negative future is envisioned.

Further, process-oriented research on future-oriented thinking suggests that not all forms of thoughts about desired or undesired future outcomes lead equally to efforts to attain or prevent them (e.g., expectations vs. fantasies, Oettingen, 1996; see also Oettingen et al., 2005; process- vs. outcome-oriented mental simulations, Taylor, Pham, Rivkin, & Armor, 1998; possible selves, Oyserman, Bybee, & Terry, 2006). Finally, research that distinguishes various measures of future orientation and time perspective from such concepts as conscientiousness, delay of gratification, and other self-regulatory skills would greatly enhance work in this area.

Other individual differences that may influence the component activities and goals of proactive coping

Two other broad classes of individual differences have been hypothesized as predictors of proactive coping. The first consists of people's expectations about future events in general (dispositional optimism, Scheier & Carver, 1985; Scheier, Carver, & Bridges, 1994; hope, Snyder, 1994) or in specific domains (defensive pessimism, Norem & Cantor, 1986; cancer fatalism, Powe, 1995; lifespan fatalism, Borowsky, Ireland, & Resnick, 2009). The second consists of measures assessing the chronic experience of negative emotions (e.g., depression, neuroticism, McCrae & Costa, 1986; see Grant & Ashford, 2008) and/or concerns with the detection of threats to well-being (e.g., anxiety, worry; Aspinwall et al., 2005; McCaul & Mullens, 2003; Thompson & Schlehofer, 2008). In the original proactive coping model, Aspinwall and Taylor (1997) predicted that the influence of both types of individual differences would depend on the particular step in the proactive coping model being considered, with some individual differences predicting greater or more successful proactive efforts at some steps and fewer or less successful efforts at other steps.

Aspinwall (2001) used the examples of optimism and neuroticism to illustrate how proactive coping efforts might unfold quite differently as a function of these two widely studied individual differences. Specifically, in both cases, individuals may share a concern with the detection and management of future negative outcomes, but engage in the component steps of proactive coping differently and with different short- and long-term outcomes. Figure 17.2 illustrates these differences and how they may be amplified by the feedback loops of the proactive coping model. As shown in Figure 17.2, dispositional optimism has been linked to increased

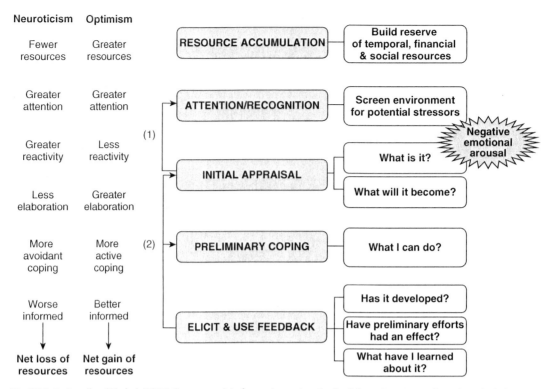

Fig. 17.2 Aspinwall and Taylor's (1997) five-step model of proactive coping. Feedback Loop 1 represents the reciprocal relations among attention/recognition, initial appraisals, and the regulation of negative emotional arousal. Feedback Loop 2 represents the reciprocal relation among appraisals, coping efforts, and information gained from one's efforts to manage an actual or potential stressor. The chart at the left illustrates how neuroticism and optimism may work at each stage of the model as people anticipate or encounter negative events and information.

attention to and elaboration of potential health threats, as well as to more active and less avoidant ways of managing problems (see Aspinwall et al., 2001, for review). These active coping efforts are more likely than avoidant coping efforts to elicit information about potential problems. As a result, optimists should have more elaborated appraisals of potential stressors and thus be more likely to engage in coping efforts that match objective features of the situation. In contrast, although neuroticism may predict greater attention to potential stressors, it may also result in greater reactivity to them and therefore greater difficulty in processing information about them. Heightened reactivity to negative events and information may also promote mood-regulation efforts that may compromise efforts to solve the problem at hand. Further, because neuroticism is consistently linked to avoidant forms of coping, people high in neuroticism may engage in coping efforts that are less likely to elicit new information about potential stressors. Over time, such avoidant coping should lead to lower-quality appraisals of potential stressors and thus to subsequent

coping efforts that may not correspond to the nature of the problem. Evidence for these predicted upward and downward spirals in information and other resources has similarly been found for the relation of positive mood and depression, respectively, to coping efforts over time (see, e.g., Fredrickson & Joiner, 2002; Pyszczynski & Greenberg, 1987; see Aspinwall, 1998, for discussion).

As our understanding not only of the component activities but also of the multiple goals served by proactivity improves, it will be important to examine the relation of particular individual differences to the goals people adopt as they anticipate potential stressors and act to manage them. For example, in a cross-sectional study of preparations for Y2K, Aspinwall et al. (2005) found that proactive coping preferences, worry about Y2K, and, to a lesser extent, dispositional optimism were independent predictors of greater information-seeking about Y2K and greater reported personal and household disaster preparations. However, optimism was uniquely related to more accommodative secondary control-oriented forms of coping, such as efforts to go with the flow or to trust a higher power among respondents who thought that the damage caused by Y2K would be severe and lasting. Of particular interest here is the finding that optimism predicted both primary and secondary control-oriented forms of anticipatory coping, while proactive coping style and worry predicted only primary control-oriented efforts to learn about and prepare for potential problems. As we saw in our review of proactive efforts to counter discrimination, these findings suggest that people may adopt multiple goals in proactive or anticipatory coping, and that some individual differences may promote multiple strategies to both prepare for problems and accommodate to their effects, while others may promote efforts focused more narrowly on preparing for the potential problem. As we will suggest in our discussion of the transactional character of proactive coping, examining how such multiple coping efforts influence not only specific outcomes but also resources and skills over time will be an important next step in elucidating the cumulative effects of specific individual differences related to proactivity.

Socioeconomic resources, demographics, and proactivity

Last but not least, researchers have begun to examine the personal and social resources involved in proactivity and, in particular, whether specific socioeconomic or demographic resources may be required for proactive coping. A particular concern is that proactivity, because it requires expending resources prior to the onset of stress, may be a luxury that can be practiced only by the relatively wealthy, well-educated, and well. If this is the case, proactivity may serve only to help the rich get richer. Worse still, the mental and physical health benefits ascribed to various measures of proactivity and planning could be due instead to these socioeconomic advantages (see Aspinwall, 2005, for discussion). An alternative perspective would be that the need for proactive coping to preserve resources and avert stressors would be greater among people with fewer resources. As the study of proactivity has expanded beyond the study of college undergraduates and new white-collar employees to examine how stigmatized, chronically ill, and otherwise disadvantaged individuals proactively manage potential stressors, some encouraging information about the frequency and success of proactive coping efforts in these groups, as well as improvements following interventions, has emerged.

SOCIOECONOMIC STATUS

In general and consistent with the idea that "the rich get richer," studies that assess measures of proactivity, future orientation, planning, and proactive competence find such preferences and skills to be consistently related to higher income and education (Aspinwall et al., 2005; Holman & Silver, 2005; Ouwehand, de Ridder, & Bensing, 2009; Prenda & Lachman, 2001). Whether these differences are accounted for by such socioeconomic advantages as relative freedom from particular economic and neighborhood stressors, parental socialization practices, or the impact of education itself on future-oriented thinking and behavior remain to be determined (see, e.g., Aspinwall & Taylor, 1997, and Taylor, Repetti, & Seeman, 1997, for reviews and discussion). It is important also to consider the possibility that income and other resources influence the nature of proactive situations that people must navigate. For example, in discussing their studies of proactivity in aging, Kahana and Kahana (2003) cautioned that their large sample of retirees consists exclusively of older adults who have the resources to move to a retirement community. Older adults who live in age-segregated versus age-integrated environments may face different situations and have access to different kinds of social resources (e.g., peers vs. younger family members).

The opportunity to participate in short-term interventions to promote proactivity may also depend on socioeconomic resources. An examination of the role of socioeconomic factors in the intervention to promote proactive self-management of diabetes in older adults indicated that participants with lower levels of education were less likely to enroll and more likely to drop out, with more than one third of nonparticipants citing specific practical barriers to participation in the intervention, such as work or transportation issues. Despite these recruitment and retention issues, it is important to note that the outcomes of the diabetes self-management intervention did not depend on education level (Thoolen et al., 2008b).

HEALTH STATUS AND EXPOSURE TO CONCURRENT STRESSORS

Another set of factors that may be influential in determining whether people can devote resources to proactive coping is the presence of poor health or other concurrent stressors. Evidence on this point is scant but suggestive. Ouwehand et al. (2009) found that physical health status was a mediator of socioeconomic status differences in self-reports of proactive coping competence, such that middle-aged and older adults with higher income and education used more proactive coping strategies in their daily lives in part because they had fewer health problems that might drain attention and other resources.

It will be important in future research to distinguish between these different explanations for the relationship of socioeconomic resources to proactivity and specifically to determine whether socioeconomic differences in proactive coping are due to differences in preferences or skills or to other factors like decreased free time, transportation issues, or greater concurrent mental and physical health stressors that influence opportunities for proactive coping and planning. Such information is essential for the development of interventions to foster proactive coping among people with relatively few resources.

Who can become proactive? Predictors of interest in and benefit from interventions to promote proactivity

Although the existing literature suggests that socioeconomic differences predict proactive coping preferences and competencies, the advent of interventions to promote proactive coping provides a unique opportunity to examine whether the potential benefits of proactivity may be available to all. The diabetes-management study we reviewed is noteworthy in its systematic examination of potential moderators of the impact of the intervention, as well as differences between adults who did or did not enroll in the intervention (Thoolen et al., 2008b; see also Bode & de Ridder, 2007, and Bode et al., 2007, for a similar analysis of the proactivity-in-aging intervention). Intervention participants were found to be lower in self-management of their disease than non-participants. Further, as noted earlier, although participants with lower education were less likely to enroll in and complete the self-management intervention, intervention outcomes were unrelated to education. Taken together, these findings suggest that proactivity interventions are appealing to people managing chronic illness and poor subjective health, but that more must be done to make participation possible for participants of low socioeconomic status.

Relevant Theoretical Issues

Continued research and application of the proactive coping concept, to more fully understand how people act in advance to avoid or reduce stress,

would likely benefit from increased attention to the three aspects of the proactive coping model we highlighted in our introduction, namely that proactive coping is forward-looking, transactional, and likely to involve at least some degree of negative affect.

Understanding the forward-looking nature of proactivity

Continued integration of theory and research on proactive coping with new developments in the study of future-oriented thinking is likely to yield new insights in research and application. In the past 10 to 15 years researchers have made major advances in understanding multiple aspects of future-oriented thinking and their implications for self-regulation in general. Three such advances—construal level theory (Liberman & Trope, 2008; Trope & Liberman, 2003), implementation intentions (Gollwitzer, 1999; Gollwitzer & Sheeran, 2006), and mental simulation and mental contrasting (Oettingen, 1996; Oettingen et al., 2005; Stadler et al., 2009; Taylor et al., 1998)—may have special importance for understanding proactivity. Some of these, alone or in combination, have already been profitably incorporated into interventions to promote proactivity, while others, such as construal level theory, have yet to be mined for their potential.

CONSTRUAL LEVEL THEORY

Construal level theory posits that thinking about current and near-future events differs in profound ways from thinking about distant-future events because of the abstract thinking capabilities necessary "to consider, evaluate, and plan situations that are removed in time or space, that pertain to others' experiences, and that are hypothetical rather than real" (Liberman & Trope, 2008, p. 1201). Specifically, Liberman and Trope posit that more temporally or psychologically distant outcomes are construed in higher-level, more abstract and decontextualized ways that emphasize superordinate goal-relevant features of events and omit incidental features. In contrast, near-future events are construed in concrete, contextualized ways that include subordinate, incidental, and goal-irrelevant features. For example, higher-level construals are more likely to include the "why" aspects of a potential action, whereas lower-level construals refer to how an action will be conducted (Trope & Liberman, 2003). Thus, in a number of ways, when we think about the future, we consider the forest, not the trees.

Construal level theory leads to a number of novel predictions regarding the impact of time on judgment that may have implications for understanding proactivity. First, predictions regarding distant-future events are more likely to be based on high-level construals and therefore to be both more confident and more accurate, because they are not thrown off by incidental (lower-level) contextual features. Second, in contrast to temporal discounting theories that predict that desired outcomes may seem less positive when removed in time, construal-level theory predicts that temporal distance shifts the overall attractiveness of an outcome closer to its higher-level construal value and away from its low-level construal value, leading to the intriguing prediction that proactivity undertaken with respect to future actions may correspond more closely to our higher-order goals and preferences. For example, Liberman and Trope (1998) demonstrated that decisions that would be implemented in the near-future were driven more by feasibility concerns, such as the ease of a course assignment, than by desirability concerns, such as its interest value, while choices that were to be implemented in the more distant future showed the opposite pattern. Although these findings suggest that planned future actions may take into account one's higher-order goals, they also suggest that such plans may lead to the relative neglect of feasibility concerns. These authors suggest that the relative underweighting of feasibility concerns in the consideration of distant-future actions accounts for the well-documented planning fallacy (Buehler, Griffin, & Ross, 1994). This phenomenon could have important implications for proactive coping if people select coping goals that have desirable outcomes, but are not necessarily fully informed by feasibility concerns (see also Sagristano, Trope, & Liberman, 2002).

It will be important to understand how ways of thinking about and preparing for potential stressors differ as a function of how far in the future such events are anticipated. For example, planning for a problematic social interaction scheduled for later in the day may differ quite fundamentally from planning for next year's family reunion or contract negotiation in that entirely different construal levels and correspondingly different weights placed on different elements of such decisions may be used to appraise the problem and different solutions to it. This phenomenon could also explain the differences between retrospective and daily diary accounts of proactive responses to discrimination obtained by Mallett and Swim (2009). When one considers a decision to confront a racist or sexist person the next time one encounters him or her, higher-level goal-relevant concerns with educating a person and sticking up for oneself should be quite salient, while lower-level feasibility concerns, such as potential costs in terms of disruption to ongoing tasks or escalating a conflict, should be less salient. On the other hand, when one is faced with the situation and must enact such plans, concerns about cost and feasibility may loom large.

IMPLEMENTATION INTENTIONS

This latter possibility—the idea that people give increasing weight to lower-level concerns as a future event becomes more temporally proximal—suggests that research on how people use implementation intentions to shield their higher-level goal pursuits from immediate lower-level concerns that might derail their efforts may be important to understanding successful proactivity (see, e.g., Gollwitzer & Sheeran, 2006). Implementation intentions refer to specific advance plans regarding how, when, and where goal-striving will be carried out in different situations. Importantly with respect to understanding proactive coping, such implementation intentions have been found to promote not only the initiation of goal-striving, but also its successful pursuit in the face of obstacles. Studying the techniques that people use in advance to regulate potential future responses to opportunities to implement proactive coping or to threats to proactive coping will continue to provide insight into how people can use such techniques to both initiate and maintain proactive coping efforts.

MENTAL SIMULATION AND MENTAL CONTRASTING

Finally, continued research on the processes of mental simulation and mental contrasting has the potential to inform our understanding of the specific kinds of thoughts about desired and undesired future outcomes that promote actions to attain or avoid them, and has particular potential to enrich our understanding of both the individual differences and component processes involved in successful and unsuccessful forms of proactivity. As noted throughout this chapter, a great deal of research on proactivity examines thoughts about the future without necessarily considering the valence or content of those thoughts. Research on mental simulation and other forms of future-oriented thinking clearly indicates that not all forms of thinking about the future lead to constructive action; that is, simply thinking about either desired future outcomes or current problems alone is insufficient to promote corresponding efforts to attain or ameliorate such states. Instead, specific thoughts about the steps one must take to achieve or avoid such outcomes (Taylor et al., 1998; Oyserman et al., 2006) and an active mental contrast between one's present situation and the envisioned future seem to be necessary to promote constructive action (see, e.g., Oettingen et al., 2001; Oettingen et al., 2005). These findings suggest that to more fully understand the links between future-oriented thinking and proactivity, we must know more about the particular future that is envisioned and how different ways of thinking about it promote proactive efforts.

Understanding the transactional nature of proactive coping

Fom the outset, we described proactive coping as a transactional process in which information acquired at one step of the model informs subsequent appraisals and coping efforts. As has been the case for the broader stress and coping literature (cf. McGrath & Tschan, 2004), this transactional character has been difficult to document with respect to proactive coping. This task is made more difficult by the fact that when proactivity is successful, not much may appear to have happened. As a result, we know relatively little about how what people learn from proactive monitoring and management of potential stressors influences their subsequent resource acquisition, attention, appraisals, and efforts, including situations in which people may decide that proactive coping will not work or is not worth the cost.

One especially important element of the proactive coping model that has been understudied is the influence of different proactive coping efforts on one's understanding of a potential stressor. The original Aspinwall and Taylor (1997) model specified at least two ways in which proactive coping efforts may influence the quantity and quality of information about potential stressors: by promoting attention to potential stressors and by leading people to take active efforts to manage them. These active efforts were predicted to be more successful than avoidant ones in eliciting information about the potential or unfolding problem. The literature on workplace proactivity, for example, suggests that people engage in active efforts to acquire information through monitoring situations for feedback, directly seeking feedback, and actively building social networks (Ashford et al., 2003; Grant &

Ashford, 2008; Morrison, 2002a,b). Similarly, the work on proactive management of discrimination (Mallett & Swim, 2005, 2009) obtained substantial evidence of heightened attention to aspects of the unfolding interaction and especially to nonverbal behavior on the part of one's interaction partner. Understanding how such proactive efforts to acquire information are related to subsequent appraisals and efforts will be an important next step in this work, as will devising paradigms with which to test the influence of active problem-solving efforts on the elicitation of information.

In our view, the emerging social psychological literature on proactive coping with stigma and discrimination has great potential to study such transactional processes as they unfold. By studying social interactions under conditions of anticipated discrimination, but in relatively controlled circumstances, measures of attention, appraisals, coping efforts, and recursive relations among them can be studied over time. Other laboratory-based paradigms, such as those involving attention to negative information in other domains (e.g., health risks, Aspinwall & Brunhart, 1996) and the allocation of effort to different kinds of problems (Aspinwall & Richter, 1999; Newby-Clark, 2004), will continue to be useful in understanding how different patterns of attention to negative information may be related both to subsequent coping efforts and the resources available for such efforts.

Understanding of the role of affect in proactive coping

As we suggested at the outset of this chapter, representations of potential future stressors are unlikely to be pallid or emotion-free, yet relatively little is known about how the specific emotions that accompany the consideration of potential stressors influence proactive coping efforts. For example, with respect to aging, we know that people may cope proactively with some of the social, physical, and financial demands of aging, but we know relatively little about how specific worries, fears, and hopes about aging influence this process. Much remains to be done to understand how different negative emotions such as worry, fear, anxiety, sadness, and anger promote or impede people's efforts to detect, appraise, and manage potential stressors, as well as respond to feedback on the success of their efforts (see Aspinwall, 2005, for discussion). Further, research on anticipated affect suggests that people's beliefs about how particular outcomes would make them feel are powerful influences on behavior, including decisions to engage in preventive or precautionary behaviors (Abramson & Sheeran, 2004; Leaf, 2008; Richard, van der Pligt, & De Vries, 1996). Indeed, the strategic activation of such considerations as anticipated regret is already being incorporated into interventions to promote proactivity in aging (Bode et al., 2007). Understanding the degree to which people accurately understand how particular outcomes would make them feel (e.g., affective forecasting, Gilbert, Pinel, Wilson, Blumberg, & Wheatley, 1998), as well as how such feelings influence decisions to attain or avoid particular outcomes, will further our understanding of the influence of both concurrent and anticipated affect on multiple steps of the proactive coping process.

Conclusion

The study of proactive coping is vibrant, documenting people's efforts to navigate and orchestrate their own outcomes in the major life domains of social interaction, health, work, and aging. Across multiple domains that present the possibility of serious threat, harm, or loss, people do appear to engage in proactive coping to prevent or otherwise limit the impact of potential stressors. Proactive coping appears to build and preserve personal and social resources, promote preparatory activities, foster the monitoring of complex stressors, and promote efforts to manage the problem and/or limit its impact on the self. Increasing evidence suggests that such efforts create measurable benefits in health and interpersonal outcomes. Further, these benefits have been documented in populations that are either disadvantaged or facing declines in resources.

Our review suggests that the search for individual differences in proactivity is at an early stage of inquiry. Researchers have examined a mixture of preferences for proactivity and planning, future temporal orientation, individual differences in the value placed on future outcomes, and other individual differences related either to the content of future-oriented thoughts or to a sensitivity to or concern with negative events and outcomes. Other approaches focus on the skills and competencies specified in the proactive coping model and related approaches to future-oriented self-regulatory efforts. Advancing our understanding in this area will require a more careful consideration of the discriminant validity of these different ways of assessing proactivity, as well as important situational moderators of their effectiveness in different domains. As this work progresses, careful attention to the particular potential stressors that people are seeking to

either prevent or offset in different domains and the particular goals adopted with respect to these proactive efforts will be essential.

A major development in the study of proactivity has been the demonstration that process-oriented short-term interventions to promote proactive approaches to maintaining health and managing chronic illness appear to create lasting gains in multiple aspects of proactive competence and measurable changes in health behaviors and outcomes. The importance of these interventions goes beyond the demonstration of the viability of the proactive coping concept and the provision of concrete evidence regarding the various skills and component processes involved in successful proactivity: By demonstrating that proactive coping competencies can be successfully taught and enacted, this work opens the door to broad-based efforts to promote proactive coping to improve life outcomes and reduce cumulative stress among all who seek such benefits, not just those favored by temperament or circumstance to possess the personal, social, and socioeconomic resources linked to successful proactivity. Understanding how to promote proactive coping methods among people who stand most to benefit—those with relatively few resources and those facing declines in resources—should provide a satisfying and challenging direction for future research.

Last, the continued integration of research on proactive coping with research on future-oriented thinking and self-regulation in general should yield insights into the processes by which decisions made with respect to future events and outcomes may differ from those made with respect to present options, by which thoughts about the future are linked to actions to attain or avoid particular future outcomes, and the ways in which people may benefit from knowledge of these mechanisms. In closing, it is particularly important to note that such an integration will likely not be a one-way exchange. By examining how people think about, prepare for, and—to the extent possible—act to alter future negative events with uncertain and potentially declining trajectories, the study of proactive coping has the potential to expand our understanding of future-oriented thinking and self-regulatory efforts beyond the achievement setting to a variety of important life domains.

Future Directions

Most research on proactive coping has focused on how individual actors navigate their own potential stressors in health, work, aging, or social relations. With the exception of studies of proactivity in the workplace (Ashford et al., 2003; Morrison, 2002a,b; Thompson, 2005) and in aging (Kahana & Kahana, 2003), relatively little research to date has emphasized the social aspects of proactive coping, including such obvious candidates as the role of social support in proactive appraisals and coping efforts. Particularly understudied are the interpersonal, dyadic, and familial aspects of proactivity, including the social-developmental antecedents of proactivity. Missing also is an understanding of collective forms of proactive coping undertaken to accomplish group (McGrath & Tschan, 2004) or societal-level goals, such as responding to the threats of global warming or other large-scale economic, environmental, or health problems. In the following sections, we suggest three directions for future research to address these gaps.

Extending the study of proactive coping with interpersonal stressors to close relationships

Our review of the literature on proactive coping with discrimination revealed multiple goals and some unique challenges inherent to the management of problematic social interactions, including the multiple priorities people may juggle in deciding whether to engage in proactive efforts and to what end. Continued research in this area is likely to reveal potential boundary conditions to proactive efforts to prevent certain kinds of stressful interpersonal situations and to identify situations in which proactive efforts may be directed primarily toward protecting the self from further harm. These parameters may well be different, however, in close relationships, where there is typically a premium on maintaining the relationship and where strategies such as avoidance are known to be harmful. Understanding when and how people try to detect, prevent, or otherwise respond to incipient stressors in relationships with friends, family members, and romantic partners will likely provide important information about relationship maintenance strategies (Canary, Stafford, & Semic, 2002) and both adaptive and maladaptive forms of proactive coping with perceived relationship stressors (Aspinwall, 1997a; Downey & Feldman, 1996).

Understanding the social-developmental antecedents of proactive coping

The documentation of frequently enacted, complex, and often successful forms of proactive coping among members of stigmatized groups suggests that it may be fruitful to examine some of the socialization processes and other social-developmental experiences that contribute to such efforts (see, e.g., Phinney & Chavira, 1995). For example, examining how stigmatized communities (at the level of families, schools, churches and other community organizations, and both formal and informal support groups) prepare their members to anticipate and manage discrimination would be an interesting avenue for future research, as would the incorporation of insights from such findings to the development of interventions to help people proactively detect and manage such treatment (Mallett & Swim, 2005).

Similarly, an enhanced understanding of the social-developmental origins of proactive approaches to maintaining physical and mental health would likely provide insight into the different ways that people respond to potential stressors. Such behaviors are likely modeled in families, and they may also be acquired and refined through social comparison processes as people learn from others' experiences about the likely trajectories of future stressors and the potential outcomes of different ways of managing them (see, e.g., Aspinwall, 1997b; Aspinwall, Hill, & Leaf, 2002).

Understanding dyadic and collective forms of proactivity

Although almost all of the research reviewed in this chapter portrayed proactive coping as an individual activity, recent approaches suggest that many threats to health and well-being (for example, a family member's chronic illness) are appraised as shared or collective stressors and managed accordingly by couples and families (Berg, Skinner, Ko, Butler, Palmer, Butner, & Wiebe, 2009; Berg & Upchurch, 2007; Berg, Wiebe, Butner, Bloor, Bradstreet, Upchurch, et al. 2008; Meegan & Berg, 2001; see also Revenson & DeLongis, Chapter 6 in the present volume). Insights from these new approaches may improve our understanding of proactive coping in such domains as familial disease, aging, economic setbacks, and other stressors in which it is unlikely that members of a couple or family engage in separate, uncoordinated coping efforts. A focus on shared appraisals and collective efforts may also elucidate cultural differences in the process of proactive coping, such as those stemming from independent versus interdependent views of the self (Markus & Kitayma, 1991).

Last, there are also particular large-scale proactive coping problems for which only collective action will be successful, notably global climate change (American Psychological Association Task Force on the Interface Between Psychology and Global Climate Change, 2009; see also Joireman, 2005). Understanding how people conceptualize their collective risks, responsibilities, and coping options at various levels (e.g., household, neighborhood, workplace, corporation, nation, region, planet) and translate these to individual responsibilities and coping efforts will be essential to understanding ways in which people may mobilize and coordinate a timely and effective response to this incipient stressor before it is fully realized.

Author Note

The assistance of Angela Newman in the preparation of this manuscript and Watcharaporn Pengchit in the preparation of the figures is gratefully acknowledged.

References

Abraham, C., & Sheeran, P. (2004). Deciding to exercise: The role of anticipated regret. *British Journal of Health Psychology, 9*, 269–78.

American Cancer Society. Cancer facts and figures 2008. [cited 2008 Mar 3]. Available from: http://www.cancer.org/downloads/STT/2008CAFFfinalsecured.pdf

American Psychological Association Task Force on the Interface Between Psychology and Global Climate Change (2009). *Psychology and global climate change: Addressing a multi-faceted phenomenon and set of challenges.* Washington, DC: Author. Retrieved from http://www.apa.org/releases/climate-change.pdf

Ashford, S. J., & Black, J. S. (1996). Proactivity during organizational entry: The role of desire for control. *Journal of Applied Psychology, 81*, 199–214.

Ashford, S. J., Blatt, R., & VandeWalle, D. (2003). Reflections on the looking glass: A review of research on feedback-seeking behavior in organizations. *Journal of Management, 29*, 773–99.

Ashford, S. J., & Cummings, L. L. (1983). Feedback as an individual resource: Personal strategies for creating information. *Organizational Behavior and Human Performance, 32*, 370–89.

Ashford, S. J., & Cummings, L. L. (1985). Proactive feedback seeking: The instrumental use of the information environment. *Journal of Occupational Psychology, 58*, 67–79.

Aspinwall, L. G. (1997a). Where planning meets coping: Proactive coping and the detection and management of potential stressors. In S. L. Friedman & E. K. Scholnick (Eds.), *The developmental psychology of planning: Why, how, and when do we plan?* (pp. 285–320). Hillsdale, NJ: Erlbaum.

Aspinwall, L. G. (1997b). Future-oriented aspects of social comparisons: A framework for studying health-related comparison activity. In B. P. Buunk & F. X. Gibbons (Eds.), *Health, coping, and well-being: Perspectives from social comparison theory* (pp. 125–165). Mahwah, NJ: Erlbaum.

Aspinwall, L. G. (1998). Rethinking the role of positive affect in self-regulation. *Motivation and Emotion, 22*, 1–32.

Aspinwall, L. G. (2001). Dealing with adversity: Self-regulation, coping, adaptation, and health. In A. Tesser & N. Schwarz (Eds.), *Blackwell handbook of social psychology: Intraindividual processes* (pp. 591–614). Malden, MA: Blackwell Publishers.

Aspinwall, L. G. (2005). The psychology of future-oriented thinking: From achievement to proactive coping, adaptation, and aging. *Motivation and Emotion, 29*, 203–35.

Aspinwall, L. G., & Brunhart, S. M. (1996). Distinguishing optimism from denial: Optimistic beliefs predict attention to health threats. *Personality and Social Psychology Bulletin, 22*, 993–1003.

Aspinwall, L. G., Hill, D. L., & Leaf, S. L. (2002). Prospects, pitfalls, and plans: A proactive perspective on social comparison activity. *European Review of Social Psychology, 12*, 267–98.

Aspinwall, L. G., Leaf, S. L., Dola, E. R., Kohlmann, W., & Leachman, S. A. (2008). *CDKN2A/p16* genetic test reporting improves early detection intentions and practices in high-risk melanoma families. *Cancer Epidemiology, Biomarkers, Prevention, 17*, 1510–9.

Aspinwall, L. G., Leaf, S. L., Kohlmann, W., Dola, E. R., & Leachman, S. A. (2009). Patterns of photoprotection following *CDKN2A/p16* genetic test reporting and counseling. *Journal of the American Academy of Dermatology, 60*, 719–896.

Aspinwall, L. G., & Richter, L. (1999). Optimism and self-mastery predict more rapid disengagement from unsolvable tasks in the presence of alternatives. *Motivation and Emotion, 23*, 221–45.

Aspinwall, L. G., Richter, L., & Hoffman, R.R. (2001). Understanding how optimism "works": An examination of optimists' adaptive moderation of belief and behavior. In E. C. Chang (Ed.), *Optimism and pessimism: Theory, research, and practice* (pp. 217–38). Washington, DC: American Psychological Association.

Aspinwall, L. G., Sechrist, G. B., & Jones, P. (2005). Expect the best and prepare for the worst: Anticipatory coping and preparations for Y2K. *Motivation and Emotion, 29*, 357–88.

Aspinwall, L. G., Taber, J. M., & Leachman, S. A. (2010). Genetic Testing and the Proactive Management of Familial Cancer Risk. *Annals of Behavioral Medicine, 39* (Suppl), s126.

Aspinwall, L. G., & Taylor, S. E. (1997). A stitch in time: Self-regulation and proactive coping. *Psychological Bulletin, 121*, 417–36.

Baltes, P. B., & Baltes, M. M. (1990). Psychological perspectives on successful aging: The model of selective optimism with compensation. In P. B. Baltes & M. M. Baltes (Eds.), *Successful aging: Perspectives from the behavioral sciences* (pp. 1–34). Cambridge, MA: Cambridge University Press.

Bateman, T. S., & Crant, J. M. (1993). The proactive component of organizational behavior: A measure and correlates. *Journal of Organizational Behavior, 14*, 103–18.

Berg, C. A., Skinner, M., Ko, K., Butler, J. M., Palmer, D. L., Butner, J., & Wiebe, D. J. (2009). The fit between stress appraisal and dyadic coping in understanding perceived coping effectiveness for adolescents with Type 1 diabetes. *Journal of Family Psychology, 23*, 521–30.

Berg, C. A., & Upchurch, R. (2007). A developmental-contextual model of couples coping with chronic illness across the adult lifespan. *Psychological Bulletin, 133*, 920–54.

Berg, C. A., Wiebe, D. J., Butner, J., Bloor, L., Bradstreet, C., Upchurch, R., Hayes, J., Stephenson, R., Nail, L., & Patton, G. (2008). Collaborative coping and daily mood in couples dealing with prostate cancer. *Psychology and Aging, 23*, 505–16.

Bishop, D. T., Demenais, F., Goldstein, A. M., Bergman, A. M., Bergman, W., Bishop, J. N., et al. (2002). Geographical variation in the penetrance of CDKN2A mutations for melanoma. *Journal of the National Cancer Institute, 94*, 894–903.

Bode, C., & de Ridder, D. T. D. (2007). Investing in the future—identifying participants in an educational program for middle-aged and older adults. *Health Education Research, 22*, 473–82.

Bode, C., de Ridder, D. T. D., & Bensing, J. M. (2006). Preparing for aging: Development, feasibility and preliminary results of an educational program for midlife and older based on proactive coping theory. *Patient Education and Counseling, 61*, 272–8.

Bode, C., de Ridder, D. T. D., Kuijer, R. G., & Bensing, J. M. (2007). Effects of an intervention promoting proactive coping competencies in middle and late adulthood. *The Gerontologist, 47*, 42–51.

Borowsky, I. W., Ireland, M., & Resnick, M. D. (2009). Health status and behavioral outcomes for youth who anticipate a high likelihood of early death. *Pediatrics, 124*(1), e81–e88.

Botkin, J. R., Smith, K. R., Croyle, R. T., Baty, B. J., Wylie, J. E., Dutson, D., et al. (2003). Genetic testing for a *BRCA1* mutation: Prophylactic surgery and screening behavior in women 2 years post testing. *American Journal of Medical Genetics, 118*, 201–9.

Boyd, J. N., & Zimbardo, P. G. (2005). Time perspective, health, and risk taking. In A. Strathman & J. Joireman (Eds.), *Understanding behavior in the context of time: Theory, research, and application* (pp. 85–107). Mahwah, NJ: Lawrence Erlbaum Associates.

Buehler, R., Griffin, D., & Ross, M. (1994). Exploring the "planning fallacy": Why people underestimate their task completion times. *Journal of Personality and Social Psychology, 67*, 366–81.

Canary, D. J., Stafford, L., & Semic, B. A. (2002). A panel study of the associations between maintenance strategies and relational characteristics. *Journal of Marriage and Family, 64*, 395–406.

Carver, C. S., & Scheier, M. F. (Eds.). (1998). *On the self-regulation of behavior*. New York: Cambridge University Press.

Chan, D. (2006). Interactive effects of situational judgment effectiveness and proactive personality on work perceptions and work outcomes. *Journal of Applied Psychology, 91*, 475–81.

Clark, R., Anderson, N. B., Clark, V. R., & Williams, D. R. (1999). Racism as a stressor for African-Americans: A biopsychosocial model. *American Psychologist, 54*, 805–16.

Cole, S. W., Kemeny, M. E., Taylor, S. E., Visscher, B. R., & Fahey, J. L. (1996). Accelerated course of human immunodeficiency virus infection in gay men who conceal their homosexual identity. *Psychosomatic Medicine, 58*, 219–31.

Crant, J. M. (2000). Proactive behavior in organizations. *Journal of Management, 26*, 435–62.

Ditto, P. H., Hawkins, N. A., & Pizarro, D. A. (2005). Imagining the end of life: On the psychology of advance medical decision making. *Motivation and Emotion, 29*, 481–502.

Downey, G., & Feldman, S. I. (1996). Implications of rejection sensitivity for intimate relationships. *Journal of Personality and Social Psychology, 70*, 1327–43.

Fiksenbaum, L. M., Greenglass, E. R., & Eaton, J. (2006). Perceived social support, hassles, and coping among the elderly. *Journal of Applied Gerontology, 25*, 17–30.

Fiske, S. T., & Taylor, S. E. (1991). *Social cognition* (2nd ed.). New York: McGraw-Hill.

Florell, S. R., Boucher, K. M., Garibotti, G., Kerber, J. A. R., Mineau, G., Wiggins, C., et al. (2005). Population-based analysis of prognostic factors and survival in familial melanoma. *Journal of Clinical Oncology, 23*, 7168–77.

Folkman, S., & Lazarus, R. S. (1985). If it changes, it must be a process: Study of emotion and coping during three stages of a college examination. *Journal of Personality and Social Psychology, 48*, 150–70.

Frable, D. E. S., Blackstone, T., & Scherbaum, C. (1990). Marginal and mindful: Deviants in social interactions. *Journal of Personality and Social Psychology, 59*, 140–9.

Frederickson, B. L., & Joiner, T. (2002). Positive emotions trigger upward spirals toward emotional well-being. *Psychological Science, 13*, 172–5.

Frese, M., Kring, W., Soose, A., & Zempel, J. (1996). Personal initiative at work: Differences between East and West Germany. *Academy of Management Journal, 39*, 37–63.

Gilbert, D. T., Pinel, E. C., Wilson, T. D., Blumberg, S. J., & Wheatley, T. P. (1998). Immune neglect: A source of durability bias in affective forecasting. *Journal of Personality and Social Psychology, 75*, 617–38.

Goldstein, A. M., Chan, M., Harland, M., Hayward, N. K. Demenais, F., Bishop, D. T., et al. (2007). Features associated with germline *CDKN2A* mutations: a GenoMEL study of melanoma-prone families from three continents. *Journal of Medical Genetics, 44*, 99–106.

Gollwitzer, P. M. (1999). Implementation intentions: Strong effects of simple plans. *American Psychologist, 54*, 493–503.

Gollwitzer, P. M., & Sheeran, P. (2006). Implementation intentions and goal achievement: A meta-analysis of effects and processes. In M. P. Zanna (Ed.), *Advances in experimental social psychology* (Vol. 38, pp. 69–119). San Diego, CA: Elsevier Academic Press.

Grant, A. M., & Ashford, S. J. (2008). The dynamics of proactivity at work. *Research in Organizational Behavior, 28*, 3–34.

Greenglass, E. (2002). Proactive coping. In E. Frydenberg (Ed.), *Beyond coping: Meeting goals, vision, and challenges* (pp. 37–62). London: Oxford University Press.

Greenglass, E. R., Schwarzer, R., & Tauber, S. (1999). *The Proactive Coping Inventory (PCI): A multidimensional research instrument*. Retrieved July 15, 2009 [On-line publication]. Available at: http://userpage.fu-berlin.de/~health/greenpci.htm

Greenglass, E. R., Marques, S., deRidder, M., & Behl, S. (2005). Positive coping and mastery in a rehabilitation setting. *International Journal of Rehabilitation Research, 28*, 331–9.

Higgins, E. T. (1997). Beyond pleasure and pain. *American Psychologist, 52*, 1280–300.

Hobfoll, S. E. (1989). Conservation of resources: A new attempt at conceptualizing stress. *American Psychologist, 44*, 513–24.

Hobfoll, S. E. (2011). Conservation of resources theory: Its implication for stress, health, and resilience. In Folkman, S. (Ed.), *The Oxford handbook of stress, health, and coping*. New York: Oxford University Press.

Holman, E. A., & Silver, R. C. (2005). Future-oriented thinking and adjustment in a nationwide longitudinal study following the September 11th terrorist attacks. *Motivation and Emotion, 29*, 389–410.

Huebner, D. M., Rebchook, G. M., & Kegeles, S. M. (2004). Experiences of harassment, discrimination, and physical violence among young gay and bisexual men. *American Journal of Public Health, 94*, 1200–3.

Hyers, L. L. (2007). Resisting prejudice every day: Exploring women's assertive responses to anti-Black racism, anti-Semitism, heterosexism, and sexism. *Sex Roles, 56*, 1–12.

Joireman, J., Strathman, A., & Balliet, D. (2006). Considering future consequences: An integrative model. In L. J. Sanna & E. C. Chang (Eds.), *Judgments over time: The interplay of thoughts, feelings, and behaviors* (pp. 82–99). New York: Oxford University Press.

Joireman, J. (2005). Environmental problems as social dilemmas: The temporal dimension. In A. Strathman & J. Joireman (Eds.), *Understanding behavior in the context of time: Theory, research, and application* (pp. 289–304). Mahwah, NJ: Lawrence Erlbaum Associates.

Jones, J. M. (1988). Cultural differences in temporal perspectives: Instrumental and expressive behaviors in time. In J. McGrath (Ed.), *The social psychology of time: New perspectives* (pp. 21–38). Thousand Oaks, CA: Sage Publications.

Kahana, E., & Kahana, B. (1996). Conceptual and empirical advances in understanding aging well through proactive adaptation. In V. Bengtson (Ed.), *Adulthood and aging: Research on continuities and discontinuities* (pp. 13–40). New York: Springer Publishing.

Kahana, E., & Kahana, B. (2003). Contextualizing successful aging: New directions in an age-old search. In R. Settersten, Jr. (Ed.), *Invitation to the life course: A new look at old age* (pp. 225–55). Amityville, NY: Baywood Publishing Company.

Kahana, E., Lawrence, R. H., Kahana, B., Kercher, K., Wisniewski, A., Stoller, E., Tobin, J., & Stange, K. (2002). Long-term impact of preventive proactivity on quality of life of the old-old. *Psychosomatic Medicine, 64*, 382–94.

Kahana, E., Kahana, B., & Kercher, K. (2003). Emerging lifestyles and proactive options for successful ageing. *Ageing International, 28*, 155–80.

Kahana, E., Kahana, B., & Zhang, J. (2005). Motivational antecedents of preventive proactivity in late life: Linking future orientation and exercise. *Motivation and Emotion, 29*, 443–64.

Kahana, E., Kahana, B., & Kelly-Moore, J. (2005, August). Coping with disability in late life: A longitudinal study of proactive adaptations. Paper presented at the annual meeting of the American Sociological Association, Philadelphia.

Kaiser, C. R., & Miller, C. T. (2004). A stress and coping perspective on confronting sexism. *Psychology of Women Quarterly*, 28, 161–78.

Kawakami, K., Dunn, E., Karmali, F., & Dovidio, J. F. (2009). Mispredicting affective and behavioral responses to racism. *Science, 323*, 276–8.

Lasane, T. P., & O'Donnell, D. A. (2005). Time orientation measurement: A conceptual approach. In A. Strathman & J. Joireman (Eds.), *Understanding behavior in the context of time: Theory, research, and application* (pp. 11–30). Mahwah, NJ: Lawrence Erlbaum Associates.

Lazarus, R. S. (1990). Theory-based stress measurement (target article). *Psychological Inquiry, 1*, 3–13.

Lazarus, R. S., & Folkman, S. (1984). *Stress, appraisal, and coping*. New York: Springer.

Leaf, S. L. (2008). Do the right thing: Anticipated affect as a guide to behavioral choice. Unpublished doctoral dissertation, University of Utah.

Leaf, S. L., Aspinwall, L. G., & Leachman, S. A. (2010). God and agency in the era of molecular medicine: Religious beliefs predict sun-protection behaviors following melanoma genetic test reporting. *Archive for the Psychology of Religion, 32*, 87–112.

Leith, K. P., & Baumeister, R. F. (1996). Why do bad moods increase self-defeating behavior? Emotion, risk taking, and self-regulation. *Journal of Personality and Social Psychology, 71*, 1250–67.

Liberman, N., & Trope, Y. (1998). The role of feasibility and desirability considerations in near and distant future decisions: A test of Temporal Construal Theory. *Journal of Personality and Social Psychology, 75*, 5–18.

Liberman, N., & Trope, Y. (2008). The psychology of transcending the here and now. *Science, 322*, 1201–5.

Magnan, R. E., Köblitz, A. R., Zielke, D. J., & McCaul, K. D. (2009). The effects of warning smokers on perceived risk, worry, and motivation to quit. *Annals of Behavioral Medicine, 37*, 46–57.

Mallett, R. K., & Swim, J. K. (2005). Bring it on: Proactive coping with discrimination. *Motivation and Emotion, 29*, 411–41.

Mallett, R. K., & Swim, J. K. (2009). Making the best of a bad situation: Proactive coping with racial discrimination. *Basic and Applied Social Psychology, 31*, 304–316.

Markus, H. R., & Kitayama, S. (1991). Culture and the self: Implications for cognition, emotion, and motivation. *Psychological Review, 98*, 224–53.

Marlatt, G. A., & Gordon, J. R. (Eds.). (1985). *Relapse prevention: Maintenance strategies in the treatment of addictive behaviors*. New York: Guilford.

Marteau, T. M., & Weinman, J. (2006). Self-regulation and the behavioural response to DNA risk information: A theoretical analysis and framework for future research. *Social Science & Medicine, 62*, 1360–8.

McCaul, K. D., & Mullens, A. B. (2003). Affect, thought and self-protective health behavior: The case of worry and cancer screening. In J. Suls & K. A. Wallston (Eds.), *Social psychological foundations of health and illness* (pp. 137–68). Malden, MA: Blackwell Publishers.

McCrae, R. R., & Costa, P. T., Jr. (1986). Personality, coping, and coping effectiveness in an adult sample. *Journal of Personality and Social Psychology, 54*, 385–405.

McGrath, J. E., & Beehr, T. A. (1990). Time and the stress process: Some temporal issues in the conceptualization and measurement of stress. *Stress Medicine, 6*, 93–104.

McGrath, J. E., & Tschan, F. (2004). *Temporal matters in social psychology: Examining the role of time in the lives of groups and individuals*. Washington, DC: American Psychological Association.

Meegan, S. P., & Berg, C. A. (2001). Whose life task is it anyway? Social appraisal and life task pursuit. *Journal of Personality, 69*, 363–89.

Meyer, I. H. (2003). Prejudice, social stress and mental health in lesbian, gay, and bisexual populations: Conceptual issues and research evidence. *Psychological Bulletin, 129*, 674–97.

Midlarsky, E., & Kahana, E. (2007). Altruism, well-being, and mental health in late life. In S. G. Post (Ed.), *Altruism and health: Perspectives from empirical research* (pp. 56–69). New York: Oxford University Press.

Miller, C. T., & Major, B. (2000). Coping with stigma and prejudice. In T. F. Heatherton, R. E. Kleck, M. R. Hebl, & J. G. Hull (Eds.), *The social psychology of stigma* (pp. 243–72). New York: Guilford University Press.

Miller, C. T., & Myers, A. M. (1998). Compensating for prejudice: How heavyweight people (and others) control outcomes despite prejudice. In J. K. Swim & C. Stangor (Eds.), *Prejudice: The target's perspective* (pp. 191–218). San Diego, CA: Academic Press.

Miller, C. T., Rothblum, E. D., Felicio, D., & Brand, P. (1995). Compensating for stigma: Obese and nonobese women's reactions to being visible. *Personality and Social Psychology Bulletin, 21*, 1093–106.

Miller, S. M., Bowen, D. J., Croyle, R. T., & Rowland, J. H. (2009). *Handbook of cancer control and behavioral science: A resource for researchers, practitioners, and policymakers.* Washington, DC: American Psychological Association.

Morrison, E. W. (1993a). Newcomer information seeking: Exploring types, modes, sources, and outcomes. *Academy of Management Journal, 36*, 557–89.

Morrison, E. W. (1993b). Longitudinal study of the effects of information seeking on newcomer socialization. *Journal of Applied Psychology, 78*, 173–83.

Morrison, E. W. (2002a). Information seeking within organizations. *Human Communication Research, 28*, 229–42.

Morrison, E. W. (2002b). Newcomers' relationships: The role of social network ties during socialization. *Academy of Management Journal, 45*, 1149–60.

Newby-Clark, I. R. (2004). Getting ready for the bad times: Self-esteem and anticipatory coping. *European Journal of Social Psychology, 34*, 309–16.

Norem, J. K., & Cantor, N. (1986). Defensive pessimism: "Harnessing" anxiety as motivation. *Journal of Personality and Social Psychology, 51*, 1208–17.

Nurmi, J.-E. (2005). Thinking about and acting upon the future: Development of future orientation across the life span. In A. Strathman & J. Joireman (Eds.), *Understanding behavior in the context of time: Theory, research, and application* (pp. 31–57). Mahwah, NJ: Lawrence Erlbaum Associates.

Oettingen, G. (1996). Positive fantasy and motivation. In P. M. Gollwitzer & J. A. Bargh (Eds.), *The psychology of action* (pp. 236–59). New York: Guilford.

Oettingen, G., Pak, H., & Schnetter, K. (2001). Self-regulation of goal setting: Turning free fantasies about the future into binding goals. *Journal of Personality and Social Psychology, 80*, 736–53.

Oettingen, G., Mayer, D., Thorpe, J. S., Janetzke, H., & Lorenz, S. (2005). Turning fantasies about positive and negative futures into self-improvement goals. *Motivation and Emotion, 29*, 237–67.

Ouwehand, C. (2005). Proactive coping and successful aging: What role do resources and strategies play in the preparation for potential goal threats associated with aging? Dissertation, University of Utrecht.

Ouwehand, C., de Ridder, D. T. D., & Bensing, J. M. (2006). Situational aspects are more important in shaping proactive coping behavior than individual characteristics: A vignette study among adults preparing for ageing. *Psychology and Health, 21*, 809–25.

Ouwehand, C., de Ridder, D. T. D., & Bensing, J. M. (2009). Who can afford to look to the future? The relationships between socio-economic status and proactive coping. *European Journal of Public Health, 19*(4), 412–7.

Ouwehand, C., de Ridder, D. T. D., & Bensing, J. M. (2007). A review of successful aging models: Proposing proactive coping as an important additional strategy. *Clinical Psychology Review, 27*, 873–84.

Oyserman, D., Bybee, D., & Terry, K. (2006). Possible selves and academic outcomes: How and when possible selves impel action. *Journal of Personality and Social Psychology, 91*, 188–204.

Pachankis, J. E. (2007). The psychological implications of concealing a stigma: A cognitive-affective-behavioral model. *Psychological Bulletin, 133*, 328–45.

Pascoe, E. A., & Smart Richman, L. (2009). Perceived discrimination and health: A meta-analytic review. *Psychological Bulletin, 135*, 531–54.

Powe, B. D. (1995). Cancer fatalism among elderly Caucasians and African Americans. *Oncology Nursing Forum, 22*, 1355–9.

Phinney, J. S., & Chavira, V. (1995). Parental ethnic socialization and adolescent coping with problems related to ethnicity. *Journal of Research on Adolescence, 5*, 31–53.

Prenda, K. M., & Lachman, M. E. (2001). Planning for the future: A life management strategy for increasing control and life satisfaction in adulthood. *Psychology and Aging, 16*, 206–16.

Pyszczynski, T., & Greenberg, J. (1987). Self-regulatory perseveration and the depressive self-focusing style: A self-awareness theory of reactive depression. *Psychological Bulletin, 102*, 122–38.

Revenson, T., & DeLongis, A. (2011). Couples coping with chronic illness. In Folkman, S. (Ed.), *The Oxford handbook of stress, health, and coping.* New York: Oxford University Press.

Richard, R., van der Pligt, J., & De Vries, N. (1996). Anticipated regret and time perspective: Changing sexual risk-taking behavior. *Journal of Behavioral Decision Making, 9*, 185–99.

Roesch, S. C., Aldridge, A. A., Huff, T. L. P., Langner, K., Villodas, F., & Bradshaw, K. (2009). On the dimensionality of the Proactive Coping Inventory: 7, 5, 3 factors? *Anxiety, Stress & Coping, 22*(3), 327–39.

Rothspan, S., & Read, S. J. (1996). Present versus future time perspective and HIV risk among heterosexual college students. *Health Psychology, 15*, 131–4.

Sagristano, M. D., Trope, Y., & Liberman, N. (2002). Time-dependent gambling: Odds now, money later. *Journal of Experimental Psychology, 131*, 364–76.

Sansone, C., & Berg, C. A. (1993). Adapting to the environment across the life span: Different process or different inputs? *International Journal of Behavioral Development, 16*, 379–90.

Scheier, M. F., & Carver, C. S. (1985). Optimism, coping, and health: Assessment and implications of generalized outcome expectancies. *Health Psychology, 4*, 219–47.

Scheier, M. F., Carver, C. S., & Bridges, M. W. (1994). Distinguishing optimism from neuroticism (and trait anxiety, self-mastery, and self-esteem): A reevaluation of the Life Orientation Test. *Journal of Personality and Social Psychology, 67*, 1063–78.

Schwarzer, R. (2000). Manage stress at work through preventive and proactive coping. In E. A. Locke (Ed.), *The Blackwell handbook of principles of organizational behavior* (pp. 342–55). Oxford, UK: Blackwell.

Schwarzer, R., & Knoll, N. (2003). Positive coping: Mastering demands and searching for meaning. In S. J. Lopez, J. Shane & C. R. Snyder (Eds.), *Positive psychological assessment: A handbook of models and measures* (pp. 393–409). Washington, DC: American Psychological Association.

Sellers, R. M., & Shelton, J. N. (2003). Racial identity, discrimination, and mental health among African Americans. *Journal of Personality and Social Psychology, 84*, 1079–92.

Senior, V., Marteau, T. M., & Weinman, J. (2000). Impact of genetic testing on causal models of heart disease and arthritis: An analogue study. *Psychology & Health, 14*, 1077–88.

Shelton, J. N., Richeson, J. A., & Salvatore, J. (2005). Expecting to be the target of prejudice: Implications for interethnic interactions. *Personality and Social Psychology Bulletin, 31*(9), 1189–202.

Shepperd, J. A., Ouellette, J. A., & Fernandez, J. K. (1996). Abandoning unrealistic optimism: Performance estimates and the temporal proximity of self-relevant feedback. *Journal of Personality and Social Psychology, 70*, 844–55.

Snyder, C. R. (1994). *The psychology of hope: You can get there from here*. New York: Free Press.

Sohl, S. J., & Moyer, A. (2009). Refining the conceptualization of a future-oriented self-regulatory behavior: Proactive coping. *Personality and Individual Differences, 47*, 139–44.

Stadler, G., Oettingen, G., & Gollwitzer, P. M. (2009). Physical activity in women: Effects of a self-regulation intervention. *American Journal of Preventive Medicine, 36*, 29–34.

Strathman, A., Gleicher, F., Boninger, D. S., & Edwards, C. S. (1994). The consideration of future consequences: Weighing immediate and distant outcomes of behavior. *Journal of Personality and Social Psychology, 66*, 742–52.

Swim, J. K., & Thomas, M. A. (2006). Responding to everyday discrimination: A synthesis of research on goal directed, self-regulatory coping behaviors. In S. Levin & C. Van Laar (Eds.), Stigma and group inequality: Social psychological perspectives (The Claremont Symposium on Applied Social Psychology) (pp. 127–51). Mahwah, NJ: Lawrence Erlbaum Associates.

Swim, J. K. & Stangor, C. (Eds). (1998). Prejudice: The target's perspective. New York: Academic Press.

Taber, J. M., Aspinwall, L. G., Kohlmann, W., Dow, R., & Leachman, S. A. (in press). Parental preferences for *CDKN2A/p16* genetic testing of minors. *Genetics in Medicine.*

Taylor, S. E., Pham, L. B., Rivkin, I. D., & Armor, D. A. (1998). Harnessing the imagination: Mental simulation, self-regulation, and coping. *American Psychologist, 53*, 429–39.

Taylor, S. E., Repetti, R. L., & Seeman, T. (1997). Health psychology: What is an unhealthy environment and how does it get under the skin? *Annual Review of Psychology, 48*, 411–47.

Thompson, J. A. (2005). Proactive personality and job performance: A social capital perspective. *Journal of Applied Psychology, 90*, 1011–7.

Thompson, S. C., & Schlehofer, M. M. (2008). Control, denial, and heightened sensitivity reactions to personal threat: Testing the generalizability of the threat orientation approach. *Personality and Social Psychology Bulletin, 34*, 1070–83.

Thoolen, B. (2007). Beyond good intentions: The effectiveness of a proactive self-management intervention in patients with screen-detected Type 2 diabetes. Dissertation, University of Utrecht.

Thoolen, B., de Ridder, D., Bensing, J., Gorter, K., & Rutten, G. (2008a). No worries, no impact? A systematic review of emotional, cognitive, and behavioural responses to the diagnosis of type 2 diabetes. *Health Psychology Review, 2*, 65–93.

Thoolen, B., de Ridder, D., Bensing, J., Gorter, K., & Rutten, G. (2008b). Beyond good intentions: The development and evaluation of a proactive self-management course for patients recently diagnosed with Type 2 diabetes. *Health Education Research, 23*, 53–61.

Thoolen, B. J., de Ridder, D., Bensing, J., Gorter, K., & Rutten, G. (2009). Beyond good intentions: The role of proactive coping in achieving sustained behavioural change in the context of diabetes management. *Psychology & Health, 24*, 237–54.

Thoolen, B., de Ridder, D., Bensing, J., Maas, C., Griffin, S., Gorter, K., & Rutten, G. (2007). Effectiveness of a self-management intervention in patients with screen-detected type 2 diabetes. *Diabetes Care, 30*, 2832–7.

Trope, Y., & Liberman, N. (2003). Temporal construal. *Psychological Review, 110*, 403–21.

Umaña-Taylor, A. J., Vargas-Chanes, D., Garcia, C. D., & Gonzales-Backen, M. (2008). A longitudinal examination of Latino adolescents' ethnic identity, coping with discrimination and self-esteem. *Journal of Early Adolescence, 28*, 16–50.

Wills, T. A., Sandy, J. M., & Yaeger, A. M. (2001). Time perspective and early-onset substance use: A model based on stress-coping theory. *Psychology of Addictive Behaviors, 15*, 118–25.

Zimbardo, P. G., & Boyd, J. N. (1999). Putting time in perspective: A valid, reliable individual-difference metric. *Journal of Personality and Social Psychology, 77*, 1271–88.

PART 6

Assessing Coping: New Technologies and Concepts

Regulating Emotions during Stressful Experiences: The Adaptive Utility of Coping through Emotional Approach

Annette L. Stanton

Abstract

Coping through emotional approach is a construct involving two component processes, both conceptualized as intentional attempts to manage demands during stressful experiences: emotional processing (i.e., attempts to acknowledge, explore, and understand emotions) and emotional expression (i.e., verbal and/or nonverbal efforts to communicate or symbolize emotional experience). Recent cross-sectional, longitudinal, and experimental research reveals that when assessed with indicators that are not confounded with distress or self-deprecatory content, emotional processing and expression can promote well-being and health during a range of stressful circumstances. The nature of the stressor and concomitant cognitive appraisals, the interpersonal context, and individual differences condition the effects of coping through emotional approach. Mechanisms for the utility of coping through emotional approach are being specified. An understanding of who benefits from coping through emotional approach in which contexts and how these effects accrue will require continued integration of findings from stress and coping research, emotion science, and clinical intervention trials. Such research will inform clinical interventions directed toward enhancing emotion regulation skills.

Keywords: emotion, emotional approach, coping, stress, emotion regulation

Even under the most dire circumstances, most individuals are able to maintain or recover psychological equilibrium (e.g., Bonanno, Galea, Bucciarelli, & Vlahov, 2006; Ozer, Best, Lipsey, & Weiss, 2008). Historically, we have learned much more from the stress and coping literature about what places people who undergo stressful or traumatic experiences at risk for bad outcomes than about the factors that serve to protect or restore well-being and health. However, researchers in this area increasingly have turned attention toward preventive and restorative processes, as evidenced by a number of chapters in this handbook. In this chapter, I evaluate the evidence for the potential benefits and costs of coping through processing and expressing emotions during stressful encounters (i.e., coping through emotional approach). After a brief description of the impetus for studying the adaptive value of coping through emotional approach and the development of a measure to assess the construct, this chapter contains an examination of recent research addressing the consequences of coping through processing and expressing emotions related to stressors, the conditions under which and the mechanisms through which emotional approach promotes or hinders psychological adjustment and physical health, and evidence pertinent to psychosocial interventions designed to influence emotional processing and expression.

The chapter concludes with remaining questions and directions for research.

History of the Construct

Our concentration on coping with adverse circumstances through intentionally processing and expressing emotions emerged from an effort to reconcile several lines of theory and research on stress, coping, and emotion. Some theorists have characterized the experience and expression of intense emotion as dysfunctional and as an obstacle to rational thought (see Averill, 1990, for a review). Moreover, in the empirical literature on stress and coping through the 1990s, measures of attempts to manage emotions surrounding stressors (i.e., emotion-focused coping; Lazarus & Folkman, 1984) yielded consistent relations with untoward psychological outcomes. An illustrative review of the PsycInfo database from 1995 through 1998 yielded more than 100 studies in which the relation between emotion-focused coping and adjustment was examined in an adult or adolescent sample (Stanton, Parsa, & Austenfeld, 2002). Three measures containing emotion-focused coping content were used most frequently: the Ways of Coping Questionnaire (Lazarus & Folkman, 1984), the COPE (Carver, Scheier, & Weintraub, 1989), and the Coping Inventory for Stressful Situations (CISS; Endler & Parker, 1990, 1994). Narrowed to studies including the two subscales most relevant to processing and expressing emotions (i.e., CISS Emotion-Oriented Coping scale and COPE Focus on and Venting of Emotion scale), the review revealed a consistent (albeit primarily cross-sectional) association of those scales and such indicators of poor adjustment as depressive symptoms, anxiety, neuroticism, and life dissatisfaction. Similarly, Coyne and Racioppo (2000) concluded in a review that the relation of emotion-focused coping and distress is "perhaps the most consistent finding in the coping literature" (p. 657).

In contrast, functionalist theories of emotion highlight its organizing, effective elements. For example, Levenson (1994) argued that emotions "alter attention, shift certain behaviors upward in response hierarchies, and activate relevant associative networks in memory," as well as create "a bodily milieu that is optimal for effective response" (p. 123). Experimental research on the consequences of expressive disclosure for health and well-being (see Frattaroli, 2006; Smyth, 1998, for reviews), clinical approaches such as emotion-focused therapy (e.g., Greenberg & Watson, 2006), and the literature on emotion regulation (e.g., Gross, 2007) also point to the potential value of processing and expressing emotions for health and well-being. These bodies of work led us to question the validity of the research suggesting the hazards of emotion-focused approaches in the stress and coping literature.

When we closely examined the research on emotion-focused coping, we discovered that the manner in which emotion-focused coping has been operationalized in coping measures was likely to account in part for the relation of emotion-focused coping with dysfunctional outcomes (Stanton, Danoff-Burg, Cameron, & Ellis, 1994; Stanton, Kirk, Cameron, & Danoff-Burg, 2000). Emotion-focused coping is a broad construct, involving behaviors oriented toward both approaching and avoiding the stressor and concomitant emotions. Accordingly, wide latitude is evident in items designed to reflect emotion-focused coping (e.g., "I let my feelings out," "I blame myself for becoming too emotional," "I say to myself 'this isn't real'"), some of which are inversely correlated (Scheier, Weintraub, & Carver, 1986). A related point is that researchers sometimes refer to "emotion-focused coping" rather than to a specific facet (e.g., avoidance) of that construct when they advance conclusions about its adaptiveness. Avoidance of stressor-related thoughts and feelings can carry very different consequences for well-being and health than does intentionally approaching the stressor through processing and expressing emotion, seeking social support, or reappraising the stressor's meaning. Behaviors aggregated under the rubric of emotion-focused coping must be disentangled in order to elucidate their distinct consequences.

Another issue in the measurement of emotion-focused coping is that a number of emotion-focused coping items across several instruments contain expressions of distress (e.g., "Become very tense") or self-deprecation (e.g., "Focus on my general inadequacies"). It is difficult to imagine that such items would not be related to indicators of maladjustment. The contention that coping measures are confounded with negative adjustment is supported by the finding that clinical psychologists rate most published, emotion-oriented coping items as symptomatic of psychopathology (Stanton et al., 1994, Study 1). Further, coping items written specifically to exclude expressions of distress and self-deprecation evidence discriminant validity with adjustment measures, whereas confounded items overlap significantly with measures of poor functioning (Stanton et al., 1994, Study 2). These limitations in the conceptualization and operationalization of emotion-focused coping catalyzed our efforts to create alternative measures of coping through identifying, processing, and expressing emotions under stressful conditions.

Assessment of Coping Through Emotional Approach

Emotion regulation involves "processes that individuals use to influence which emotions they generate, when they do so, and how these emotions are experienced or expressed" (Ochsner & Gross, 2005, p. 243). A range of self-report measures are available relevant to emotion regulation (e.g., Berkeley Expressivity Questionnaire, Gross & John, 1995; Emotion Regulation Questionnaire, Gross & John, 2003; Emotional Expressiveness Questionnaire and Ambivalence over Emotional Expressiveness Questionnaire, King & Emmons, 1990; Levels of Emotional Awareness Scale, Lane, Quinlan, Schwartz, Walker, & Zeitlin, 1990). However, they are not designed specifically to assess emotional processing and expression as coping processes elected during stressful experiences—hence our effort to develop such a measure free of content indicating distress or self-deprecation (Stanton et al., 1994; Stanton, Kirk et al., 2000). In four scale development studies with young adults (Stanton, Kirk et al., 2000), exploratory (Study 1) and confirmatory (Study 3) factor analyses yielded two distinct facets of emotional approach coping: emotional processing (EP) and emotional expression (EE). The EP items reflect active attempts to acknowledge, explore, and come to understand one's stressor-related emotions (e.g., "I acknowledge my emotions," "I take time to figure out what I'm really feeling"). The EE items represent active verbal and/or nonverbal efforts to communicate or symbolize emotional experience (e.g., "I feel free to express my emotions," "I take time to express my emotions").

The emotional approach coping (EAC) scales have been examined in both a situational version (i.e., instruction set specific to the stressor) and a dispositional version (i.e., "indicate what you generally do, feel, and think when you experience stressful situations"). Uncorrelated with social desirability (Stanton, Kirk et al., 2000, Study 1 and 3; Segerstrom, Stanton, Alden, & Shortridge, 2003), the scales also demonstrate adequate internal consistency reliability and test–retest reliability at 4 weeks in both versions (see Austenfeld & Stanton, 2004, for a review of psychometric properties and descriptive statistics). EP and EE are conceptualized as approach-oriented coping processes, and the scales

correlate moderately with other approach-oriented strategies such as problem-focused coping and positive reframing (Stanton, Danoff-Burg et al., 2000; Stanton, Kirk et al., 2000, Study 1 and 3). The scales are uncorrelated (Stanton, Danoff-Burg et al., 2000; Stanton, Kirk et al., 2000) or negatively correlated (Smith, Lumley, & Longo, 2002) with avoidance-oriented coping processes such as mental disengagement. Although the EP and EE subscales are moderately to highly intercorrelated, they demonstrate distinct relations with other variables. The EE scale correlates more highly with self-report measures of dispositional emotional expressiveness and family expressiveness than does the EP scale (Stanton, Kirk et al, 2000, Study 1, Study 3). Family members are better able to estimate each other's presumably more observable coping through EE than their EP (Stanton, Kirk et al., 2000, Study 2).

The EAC scales are related to measures of coping through seeking social support (Stanton, Kirk et al., 2000, Study 1 and 3) and other measures pertaining to interpersonal relationships. Pakenham, Rattan, and Smith (2007) found that EAC regarding pregnancy was correlated with higher maternal care (but not paternal care) and lower maternal overprotection on a measure of extent of bonding with the family of origin. Pregnancy-related EAC also was related to perceived availability of general and pregnancy-related support from the partner and potential support persons outside the family. Also studying pregnant women, Rini, Dunkel Schetter, Hobel, Glynn, and Sandman (2006) found that coping through EE was associated with secure attachment in romantic relationships, high social network orientation, skill at conflict management, support-seeking, kin collectivism, and relationship quality with the partner. That the magnitudes of the relations between the EAC scales and interpersonal indicators in these studies are not high suggest that the measure is not simply a proxy for social support (also see the section on mechanisms for the effects of EAC below).

Women and men differ significantly in their endorsement of emotional approach in some samples (see Austenfeld & Stanton, 2004), with women reporting greater use of EP and/or EE than men, whereas other studies have not identified a gender difference (e.g., Smith et al., 2002). Relations of the scales with personality attributes tend to vary by gender in young adults. In undergraduate women, EP is positively associated with adaptive traits such as self-esteem, hope, and instrumentality and negatively correlated with personality variables such as neuroticism. In undergraduate men, EP is associated with ruminative and distracting reactions to depressive symptoms and unrelated to positive personality characteristics (Stanton, Kirk et al., 2000, Study 1, Study 3). In another study (Segerstrom et al., 2003, Study 1), significant gender differences did not emerge in the relationship of EP to rumination and other forms of repetitive thought in young adults, but EP was distinct from measures of negatively valenced repetitive thought, including depressive rumination and pervasive worry. Similarly, Rude, Maestas, and Neff (2007) found that the EP scale was correlated more strongly with items pertaining to reflection on feelings that contained no indication of negative judgment than with items containing negative judgment.

Emotional regulation constructs are especially relevant to coping through emotional approach. In an analysis of relationships among measures of emotional intelligence, alexithymia, and EAC, Lumley, Gustavson, Partridge, and Labouvie-Vief (2005) found moderate, positive associations of dispositional versions of EAC scales with self-report measures of attention to feelings, clarity of feelings, and mood repair, which are aspects of emotional intelligence (Salovey, Mayer, Goldman, Turvey, & Palfai, 1995), and lower correlations ($r \approx .20$) with a performance-based measure of emotional intelligence. The EAC scales evidenced moderate, negative correlations with a self-report measure of alexithymia (Bagby, Parker, & Taylor, 1994), a construct reflecting difficulties with identifying and describing feelings. In a study of 162 African American adults, Peters (2006) also found a moderate, negative association of EAC with alexithymia.

In that coping through emotional approach represents a tendency to approach stressful experiences actively, an assumption (Stanton & Franz, 1999) is that it might be subsumed under a broader, biologically mediated approach system (e.g., Allen & Kline, 2004; Fox, 1991; Sutton & Davidson, 1997). Individual differences in the approach system are associated with greater resting activation of the left prefrontal cortex, a region involved in the coordination of goal-directed behavior and self-regulation (e.g., Amodio et al., 2008; Coan & Allen, 2003; Harmon-Jones & Sigelman, 2001). In a study of healthy young adults (Master et al., 2009), dispositional EE was correlated significantly with resting left frontal electroencephalography (EEG) asymmetry. Controlling for scores on a generalized dispositional approach orientation measure (Carver & White, 1994) did not alter this significant relation.

The correlation of left frontal EEG asymmetry with EP was positive but not significant. In addition to providing evidence that EAC is an indicator of the approach system and, as such, is a mechanism involved in self-regulation, this finding is important because left frontal asymmetry also is related to healthier psychological and biological profiles, including lower depression and less negative psychological reactivity to particular stressors, as well as lower cortisol levels and stronger immunocompetence (see Master et al., 2009, for a brief review).

Taken together, findings provide support for the satisfactory psychometric properties of the EAC scales, as well as their convergent and discriminant validity. Evidence also suggests that coping through emotional approach can be considered a facet of a broader approach-oriented motivational system. The next section summarizes research on the important question of whether coping through EP and EE can enhance psychological and physical health.

Coping Through Emotional Approach as a Contributor to Psychological and Physical Health

Since the publication of the EAC scales (Stanton, Kirk et al., 2000), a number of studies have been conducted to examine the adaptive correlates and consequences of coping through emotional approach. This section contains a review of that literature, focusing first on cross-sectional studies and then on longitudinal designs. Research on moderators of and mechanisms for the effects of emotional approach coping also are addressed. Except where specifically noted, the researchers used the EAC scales.

Cross-sectional research

Cross-sectional studies provide evidence that coping through emotional approach is related to indicators of positive psychological adjustment, at least under particular conditions (addressed in the section below on moderated relations). In the original research conducted during scale development, young women who reported higher dispositional EP had higher life satisfaction and lower depressive symptoms and anxiety than women low in EP (note that EE was not related significantly to those variables in women; Stanton, Kirk et al., 2000). For young men, the only significant relation of dispositional EAC and adjustment was between EE and greater life satisfaction. In other research (Kashdan, Zvolensky, & McLeish, 2008), 248 young adults with higher dispositional EE reported fewer anhedonic depressive symptoms than individuals low in EE, and

EAC was negatively related to depressive symptoms and trait anxiety and anger in a community sample of 162 African American adults (Peters, 2006). In a sample of 79 undergraduate students who reported at least one uncued panic attack within the preceding year, Tull, Gratz, and Lacroce (2006) found that individuals reporting high dispositional EAC had lower depressive symptoms, anxiety sensitivity, and panic-related disability and symptom severity than participants with low EAC (EP and EE were not reported separately). When panic symptom severity, disability, and frequency were controlled in a regression analysis, high EAC and low fear of cognitive dyscontrol were unique predictors of low depressive symptoms.

Several cross-sectional studies have been conducted in clinical or medical populations. Simon and colleagues (2007) studied the relations of dispositional EAC and other variables with a comprehensive measure of suicidal ideation and behavior in a sample of 98 patients diagnosed with bipolar disorder an average of 27 years earlier. EP was related to significantly lower anxiety on several measures (i.e., fear, worry, panic, anxiety sensitivity) but not to depressive rumination or fear of negative evaluation; relations of EE with those measures were in the same direction but not statistically significant. In stepwise regression analyses controlling for age, gender, bipolar subtype, and bipolar recovery status, the anxiety variables were not associated significantly with suicidal ideation/behavior. Rather, lower EE and higher depressive rumination accounted for 13% of the variance in suicidal ideation/behavior. In separate analyses with men and women, men's (n = 42) higher EP and women's (n = 56) higher EE were associated with lower suicidal ideation/behavior.

Regarding medical populations, a small study (n = 31) of women with a maternal history of breast cancer revealed a significant relation of cancer-related EP with greater post-traumatic growth (Mosher, Danoff-Burg, & Brunker, 2006). In 80 adults living with chronic myofascial pain, Smith et al. (2002) found that EAC (total score and EP) specific to coping with pain was associated with lower negative affect. Even when negative affect, education, marital status, and passive pain-related coping were controlled, greater use of EAC (total score) was related significantly to lower affective pain and depressive symptoms, accounting for approximately 4% of unique variance in each dependent variable. In men with chronic pain, EE also was associated with lower physical impairment and

sensory pain. In a sample of 183 men (M age = 68 years) being treated for various cancers (Hoyt, 2009), structural equation modeling revealed that men who reported lower gender role conflict were more likely to cope through EE related to their cancer, which in turn was associated with lower psychological distress (a latent construct indicated by depressive symptoms, negative affect, and cancer-related thought intrusion).

Although cross-sectional analyses in both young adult or community samples and medical or clinical samples suggest that EAC or its component processes are associated with favorable psychological adjustment, the relations are not entirely consistent. In EAC scale development (Stanton, Kirk, et al., 2000, Study 1), significant sex differences emerged, such that dispositional EP was associated with indicators of positive adjustment more strongly for young women than for young men. Similarly, in the Hoyt (2009) study of men with cancer, greater cancer-related EP was associated with higher distress (and separate analyses suggested that this relation was stronger for younger men). Some studies reveal no reliable relations between EAC and psychological adjustment. For example, in the small study of women with a maternal breast cancer history, cancer-related EAC was not related to post-traumatic stress symptoms (Mosher, Danoff-Burg, & Brunker, 2005). In a study of 242 women in their third trimester of pregnancy (Pakenham et al., 2007), pregnancy-related EAC was not significantly related to depressive symptoms; rather, higher depressive symptoms were related to reports of more stressful life events, threat appraisal, and coping with pregnancy through wishful thinking. Other studies suggest that EAC is related to adjustment only under particular conditions (see section on moderated relations below).

Longitudinal research
Longitudinal research, in which EP and EE are examined as predictors of change in adjustment over time, allows for stronger causal inference regarding their relations. The benefits of EAC have been demonstrated in individuals coping with an array of experiences, including sexual assault, disclosure of sexual orientation, infertility, and breast cancer. In the original scale development research with young adults coping with self-nominated stressors, high scores on a preliminary EAC scale predicted an increase in life satisfaction and a decline in depressive symptoms for young women, whereas high EAC predicted a decline in adjustment on

those indices for young men (Stanton et al., 1994, Study 2). EAC did not predict physical symptoms. In a second longitudinal study of young adults coping with self-nominated stressors (Stanton, Kirk, et al., 2000, Study 3), high EP and EE were beneficial with regard to improved depressive symptoms and life satisfaction when used alone, but their advantage was not additive. The simultaneous endorsement of low EP and EE or high EP and EE predicted poorer adjustment over time, perhaps suggesting the adaptiveness of their sequential use.

Frazier, Mortensen, and Steward (2005) conducted a 12-month longitudinal study of 171 women who reported sexual assault in an emergency room visit and elected at least one subsequent counseling session. An increase in coping with the assault through expressing emotions, as assessed with the Coping Strategies Inventory (Tobin Holroyd, & Reynolds, 1984) with distress-confounded items removed, was associated with an increase in feelings of control over the recovery process, and such feelings of control were associated with decreasing distress following the assault. However, EE did not significantly mediate the relation between perceived control and distress; rather, greater use of coping through cognitive restructuring and less use of social withdrawal mediated the control–distress relation. In a separate report (Frazier, Tashiro, Berman, Steger, & Long, 2004), an increase in approach-oriented coping (a composite of EE and cognitive restructuring) was related to increasing perceptions of positive life change associated with the assault experience over time, and coping partially mediated the relations of social support with positive change trajectories.

Beals, Peplau, and Gable (2009) investigated the consequences of EP during daily experiences of the opportunity to disclose sexual orientation in a 14-day experience-sampling design with 84 lesbians and gay men (note that EE was not measured). On average, participants reported three disclosure opportunities over the 2 weeks. Participants disclosed their sexual orientation during 64% of opportunities, and disclosure (vs. concealment) was accompanied by greater well-being (i.e., positive affect, self-esteem, life satisfaction) on those days. Although not completely consistent across dependent variables, mediators of the association between disclosure and higher daily well-being were greater perceived social support and more EP regarding sexual orientation. Greater suppression of feelings about sexual orientation mediated the association of concealment of orientation with lower daily life satisfaction. When putative

mediators were tested simultaneously as predictors of daily well-being, EP was a unique predictor of higher daily positive affect and satisfaction with life, suggesting that its effects were unique vis à vis effects of social support. Daily EP did not predict well-being 2 months later.

Two longitudinal studies with infertile samples suggest the benefits of EAC when confronting a cherished, blocked goal over which one has only a modicum of control. EP and EE regarding infertility each protected against depressive symptoms in both members of 43 heterosexual, infertile couples following an unsuccessful insemination attempt (Berghuis & Stanton, 2002). When the interaction of partners' EAC was examined, women high in EAC had low predicted depressive symptoms after the disappointing insemination attempt, regardless of their partners' coping. However, for women low in EAC, high infertility-related EP and EE by their partners was protective against women's depressive symptomatology. Thus, their partners' use of EAC appeared to compensate for women's low EAC. When both partners were low in EAC, women's predicted scores on a standard depression measure exceeded the cutoff suggestive of clinical depression after the disappointing fertility attempt. In a sample of women coping with infertility, Terry and Hynes (1998) also found that expressive coping predicted favorable psychological adjustment over time (note that their expressive coping measure included items related to social support).

The adaptive utility of EAC also has been examined in the context of breast cancer, where the most consistent evidence emerges for EE as a contributor to psychological health. In a 3-month longitudinal study of 92 women who recently had completed primary medical treatments for breast cancer, Stanton, Danoff-Burg, and colleagues (2000) examined the predictive utility of EAC. After initial values on dependent variables, participant age, and coping strategies other than emotional approach were controlled, women who were more expressive regarding their experience of breast cancer evidenced an increase in vigor and a decline in distress 3 months later. For women who perceived their social environment as highly receptive to their cancer-related expression, coping through EE also predicted improved quality of life. Manne, Ostroff, and colleagues (2004) demonstrated that coping through EE approximately 4 months following breast cancer diagnosis predicted an increase in post-traumatic growth over the next 18 months for women with breast cancer. Women also evidenced more post-traumatic growth when their partners reported high use of EE. In contrast, no significant association emerged between EE and finding benefit in the breast cancer experience at approximately 2 months after surgery or at 5-year follow-up in a study by Lechner, Carver, Antoni, Weaver, and Phillips (2006, Study 2).

In longitudinal studies with breast cancer patients, the adaptive utility of EP, in contrast to EE, is less consistently demonstrated. Demonstrating that EP can carry positive effects, Manne, Ostroff et al. (2004) found that higher EP by partners (but not breast cancer patients) at approximately 4 months after cancer diagnosis predicted maintenance of their own post-traumatic growth over time, whereas lower EP predicted declining post-traumatic growth. Lechner et al. (2006, Study 2) reported a concurrent relation of cancer-related EP and finding benefit in the cancer experience at 2 months after surgery, but early EP did not predict benefit-finding at 5 years. In the Stanton, Danoff-Burg et al. (2000) longitudinal study of breast cancer patients, EP was related to better adjustment in zero-order correlations, but it predicted an increase in distress in regression analyses, when EE was controlled statistically. As the researchers speculated, EP might promote diminished distress to the extent that it is channeled through EE. Furthermore, the variance unique to EP might represent a ruminative component, particularly when processing continues long after stressor onset (note that women entered the study approximately 6 months after diagnosis).

One longitudinal study suggests that EP might be maladaptive in breast cancer patients when the disease is chronic and likely to be life-limiting. In a 3-month longitudinal study of 103 women with metastatic disease (Stanton & Low, under review), greater endorsement of coping through cancer-related EP at study entry predicted an increase in depressive symptoms and cancer-related intrusive thoughts. Again, perhaps the effects of EP depend on the stressor trajectory, such that attempts to acknowledge and understand emotions are more adaptive when they occur relatively early in the stressful experience, promoting efficient EE and goal pursuit (see also Stanton, Kirk et al., 2000, Study 3). As time passes or the stressor becomes chronic, however, sustained EP might become ruminative. The timing of use of EP and EE over the course of stressors requires study.

There is some longitudinal evidence that the benefits of EAC extend to the domain of physical health. Emotionally expressive breast cancer patients had fewer medical appointments for cancer-related morbidities over 3 months, as well as improved self-reported physical health in a study by Stanton, Danoff-Burg et al. (2000). One longitudinal epidemiological study revealed that a different measure of coping through EE during the first month after diagnosis of breast cancer predicted longer survival at 8-year follow-up for African American and European American women, particularly for those who also reported available emotional support (Reynolds et al., 2000).

Moderators of the relations between EAC and outcomes

Some of the findings in the previous sections hinted at the likelihood that coping through EP and EE is not uniformly beneficial, but rather that personal and environmental attributes condition the effectiveness of those strategies. The original contention of Lazarus and Folkman (1984) that coping strategies are neither inherently maladaptive nor adaptive applies in the case of EAC.

Receptiveness of the interpersonal milieu in which the individual processes and expresses stressor-related emotions may influence the benefits derived from EAC (e.g., Lepore, Silver, Wortman, & Wayment, 1996). Quality of life improved for women who coped with breast cancer through EE if they perceived their social contexts to be receptive to cancer-related expression in the longitudinal study by Stanton, Danoff-Burg et al. (2000). Similarly, in Hoyt's (2009) cross-sectional study of men with cancer, more cancer-related EE was related to lower distress in men who reported low social constraint in communicating with close others about their cancer (e.g., "How often in the past week has your spouse changed the subject when you tried to discuss your illness?"; Lepore & Ituarte, 1999) and to higher distress in men in highly socially constrained environments. Support from the social environment appears to be a facilitative but not a necessary condition for EAC to confer benefit, in that EAC is related to positive adjustment even when social support is statistically controlled (e.g., Stanton et al., 1994; Stanton, Danoff-Burg et al., 2000; Stanton, Kirk et al., 2000). Because the acceptability of the experience and expression of particular emotions varies as a function of cultural contexts, social factors deserve greater empirical attention in understanding the costs and benefits of EAC.

The nature of the stressor as appraised by the individual can influence the likelihood that individuals will use EAC as well as its consequences. For example, Park, Armeli, and Tennen (2004a) asked undergraduates to rate the controllability of and coping strategies used during the day's most stressful event. Students used more EAC in response to stressors perceived as uncontrollable. There also is some evidence that EAC might have a more potent influence on favorable adjustment to uncontrollable situations than to more mutable stressors (Stanton et al., 1994, Study 2). The larger stressful context also might influence the adaptiveness of EAC. Low, Stanton, Thompson, Kwan, and Ganz (2006) found that a greater use of EP, EE, and seeking social support (composite index) specifically in response to breast cancer predicted more favorable adjustment 6 and 12 months later in women when their contextual life stress was low, but not when they were experiencing other major life stressors.

Individual differences can condition the effects of EAC. Although some evidence suggests that effects of EAC vary as a function of gender (Stanton et al., 1994), with young women deriving more benefit than men, other research has suggested that EAC or its component processes also can be useful for men (Berghuis & Stanton, 2002; Hoyt, 2009). Benefits of EP and EE might be compromised in individuals with dispositional vulnerabilities that bear on emotion regulation. For such individuals, EP and EE might become ruminative, be experienced as uncontrollable, amplify negative emotions, deplete social resources, or fail to reduce barriers to life goals, among other consequences.

Several relevant personality attributes have been examined in single investigations. In a cross-sectional study of 248 young adults (Kashdan et al., 2008), participants with higher dispositional EE had lower agoraphobic cognitions if their anxiety sensitivity was low, but highly anxiety-sensitive individuals had higher agoraphobic cognitions (but not anxious arousal or worry) if they reported high EE (EP was not assessed). Zuckerman, Knee, Kieffer, and Gagne (2004) found that holding highly unrealistic control beliefs was related to lower use of EP and EE. The researchers argued that individuals who cling to unrealistic notions of control are reluctant to cope through EP because careful evaluation of situations might require relinquishing illusions of control. Stanton, Danoff-Burg et al. (2000) found that breast cancer patients' EE coping was beneficial for women high in dispositional hope (i.e., goal-directed determination and ability to generate plans to achieve goals) with regard to distress and medical appointments for cancer-related morbidities

and was unrelated to outcomes for women low in hope. Moderated effects also emerged in a daily process study (Park, Armeli, & Tennen, 2004b). For undergraduates high in social enhancement motives and low in sensation-seeking who also had a family history of alcohol abuse, EAC was related to greater alcohol use. Taken together, findings suggest that individuals who have more robust intrapersonal resources might be more likely to glean benefit from the use of EP and EE in coping with stressors relative to more dispositionally vulnerable individuals.

Two studies have addressed specific facets of dispositional emotion regulation in interaction with EAC. van Middendorp et al. (2007) conducted a cross-sectional study of 403 women with fibromyalgia. Dispositional affect intensity interacted significantly with EP on pain and fatigue, such that fibromyalgia patients with high dispositional affect intensity but low EP reported high fatigue and pain relative to women whose dispositional and situational emotion regulation were more congruent. The authors suggested that intensely experiencing emotions is not maladaptive unless the emotions are not adequately processed.

In their longitudinal study of metastatic breast cancer patients, Stanton and Low (under review) found that, by itself, cancer-related EE did not predict change in adjustment outcomes. However, in the context of high dispositional affect intensity or high negative or positive dispositional expressivity, an increase in EE predicted improvements in depressive symptoms and life satisfaction. As in van Middendorp et al. (2008), congruence between high dispositional affect intensity and expressivity and situation-specific expression was adaptive. Findings for EP were less consistent. Cancer-related EP at study entry predicted increases in depressive symptoms and cancer-related intrusive thoughts, as well as declining life satisfaction among highly dispositionally expressive women. An increase in EP over time, however, predicted improvements in depressive symptoms in the context of high dispositional expressivity. Sustained EP in the context of chronic stressors (on average, women had received the metastatic diagnosis nearly 2 years previously) and of high dispositional expressivity might tax psychological resources, involve a ruminative component, or indicate lack of resolution of emotional challenges. The exception for women with high positive expressivity might be explained by their EP promoting positive reappraisal or resulting in more effective goal clarification and pursuit. High EP by individuals high in positive expressivity also might promote more balanced emotional experience and expression and hence might be unlikely to erode vital intrapersonal and interpersonal resources.

Mechanisms for the effects of EAC

What are the pathways through which EAC might promote positive outcomes? First, EAC might facilitate effective goal clarification and pursuit (Stanton & Franz, 2000; Stanton, Parsa, & Austenfeld, 2002). In a longitudinal study of breast cancer patients, coping with the cancer experience through EE partially mediated the relations of dispositional hope, a construct related to positive goal orientation, with improvements in vigor and self-reported health. Thus, EAC may assist in directing attention toward important goals (i.e., a signaling function, Frijda, 1994), identifying barriers to goal achievement, and generating new pathways to reaching them. This interpretation is consistent with findings linking EAC with problem-focused coping (Pakenham et al., 2007; Stanton, Kirk et al., 2000).

Second, effects of EAC might stem from sustained exposure to the stressful event involved in actively processing and expressing emotions. Research indicates that exposure through EP and EE can promote physiological habituation to (e.g., Low, Stanton, & Danoff-Burg, 2006; Stanton, Kirk et al., 2000, Study 4) and cognitive reappraisal of stressors and one's ability to manage them (e.g., Creswell et al., 2007; Pakenham et al., 2007; Pennebaker, Mayne, & Francis, 1997). If EAC proves salutary for physical health, an important question regards specification of the relevant physiological pathways. In addition to providing evidence that EAC (and particularly EE) is related to left frontal EEG asymmetry, which itself is associated with positive health indicators, Master and colleagues (2009) addressed this question by examining biological stress responses. For 22 of the 46 young adult participants, an acute laboratory stressor was administered (Trier Social Stress Test; Kirschbaum et al., 1993), accompanied by assessment of proinflammatory cytokines (sTNFαRII and interleukin [IL]-6) and salivary cortisol. Participants who reported coping with stressors through processing and expressing emotions had lower sTNFαRII responses 25 minutes after onset of the induced stressor than those lower on emotional approach. Specifically, partial correlations controlling for baseline cytokine levels between sTNFαRII and EAC were $-.50$, $p < .05$, for the total EAC score, $-.48$, $p < .05$, for EP, and $-.41$, $p < .06$, for EE. Controlling for measures

of depressive symptoms and dispositional approach motivation did not alter these relations; controlling for health behaviors attenuated the correlations slightly. Findings were similar although not statistically significant at 55 minutes after stressor onset. EAC was not significantly related to changes in cortisol or IL-6.

Research provides suggestive evidence that EAC might modulate physiological responses to stress. Over repeated stressful occasions, coping through processing and expressing emotions might protect against chronic inflammatory processes, which have been associated with several adverse health outcomes. Additional research is needed on the potential of EAC to affect biological stress responses and, ultimately, important physical health outcomes.

Third, EAC may help individuals select and maximally draw upon their interpersonal milieu (e.g., Carstensen, 1998; Manne, Ostroff et al., 2004). In 18 couples including individuals recently diagnosed with malignant melanoma or dysplastic nevi (a potential precursor to melanoma) and their partners, patients' greater use of EAC (and specifically EP) was associated with higher correspondence between patients' received and partners' provided support, suggesting that patients high in EAC might have been better able to formulate and convey their needs for support (Lichtenthal, Cruess, Schuchter, & Ming, 2003). In addition, partners' EE and EP were significantly associated with their empathic concern. Rini and colleagues (2006) demonstrated a relationship between EE and diminished anxiety in a study of pregnant women and their partners, mediated by interpersonal variables. Along with other variables such as secure attachment, greater coping through EE in pregnant women formed a latent construct reflecting interpersonal orientation. Interpersonal orientation was related to stronger marital quality and greater effectiveness of social support, which in turn predicted reduction in anxiety over the course of pregnancy (also see Huizink, de Medina, Mulder, & Visser, 2002). EAC is related to coping through seeking social support (Stanton, Kirk et al., 2000, Study 1 and Study 3), and a cross-sectional study of pregnant women in their third trimester (Pakenham et al., 2007) revealed that greater coping with pregnancy through emotional approach was related to stronger perceived availability of social support from the partner and non-family (but not family) members. Thus, the benefits of EAC may derive from both intrapersonal and interpersonal pathways.

Interventions to Promote Emotional Processing and Expression

As contemporary emotion science increasingly informs research in psychopathology and psychotherapy, a disturbance in core affective processing has been acknowledged as a shared characteristic of many psychological disorders (e.g., Barrett, Mesquita, Ochsner, & Gross, 2007). Moreover, emotion regulation has emerged as a unifying construct in therapeutic approaches (e.g., Moses & Barlow, 2006) and is acknowledged as vital to positive change across a number of psychotherapeutic traditions (see Whelton, 2004, for a review). An example of an approach in which EP and EE are central is the emotion-focused therapy (EFT) of Greenberg and colleagues (e.g., Greenberg & Watson, 2006). In accordance with the assumptions that awareness, tolerance, and utilization of negative emotions, as well as awareness and active enjoyment of positive emotions, are essential to psychological adjustment, EFT uses a number of techniques designed to promote emotional processing. A meta-analysis of four randomized, controlled studies of EFT in married couples yielded significant improvement in marital distress (Johnson, Hunsley, Greenberg, & Schindler, 1999). Greater depth of emotional processing, as indicated by the Experiencing Scale (Klein, Mathieu-Coughlan, & Kiesler, 1986), predicts favorable outcomes in the related process-experiential therapy as a treatment for depression (Pos, Greenberg, Goldman, & Korman, 2003; Watson & Bedard, 2006). Therapies that encourage stressor-related emotional processing and expression also have produced positive psychological effects in medical populations (e.g., Giese-Davis et al., 2002; Spiegel, Bloom, Kraemer, & Gottheil, 1989). Compared with a randomized control group, women with metastatic breast cancer in group supportive-expressive therapy demonstrated improvement in domains of emotion regulation, with a decline in suppression of negative affect and increases in restraint of aggressive, impulsive, inconsiderate, and irresponsible behavior (Giese-Davis et al., 2002). Acceptance and commitment therapy (e.g., Hayes, Luoma, Bond, Masuda, & Lillis, 2006) and dialectical behavior therapy (e.g., Lynch, Chapman, Rosenthal, Kuo, & Linehan, 2006) are additional therapeutic modalities in which attention to and regulation of emotion are central components.

Although not designed to be a therapeutic intervention, experimental trials of expressive disclosure, in which participants are randomly assigned to write (or talk) about their deepest feelings and thoughts regarding a stressor over several sessions or to comparison or control writing conditions (Pennebaker & Beall, 1986), provide evidence regarding the utility of EP and EE. Meta-analyses demonstrate the positive effects of processing and expressing emotions regarding stressful experiences through writing (Frattaroli, 2006; Smyth, 1998). For example, in a meta-analysis of 146 experiments, Frattaroli (2006) reported that expressive writing demonstrated significant benefits on both psychological outcomes (e.g., distress, depressive symptoms, anxiety, positive functioning) and physical health (e.g., illness behaviors such as medical visits, specific disease outcomes). Experimental studies also demonstrate that inducing individuals to experience emotions in a fully accepting way promotes recovery from negative affect in anxiety-inducing situations, relative to emotional suppression (Campbell-Sills, Barlow, Brown, & Hofmann, 2006; Levitt, Brown, Orsillo, & Barlow, 2004). In another experimental study (Low, Stanton, & Bower, 2008), writing about stressor-related emotions in an accepting way led to more efficient heart rate habituation and recovery than did evaluating the appropriateness of stressor-related emotions.

Also relevant to the utility of coping through emotional approach are comparisons of interventions targeting emotion-focused and problem-focused coping skills, in which the emotion-focused interventions typically include emotional approach strategies. In a controlled comparison of problem-focused with emotion-focused counseling for bereavement (Schut, Stroebe, van den Bout, & de Keijser, 1997), problem-focused counseling was more beneficial for women, whereas emotion-focused counseling was more beneficial for men (at 7 months after treatment). In a controlled trial of problem-focused versus emotion-focused group treatment for infertile women (McQueeney, Stanton, & Sigmon, 1997), both treatment groups evidenced a decline in general distress at treatment completion relative to controls, but the emotion-focused group also evidenced enhanced adjustment at 1-month follow-up. The problem-focused group was more likely to attain parenthood at 18-month follow-up than the other two groups, perhaps reflecting more persistent efforts to become parents. In another controlled trial, Bond and Bunce (2000) compared problem-focused and emotion-focused group interventions to alleviate worksite stress. Based on Acceptance and Commitment Therapy (ACT; Hayes et al., 2006), the emotion-focused intervention facilitated emotional approach and acceptance, whereas the problem-focused treatment trained workers to identify and lessen workplace stressors. Both treatments improved psychological adjustment and propensity to innovate at work, but via different mechanisms: ACT enhanced acceptance of negative emotions and thoughts, whereas the problem-focused treatment increased direct attempts to modify work stressors. One intervention that integrates, rather than compares, both emotion-focused and problem-focused skills is Folkman and colleagues' Coping Effectiveness Training (CET; 1991), in which participants learn to select specific coping approaches for particular aspects of stressful situations. In HIV-positive men, CET improved perceived stress, burnout, and anxiety (but not depressive symptoms) relative to a control condition, and coping self-efficacy mediated intervention effects on stress and burnout (Chesney, Chambers, Taylor, Johnson, & Folkman, 2003).

Emotional approach coping as a mediator of intervention effects

To the extent that emotional processing and expression are targeted in intervention approaches, increases in their use might act as mechanisms for positive intervention effects. In a first trial of a 10-week cognitive-behavioral stress management (CBSM) group intervention (also see Chapter 21 in this volume), which promotes EP and EE, Antoni and colleagues (2001) found that CBSM reduced the prevalence of moderate depressive symptoms and increased benefit-finding and optimism for women with early-stage breast cancer relative to a control group, effects that were maintained at 3-month follow-up. Although EAC increased in CBSM relative to the control condition, and it was correlated with increased benefit-finding during and after CBSM, it did not meet criteria to act as a significant mediator of the relation between CBSM and benefit-finding. In a second trial, Antoni and colleagues (Antoni, Lechner et al., 2006; Antoni, Wimberly et al., 2006) tested the effects of CBSM against a control condition (one-day educational seminar) in 199 women recently diagnosed with nonmetastatic breast cancer. Relative to the control condition, CBSM produced a number of significant positive effects on dependent variables (i.e., cancer-related intrusive thoughts, negative affect, anxiety, social disruption, emotional well-being, positive states of mind, cancer-related benefit-finding, positive affect) for up to 12 months. Confidence in one's ability to relax mediated the effects of the intervention (Antoni, Lechner et al., 2006; Antoni, Wimberly et al., 2006). CBSM also increased participants' cancer-related coping through EE, which in turn mediated the relation of the intervention with the decline in negative affect and increases in positive states of mind and benefit-finding (Antoni, Carver, & Lechner, 2006).

Other trials have not revealed EP and EE to be significant mediators of effects. In a small sample of women with breast cancer ($n = 39$), a four-session creative arts intervention, which was intended to increase EE, reduced negative affect relative to a control group but did not alter EE (Puig, Lee, Goodwin, & Sherrard, 2006). Manne, Babb, Pinover, Horwitz, and Ebbert (2004) tested a psychoeducational group intervention for wives of men with prostate cancer and found no significant differences between the treatment and control groups on either post-treatment distress or EAC (although the treatment group evidenced a nonsignificant trend toward more EAC). The researchers noted, however, that distress declined over time in the control group, and the study had limited power to detect differences in distress. Manne and colleagues (2008) also tested mediators of an intervention designed to enhance communication and coping skills versus a supportive counseling intervention in 353 gynecological cancer patients in active medical treatment. Both interventions produced a significant decline in depressive symptoms at 6- and 9-month follow-up assessments relative to a usual care control. The two interventions significantly increased EP and EE (marginally significant for the communication intervention), and the effect of the communication intervention on depressive symptoms was no longer significant when EP was controlled. However, other mediators, such as positive reappraisal, were more reliably associated with effects of both interventions.

At present, relatively little evidence has emerged for EAC as a mechanism for psychosocial intervention effects (Antoni, Carver, & Lechner, 2006). Perhaps active attempts to process and express emotions surrounding a stressor subside once they have been successful in resolving the associated emotions. Thus, expressive coping efforts might increase during psychosocial intervention but actually might diminish after effective resolution. Another possibility is that increases in EE prompted by a therapeutic intervention might meet with unsupportive responses in the individual's natural environment, thus dampening its potentially positive effects (Manne et al., 2008). It also is possible that EAC may be most effective for subsets of intervention samples (e.g., individuals in highly supportive environments or with more personal resources), and therefore the action of EAC may be more reliably identified through analyses of interaction with individual difference or contextual variables. EAC itself also might moderate the effects of interventions on outcomes, a possibility for which there is emerging evidence.

Emotional approach coping as a moderator of expressive intervention effects

Evidence is accumulating that naturally elected coping approaches, and EAC specifically, can moderate the effects of experimentally induced expressive disclosure. Stanton, Kirk, and colleagues (2000, Study 4) randomly assigned undergraduates who were coping with a parent's psychological or physical health problem to talk with a neutral interviewer about either their emotions related to their parent's disorder or the facts of their parent's disorder over two sessions. At the second session, naturally elected coping interacted significantly with experimental condition: participants who reported high baseline EE with regard to their parent's disorder displayed lower physiological arousal (heart rate) and negative affect when assigned to talk about their emotions relative to participants in other conditions.

Four trials of written expressive disclosure also suggest that naturally elected emotional processing and expression can condition responses to experimentally imposed instructions promoting emotion regulation. In an expressive disclosure trial with medical students writing about their clinical clerkships (Austenfeld, Paolo, & Stanton, 2006), participants with high baseline EE or EP related to stressful medical school experiences evidenced fewer depressive symptoms 3 months later if they were randomized to three sessions of writing about their deepest thoughts and feelings regarding upsetting medical clerkship experiences, whereas those low in EE or EP had lower depressive symptoms if they wrote about the future as if all their goals had been realized (i.e., best possible self). Control participants, who wrote objectively about activities in the past 24 hours in the clerkship, evidenced relatively high depressive symptoms that did not vary as a function of EAC. In addition, individuals low in EP assigned to the best-possible-self condition had fewer health care visits at 3 months compared to low-EP participants in the other conditions. In a similar study of undergraduate participants, Austenfeld and Stanton (2008) found that high-EP participants evidenced a decline in hostility (but not depressive symptoms or medical visits) at a 1-month follow-up in the emotional disclosure condition, whereas low-EP participants benefitted more in the best-possible-self condition on both hostility and medical visits.

In another trial, Kraft, Lumley, D'Souza, and Dooley (2008) compared written expressive disclosure to audiotaped relaxation training and a time-management control condition in individuals with migraine headaches. Assessed at baseline and 3-month follow-up, dependent variables were headache frequency, pain severity, functional and emotional disability from headache, and negative and positive affect. Greater dispositional EAC (combined EE and EP) predicted improvement on all measures following expressive disclosure (vs. the relaxation or control conditions), and EAC significantly moderated effects of expressive disclosure versus the control group on headache frequency and disability (and marginally on pain severity and negative affect). EAC significantly moderated the effects of expressive disclosure versus the relaxation intervention on headache frequency and positive affect. Patterns were similar for EE and EP as moderators. Thus, EAC specifically predicted improvement following expressive disclosure. The researchers suggested that "People with limited motivation or ability to process and express emotions may find WED [written expressive disclosure] unappealing, or struggle to identify stressors, disclose feelings, and generate cognitive or affective changes" (p. 70). Finally, investigating effects of a single session of written expressive disclosure regarding a stressful experience as compared with a session of interpersonal disclosure to a nondirective, empathic listener and a written time-management control, Cohen, Sander, Slavin, and Lumley (2008) found that high dispositional EP predicted a decline in negative affect immediately after the session for those in the expressive writing condition, whereas high EP predicted an increase in stressor-specific thought intrusion and avoidance at 6 weeks for participants in the interpersonal disclosure condition. The researchers speculated that high emotional processors might have benefitted from a more active interpersonal intervention rather than their employed nondirective intervention.

Written expressive disclosure is an approach that requires self-directed focus on processing and expressing emotions and that typically entails fewer than 90 total minutes of expression. Individuals who naturally elect to actively approach emotions when they confront stressful encounters are likely to make more effective use of EP and EE when imposed in an experimental context than are individuals who eschew those strategies. However, there is evidence from an intervention trial by Manne, Ostroff, and Winkel (2007) that individuals who endorse EAC also glean greater benefit from more intensive therapeutic interventions. Those researchers conducted a trial of a couple-focused group intervention compared with usual care in a sample of 238 women within 6 months of diagnosis with early-stage breast cancer. Conducted in six, 90-minute sessions, the intervention focused on bolstering couples' understanding of the impact of cancer on their relationship and enhancing communication and support. Assessed at pre-intervention and 1 week and 6 months after the intervention, dependent variables were depressive symptoms, anxiety, well-being, loss of behavioral/emotional control, and cancer-specific distress.

Intent-to-treat analyses revealed that women who were high on coping with their cancer through EP or EE at baseline had declining depressive symptoms in the intervention versus the control group (Manne et al., 2007). Analyses also were conducted to examine differences among those randomly assigned to the intervention who did not attend any sessions ($n = 42$), those who attended at least one intervention session ($n = 78$), and the usual care group ($n = 118$). Coping through processing and coping through expressing cancer-related emotions also were moderators of intervention effects in those analyses, such that women high on EE or EP who attended at least one intervention session benefitted from the intervention on depressive symptoms and anxiety (and well-being for women high on EP) relative to women who were offered but did not attend the intervention and control group participants. EAC was a stronger and more consistent moderator of intervention effects than was use of protective buffering toward the partner or coping with cancer through active acceptance. In a previous paper, Manne and colleagues (Manne, Ostroff, Winkel, Fox, Grana, Miller, Ross, & Frazier, 2005) reported that the intervention also was more beneficial for women who had unsupportive partners.

Summary of experimental intervention findings

A number of psychosocial interventions and experimental inductions that promote EP and EE have yielded positive effects on a range of dependent variables. Although a different indicator of EP (Klein et al., 1986) has been demonstrated to mediate the effectiveness of such interventions (Pos et al., 2003; Watson & Bedard, 2006), minimal evidence

has emerged for emotional approach coping as assessed by the EAC scales as a mechanism for effects (Antoni, Carver et al., 2006). However, findings from experimental research involving both relatively brief experimental inductions and a more intensive therapeutic intervention that encourage EP and EE reveal that congruence between the naturally elected level of emotional approach and the extent of processing and expression promoted in the intervention carries salutary effects. In conjunction with the evidence for moderated effects in longitudinal studies, these findings highlight the importance of the interplay of person attributes and environmental contingencies when evaluating the utility of coping through emotional approach and other strategies to regulate emotion under stressful conditions.

Remaining Questions and Directions for Research

In stimulating research on the construct of coping through emotional approach, we hoped to make three contributions to the stress and coping literature. Our central goal was to challenge the "bad reputation" of emotion-focused coping by providing a fair test of whether coping through processing and expressing emotions during stressful experiences can confer benefit for well-being and health. To that end, our second goal was to provide a measure of coping through emotional approach that is not confounded with distress and self-deprecatory content. Finally, we hoped to contribute to the understanding of the conditions under which coping through emotional approach could generate benefit (or harm) and of the mechanisms underlying its effects. In our view, we and other researchers have made progress toward these goals.

With regard to our first goal, evidence accumulated over the past two decades convincingly demonstrates that coping through processing and expressing emotions can promote psychological and physical health. The cross-sectional, longitudinal, and experimental research specific to coping through emotional approach that is described in this chapter joins the experimental research on expressive disclosure and controlled trials of relevant therapeutic approaches to support this conclusion. Of course, this conclusion does not imply that coping through emotional approach invariably is adaptive: Some of the work described in this chapter suggests that such coping can be maladaptive or inconsequential, as do many other examples in the broader literature (e.g., Bonanno, Papa, Lalande, Zhang, & Noll, 2005;

Seery, Silver, Holman, Ence, & Chu, 2008). The ability to respond flexibly to intrapersonal and interpersonal exigencies with regard to approaching one's emotions might yield the most favorable outcomes (e.g., Bonanno, Papa, Lalande, Westphal, & Coifman, 2004). In future research, it will be important to investigate the consequences of processing and expressing specific negative emotions such as sadness, anger, and fear (e.g., Lieberman & Goldstein, 2006; Trierweiler, Eid, & Lischetzke, 2002), the role of the experience and expression of positive emotions in the coping process (e.g., Folkman & Moskowitz, 2004; Fredrickson, 2001), and the influence of coping through emotional approach on a broader range of physical health and behavioral outcomes.

With regard to our second goal of offering a self-report measure of coping through emotional approach, the resulting scales (Stanton, Kirk et al., 2000) are seeing use in our and others' laboratories. When should the EAC scales be used? If the researcher is seeking an indicator of the intentional tendency to process and express emotions during stressful experiences in general or during specific stressors that is brief, psychometrically sound, and has evidence of predictive utility, the EAC scales are a good choice. In that they do not contain content that indicates distress or self-deprecation, they represent an advance over several published scales of emotion-focused coping. They easily can be added to other self-report coping measures (e.g., Carver et al., 1989) if the goal is to assess a broader range of coping processes (e.g., seeking social support, positive reappraisal, avoidance). Moreover, research demonstrates that the EAC scales are useful indicators of stress-related EP and EE in investigations of determinants of psychological and physical health outcomes across a range of naturalistic stressors and of who stands to benefit from psychosocial interventions that promote emotion regulation. However, the EAC scales simply are not sufficiently nuanced to capture the intricacies of EP and EE. For example, several qualities distinguish EP or EE that facilitates effective goal pursuit and resolution of stressors and that which devolves into unproductive rumination or counterproductive emotional discharge (see Kennedy-Moore & Watson, 2001; Nolen-Hoeksema, Wisco, & Lyubomirsky, 2008; Watkins, 2008 for illustrative reviews). More fine-grained assessment and experimental research are necessary to refine the conclusions allowed from research with the EAC scales.

With regard to our third goal, some progress is evident in delineating the conditions under which coping through emotional approach confers benefit and the pathways for its effects. Thus far, research suggests that the utility of emotional approach is conditioned by characteristics of the stressor and concomitant cognitive appraisals (e.g., controllability, stressor trajectory), the interpersonal context, and dispositional characteristics that affect emotion regulation (e.g., gender-related attributes, affect intensity). Basic and applied investigations provide some evidence for the adaptive utility of congruence between naturally elected emotional approach strategies and skills promoted in therapeutic interventions, as well as between dispositional emotion regulation tendencies and situation-specific emotional approach coping processes. Mechanisms through which emotional approach carries its effects include goal clarification and pursuit, cognitive reappraisal and psychological habituation, physiological habituation and other biological stress-moderating responses, and interpersonal processes that promote stressor resolution. The body of research on moderators and mediators of the effects of coping through emotional approach is small, however, and continued longitudinal and experimental investigations are needed. Future research on the adaptive implications of engaging in EP and EE in tandem or in sequence also could be useful. Increasingly precise understanding of for whom, under what circumstances, and how coping through processing and expressing emotions in stressful contexts is effective will be vital next steps in this line of research and will inform clinical interventions to enhance skills in emotion regulation.

Author Note

I thank Sarah Sullivan and Jennifer Austenfeld for their collaboration on an earlier chapter regarding coping through emotional approach (Stanton, Sullivan, & Austenfeld, 2009).

References

Allen, J. J. B., & Kline, J. P. (2004). Frontal EEG asymmetry, emotion and psychopathology: The first, and next 25 years. *Biological Psychology, 67*, 1–5.

Amodio, D. M., Master, S. L., Yee, C. M., & Taylor, S.E. (2008). Neurocognitive components of the behavioral inhibition and activation systems: implications for theories of self-regulation. *Psychophysiology, 45*, 11–9.

Antoni, M. H., Carver, C. S., & Lechner, S. C. (March, 2006). Stress management intervention effects on benefit finding, positive adaptation and physiological regulation for women treated for breast cancer. In A. L. Stanton (Chair). Finding benefits in adversity: Psychological and physiological processes. Symposium presented at the annual meeting of the American Psychosomatic Society, Denver.

Antoni, M. H., Lechner, S. C., Kazi, A., Wimberly, S. R., Sifre, T., Urcuyo, K. R., et al. (2006). How stress management improves quality of life after treatment for breast cancer. *Journal of Consulting and Clinical Psychology, 74*, 1143–52.

Antoni, M. H., Lehman, J. M., Kilbourn, K. M., Boyers, A. E., Culver, J. L., Alferi, S. M., et al. (2001). Cognitive-behavioral stress management intervention decreases the prevalence of depression and enhances benefit finding among women under treatment for early-stage breast cancer. *Health Psychology, 20*, 20–32.

Antoni, M. H., Wimberly, S. R., Lechner, S. C., Kazi, A., Sifre, T., Urcuyo, K. R., et al. (2006). Reduction of cancer-specific thought intrusions and anxiety symptoms with a stress management intervention among women undergoing treatment for breast cancer. *American Journal of Psychiatry, 163*, 1791–7.

Austenfeld, J. L., Paolo, A. M., & Stanton, A. L. (2006). Effects of writing about emotions versus goals on psychological and physical health among third-year medical students. *Journal of Personality, 74*, 267–86.

Austenfeld, J. L., & Stanton, A. L. (2004). Coping through emotional approach: A new look at emotion, coping, and health-related outcomes. *Journal of Personality, 72*, 1335–63.

Austenfeld, J. L., & Stanton, A. L. (2008). Writing about emotions versus goals: Effects on hostility and medical care utilization moderated by emotional approach coping processes. *British Journal of Health Psychology, 13*, 35–8.

Averill, J. R. (1990). Inner feelings, works of the flesh, the beast within, diseases of the mind, driving force, and putting on a show: Six metaphors of emotion and their theoretical extensions. In D. E. Leary (Ed.), *Metaphors in the history of psychology* (pp. 104–32). New York: Cambridge University Press.

Bagby, R. M., Parker, J. D. A., & Taylor J. G. (1994). The twenty-item Toronto Alexithymia Scale: I. Item selection and cross-validation of the factor structure. *Journal of Psychosomatic Research, 38*, 23–32.

Barrett, L. F., Mesquita, B., Ochsner, K. N., & Gross, J. J. (2007). The experience of emotion. *Annual Review of Psychology, 58*, 373–403.

Beals, K. P., Peplau, L. A., & Gable, S. L. (2009). Stigma management and well-being: The role of perceived social support, emotional processing, and suppression. *Personality and Social Psychology Bulletin, 35*, 867–79.

Berghuis, J. P., & Stanton, A. L. (2002). Adjustment to a dyadic stressor: A longitudinal study of coping and depressive symptoms in infertile couples over an insemination attempt. *Journal of Consulting and Clinical Psychology, 70*, 433–8.

Bonanno, G. A., Galea, S., Bucciarelli, A., & Vlahov, D. (2006). Psychological resilience after disaster: New York City in the aftermath of the September 11th terrorist attack. *Psychological Science, 17*, 181–6.

Bonanno, G. A., Papa, A., Lalande, K., Westphal, M., & Coifman, K. (2004). The importance of being flexible: The ability to both enhance and suppress emotional expression predicts long-term adjustment. *Psychological Science, 15*, 482–7.

Bonanno, G. A., Papa, A., Lalande, K., Zhang, N., & Noll, J. G. (2005). Grief processing and deliberate grief avoidance: A prospective comparison of bereaved spouses and parents in the United States and the People's Republic of China. *Journal of Consulting and Clinical Psychology, 73*, 86–98.

Bond, F. W., & Bunce, D. (2000). Mediators of change in emotion-focused and problem-focused worksite stress management interventions. *Journal of Occupational Health Psychology, 5*, 156–63.

Campbell-Sills, L., Barlow, D. H., Brown, T. A., & Hofmann, S. G. (2006). Effects of suppression and acceptance on emotional responses of individuals with anxiety and mood disorders. *Behaviour Research and Therapy, 44*, 1251–63.

Carstensen, L. L. (1998). A life-span approach to social motivation. In J. Heckhausen & C. S. Dweck (Eds.), *Motivation and self-regulation across the life span* (pp. 341–64). Cambridge, England: Cambridge University Press.

Carver, C. S., Scheier, M. F., & Weintraub, J. K. (1989). Assessing coping strategies: A theoretically based approach. *Journal of Personality and Social Psychology, 56*, 267–83.

Carver, C. S., & White, T. L. (1994). Behavioral inhibition, behavioral activation, and affective responses to impending reward and punishment: the BIS/BAS scales. *Journal of Personality and Social Psychology, 67*, 319–33.

Chesney, M. A., Chambers, D. B., Taylor, J. M., Johnson, L. M., & Folkman, S. (2003). Coping effectiveness training for men living with HIV: Results from a randomized clinical trial testing a group-based intervention. *Psychosomatic Medicine, 65*, 1038–46.

Coan, J. A., & Allen, J. J. B. (2003). Frontal EEG asymmetry and the behavioral activation and inhibition systems. *Psychophysiology, 40*, 106–14.

Cohen, J. L., Sander, L. M., Slavin, O. M., & Lumley, M. A. (2008). Different methods of single-session disclosure: What works for whom? *British Journal of Health Psychology, 13*, 23–6.

Coyne, J. C., & Racioppo, M. W. (2000). Never the twain shall meet? Closing the gap between coping research and clinical intervention research. *American Psychologist, 55*, 655–64.

Creswell, J. D., Lam, S., Stanton, A. L., Taylor, S. E., Bower, J. E., & Sherman, D. K. (2007). Does self-affirmation, cognitive processing, or discovery of meaning explain cancer-related health benefits of expressive writing? *Personality and Social Psychology Bulletin, 33*, 238–50.

Endler, N. S., & Parker, J. D. A. (1990). *Coping Inventory for Stressful Situations (CISS): Manual.* Toronto: Multi-Health Systems.

Endler, N. S., & Parker, J. D. A. (1994). Assessment of multidimensional coping: Task, emotion, and avoidance strategies. *Psychological Assessment, 6*, 50–60.

Folkman, S., Chesney, M., McKusick, L., Ironson, G., Johnson, D. S., & Coates, T. J. (1991). Translating coping theory into intervention. In J. Eckenrode (Ed.), *The social context of coping* (pp. 239–59). New York: Plenum.

Folkman, S., & Moskowitz, J. T. (2004). Coping: Pitfalls and promise. *Annual Review of Psychology, 55*, 745–74.

Fox, N. A. (1991). If it's not left, it's right: Electroencephalograph asymmetry and the development of emotion. *American Psychologist, 46*, 863–72.

Frattaroli, J. (2006). Experimental disclosure and its moderators: A meta-analysis. *Psychological Bulletin, 132*, 823–65.

Frazier, P. A., Mortensen, H., & Steward, J. (2005). Coping strategies as mediators of the relations among perceived control and distress in sexual assault survivors. *Journal of Counseling Psychology, 52*, 267–78.

Frazier, P., Tashiro, T., Berman, M., Steger, M., & Long, J. (2004). Correlates of levels and patterns of positive life changes following sexual assault. *Journal of Consulting and Clinical Psychology, 72*, 19–30.

Fredrickson, B. L. (2001). The role of positive emotions in positive psychology: The broaden-and-build theory of positive emotions. *American Psychologist, 56*, 218–26.

Giese-Davis, J., Koopman, C., Butler, L. D., Classen, C., Cordova, M., Fobair, P., et al. (2002). Change in emotion-regulation strategy for women with metastatic breast cancer following supportive-expressive group therapy. *Journal of Consulting and Clinical Psychology, 70*, 916–25.

Greenberg, L. S., & Watson, J. C. (2006). *Emotion-focused therapy for depression*. Washington, DC: American Psychological Association.

Gross, J. J. (Ed.). (2007). *Handbook of emotion regulation*. New York: Guilford Press.

Gross, J. J., & John, O. P. (1995). Facets of emotional expressivity: Three self-report factors and their correlates. *Personality and Individual Differences, 19*, 555–68.

Gross, J. J., & John, O. P. (2003). Individual differences in two emotion regulation processes: Implications for affect, relationships, and well-being. *Journal of Personality and Social Psychology, 85*, 348–62.

Harmon-Jones, E., & Sigelman, J. (2001). State anger and prefrontal brain activity: Evidence that insult-related relative left-prefrontal activation is associated with experienced anger and aggression. *Journal of Personality and Social Psychology, 80*, 797–803.

Hayes, S. C., Luoma, J. B., Bond, F. W., Masuda, A., & Lillis, J. (2006). Acceptance and commitment therapy: Model, processes and outcomes. *Behaviour Research and Therapy, 44*, 1–25.

Hoyt, M. A. (2009). Gender role conflict and emotional approach coping in men with cancer. *Psychology and Health, 24*, 981–96.

Huizink, A. C., de Medina, P. G. R., Mulder, E. J. H., & Visser, G. H. A. (2002). Coping in normal pregnancy. *Annals of Behavioral Medicine, 24*, 132–40.

Johnson, S. M., Hunsley, J., Greenberg, L., & Schindler, D. (1999). Emotionally focused couples therapy: Status and challenges. *Clinical Psychology: Science and Practice, 6*, 67–79.

Kashdan, T. B., Zvolensky, M. J., & McLeish, A. C. (2008). Anxiety sensitivity and affect regulatory strategies: Individual and interactive risk factors for anxiety-related symptoms. *Journal of Anxiety Disorders, 22*, 429–40.

Kennedy-Moore, E., & Watson, J. C. (2001). How and when does emotional expression help? *Review of General Psychology, 5*, 187–212.

King, L. A., & Emmons, R. A. (1990). Conflict over emotional expression: Psychological and physical correlates. *Journal of Personality and Social Psychology, 58*, 864–77.

Kirschbaum, C., Pirke, K. M., & Hellhammer, D. H. (1993). The 'Trier Social Stress Test'—a tool for investigating psychobiological stress responses in a laboratory setting. *Neuropsychobiology, 28*, 76–81.

Klein, M. H., Mathieu-Coughlan, P., & Kiesler, D. J. (1986). The Experiencing Scales. In L. S. Greenberg & W. Pinsof (Eds.), *The psychotherapeutic process: A research handbook* (pp. 27–71). New York: Guilford Press.

Kraft, C. A., Lumley, M. A., D'Souza, P. J., & Dooley, J. A. (2008). Emotional approach coping and self-efficacy moderate the effects of written emotional disclosure and relaxation training for people with migraine headaches. *British Journal of Health Psychology, 13*, 67–71.

Lane, R. D., Quinlan, D. M., Schwartz, G. E., Walker, P. A., & Zeitlin, S. B. (1990). The levels of emotional awareness scale: A cognitive-developmental measure of emotion. *Journal of Personality Assessment, 55*, 124–34.

Lazarus, R. S., & Folkman, S. (1984). *Stress, appraisal, and coping*. New York: Springer.

Lechner, S. C., Carver, C S., Antoni, M. H., Weaver, K. E., & Phillips, K. M. (2006). Curvilinear associations between benefit finding and psychosocial adjustment to breast cancer. *Journal of Consulting and Clinical Psychology, 74*, 828–40.

Lepore, S. J., & Ituarte, P. H. G. (1999). Optimism about cancer enhances mood by reducing negative social interactions. *Cancer Research, Therapy and Control, 8*, 165–74.

Lepore, S. J., Silver, R. C., Wortman, C. B., & Wayment, H. A. (1996). Social constraints, intrusive thoughts, and depressive symptoms among bereaved mothers. *Journal of Personality and Social Psychology, 70*, 271–82.

Levenson, R. W. (1994). Human emotion: A functional view. In P. Ekman & R. J. Davidson (Eds.), *The nature of emotion: Fundamental questions* (pp. 123–6). New York: Oxford University Press.

Levitt, J. T., Brown, T. A., Orsillo, S. M., & Barlow, D. H. (2004). The effects of acceptance versus suppression of emotion on subjective and psychophysiological response to carbon dioxide challenge in patients with panic disorder. *Behavior Therapy, 35*, 747–66.

Lichtenthal, W. G., Cruess, D. G., Schuchter, L. M., & Ming, M. E. (2003). Psychosocial factors related to the correspondence of recipient and provider perceptions of social support among patients diagnosed with or at risk for malignant melanoma. *Journal of Health Psychology, 8*, 705–19.

Lieberman, M. A., & Goldstein, B. A. (2006). Not all negative emotions are equal: The role of emotional expression in online support groups for women with breast cancer. *Psycho-Oncology, 15*, 160–8.

Low, C. A., Stanton, A. L., & Bower, J. E. (2008). Effects of acceptance-oriented versus evaluative emotional processing on heart rate recovery and habituation. *Emotion, 8*, 419–24.

Low, C. A., Stanton, A. L., & Danoff-Burg, S. (2006). Expressive disclosure and benefit finding among breast cancer patients: Mechanisms for positive health effects. *Health Psychology, 25*, 181–9.

Low, C. A., Stanton, A. L., Thompson, N., Kwan, L., & Ganz, P. A. (2006). Contextual life stress and coping strategies as predictors of adjustment to breast cancer survivorship. *Annals of Behavioral Medicine, 32*, 235–44.

Lumley, M. A., Gustavson, B. J., Partridge, R. T., & Labouvie-Vief, G. (2005). Assessing alexithymia and related emotional ability constructs using multiple methods: Interrelationships among measures. *Emotion, 5*, 329–42.

Lynch, T. R., Chapman, A. L., Rosenthal, M. Z., Kuo, J. R., & Linehan, M. M. (2006). Mechanisms of change in dialectical behavior therapy: Theoretical and empirical observations. *Journal of Clinical Psychology, 62*, 459–80.

Manne, S. L., Ostroff, J. S., Winkel, G., Fox, K., Grana G., Miller, E., et al. (2005). Couple-focused group intervention for women with early stage breast cancer. *Journal of Consulting and Clinical Psychology, 73*, 634–46.

Manne, S. L., Winkel, G., Rubin, S., Edelson, M., Rosenblum, N., Bergman, C., et al. (2008). Mediators of a coping and communication-enhancing intervention and a supportive counseling intervention among women diagnosed with gynecological cancers. *Journal of Consulting and Clinical Psychology, 76,* 1034–45.

Manne, S., Babb, J., Pinover, W., Horwitz, E., & Ebbert, J. (2004). Psychoeducational group intervention for wives of men with prostate cancer. *Psycho-Oncology, 13,* 37–46.

Manne, S., Ostroff, J. S., & Winkel, G. (2007). Social-cognitive processes as moderators of a couple-focused group intervention for women with early stage breast cancer. *Health Psychology, 26,* 735–44.

Manne, S., Ostroff, J., Winkel, G., Goldstein, L., Fox, K., & Grana, G. (2004). Posttraumatic growth after breast cancer: Patient, partner, and couple perspectives. *Psychosomatic Medicine, 66,* 442–54.

Master, S. L., Amodio, D. M., Stanton, A. L., Yee, C. M., Hilmert, C. J., & Taylor, S. E. (2009). Neurobiological correlates of coping through emotional approach. *Brain, Behavior, and Immunity, 23,* 27–35.

McQueeney, D. A., Stanton, A. L., & Sigmon, S. (1997). Efficacy of emotion-focused and problem-focused group therapies for women with fertility problems. *Journal of Behavioral Medicine, 20,* 313–31.

Moses, E. B., & Barlow, D. H. (2006). A new unified treatment approach for emotional disorders based on emotion science. *Current Directions in Psychological Science, 15,* 146–50.

Mosher, C. E., Danoff-Burg, S., & Brunker, B. (2005). Women's posttraumatic stress responses to maternal breast cancer. *Cancer Nursing, 28,* 399–405.

Mosher, C. E., Danoff-Burg, S., & Brunker, B. (2006). Posttraumatic growth and psychosocial adjustment of daughters of breast cancer survivors. *Oncology Nursing Forum, 33,* 543–51.

Nolen-Hoeksema, S., Wisco, B. E., & Lyubomirsky, S. (2008). Rethinking rumination. *Perspectives on Psychological Science, 3,* 400–24.

Ochsner, K. N., & Gross, J. J. (2005). The cognitive control of emotion. *Trends in Cognitive Science, 9,* 242–9.

Ozer, E. J., Best, S. R., Lipsey, T. L., & Weiss, D. S. (2008). Predictors of posttraumatic stress disorder and symptoms in adults: A meta-analysis. *Psychological Trauma: Theory, Research, Practice, and Policy, S*(1), 3–36.

Pakenham, K. I., Smith, A., & Rattan, S. L. (2007). Application of a stress and coping model to antenatal depressive symptomatology. *Psychology, Health, & Medicine, 12,* 266–77.

Park, C. L., Armeli, S., & Tennen, H. (2004a). Appraisal-coping goodness of fit: A daily Internet study. *Personality and Social Psychology Bulletin, 30,* 558–69.

Park, C. L., Armeli, S., & Tennen, H. (2004b). The daily stress and coping process and alcohol use among college students. *Journal of Studies on Alcohol, 65,* 126–35.

Pennebaker, J. W., & Beall, S. (1986). Confronting a traumatic event: Toward an understanding of inhibition and disease. *Journal of Abnormal Psychology, 95,* 274–81.

Pennebaker, J. W., Mayne, T. J., & Francis, M. E. (1997). Linguistic predictors of adaptive bereavement. *Journal of Personality and Social Psychology, 72,* 863–71.

Peters, R. M. (2006). The relationship of racism, chronic stress emotions, and blood pressure. *Journal of Nursing Scholarship, 38,* 234–40.

Pos, A. E., Greenberg, L. S., Goldman, R. N., & Korman, L. M. (2003). Emotional processing during experiential treatment of depression. *Journal of Consulting and Clinical Psychology, 71,* 1007–16.

Puig, A., Lee, S. M., Goodwin, L., Sherrard, P. A. D. (2006). The efficacy of creative arts therapies to enhance emotional expression, spirituality, and psychological well-being of newly diagnosed Stage I and Stage II breast cancer patients: A preliminary study. *The Arts in Psychotherapy, 33,* 218–28.

Reynolds, P., Hurley, S., Torres, M., Jackson, J., Boyd, P., Chen, V. W., & the Black/White Cancer Survival Study Group (2000). Use of coping strategies and breast cancer survival: Results from the Black/White Cancer Survival Study. *American Journal of Epidemiology, 152,* 940–9.

Rini, C., Dunkel Schetter, C., Hobel, C. J., Glynn, L. M., & Sandman, C. A. (2006). Effective social support: Antecedents and consequences of partner support during pregnancy. *Personal Relationships, 13,* 207–29.

Rude, S. S., Maestas, K. L., & Neff, K. (2007). Paying attention to distress: What's wrong with rumination? *Cognition and Emotion, 21,* 843–64.

Salovey, P., Mayer, J. D., Goldman, S. L., Turvey, C., & Palfai, T. (1995). Emotional attention, clarity, and repair: Exploring emotional intelligence using the Trait Meta-Mood Scale. In J. W. Pennebaker (Ed.), *Emotion, disclosure, and health* (pp. 125–54). Washington, DC: American Psychological Association.

Salovey, P., Stroud, L. R., Woolery, A., & Epel, E. S. (2002). Perceived emotional intelligence, stress reactivity, and symptom reports: Further explorations using the trait meta-mood scale. *Psychology and Health, 17,* 611–27.

Scheier, M. F., Weintraub, J. K., & Carver, C. S. (1986). Coping with stress: Divergent strategies of optimists and pessimists. *Journal of Personality and Social Psychology, 51,* 1257–64.

Schut, H. A. W., Stroebe, M. S., van den Bout, J., & de Keijser, J. (1997). Intervention for the bereaved: Gender differences in the efficacy of two counselling programmes. *British Journal of Clinical Psychology, 36,* 63–72.

Seery, M. D., Silver, R. C., Holman, E. A., Ence, W. A., Chu, T. Q. (2008). Expressing thoughts and feelings following a collective trauma: Immediate responses to 9/11 predict negative outcomes in a national sample. *Journal of Consulting and Clinical Psychology, 76,* 657–67.

Segerstrom, S. C., Stanton, A. L., Alden, L. E., & Shortridge, B. E. (2003). A multidimensional structure for repetitive thought: What's on your mind, and how, and how much? *Journal of Personality and Social Psychology, 85,* 909–21.

Simon, N. M., Pollack, M. H., Ostacher, M. J., Zalta, A. K., Chow, C. W., Fischmann, D., et al. (2007). Understanding the link between anxiety symptoms and suicidal ideation and behaviors in outpatients with bipolar disorder. *Journal of Affective Disorders. 97,* 91–9.

Smith, J. A., Lumley, M. A., & Longo, D. J. (2002). Contrasting emotional approach coping with passive coping for chronic myofascial pain. *Annals of Behavioral Medicine, 24,* 326–35.

Smyth, J. M. (1998). Written emotional expression: Effect sizes, outcome types, and moderating variables. *Journal of Consulting and Clinical Psychology, 66,* 174–84.

Spiegel, D., Bloom, J. R., Kraemer, H. C., & Gottheil, E. (1989). Effect of psychosocial treatment on survival of patients with metastatic breast cancer. *Lancet, ii,* 888–891.

Stanton, A. L., Danoff-Burg, S., Cameron, C. L., Bishop, M. M., Collins, C. A., Kirk, S. B., et al. (2000). Emotionally expressive coping predicts psychological and physical adjustment to breast cancer. *Journal of Consulting and Clinical Psychology, 68,* 875–82.

Stanton, A. L., Danoff-Burg, S., Cameron, C. L., & Ellis, A. P. (1994). Coping through emotional approach: Problems of conceptualization and confounding. *Journal of Personality and Social Psychology, 66,* 350–62.

Stanton, A. L., & Franz, R. (1999). Focusing on emotion: An adaptive coping strategy? In C. R. Snyder (Ed.), *Coping: The psychology of what works* (pp. 90–118). New York: Oxford University Press.

Stanton, A. L., Kirk, S. B., Cameron, C. L., & Danoff-Burg, S. (2000). Coping through emotional approach: Scale construction and validation. *Journal of Personality and Social Psychology, 74*, 1078–92.

Stanton, A. L., & Low, C. A. (under review). Dispositional and situational emotion regulation in the context of a chronic, life-limiting stressor.

Stanton A. L., Parsa, A., & Austenfeld, J. L. (2002). The adaptive potential of coping through emotional approach. In C. R. Snyder & S. J. Lopez (Eds.), *Handbook of positive psychology* (pp. 148–58). New York: Oxford University Press.

Stanton, A. L., Sullivan, S. J., & Austenfeld, J. L. (2009). Coping through emotional approach: Emerging evidence for the utility of processing and expressing emotions in responding to stressors. In C. R Snyder & S. J. Lopez (Eds.), *Oxford handbook of positive psychology* (2nd ed.) (pp. 225–36). New York: Oxford University Press.

Sutton, S. K., & Davidson, R. J. (1997). Prefrontal brain asymmetry: A biological substrate of the behavioral approach and inhibition systems. *Psychological Science, 8*, 204–10.

Terry, D. J., & Hynes, G. J. (1998). Adjustment to a low-control situation: Reexamining the role of coping responses. *Journal of Personality and Social Psychology, 74*, 1078–92.

Tobin, D. L., Holroyd, K. A., & Reynolds, R. V. C. (1984). *User's manual for the Coping Strategies Inventory.* Department of Psychology, Ohio University.

Trierweiler, L. I., Eid, M., & Lischetzke, T. (2002). The structure of emotional expressivity: Each emotion counts. *Journal of Personality and Social Psychology, 82*, 1023–40.

Tull, M. T., Gratz, K. L., & Lacroce, D. M. (2006). The role of anxiety sensitivity and lack of emotional approach coping in depressive symptom severity among a non-clinical sample of uncued panickers. *Cognitive Behaviour Therapy, 35*, 74–87.

van Middendorp, H., Lumley, M. A., Jacobs, J. W. G., van Doornen, L. J. P., Bijlsma, J. W. J., & Geenen, R. (2008). Emotions and emotional approach and avoidance strategies in fibromyalgia. *Journal of Psychosomatic Research, 64*, 159–67.

Watkins, E. R. (2008). Constructive and unconstructive repetitive thought. *Psychological Bulletin, 134*, 163–206.

Watson, J. C., & Bedard, D. L. (2006). Clients' emotional processing in psychotherapy: A comparison between cognitive-behavioral and process-experiential therapies. *Journal of Consulting and Clinical Psychology, 74*, 152–9.

Whelton, W. J. (2004). Emotional processes in psychotherapy: Evidence across therapeutic modalities. *Clinical Psychology and Psychotherapy, 11*, 58–71.

Zuckerman, M., Knee, C. R., Kieffer, S. C., & Gagne, M. (2004). What individuals believe they can and cannot do: Explorations of realistic and unrealistic control beliefs. *Journal of Personality Assessment, 82*, 215–32.

The Dynamics of Stress, Coping, and Health: Assessing Stress and Coping Processes in Near Real Time

Mark D. Litt, Howard Tennen, *and* Glenn Affleck

Abstract

The idea of coping has been central to our understanding of adaptation to stressors for more than 30 years. Models of coping have included factors such as traits or other dispositions, appraisals, expectancies, moods, characteristics of the situation, and health outcomes themselves. Despite the fact that coping theory was initially construed as dynamic and transactional in nature, most models of coping have been unidirectional, and have treated coping as a static outcome of the constituent factors. In this chapter we argue that unidirectional models of coping and adaptation have come about as a result of our difficulty in measuring coping as a dynamic process that unfolds over time, and that coping changes moment to moment or day to day depending on the situational determinants and the coping processes that have occurred before. Daily process and momentary assessment technologies, allied with multi-level statistical techniques, are now allowing a more detailed understanding of coping and its complexities. In this chapter we review the development of new coping models and how intensive measurement is enhancing our view of how coping works.

Keywords: coping, daily process, stress, experience sampling, Ecological Momentary Assessment

Introduction

The advent of multi-determined and biopsychosocial models of health and well-being signaled a breakthrough in conceptualizing the relationship among physical vulnerabilities, external stressors, and biological and emotional consequences. At the center of the stress–illness relationship was the process of *coping*; the cognitive and behavioral efforts of the person in response to stressors that determine how those stressors will affect physical and emotional well-being (Lazarus & Folkman, 1984). Research on coping typically reflects the belief that the relationship between stress and indicators of psychological or physical health is mediated or moderated by coping processes. But the relationships among stress, coping, and health indicators were initially construed as dynamic (Folkman, Lazarus, Gruen, & DeLongis, 1986). In this conceptualization the coping responses made by the individual at any given moment in response to stressors can feed back to alter those environmental stressors, as well as one's internal state, and in turn alter appraisals and the choice of subsequent coping responses.

We will argue in this chapter that limitations on our ability to measure complex dynamic relationships in temporally meaningful ways has limited our understanding of coping and adaptational processes in situations involving threats to psychological or physical health. We will also argue that conceptual, technical, and statistical advances in recent years now allow us to see a fuller and more accurate picture of how people cope and respond to stresses, and can help us devise more effective means to help people adapt.

Coping as a Dynamic Process

In 1978 Bandura described a perspective on psychosocial functioning that he called "reciprocal determinism." According to this view, "functioning involves a continuous reciprocal interaction between behavioral, cognitive, and environmental influences" (p. 344). Social learning theory, and consequently stress and coping theory, represented a departure from extant unidirectional models of human behavior that emphasized forces, either internal (e.g., needs, desires) or external (environmental contingencies), that determine behavior. In contrast, social learning theory proposed that internal or external forces that elicit behavioral and cognitive responses would in turn be altered by those responses. Once a person emits a coping response, the entire dynamic changes. According to Lazarus and Folkman and colleagues, coping theory "is transactional in that the person and the environment are viewed as being in a dynamic, mutually reciprocal, bidirectional relationship" (Folkman et al., 1986, p. 572).

In the domain of health there are numerous examples of reciprocal forces at work. Turk, Meichenbaum, and Genest (1983), for example, offered a scenario in which a man awakens with a headache. Depending on his history and other influences he may appraise the headache as a short-term irritant, the result of his night of drinking, or as a brain tumor. The actions he takes based on that appraisal will influence not only his subsequent internal state (e.g., his emotions), but also the physiological sensation itself, and the reactions of other people in his environment. Those changes in turn may cause a reappraisal; if the aspirin the man takes for his hangover doesn't work maybe he will reconsider the brain tumor theory.

The same processes, over a much longer timeline, occur in chronic illnesses. Manne and Zautra (1992) surveyed factors that influence coping choice among individuals living with chronic pain, including cognitive appraisals, disease activity, interpersonal relationships, and personality disposition. Appraisals and expectancies such as self-efficacy were implicated in determining choice of coping strategies, which in turn partly predicted subsequent pain outcomes. The background factors of personality disposition and disease status also influenced coping choice and outcomes. Manne and Zautra (1990) found that interpersonal relationships, too, are linked to coping. For example, among women with rheumatoid arthritis, those whose spouses made critical remarks were more likely to engage in maladaptive coping, whereas those whose spouses were supportive used more adaptive strategies.

The Manne and Zautra (1992) review also hinted at a more dynamic process. Successful coping strategies offer relief, leading to increases in self-efficacy for pain control, leading to further adaptive coping efforts. Improvements in management may lead to improvements in disease status. Adaptive coping efforts may also improve relationships with family members, further improving mood and bolstering the person's confidence, improving appraisals of the illness as controllable, and so on. Alternatively, coping failure may lead to loss of confidence, negative reactions from spouses, and increased appraisals of loss of control.

The dynamic nature of coping is evident even in a single, time-limited stressful encounter. Litt (1996) discussed the processes involved in coping and adaptation with a painful dental procedure. Distress at any given moment during the stressful procedure is a product of situational factors such as current anxiety, appraisal of the situation along dimensions of threat and controllability, self-efficacy, specific coping skills, and dentist behaviors, as well as dispositional factors such as pain sensitivity, general appraisal processes (e.g., optimism), experience with the stressor, and general coping style. Figure 19.1 depicts the processes involved in determining distress during an invasive procedure. Litt makes the case that a reduction in distress will feed back to increase self-efficacy, decrease the appraisal of threat, lower anxiety, and cause the person to relax, which in turn will reduce the anxiety level of the dentist, improving performance of the procedure, and so on. In this schema, dispositional factors set gross limits on the variability of the situational factors (see Bolger & Zuckerman, 1995), but considerable variability in appraisals, coping behaviors, and momentary affects is possible. The result is a highly dynamic model of coping and adaptation. Litt (1996) noted that although the instruments to measure all of the constructs in the process model were available, the ability to capture momentary changes in these processes was not.

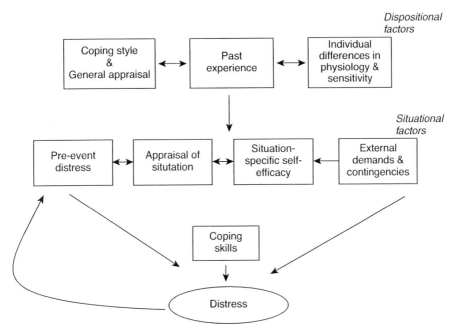

Fig. 19.1 Multi-level, multivariate model depicting the situational and dispositional contributors to acute dental distress. Double-headed arrows imply reciprocal relationships between variables, such that a change in one will engender a change in the others. Curving arrow from "Distress" back to the situational-level variables suggests a feedback mechanism whereby changes in distress will prompt changes in situational variables. "External demands and contingencies" refers to behavior on the part of the practitioner, whose behavior may change as a function of how composed the patient is at any given moment.

(From Litt, M. D. [1996]. A model of pain and anxiety in response to acute stressors: The case of dental procedures. *Behaviour Research and Therapy, 34,* 459–476. Copyright 1996, Elsevier. Adapted with permission.)

Limitations of Current Research on Coping

The unidirectional perspective

Despite the recognition by Bandura (1978) and Lazarus and Folkman (1984; Folkman et al., 1986) that coping theory is dynamic, most research in the area of coping and health treats coping in a unidirectional, static and deterministic way. In most research individuals facing a health-related stressor appraise the stressor, cope more or less effectively, and adapt. One or more health outcomes at a given point in time, or at several points in time, serve as the dependent variable(s). Coping is typically measured once, or at distant intervals (e.g., pretreatment and post-treatment). There is little recognition that changes in coping lead to changes in adaptational outcomes, which in turn may lead to changes in subsequent appraisals, coping, or external contingencies on behavior. The transactional nature of coping is not captured.

There have been exceptions. The increased popularity of structural equation modeling (SEM) has improved our ability to evaluate reciprocal processes over time. Wong et al. (2004), for example, examined the reciprocal relationship between self-efficacy

for effective coping and abstinence in cocaine-dependent outpatients. Self-efficacy and abstinence were measured at treatment entry, after 6 months of treatment, and again a year after study entry. Social learning theory predicts that coping self-efficacy should contribute to treatment success, and that treatment success in turn predicts greater self-efficacy at the next time point (Bandura, 1999; Larimer, Palmer, & Marlatt, 1999). However, results of SEM indicated that early self-efficacy predicted later self-efficacy, but not later abstinence, whereas early abstinence predicted later abstinence and self-efficacy. The authors interpreted their findings as supporting a view of drug abstinence in which prior abstinence is the primary determinant, and self-efficacy plays almost no role.

In view of the extensive literature documenting the predictive power of self-efficacy in substance use (e.g., Adamson, Sellman, & Frampton, 2009), Wong et al.'s (2004) results were surprising. Perhaps the long intervals between assessments, and a host of intervening events, attenuated the relationship between self-efficacy expectancies and later outcomes. A more extensive study of coping and change processes in substance abuse treatment was conducted by Litt, Kadden, Kabela-Cormier, and Petry (2009). Alcohol-dependent men and women were treated on an outpatient basis in a trial testing social network-based approaches to treatment and were followed every 3 months for 27 months. Latent growth modeling indicated that treatment led to adaptive changes in the social network, as planned. Social network changes in turn predicted increases in self-efficacy and coping at 15 months, which in turn predicted drinking outcomes at 27 months. Also, post-treatment outcome influenced both self-efficacy and coping behavior. Greater abstinence predicted both increased coping and increased self-efficacy in the future, illustrating something of the dynamic relations among behavioral outcomes, coping, and expectancies.

Although Litt et al.'s (2009) findings are more consistent with theory than were those of Wong et al. (2004), they raise as many questions as they answer. How, for example, did changes in the social network lead to changes in self-efficacy and coping abilities? What did patients actually do differently to improve their chances of success? Conventional research protocols have difficulty answering such questions.

Coping as a trait

Another attribute of current coping research is the tendency to treat coping as a trait, as the manifestation of a trait, or as a classifiable disposition. Folkman et al. (1986) discussed four conceptualizations of coping that highlight this problem. In the first approach, personality characteristics are viewed as disposing the person to cope in certain characteristic ways. Different theorists have focused on different personality characteristics: Bolger (1990) focused on neuroticism, Wheaton (1983) on fatalism, and Kobasa (1979) on hardiness.

The second approach noted by Folkman et al. (1986) makes no claims for personality *per se* but does assume that the way a person copes in one or more stressful events is the way he or she will cope with all stressful events. This approach is exemplified in the Coping Responses Inventory (Billings & Moos, 1984) and several subsequent coping inventories that require research participants to report how they coped with a current, supposedly representative, stressful event.

The third approach focuses on the nature of the stressor itself as a determinant of coping. In these conceptualizations maladaptive coping is determined by repeated encounters with stressors that are uncontrollable or otherwise touch on a vulnerability.

A fourth perspective was that by Pearlin and Schooler (1978), and endorsed by Suls and David (1996), who considered the relative contributions of personality characteristics and coping responses to well-being in the face of different types of stressors. In this formulation, coping in situations characterized by less controllable stressors is determined by personality factors. But in situations in which the stressor is controllable, specific situational coping responses are better predictors of adaptation. This combined model represented an advance over what had come before it.

Bolger and Zuckerman (1995) suggested another variation on the deterministic model of coping. They introduced a differential coping choice-effectiveness model that held that personality partly determines both how one copes with stress and the effectiveness of the coping response. Students in their study provided daily ratings of their exposure to interpersonal conflicts, their coping choices, and their emotional states over a 14-day period. Analyses were conducted linking coping with negative affect reactivity on the next day. Results showed that high-neuroticism participants experienced both greater exposure to interpersonal conflicts and more emotional reactivity to such conflicts. Furthermore, high- and low-neuroticism participants differed both in their choice of coping efforts and in the effectiveness of those efforts. Interestingly, individuals high in neuroticism were more likely than their low-neuroticism counterparts to use planful problem-solving, self-control, seeking social support, and escape-avoidance to cope with conflicts. Also, both coping choice and coping effectiveness differed by level of neuroticism depending on which outcome was examined—anxiety, anger, or depression. This model is one of several influential models that sought to incorporate dispositions and situational coping.

Carver and Scheier (Carver, Scheier & Weintraub, 1989; Carver & Scheier, 1994) likewise endorsed a dispositional-situational view of coping, and made efforts to capture changes in coping as the nature of the stressor changed over time. Carver, Scheier, and colleagues conjectured that personality traits or other enduring dispositions might predispose a person to engage in one or another type of coping, but situational constraints would ultimately decide the specific coping action used. The means by which they tested this model, however, may not have clearly captured situation-specific coping. Carver and Scheier (1994) employed a version of the COPE coping checklist in which respondents were asked to indicate the extent to which they had been engaging in each coping response during a particular period of time, with respect to a particular stressor. Instead of being phrased in the past tense, items were phrased in the present tense (e.g., "I am making a plan of action"), and referred to a stressor in the recent past, or one that was ongoing.

The respondents in this study were college students, and the stressor was an examination. Students were assessed 2 days before the exam, after the exam but before grades were posted, and after grades were posted. Pre-exam coping was dominated by planning, suppression of competing activities, and acceptance. Both post-exam coping and post-grades coping were characterized by acceptance and positive reframing. These results were theoretically interesting and the methodology was elegant and useful, but they still do not capture all the complexity of coping with this ongoing exam stressor.

Each of the models discussed here has proven useful and comprises personality factors, characteristics of the stressor, exposure to stressors, reactivity to stressors, coping choice, and coping effectiveness. The models described by Carver and Scheier and by Bolger and Zuckerman, employing daily diaries, were even temporally dynamic. These models, and the methods used by Bolger and Zuckerman in particular, represented an advance in thinking about coping. However, each of these models treats coping as a function of personality, and each operates in one direction: personality determines coping, coping leads to outcomes. The transactional quality of coping and environment, championed by Folkman, Lazarus, and colleagues, is still not captured. Furthermore, the view of coping-as-personality has tended to dominate thinking about coping and adaptation, despite repeated findings that situational appraisals of control are not stable, and that coping responses themselves are more situationally determined than stable (e.g., Carver, Scheier, & Weintraub, 1989; Folkman et al., 1986; Mischel, 1968, 1973).

Limitations on Our Measurement of Coping

"We shape our tools and afterwards our tools shape us."
(Marshall McLuhan)

To a large extent the somewhat static and unidirectional view of coping is a function of the way we measure it. In a very real sense, to borrow from Marshall McLuhan, our measurement tools have shaped our perspective on coping.

Measurement is cross-sectional

We typically measure coping with questionnaires. Invariably, these questionnaires require the respondent to imagine or recall a stressful event during some period of time, such as the last few days, the last month (Ways of Coping Checklist [WCCL]; Folkman & Lazarus, 1980, 1985), or the last year (Coping Response Inventory; Moos, 1988/1992), and to indicate what strategies were used to manage the situation. The COPE (Carver et al., 1989) employs all of these time frames. These inventories tend to provide a snapshot of coping behavior. Because they typically yield only a single measure at a single moment, they encourage the view that the way people respond at any moment defines their coping style.

To be sure, what little data exist do suggest that people respond quite similarly on measures like the WCCL from one time to another. Hatton et al. (1995), for example, administered the WCCL to parents of Down syndrome children when their children were first evaluated and 3 years later. Mothers' and fathers' scores on coping strategy subscales did not change substantially over the 3-year period. Whereas the test–retest reliability of the measure may be reassuring in a way, one is forced to wonder whether that level of reliability is desirable in a measure that is supposed to capture people's reactions to specific situations. The temporal stability of coping measures approaches that of trait measures.

The Hatton et al. (1995) study highlights the inability of current coping measures to capture the dynamic effects of coping on adaptive outcomes, and vice versa. If the Hatton et al. results are accepted at face value, parents of children with Down syndrome were coping *in virtually the same way* 3 years after their child was first assessed: Apparently there was no learning of additional skills, and changes in adaptational outcomes did not lead to changes in coping.

Coping is general

Another characteristic of coping as it is typically measured is that it is very general, again consistent with a trait or dispositional view of coping. Thus people are classified as adaptive or maladaptive copers, or as using one or another class of strategy (e.g., problem-focused or emotion-focused) in the face of particular stressors. Whereas this general classification of coping may be theoretically useful, it offers little information as to what a person will actually *do* during a specific stressful encounter.

Coping inventory scores will not tell us, for example, whether an alcohol-dependent individual who is trying to quit drinking will or will not turn down a drink offered at the office party, or whether the person with rheumatoid arthritis will rest at prescribed intervals to help manage intractable joint pain. As noted by Lazarus and Folkman (1984), with the trait approach taken by most assessments of coping, "what is *actually* done is not examined, because the person is asked what he or she usually does, which is an abstraction or at best a synthesis of many specific acts, not a description of a particular act or set of acts" (pp. 297–8).

Measurement is retrospective

Nearly all measures of coping are retrospective. Retrospective self-report measures of coping tend to be overly general and fairly crude (Coyne & Racioppo, 2000). This is not just a problem of specificity, however, but also of validity. In studies of determinants of substance use, for example, comparisons of retrospective versus prospective measurement (i.e., through the use of paper or electronic diaries) has indicated that even the occurrence of substance use is subject to recall error (Shiffman et al., 1997; Whitty & Jones, 1992).

Retrospective reports of coping are subject to attributional biases and the demand characteristics of the situation when people are asked to reconstruct memories and to explain their actions and their reasons for them (Monroe & McQuaid, 1994). Hammersley (1994), for example, suggested that memories of events in addiction research are "biased narratives" rather than true recollections of events. These narratives are influenced by the person's need to explain his or her actions, or to simply make coherent a set of poorly connected memories (Bradburn, Rips, & Shevell, 1987; Coyne & Gottlieb, 1996; Mandler & Johnson, 1977). Related to this phenomenon is the concept of retrospective bias, or "effort after meaning" (Brown & Harris, 1978). That is, reports of coping with events that have already taken place could be distorted by knowledge of the resolution of the event (i.e., success or failure). Finally, recollections of events are often dominated by the atypical or dramatic (Mandler & Johnson, 1977; Reiser, Black, & Abelson, 1985) and are influenced by both intervening events and contemporary moods and cognitions (e.g., Loftus, 1979).

Studies that have directly compared retrospective and near-real-time coping reports underscore the limits of the predominant retrospective methodology.

Ptacek, Smith, Espe, and Raffety (1994) had college students record ways in which they coped with an anticipated course examination every day for a week prior to the exam. Five days following the exam, these students used the same coping measure to describe how they had coped with the examination during the time when they had completed daily coping reports. The observed correlations revealed limited correspondence between daily coping reports and recalled coping. Stone et al. (1998) compared momentary coping reports recorded over a 48-hour period and retrospective reports of coping over this period. Again, correlations were of only moderate strength. Todd, Tennen, Carney, Armeli, and Affleck (2004) found weak concordance between global and daily coping reports, and Schwartz, Neale, Marco, Shiffman, and Stone (1999) reported very limited overlap between dispositional coping scores and the trait-like component of momentary coping reports. Overall, there is rather compelling evidence that recalled coping reports are inaccurate and possibly biased, yet this remains the preferred measurement method.

Coping is almost always adaptive

A survey of most coping checklists suggests that coping is lopsidedly adaptive. Most researchers have made some effort to capture maladaptive efforts to cope (e.g., alcohol and drug items on the revised COPE; Carver & Scheier, 1994), but these items are often swamped by adaptive ones. Some serious types of maladaptive coping behaviors, such as IV drug use and interpersonal violence, are almost never assessed, despite the fact that these actions are used to cope by some individuals (e.g., Aymer, 2008). Other types of maladaptive coping, such as reframing controllable situations as uncontrollable, are also seldom tapped.

As Coyne and Gottlieb (1996) noted in their critique of coping checklists,

> as they are currently employed, conventional checklists render an incomplete and distorted portrait of coping. Specifically, these checklists are grounded in too narrow a conception of coping; the application and interpretation of checklists in the typical study are not faithful to a transactional model of stress and coping; statistical controls cannot eliminate the effects of key person and situation variables on coping; and no consistent interpretation can be assigned to coping scale scores. (p. 959)

Attempts have been made to remedy some of the defects in standard assessments of coping.

For example, it has been suggested that role-play tests of coping, like the Situational Competency Test (SCT; Chaney, O'Leary & Marlatt, 1978) or the Alcohol-Specific Role-Play Test (ASRPT; Abrams et al., 1991), may solve some of the problems discussed. Our experience, however, is that these procedures are cumbersome and highly artificial, and may not be valid indicators of subjects' behavior in the natural environment (Kadden et al., 1992).

Keeping in mind the many serious methodological limitations of current stress and coping research, and the failure of current methods and study designs to capture the inherently dynamic nature of coping, we now turn to what we view as the most promising alternative: near-real-time assessment of stress, coping, and health processes, and intensive micro-longitudinal study designs.

Daily and Momentary Assessment of Stress, Coping, and Health
Assessment of human experience in near real time

To avoid many of the problems of retrospective reports, researchers have adopted diary methodologies that collect experiential data daily or multiple times per day. These methods avoid many of the problems associated with reconstructing events and actions over many days or weeks, and capture associations among events, cognitions, affects, and behavioral responses that the individual can neither recognize nor report retrospectively (Csikszentmihalyi & Larson, 1987).

Early efforts to assess human experience in a more contemporaneous way employed pencil-and-paper methods. In 1978 Klinger devised a procedure for sampling thoughts in the natural environment: Subjects carried a beeper that signaled them at random intervals to record their thoughts, feelings, and behaviors during daily activities. In the early 1980s, Csikszentmihalyi and Larson (Csikszentmihalyi & Graef, 1980; Csikszentmihalyi & Larson, 1987; Larson & Csikszentmihalyi, 1983) developed the Experience Sampling Method (ESM), in which subjects carried electronic pagers and recorded thoughts and activities as they were happening.

Data have since accumulated indicating that paper diaries are vulnerable to faked compliance and falsification of data (Broderick et al., 2003; Litt, Cooney & Morse, 1998; Stone et al., 2002; see Tennen, Affleck, Coyne, Larsen, & DeLongis, 2006, for a discussion of the relative strengths and weaknesses of paper diaries). ESM and daily process methodologies have thus been updated using electronic devices to capture daily or momentary data. An example is the methodology of Ecological Momentary Assessment (EMA; Stone & Shiffman, 1994). The hallmark of these methods is the use of technology that can store event records with a time-and-date stamp automatically, and that are resistant to tampering by the respondent. Among the devices used are palm-top computers or personal digital assistants, Internet-capable devices linked to Web-based data capture applications, and telephone-based interactive voice response (IVR) systems.

The rapidly expanding use of electronic devices capable of reliably recording daily or momentary data has expanded our understanding of coping and the types of coping models we can test. One influential model is that of Kenny and Zautra (1995), who outlined a multi-level model of coping that entails examining a person's status over many points in time. As did Carver and Scheier (Carver, Scheier, & Weintraub, 1989) and Bolger (1990), they posited a dispositional-situational model of coping behavior. According to this "state-trait" model, a person's standing on a given variable at a given time is a function of (at least) three sources of variance: a trait term that does not change over time, a state term that changes with circumstances, and a random error term. In this model a full understanding of coping and adaptation can best be understood by taking into account trait or *dispositional* level variables (e.g., personality traits, stable individual difference variables, genotypes) as well as state or *situational* level variables (including situational characteristics and coping strategies used). The model further suggests that the situational variables should be measured as close in time as possible to the event of interest.

Daily process and experience sampling methodology are ideally suited to examining models of this type. Highly variable and fleeting phenomena, such as episodic pain or urges to smoke or drink, can be measured multiple times per day, along with associated situational characteristics and coping behaviors. Less variable behaviors or events, such as daily calorie intake or daily drinking, may be measured on a daily basis. Daily and momentary methods of data collection are now being used in conjunction with multi-level statistical designs that allow the evaluation of the influence of the dispositional variables on the trajectories of daily or momentary events. These methodologies have introduced new ways of thinking about stress, coping, and adaptation.

Promising Applications of Daily Process and Experience Sampling Methods to Coping Research

We now describe several promising applications of near-real-time ambulatory assessment and intensive micro-longitudinal study designs of stress, coping, and health processes. These new applications span gene–stress interactions, coping vulnerability, and resilience as 'behavioral signatures,' the application of flexible time windows to study coping as it develops in everyday life, the study of momentary coping to capture feed-forward processes, and the mechanisms of action of behavior change interventions. Each of these recent applications is founded on the premise that stress, coping, and adaptation are temporally unfolding dynamic processes.

Refining the measurement of behavioral and emotional correlates of genetic variation

One way in which intense daily or momentary measurement has started to inform stress and coping research is by refining the conceptualization and assessment of behavioral and emotional correlates of genetic variation in studies of gene–stress interactions. Behavioral geneticists and clinical neuroscientists have become increasingly aware that imprecise measurement is a limiting factor in evaluating genetic vulnerability and resilience models, and that replicable findings demand precise characterization of target behaviors and emotional experiences. Questionnaire and interview-based assessments of emotional symptoms, like retrospective questionnaire-based coping reports, are typically infused with recall error and bias. To obtain more precise emotional symptom markers, some behavioral geneticists have turned to the candidate symptom approach (Leboyer et al., 1998). Recent evidence suggests that intensive micro-longitudinal study designs (Walls, 2006) that measure behavior and emotions daily or several times a day during participants' everyday lives may provide unusually precise indicators with which to evaluate genetic vulnerability and resilience and, most relevant to this chapter, test gene–stress interactions.

These daily process markers offer three advantages over questionnaire and interview-based indicators: (1) as mentioned above, by measuring near-time behavior and experience, daily methods limit recall error and bias (Tennen et al., 2000); (2) by aggregating repeated assessments of the behavior or emotional symptom across time and situations, these methods yield highly reliable markers (Epstein, 1983); and (3) by measuring stressful encounters, behaviors, and emotional responses as they occur over time, this approach offers the opportunity to capture the *if–then* nature of stress–behavior associations (Shoda, Mischel, & Wright, 1994), thereby creating the opportunity to examine how an hypothesized genetic vulnerability or resilience factor modifies the contingency between a stressful encounter and the behavioral or emotional symptom of interest.

In a recent study of college student alcohol use in response to stress, Covault et al. (2007) demonstrated the potential benefits of aggregating repeated near-time behavioral measures, specifically the tendency to use alcohol or drugs in response to stressors. These investigators recruited a large group of college students who reported their last year's major life stressors and then each day for 30 days recorded their alcohol and non-prescription drug use. The same procedure was repeated the next year with the same study participants. Covault et al. found that the serotonin transporter 5-HTTLPR polymorphism interacted with life events to predict subsequent alcohol and drug use, such that the drinking and drug use of students with two short alleles (s/s) and that of students with two long alleles (l/l) was indistinguishable at low levels of life stress. At high levels of life stress, however, s/s students were considerably more likely than their l/l counterparts to use alcohol and drugs frequently. These findings point to the promise of including daily assessments of self-reported behavior in evaluating how gene–stress interactions influence health behaviors.

The ability of intensive micro-longitudinal designs to capture daily dynamic emotional sequences, including daily stress–distress sequences, was demonstrated by Gunthert et al. (2007), who noted that although numerous studies have attempted to identify specific genes that predispose people to anxiety-related outcomes, studies of the relationship between the 5-HTTLPR polymorphism and anxiety-related personality traits have produced mixed results. These investigators reasoned that one possible explanation for the mixed results is that genetic vulnerability might be revealed in reports of anxiety, but only when activated by stress. Indeed, animal research and functional magnetic resonance imaging (fMRI) studies in humans indicate that 5-HTTLPR differences in anxiety may be best observed under conditions of immediate threat. Whereas most correlational studies investigating the gene–environment interplay, including Covault et al.'s (2007) study, have focused on "macro-level" stressors (i.e., major life events), Gunthert and associates reasoned that vulnerability–stress processes might also occur in the context of "micro-level" stressors that occur during day-to-day encounters.

Using the same student sample as Covault et al. (2007), Gunthert et al. found support for the hypothesis that allelic variation in the gene encoding 5-HTT acts as a genetic diathesis for the experience of anxious mood in response to daily stressors. On days with more intense stressors, short allele student carriers reported elevated feelings of anxiety, compared to long allele students. This gene–stress interaction was *not* replicated when measures of trait anxiety and neuroticism were substituted for the marker of daily anxiety reactivity. For investigators interested in gene–environment interactions, these findings complement emerging research regarding the role of environmental circumstances in the expression of genetic differences. They also suggest that by virtue of their ability to capture affective states in close temporal proximity to daily stressors, daily indicators may be more sensitive than one-time trait reports for detecting the subjective correlates of genetic variation. For investigators involved more broadly in stress and coping research, these findings suggest that intensive longitudinal sampling of acute affective reactions in daily life, daily stressors, and coping efforts may offer unique opportunities to examine stress and coping in the spirit of Folkman and Lazarus's (1985) conception of coping as a temporally unfolding process.

Identifying hidden vulnerabilities, resilience, and coping "signatures"

Most studies in the stress and coping literature assess individuals' reports of their coping efforts by asking them what they think and do in response to a particular stressor. But if coping is a dynamic process, as Folkman and her colleagues have asserted, coping strategies should change in response to changes in the stressful encounter, and we should be able to identify individual differences in the contingent relationship between changes in the stressor and changes in coping behavior over time. In the personality literature, Shoda et al. (1994) introduced the notion of "behavioral signatures," which are "*if–then*" behavioral contingencies. Intensive longitudinal methods are well suited to study the

inherently idiographic nature of behavioral signatures. Two studies have examined "coping signatures" as a way to identify otherwise hidden coping vulnerabilities among formerly depressed individuals living with chronic pain.

Tennen, Affleck, and Zautra (2006) hypothesized that an episode of major depression leaves an individual with affective and coping deficits or scars that manifest themselves even years after the depressive episode is resolved. They reasoned that the distinctly mixed results in the literature regarding the "scar hypothesis" (Lewinsohn, Steinmetz, Larson, & Franklin, 1981) might reflect the fact that these depression-related coping deficits emerge as behavioral signatures (i.e., *if–then* contingent sequences) rather than as the personality traits, attitudes, and appraisal styles that are typically assessed in the literature. For example, among chronic pain patients, on a day when pain worsens, individuals with a prior depression might view that day's coping strategies as particularly ineffective. Such daily sequences could be captured only through daily methods.

Tennen et al. (2006) asked women diagnosed with primary fibromyalgia to report in nightly paper diaries (time-stamped via postmarks) their perceived pain control, their preoccupations with the worst possible outcomes of a pain episode (i.e., catastrophizing), how they coped with that day's pain, and the efficacy of that day's coping efforts. They also assessed current levels of pain and depressive symptoms three times a day with palm-top computers programmed as electronic interviewers.

The study findings supported the notion that formerly depressed individuals continue to exhibit coping deficits years after their most recent depressive episode, which in this sample was more than 4 years prior to study participation. Each of these deficits took the form of a behavioral signature. Specifically, formerly depressed participants did not differ from their never-depressed counterparts on overall affective experience, catastrophizing tendencies, coping strategies, or how they appraised the effectiveness of those strategies. However, for individuals with a depression history, a rise in daily pain was more strongly associated with a decline in perceived coping efficacy than it was for those who had never been depressed. Similarly, for participants with a depression history, the tendency to vent emotions on a more painful day was more likely than it was for those without a depression history. Finally, for individuals without a previous depression, the experience of current depressive symptoms played little part in the relation between daily pain and daily pleasant mood. In contrast, for participants with a depression history, higher levels of current depressive symptoms accentuated the drop in pleasant mood on a more painful day. Had these investigators not examined *if–then* coping and affective contingencies through their intensive longitudinal study design and daily diary methods, they would have joined other investigators in asserting that there was no support for the scar hypothesis.

Conner, Tennen, Zautra, Affleck, Armeli, and Fifield (2006) examined whether these coping signatures emerged among individuals with rheumatoid arthritis (RA). They found that on higher pain days, RA patients with a past depressive episode were more likely to cope by venting their emotions and to show steeper declines in mood. In fact, venting emotions as a coping strategy and negative mood were twice as strongly yoked to daily pain for individuals with a history of depression. To the extent that psychological health and coping success is reflected in the ability to regulate emotions in the face of changing circumstances (John & Gross, 2004), especially in the context of chronic pain (Hamilton et al., 2005), individuals with a history of depression appear less able to maintain their emotional well-being and coping efficacy in the face of challenging changes in their physical state.

The influence of history of depression and depressed mood in drinking was evaluated on a momentary basis in treated alcoholics. Litt et al. (2000) followed 26 alcoholics for 2 weeks after extensive outpatient treatment using an experience sampling protocol in which they were signaled eight times per day to record urges to drink, moods, situations, and drinking on a palm-top computer. Results indicated that those patients who were depressed reported craving and relapse, but only while in drinking-related milieus and during negative mood states. The field recordings also indicated that those who did not report craving and did not relapse were more often those who avoided drinking-related situations and engaged in activities incompatible with drinking (e.g., going to AA meetings, going to church). In fact, about half of the sample elected to change living situation and/or engage in activities that were not drinking-related in order to avoid drinking (i.e., they engaged in anticipatory coping). In this study, then, the intensive recording revealed several patterns: (1) depression made patients vulnerable to craving, but only while they were in a depressed mood; (2) coping was affected by situational determinants (e.g., presence of others drinking); and (3) situational exposure was affected by coping (e.g., intentional avoidance). This study highlighted some of the transactional nature of the coping process. To capture the day-to-day within-person dynamics inherent in such self-regulatory and coping processes, we assert that investigators must turn to daily or more frequent measurement strategies and intensive longitudinal study designs.

Moving beyond fixed intervals in the study of coping behavior

Most diary-based coping research relies on fixed intervals and fixed interval analytic methods to examine stress-coping associations. In the typical diary study an investigator examines the same-day association between stress exposure and coping efforts, and whether this association varies across individuals. Less frequently, within-day lagged associations or cross-day lags are examined (i.e., does stress exposure at time t anticipate a particular coping strategy at $t+1$?). Each of these approaches relies on fixed intervals. However, in everyday life some coping strategies cannot be applied on the day a stressor occurs, and the use of a particular strategy might vary across exposures. Daily methods allow investigators to examine such variability in coping responses and to test more sophisticated hypotheses linking daily stress exposure and coping efforts. Among these are "time to coping behavior" models.

Researchers interested in individual differences in drinking to cope with negative moods have begun to turn to the intensive longitudinal study designs we have described. Several of these studies have evaluated the prediction that individuals with drink to cope (DTC) motivations (i.e., the preference for using alcohol to reduce the effects of stress and negative mood; Cooper, 1994) drink more following stressful encounters or negative mood episodes. Surprisingly, these studies have not been consistent in their support for the premise that individuals with stronger DTC motives drink relatively more on days during which they experience more negative mood (e.g., Hussong et al., 2005; Mohr et al., 2005; Todd et al., 2003). However, constraints on drinking due to work-related demands or school-related responsibilities may not allow individuals to drink as a way to deal with a negative mood. Moreover, some models of stress-related drinking (e.g., Volpicelli, 1987) predict that alcohol use is more likely only after a stressful situation has resolved. The commonly used fixed interval approach cannot adequately capture these situational constraints and hypothesized delays in the use of alcohol as a coping strategy.

In response to these limitations, Armeli et al. (2008) demonstrated how an alternative drinking outcome, immediacy of drinking within the weekly cycle, can be applied in daily diary studies of alcohol use to deal with the likelihood that the temporal lag between negative mood and alcohol use may vary, and that the endorsement of DTC motives is more likely to predict time to initiate alcohol use than drinking on the negative-mood day. Indeed, using a 30-day electronic diary during each of two successive years, Armeli et al. (2008) found that among college students with stronger DTC motives, drinking was initiated relatively earlier on high- compared to low-anxiety weeks, whereas among students with weaker DTC motives, drinking was initiated relatively later on high- compared to low-anxiety weeks. This interaction between anxiety and coping motives could not be detected using the fixed interval approach.

More recently, Todd et al. (2009) applied similar time-to-drinking models to drinking *within a day* in response to daily stress and negative mood. These investigators reasoned that drinking initiation more proximal to the experience of stressors and negative affect might be a more sensitive indicator of problematic coping-related alcohol use compared to covariation between negative affect and amount of alcohol consumed. Drinking that occurs soon after the experience of negative affect, especially if it violates strong social norms or disregards role responsibilities, suggests stronger motivation to use alcohol to cope. This study focused on interpersonal stressors because they are particularly common and potent stressors (Bolger & Zuckerman, 1995), and because they are thought to be relevant to stress-related drinking (Higgins & Marlatt, 1975).

Todd et al. recruited community-dwelling adults who were drinking at potentially hazardous levels. For 21 consecutive days they recorded via a palm-top computer their negative and positive moods and interpersonal problems three times a day, in the morning, afternoon, and evening. Alcohol was recorded in real time. Whereas prior analyses of these data (Todd et al., 2005) revealed no evidence for covariation between intensity of prior negative mood and amount of alcohol consumed over various fixed time intervals, the multi-level hazard models used in this study revealed an association between intensity of early-day negative mood and the immediacy of alcohol consumption within the same day. Moreover, individuals with stronger DTC motives were more likely to respond to negative mood by initiating drinking earlier in the day than those with relatively weaker DTC motives. Using similar daily methods and analytic strategies, Hussong (2007) was able to demonstrate how gender and coping motives predicted shorter sadness-to-drinking intervals among individuals who had experienced greater alcohol-related drinking consequences. Again, these patterns could be revealed *only* through near-real-time measurement and creative data analytic applications.

Capturing a moment: Momentary coping behavior and its influence on outcomes

Much of the research on coping has been limited to characterizing coping actions in rather abstract terms (e.g., seeking support, problem-solving, emotion-focused vs. problem-focused, cognitive vs. behavioral). Experience sampling and EMA methods are now making it possible to assess what people actually *do* in stressful circumstances, through the use of recording technologies that can capture the entire range of specific coping behaviors, and relate those behaviors to meaningful behavioral outcomes. Studies of coping may therefore no longer be restricted to those categories of coping behaviors that apply to "most people."

O'Connell et al. (1998), for example, used EMA methods to gather real-time quantitative and qualitative data from cigarette smokers enrolled in smoking cessation programs. The participants were issued tape recorders and palm-top computers to record episodes of coping for 3 consecutive days during their first 10 days of smoking cessation. Participants were instructed to provide a recording after engaging in coping responses, after each slip, and in response to computer-initiated prompts. The authors reported that the participants recorded 389 coping episodes, during which they employed 1,047 coping responses. This worked out to an average of 3.6 coping episodes per day and an average of 2.7 coping responses per episode. The tape recordings were content-coded to categorize coping efforts into behavioral and cognitive coping. Most of these efforts were classified into one of nine major categories of coping, but many were quite idiosyncratic, including using the recording equipment itself as a distraction, and smoking to cope with smoking urges (that is, coping failure).

Sex of the participant, location of the episode, and level of nicotine dependence were all associated with the use of specific strategies. Men were more likely to engage in cognitive distraction and self-encouragement when faced with a high smoking craving situation, whereas women were more likely to engage in behavioral distraction (e.g., drawing or keeping one's hands busy). These results linked if–then strategies of smokers to specific subgroups; different smoking subgroups displayed different behavioral "signatures" in high-risk-for-smoking situations.

In an experience sampling study of pain experience among individuals experiencing chronic temporomandibular dysfunction-related pain (TMD), Litt, Shafer, and Napolitano (2004) used multiple recordings per day to characterize the momentary dynamics of affect, self-efficacy, catastrophizing, and pain. As suggested by Kenny and Zautra (1995), the trait-state-error model was adopted to characterize patients' pain status at a given moment in time. Study participants provided recordings on a palm-top computer in response to prompts four times per day for 7 days prior to starting treatment. Multilevel linear regression analyses were used to evaluate predictors of momentary pain using dispositional measures (dispositional coping and catastrophizing) and momentary measures. By using lagged values of the momentary variables a dynamic picture was drawn of the process of episodic pain experience. Momentary pain at any given time was a function of dispositional coping and dispositional catastrophizing, and concurrent mood, self-efficacy, and catastrophizing. However, negative mood, catastrophizing, and pain in the prior 3 to 6 hours also contributed to momentary pain, and increased momentary pain, in turn, led to increased pain and more negative mood at the next time point. Thus we see in this study the beginnings of a feed-forward process whereby even episodic pain can propagate itself by altering mood and expectancies later in time. Thus what starts as a "bad day" continues as a bad day.

Momentary coping and evaluating mechanisms of treatment

One of the most promising aspects of intensive measurement of coping is its adaptation to understanding mechanisms of treatment. A number of psychosocial treatments have been able to demonstrate improvements in physical and psychosocial outcomes in a number of health domains, including treatment of addictions, pain management, medication adherence, and exercise behavior. Most of these treatments are based on theories of adaptive behavior change that are presumed to explain the effectiveness of treatment. Cognitive-behavioral

coping skills treatments, for example, are intended to teach skills to patients to better cope with particular stressors. As individuals learn these skills they become more successful at managing the stressor, and thereby their self-efficacy for coping is increased. Increased self-efficacy leads to greater persistence at coping in the face of new or recurring stressors, and the person shows a net improvement in adaptation (e.g., Marlatt & Gordon, 1985).

MECHANISMS OF TREATMENT IN CHRONIC PAIN

The difficulty with these theories is that relatively little research has been conducted to determine if treatments are in fact leading to the kinds of changes expected, and if so, whether those changes are accounting for symptom reduction. In the area of chronic pain management, for example, McCracken and Turk (2002) made some efforts to evaluate the moderators and processes of behavioral treatment for chronic pain problems. They concluded that very distressed patients fared less well overall, and that decreased negative emotional responses to pain, decreased perceptions of disability, and increased orientation toward self-management during treatment were associated with better treatment outcomes. Their review could not specifically link any adaptive changes to treatment *per se*, however.

Electronic diaries capable of recording coping strategies that people use in real situations are shedding some light on the mechanisms of effective treatment. Turner, Mancl, and Aaron (2005) employed electronic diaries to determine what changes in coping behaviors occurred in patients with chronic TMD pain after cognitive-behavioral treatment (CBT). TMD clinic patients were assigned randomly to either a brief cognitive-behavioral pain management training or to an education/attention control condition and were asked to complete electronic interviews three times daily during the 8-week treatment. Multi-level regression analyses on the daily data indicated no statistically significant difference between the study groups on the daily pain and interference measures, but consistently greater within-subject improvement in the CBT group on the daily process measures. The brief CBT resulted in decreased catastrophizing and increased perceived control over pain relative to the control treatment. The study demonstrated that coping and cognitive appraisal processes could be assessed multiple times per day, allowing us a better understanding of what changes may take place in treatment. However, the authors of this study were not able to relate changes in coping and cognitive process measures to changes in pain and interference.

A study by Litt, Shafer, Kreutzer, Ibanez, and Tawfik-Yonkers (2009) sought to clarify the links between treatment, use of coping skills, and outcomes. Patients were men and women with TMD enrolled in a study of brief standard conservative treatment or standard treatment plus CBT. Momentary affects, pain, and coping processes were recorded on a cellphone keypad four times per day for 7 days prior to treatment, and for 14 days following treatment, using an experience sampling protocol. Analyses of general retrospective measures of pain, depression, and pain-related interference with lifestyle at post-treatment indicated few effects attributable to treatment differences. However, mixed model analyses on *momentary* pain and coping recorded before and after treatment indicated that the patients who received standard treatment plus CBT reported significantly greater increases in the use of active cognitive and behavioral coping, and significantly decreased catastrophizing, than did the standard treatment patients, as well as greater decreases in momentary pain at post-treatment. Mixed model analyses of the experience sampling data indicated that post-treatment momentary pain was negatively predicted by concurrent active coping, self-efficacy, perceived control over pain, and positive high arousal affect. Concurrent catastrophizing also strongly predicted pain. The results indicated that CBT for TMD pain can help patients alter their coping behaviors, and that these changes may translate into improved outcomes.

The results also indicated something else, however. Overall, differences in momentary outcomes by treatment were not entirely accounted for by differences in coping responses. Differences in momentary pain by treatment condition persisted even when coping responses were accounted for. Changes in other aspects of pain management and pain experience, including affects and cognitions, did account for the treatment effects. The addition of CBT to standard conservative treatment resulted not only in specific improvements in some coping behaviors, but also in improvements in affects and cognitions, particularly increases in self-efficacy expectations and decreases in catastrophizing, that may have been more important than the coping changes *per se*. At least in this instance, treatment was doing more than just teaching coping skills.

MECHANISMS OF ACTION IN TREATMENT OF ADDICTIONS

The lack of data documenting actual treatment-related changes in coping behavior appears also in the addictions literature. A discussion of the role of coping in treatment outcome appears in Morgenstern and Longabaugh's (2000) evaluation of proposed mechanisms of action in CBT for alcohol dependence. The authors examined numerous studies of CBT but found only 10 that met criteria for inclusion in their analysis. Each of the 10 studies was examined in terms of three criteria: (1) Did CBT lead to better treatment outcomes than a comparison group in which coping skills were not a focus? (2) Did the CBT group demonstrate increased coping skills relative to the comparison group? and (3) Did the use of coping skills predict better treatment outcome? A fourth criterion was also examined: Did the inclusion of coping skills as a covariate in statistical analyses weaken the relationship between treatment and outcome? If so, then a mediational relationship could be said to exist (Baron & Kenny, 1986).

Morgenstern and Longabaugh (2000) found that only 1 of the 10 studies they examined even came close to establishing a mediational role for coping skills. For the remainder of the studies, one of two patterns emerged: either CBT resulted in more coping responses reported than did a comparison treatment but increased coping score was not related to outcome, or reported coping skills were related to outcome but change in coping could not be attributed to CBT. They concluded that research has not yet established the mechanisms of action for CBT. A similar test of mediation was undertaken by Litt et al. (2003). A comparison of group CBT and group interactional treatments indicated that coping skills did predict drinking outcomes, but that CBT was no better than interactional treatment at producing coping skills increases. In other words, a coping skills treatment was no better than a comparison treatment at actually producing increased coping.

To determine if the relative failure of coping skills treatment was attributable to inadequate teaching of skills, Litt, Kadden, and Kabela-Cormier (2009) sought to develop an optimal coping skills training program in which experience sampling via cellphone was used to detect those situations in which alcohol-dependent persons awaiting treatment would be most likely to drink, what coping skills they used, and what skills they most needed. The results of the experience sampling were then used to develop a highly personalized coping skills program in which the therapist identified those skills the person already had, and those that he or she needed to develop. This treatment was referred to as the Individualized Assessment and Treatment Program (IATP).

The IATP treatment yielded a higher proportion of days abstinent following treatment than did a standardized CBT. IATP also elicited more adaptive momentary coping responses (e.g., refusing a drink, waiting out the urge to drink) and less drinking, in high-risk situations, as recorded by experience sampling following treatment. Post-treatment coping response rates were, in turn, associated with decreases in drinking. The highly individualized training of coping skills made possible by the experience sampling data made the importance of coping skills more apparent. The experience sampling procedure allowed a level of measurement that was not otherwise possible. The use of voice recordings to document specific coping behaviors as they occur will further refine this treatment.

A Note on Context

For the most part, our discussion of enhanced models of coping concerned two different contexts: chronic pain and addiction. The adaptation of temporally sensitive models to these contexts illustrates to some extent the universality of the methods discussed, and their adaptability to most coping contexts. Although both managing pain and managing addiction require coping resources, the circumstances are different. In the case of addiction, the outcome to be managed is behavioral in nature and significantly controllable; people develop coping resources in order to refrain from substance use. The models studied here are thus applicable to any health problem that involves self-regulation, such as smoking, weight management, exercise, and so on.

The management of chronic pain, on the other hand, deals with an outcome over which the subject has much less direct control, the physiological/cognitive phenomenon of pain. Coping efforts are directed less at eliciting behaviors that will directly affect the outcome than they are in developing cognitive and emotional resources and behaviors that will indirectly affect the outcome. The coping processes in this context are the same as those used in any situation in which management and adaptation are the goals, such as in coping with chronic diseases like diabetes, heart disease, or cancer.

Despite the difference in goals and emphasis, many of the coping strategies applied are the same in both contexts, and we conceptualize the coping processes in much the same way in each. A person with a given condition is confronted by a stimulus that has the potential to alter his or her equilibrium (physical or emotional). The way the person responds to that stimulus (i.e., *copes*) will determine the outcome of that event, be it recurrence of drinking or increased pain. It is that process, occurring dynamically over minutes or hours or days, that interests us, and that we are only just now beginning to study.

Conclusions

Together, these studies demonstrate the flexibility of intensive longitudinal designs that include daily or within-day data capture to detect the ebb and flow of coping and coping-related processes as they emerge in people's daily lives. It would be limiting to view these studies as simply the application of sophisticated methodological and analytic strategies to daily or momentary data. Instead, they demonstrate that daily and momentary data offer investigators the opportunity to study stress and coping as temporally unfolding dynamic processes, true to the spirit of Folkman and colleagues' (Lazarus & Folkman, 1984; Folkman et al., 1986) vision of how coping works. What results is a richer, and admittedly more complicated, view of human adaptation, in which appraisals, coping, expectancies, and adaptational outcomes all may change over days or over minutes, and which in turn will set the stage for all these factors at the next moment in time.

It is likely that many processes involved in human health and adaptation do not require the level of measurement discussed in this chapter. But for those processes that do, daily process and momentary measurement techniques are opening new areas of study and providing a new understanding of the dynamics of the coping process.

Future Directions

The research reviewed in this chapter has only begun to study the intricate relationships among dispositions, appraisals, coping, and the effects of interventions to improve health. Still largely a mystery is what people actually do (think, feel, act) differently to improve their health status. Some of the questions that remain include:

1. How do treatments intended to change health behaviors actually work? Do they change expectancies? Coping? How does behavior change result?

2. Can we capitalize on dispositional tendencies to improve coping in highly stressful situations? Can we base idiographic treatments on nomothetic data?

3. How can we improve our ability to measure and analyze human experience? Are there new technologies that will better capture thoughts, feelings, and behaviors relevant to coping and health?

These questions will keep us busy for some time to come.

References

Abrams, D. B., Binkoff, J. A., Zwick, W. R., Liepman, M. R., Nirenberg, T. D., Munroe, S. M., & Monti, P. M. (1991). Alcohol abusers' and social drinkers' responses to alcohol-relevant and general situations. *Journal of Studies on Alcohol, 52*, 409–14.

Adamson, S. J., Sellman, J. D., & Frampton, C. M. (2009). Patient predictors of alcohol treatment outcome: A systematic review. *Journal of Substance Abuse Treatment, 36*, 75–86.

Armeli, S., Todd, M., Conner, T. S., & Tennen, H. (2008). Drinking to cope with negative moods and the immediacy of drinking within the weekly cycle among college students. *Journal of Studies on Alcohol and Drugs, 69*, 313–22.

Aymer, S. R. (2008). Adolescent males' coping responses to domestic violence: A qualitative study. *Children and Youth Services Review, 30*, 654–64.

Bandura, A. (1978). The self system in reciprocal determinism. *American Psychologist, 33*, 344–58.

Bandura, A. (1999). A sociocognitive analysis of substance abuse: An agentic perspective. *Psychological Science, 10*, 214–7.

Baron, R. M., & Kenny, D. A. (1986). The moderator-mediator variable distinction in social psychological research: Conceptual, strategic, and statistical considerations. *Journal of Personality and Social Psychology, 51*, 1173–82.

Billings, A. G., & Moos, R. H. (1984). Coping, stress, and social resources among adults with unipolar depression. *Journal of Personality and Social Psychology, 46*, 877–91.

Bolger, N. (1990). Coping as a personality process. *Journal of Personality and Social Psychology, 59*, 525–37.

Bolger, N., & Zuckerman, A. (1995). A framework for studying personality in the stress process. *Journal of Personality and Social Psychology, 69*, 890–902.

Bradburn, N., Rips, L., & Shevell, S. (1987). Answering autobiographical questions: The impact of memory and inference on surveys. *Science, 236*, 157–61.

Broderick, J. E., Schwartz, J. E., Shiffman, S., Hufford, M. R. & Stone, A. A. (2003). Signaling does not adequately improve diary compliance. *Annals of Behavioral Medicine, 26*, 139–48.

Brown, G. W., & Harris, T. (1978). The social origins of depression: A study of psychiatric disorder in women. New York: Free Press.

Carver, C. S., & Scheier, M. F. (1994). Situational coping and coping dispositions in a stressful transaction. *Journal of Personality and Social Psychology, 66*, 184–95.

Carver, C. S., Scheier, M. F., & Weintraub, J. K. (1989). Assessing coping strategies: A theoretically based approach. *Journal of Personality and Social Psychology, 56*, 267–83.

Chaney, E. F., O'Leary, M. R., & Marlatt, G. A. (1978). Skill training with alcoholics. *Journal of Consulting and Clinical Psychology, 46*, 1092–104.

Conner, T., Tennen, H., Zautra, A., Affleck, G., Armeli, S., & Fifield, J. (2006). Coping with rheumatoid arthritis pain in daily life: Within-person analyses reveal hidden vulnerability for the formerly depressed. *Pain, 126*, 198–209.

Cooper, M. L. (1994). Motivations for alcohol use among adolescents: Development and validation of a four-factor model. *Psychological Assessment, 6*, 117–28.

Covault, J., Tennen, H., Herman, A. I., Armeli, S., Conner, T., Cillessen, A. H. N., & Kranzler, H. R. (2007). The interactive effect of the serotonin transporter 5-HTTLPR polymorphism and stressful life events on college student drinking and drug use. *Biological Psychiatry, 61*, 609–16.

Coyne, J. C., & Gottlieb, B. H. (1996). The mismeasure of coping by checklist. *Journal of Personality, 64*, 959–91.

Coyne, J. C., & Racioppo, M. W. (2000). Never the twain shall meet? Closing the gap between coping research and clinical intervention research. *American Psychologist, 55*, 655–64.

Csikszentmihalyi, M., & Graef, R. (1980). The experience of freedom in daily experience. *American Journal of Community Psychology, 8*, 404–14.

Csikszentmihalyi, M., & Larson, R. (1987). Validity and reliability of the experience-sampling method. *Journal of Nervous and Mental Disease, 175*, 526–36.

Epstein, S. (1983). Aggregation and beyond: Some basic issues on the prediction of behavior. *Journal of Personality, 51*, 360–92.

Folkman, S., & Lazarus, R. S. (1980). An analysis of coping in a middle-aged community sample. *Journal of Health and Social Behavior, 21*, 219–39.

Folkman, S., & Lazarus, R. S. (1985). If it changes it must be a process: Study of emotion and coping during three stages of a college examination. *Journal of Personality and Social Psychology, 48*, 150–70.

Folkman, S., Lazarus, R. S., Gruen, R. J., & DeLongis, A. (1986). Appraisal, coping, health status, and psychological symptoms. *Journal of Personality and Social Psychology, 50*, 571–9.

Gunthert, K. C., Conner, T.S., Armeli, S., Tennen, H., Covault, J., & Kranzler, H. R. (2007). The serotonin transporter gene polymorphism (5-HTTLPR) and anxiety reactivity in daily life: A daily process approach to gene-environment interaction. *Psychosomatic Medicine, 69*, 762–8.

Hamilton, N. A., Zautra, A. J., & Reich, J. W. (2005). Affect and pain in rheumatoid arthritis: Do individual differences in affective regulation and affective intensity predict emotional recovery from pain? *Annals of Behavioral Medicine, 29*, 216–24.

Hammersley, R. (1994) A digest of memory phenomena for addiction research. *Addiction, 89*, 283–93.

Hatton, C., Knussen, C., Sloper, P., & Turner, S. (1995). The stability of the Ways of Coping (Revised) Questionnaire over time in parents of children with Down's syndrome: A research note. *Psychological Medicine, 25*, 419–22.

Higgins, R. L., & Marlatt, A. G. (1975). Fear of interpersonal evaluation as a determinant of alcohol consumption in male social drinkers. *Journal of Abnormal Psychology, 84*, 644–51.

Hussong, A. M. (2007). Predictors of drinking immediacy following daily sadness: An application of survival analysis to experience sampling data. *Addictive Behaviors, 32*, 1054–65.

Hussong, A. M., Galloway, C. A., & Feagans, L. A. (2005). Coping motives as a moderator of daily mood-drinking covariation. *Journal of Studies on Alcohol, 66,* 344–53.

John, O. P., & Gross, J. J. (2004). Healthy and unhealthy emotional regulation: Personality processes, individual differences, and life span development. *Journal of Personality, 72,* 1301–33.

Kadden, R. M., Litt, M. D., Cooney, N. L., & Busher, D. A. (1992). Relationship between role-play measures of coping skills and alcoholism treatment outcome. *Addictive Behaviors, 17,* 425–37.

Kenny, D. A., & Zautra, A. (1995). The trait-state-error model for multiwave data. *Journal of Consulting and Clinical Psychology, 63,* 52–9.

Kobasa, S. C. (1979). Stressful life events, personality, and health: An inquiry into hardiness. *Journal of Personality and Social Psychology, 37,* 1–11.

Klinger, E. (1978). Dimensions of thought and imagery in normal waking states. *Journal of Altered States of Consciousness, 4,* 97–113.

Larimer, M. E., Palmer, R. S., & Marlatt, G. A. (1999). Relapse prevention. An overview of Marlatt's cognitive-behavioral model. *Alcohol Research and Health, 23,* 151–60.

Larson, R., & Csikzentmihalyi, M. (1983). The experience sampling method. In H. Reis (Ed.), *New directions for naturalistic methods in the behavioral sciences* (pp. 41–56). San Francisco: Jossey-Bass.

Lazarus, R. S., & Folkman, S. (1984). *Stress, appraisal, and coping.* New York: Springer.

Leboyer, M., Leboyer, M., Bellivier, F., Jouvent, R., Nosten-Bertrand, M., Mallet, J., & Pauls, D. (1998). Psychiatric genetics: Search for phenotypes. *Trends in Neurosciences, 21,* 102–5.

Lewinsohn, P. M., Steinmetz, J. L., Larson, D. W., & Franklin, J. (1981). Depression-related cognitions: Antecedent or consequence? *Journal of Abnormal Psychology, 90,* 213–9.

Litt, M. D. (1996). A model of pain and anxiety in response to acute stressors: The case of dental procedures. *Behaviour Research and Therapy, 34,* 459–76.

Litt, M. D., Cooney, N. L., & Morse, P. (1998). Ecological Momentary Assessment (EMA) with treated alcoholics: Methodological problems and potential solutions. *Health Psychology, 17,* 48–52.

Litt, M. D., Cooney, N. L., & Morse, P. (2000). Reactivity to alcohol-related stimuli in the laboratory and in the field: Predictors of craving in treated alcoholics, *Addiction, 95,* 889–900.

Litt, M. D., Kadden, R. M., Cooney, N. L., & Kabela, E. (2003). Coping skills and treatment outcomes in cognitive-behavioral and interactional group therapy for alcoholism. *Journal of Consulting and Clinical Psychology, 71,* 118–28.

Litt, M. D., Kadden, R. M., Kabela-Cormier, E. (2009). Individualized assessment and treatment program for alcohol dependence: results of a initial study to train coping skills. *Addiction, 104,* 1837–1848.

Litt, M. D., Kadden, R. M., Kabela-Cormier, E., & Petry, N. M. (2009). Changing network support for drinking: Network Support Project two-year follow-up. *Journal of Consulting and Clinical Psychology, 77,* 229–42.

Litt, M. D., Shafer, D. M., Ibanez, C. R., Kreutzer, D. L., & Tawfik-Yonkers, Z. (2009). Momentary pain and coping in temporomandibular disorder pain: Exploring mechanisms of cognitive behavioral treatment for chronic pain. *Pain, 145,* 160–8.

Litt, M. D., Shafer, D., & Napolitano, C. (2004). Momentary mood and coping processes in TMD pain. *Health Psychology, 23,* 354–62.

Loftus, E. (1979). *Eyewitness testimony.* Cambridge, MA: Harvard University Press.

Mandler, J. M., & Johnson, N. S. (1977) Remembrance of things parsed: Story structure and recall. *Cognitive Psychology, 9,* 111–51.

Manne, S. L., & Zautra, A. J. (1990). Couples coping with chronic illness: Women with rheumatoid arthritis and their healthy husbands. *Journal of Behavioral Medicine, 13,* 327–42.

Manne, S. L., & Zautra, A. J. (1992). Coping with arthritis: Current status and critique. *Arthritis and Rheumatism, 35,* 1273–80.

Marlatt, G. A., & Gordon, J. R. (1985). Relapse prevention: Maintenance strategies in the treatment of addictive behaviors. New York: Guilford.

McCracken, L. M., & Turk, D. C. (2002). Behavioral and cognitive-behavioral treatment for chronic pain: Outcome, predictors of outcome, and treatment process. *Spine, 27,* 2564–73.

Mischel, W. (1968). *Personality and assessment.* New York: Wiley.

Mischel, W. (1973). Toward a cognitive social learning reconceptualization of personality. *Psychological Review, 80,* 252–83.

Mohr, C. D., Armeli, S., Tennen, H., Temple, M., Todd, M., Clark, J., & Carney, M. A. (2005). Moving beyond the keg party: A daily process investigation of college student drinking motivations. *Psychology of Addictive Behaviors, 19,* 392–403.

Monroe, S. M., & McQuaid, J. R. (1994). Measuring life stress and assessing its impact on mental health. In W. R. Avison & I. H. Gotlib (Eds.), *Stress and mental health* (pp. 43–76). New York: Plenum.

Moos, R. H. (1988/1992). *Coping Responses Inventory. Adult form manual.* Center for Health Care Evaluation, Stanford University and Department of Veterans Affairs Medical Center, Palo Alto, CA.

Morgenstern, J., & Longabaugh, R. (2000). Cognitive-behavioral treatment for alcohol dependence: A review of evidence for its hypothesized mechanisms of action. *Addiction, 95,* 1475–90.

O'Connell, K. A., Gerkovich, M. M., Cook, M. R., Shiffman, S., Hickcox, M., & Kakolewski, K. E. (1998). Coping in real time: Using ecological momentary assessment techniques to assess coping with the urge to smoke. *Research in Nursing & Health, 21,* 487–97.

Pearlin, L. I., & Schooler, C. (1978). The structure of coping. *Journal of Health and Social Behavior, 19,* 2–21.

Ptacek, J. T., Smith, R. E., Espe, K., & Raffety, B. (1994). Limited correspondence between daily coping reports and retrospective coping recall. *Psychological Assessment, 6,* 41–9.

Reiser, B. J., Black, J. B., & Abelson, R. P. (1985). Knowledge structures and the organization and retrieval of autobiographical memories. *Cognitive Psychology, 17,* 89–137.

Schwartz, J. E., Neale, J., Marco, C., Shiffman, S. S., & Stone, A. A. (1999). Does trait coping exist? A momentary assessment approach to the evaluation of traits. *Journal of Personality & Social Psychology, 77,* 360–9.

Shiffman, S., Hufford, M., Hickcox, M., Paty, J. A., Gnys, M., & Kassel, J. D. (1997). Remember that? A comparison of real-time vs. retrospective recall of smoking lapses. *Journal of Consulting and Clinical Psychology, 65,* 292–300.

Shoda, Y., Mischel, W., & Wright, J. (1994). Intraindividual stability in the organization and patterning of behavior: Incorporating psychological situations into the idiographic analysis of personality. *Journal of Personality and Social Psychology, 67,* 674–87.

Stone, A., & Shiffman, S. (1994). Ecological momentary assessment (EMA) in behavioral medicine. *Annals of Behavioral Medicine, 16,* 199–202.

Stone, A. A., Schwartz, J. E., Neale, J. M., Shiffman, S., Marco, C. A., Hickcox, M., et al. (1998). A comparison of coping assessed by ecological momentary assessment and retrospective recall. *Journal of Personality & Social Psychology, 74,* 1670–80.

Stone, A. A., Shiffman, S., Schwartz, J. E., Broderick, J. E., & Hufford, M. R. (2002). Patient noncompliance with paper diaries. *British Medical Journal, 324,* 1193–4.

Suls, J., & David, J. P. (1996). Coping and personality: third time's the charm? *Journal of Personality, 64,* 993–1005.

Tennen, H., Affleck, G., Armeli, S., & Carney, M. A. (2000). A daily process approach to coping: Linking theory, research and practice. *American Psychologist, 55,* 626–36.

Tennen, H., Affleck, G., Coyne, J. C., Larsen, R. J., & DeLongis, A. (2006). Paper and plastic in daily diary research. *Psychological Methods 11,* 112–8.

Tennen, H., Affleck, G., & Zautra, A. (2006). Depression history and coping with chronic pain: A daily process analysis. *Health Psychology, 25,* 370–9.

Todd, M., Armeli, S., Tennen, H., Carney, M. A., & Affleck, G. (2003). A daily diary validity test of drinking to cope measures. *Psychology of Addictive Behaviors, 17,* 303–11.

Todd, M., Armeli, S., Tennen, H., Carney, M. A., Ball, S. A., Kranzler, H. R., & Affleck, G. (2005). Drinking to cope: A comparison of questionnaire and electronic diary reports. *Journal of Studies on Alcohol, 66,* 121–9.

Todd, M., Armeli, S., & Tennen, H. (2009). Interpersonal problems and negative mood as predictors of within-day time to drinking. *Psychology of Addictive Behaviors, 23,* 205–15.

Todd, M., Tennen, H., Carney, M. A., Armeli, S., & Affleck, G. (2004). Do we know how we cope? Relating daily coping reports to global and time-limited retrospective assessments. *Journal of Personality and Social Psychology, 86,* 310–9.

Turk, D. C., Meichenbaum, D., & Genest, M. (1983). *Pain and behavioral medicine: A cognitive behavioral perspective.* New York: Guilford.

Turner, J. A., Mancl, L., & Aaron, L. A. (2005). Brief cognitive-behavioral therapy for temporomandibular disorder pain: Effects on daily electronic outcome and process measures. *Pain, 117,* 377–87.

Volpicelli, J. R. (1987). Uncontrollable events and alcohol drinking. *Addiction, 82,* 381–92.

Walls, T. A., & Schafer, J. L. (Eds.) (2006). *Models for intensive longitudinal data.* New York: Oxford University Press.

Whitty, C., & Jones, R. J. (1992) A comparison of prospective and retrospective methods of assessing alcohol use among university undergraduates. *Journal of Public Health Medicine, 14,* 264–70.

Wheaton, B. (1983). Stress, personal coping resources, and psychiatric symptoms: An investigation of interactive models. *Journal of Health and Social Behavior, 24,* 208–29.

Wong, C. J., Anthony, S., Sigmon, S. C., Mongeon, J. A., Badger, G. J., & Higgins, S. T. (2004). Examining interrelationships between abstinence and coping self-efficacy in cocaine-dependent outpatients. *Experimental and Clinical Psychopharmacology, 12,* 190–9.

PART 7

Coping Interventions

Coping Interventions and the Regulation of Positive Affect

Judith Tedlie Moskowitz

Abstract

Research in the past few decades has demonstrated that positive affect co-occurs with negative affect in the context of stressful life events, has unique beneficial consequences, and may be a useful focus of intervention. The purpose of this chapter is to provide an overview of the variety of single- and multiple-component interventions that hold promise for increasing positive affect for people experiencing serious life stress. The research shows that positive affect interventions are feasible, acceptable, and in many cases efficacious and that many different approaches hold promise for increasing positive affect. The field is relatively new, however. Future work should test these approaches in more applied settings to determine whether the findings can be translated into the "real world" with all its attendant constraints, challenges, and complexities.

Keywords: positive affect, positive emotion, interventions, coping

Decades of research leave little question that stress and the associated negative emotions have deleterious effects on psychological and physical health (Cohen, Janicki-Deverts, & Miller, 2007). Stress affects nearly every system in the body, including the immune (Segerstrom & Miller, 2004), cardiovascular (Dimsdale, 2008), and respiratory systems (Chen et al., 2006), and is associated with a higher risk of mortality in healthy and chronically ill samples (Matthews & Gump, 2002; Nielsen, Kristensen, Schnohr, & Gronbaek, 2008; Rosengren, Orth-Gomer, Wedel, & Wilhelmsen, 1993; Schulz & Beach, 1999; Turrell, Lynch, Leite, Raghunathan, & Kaplan, 2007). Psychologically, life stress is associated with subsequent depression (Brown & Harris, 1989; Hammen, 2005) and other forms of psychopathology (Dohrenwend, 2000; Johnson & Roberts, 1995). Recognition of the harmful effects of stress

has led to the development of interventions aimed at improving coping and reducing stress among physically healthy individuals coping with life stressors (e.g., Knight, Lutzky, & Macofsky-Urban, 1993; van der Klink, Blonk, Schene, & van Dijk, 2001) as well as chronically ill individuals such as those with cardiovascular disease (e.g., Blumenthal et al., 2005; Frasure-Smith & Prince, 1985; Orth-Gomer et al., 2009), cancer (e.g.,Antoni et al., 2001; Fawzy et al., 1990), HIV (e.g., Antoni, 2000; Chesney, Chambers, Taylor, Johnson, & Folkman, 2003), and diabetes (e.g., Ismail, Winkley, & Rabe-Hesketh, 2004; Surwit et al., 2002). These interventions have met with some success in terms of decreased depression and negative affect and improvements in indicators of physical health.

As evidenced by many of the chapters in this volume, however, the zeitgeist in coping research has begun to shift away from an exclusive focus on negative affect toward acknowledgement that positive affect may have a significant unique influence on psychological and physical health among people coping with life stress. A recent meta-analysis of the effects of 51 interventions explicitly targeted to positive affect outcomes indicates that, as a whole, these interventions are associated with significant increases in well-being (which included measures of positive affect, hope, life satisfaction, happiness) and decreases in depression (Sin & Lyubomirsky, 2009).

Why focus on positive affect? It may seem counterintuitive to focus on positive affect in the context of stress. Stressful life events give rise to negative affect and the goal of interventions should thus be to reduce the stress and distress. However, research in the past few decades has demonstrated that positive affect also occurs in the context of stressful life events, has unique beneficial consequences (Folkman, 1997; Folkman & Moskowitz, 2000), and may be a useful focus of intervention. Independent of the effects of negative affect, positive affect is associated with better physical health (Chida & Hamer, 2008; Pressman & Cohen, 2005) and lower risk of mortality in healthy samples (Danner, Snowdon, & Friesen, 2001; Moskowitz, Epel, & Acree, 2008; Ostir, Markides, Black, & Goodwin, 2000) as well as those with serious illness such as HIV or diabetes (Chida & Steptoe, 2008; Moskowitz, 2003; Moskowitz, Epel, & Acree, 2008). Positive affect is also uniquely predictive, independent of negative affect, of other desirable outcomes such as work success, higher income, and better social relationships (Lyubomirsky, King, & Diener, 2005).

Revised stress and coping theory (Folkman, 1997, 2008) and the broaden-and-build theory of positive emotion (Fredrickson, 1998) provide a theoretical rationale for coping interventions aimed primarily at increasing positive affect. Folkman (1997) proposed a revision to stress and coping theory that explicitly posits a role for positive affect in the coping process. According to the original theory (Lazarus & Folkman, 1984), the coping process begins when an event is appraised as threatening, harmful, or challenging. These appraisals are associated with affect (negative affect in response to threat or harm, a mix of positive and negative in response to challenge) and prompt coping. If the event is resolved favorably, a positive affective state is the result. If the event is resolved unfavorably or if it is unresolved, a negative affective state results and the coping process continues through reappraisal and another round of coping. The revised model suggests that the negative affect associated with unfavorable resolution motivates coping processes that draw on important goals and values, including positive reappraisal and goal-directed problem-focused coping. These coping processes result in positive affect, which is hypothesized to serve important coping functions. For example, positive affect may provide a psychological "time-out" from the distress associated with chronic stress and help motivate and sustain ongoing efforts to cope with the negative effects of the chronic stress (Lazarus, Kanner, & Folkman, 1980). In the context of serious life stress such as diagnosis with a chronic illness, positive affect may facilitate more adaptive coping and foster more challenge appraisals that lead to more proactive and adaptive coping efforts (Fredrickson & Joiner, 2002; Moskowitz, Folkman, Collette, & Vittinghoff, 1996).

Fredrickson (1998) proposed the "broaden-and-build" model of the function of positive emotion that complements revised stress and coping theory. In this model the "broadening" function of positive affect enables the individual to see beyond the immediate stressor and possibly come up with creative alternative solutions to problems. The "building" function helps to rebuild resources (such as self-esteem and social support) depleted by enduring stressful conditions. In contrast to the narrowing of attention and specific actions tendencies associated with negative affect, positive affect broadens the individual's attentional focus (Fredrickson & Branigan, 2005; Rowe, Hirsh, & Anderson, 2007; Wadlinger & Isaacowitz, 2006) and behavioral repertoire (Cunningham, 1988; Fredrickson & Branigan, 2005). Repeated experiences of positive affect build social, intellectual, and physical resources (Fredrickson, Cohn, Coffey, Pek, & Finkel, 2008; Fredrickson, Tugade, Waugh, & Larkin, 2003; Gable, Gonzaga, & Strachman, 2006; Gable, Reis, Impett, & Asher, 2004; Waugh & Fredrickson, 2006). Although the broaden-and-build model was not developed specifically to address positive affect in the context of stress, under stressful conditions the functions of positive affect suggested by the model become especially important (Fredrickson, Tugade, Waugh, & Larkin, 2003). In the context of stress, positive affect may prevent the individual from feeling overwhelmed, lead to more flexibility in coping efforts, and, ultimately, help build resilience to the stress (Cohn, Fredrickson, Brown, Mikels, & Conway, 2009; Moskowitz, 2010).

Review of Positive Affect Interventions

The purpose of the present chapter is to provide an overview of the variety of interventions that hold promise for increasing positive affect. The chapter is intended to be a resource for investigators wishing to design positive affect interventions for samples experiencing serious life stress. The review is comprehensive, but it is not exhaustive: It would not be feasible to include every published intervention with a positive affective outcome in a chapter format. In fact, the literatures for several of these interventions, such as meditation (Arias, Steinberg, Banga, & Trestman, 2006) and exercise (Rethorst, Wipfli, & Landers, 2009), are large enough to merit their own reviews. Further, not every intervention included here was designed to increase positive affect and not all were tested in samples experiencing serious stress, but I included them in the review because they show promise for increasing positive affect. I first review single-component interventions that focus on a single skill or behavior, and then I review the multiple-component interventions that target positive affect.

A note on the measurement of affect

Positive affect can be measured a number of different ways, which is important to keep in mind when reading this review. One of the most widely used affect measures is the PANAS (Watson, Clark, & Tellegen, 1988), which includes high arousal affects like "excited" and "enthusiastic" but not lower activation affects like "happy" or "content." Another frequently cited affect measure is the Profile of Mood States (POMS; McNair, Lorr, & Droppleman, 1971), which includes a Vigor subscale that is interpreted as positive affect. The POMS also consists mostly of high activation items like "energetic," "full of pep," and "lively" (Norcross, Guadagnoli, & Porochaska, 1984). Other less frequently used measures tap into more general well-being (Lyubomirsky, Sheldon, & Schkade, 2005), happiness (Fordyce, 1988), or life satisfaction (Endicott, Nee, Harrison, & Blumenthal, 1993). The variability of intervention effects reviewed below may be due in part to differences in the measurement of positive affect. I will return to this point in the discussion at the end of the chapter.

Single-component interventions
GRATITUDE

Gratitude is defined as a feeling of thankfulness and appreciation expressed toward other people, nature, or God. The association between intentionally noting things for which one is grateful and increased well-being is well supported empirically (Emmons, 2007). Studies with students and people with serious illness have demonstrated that keeping a gratitude journal is associated with higher positive affect (assessed with a modification of the PANAS that included some lower activation positive affects as well as gratitude-related affects like "appreciative"), lower negative affect, fewer physical symptoms, better sleep quality, and greater satisfaction with life (Emmons & McCullough, 2003) compared to control conditions. Kashdan, Uswatte, and Julian (2006) found that gratitude predicted greater daily positive affect (on a modified PANAS that also included "happy") in Vietnam war veterans with post-traumatic stress disorder, and Lyubomirsky, Sheldon, and Schkade (2005) found that college students who were asked to "count their blessings" once per week had a significant increase in well-being (a scale that combined positive affect, negative affect, and life satisfaction) over 6 weeks compared to a control group.

Froh, Sefick, and Emmons and colleagues (2008) tested a gratitude intervention in middle-school students. Middle school is a stressful transitional period for many children and thus a key point in which to conduct stress reduction interventions. Classes were randomly assigned to one of three conditions: one in which students composed gratitude lists, another in which students composed hassles lists, or a no-intervention control condition. Students were asked to engage in the gratitude or hassles list activities daily for 2 weeks. Results indicated that students in the gratitude condition had significantly greater gratitude and school satisfaction compared to the other two groups and significantly lower negative affect compared to the hassles condition. The groups did not differ on positive affect, however. It isn't clear why there was no effect on positive affect itself, but it may be a function of the positive affect measure, which was made up primarily of high activation positive affects (e.g., interested, excited, and alert), which may be less likely to change in response to gratitude interventions than other, lower activation positive affects (e.g., happy, calm).

POSITIVE EVENTS AND SAVORING
A number of studies demonstrate that positive life events are associated with increases in positive affect (Murrell & Norris, 1984; Zautra & Reich, 1983) and that engaging in recreational or social activities is associated with positive affect, but not negative affect (Mausbach, Coon, Patterson, & Grant, 2008; Mausbach, Roepke, Depp, Patterson, & Grant, 2009).

Our previous work in caregivers of partners with AIDS demonstrated that even in the midst of severe stress, people experience and note positive events and these events may help them cope with the stress (Folkman, Moskowitz, Ozer, & Park, 1997). These findings led us to hypothesize that under enduring stressful conditions, people may consciously seek out or create positive events that can increase their positive affect and, as a result, replenish their psychological resources and help to sustain their coping efforts.

It may not be enough to simply notice the positive events, however. Savoring (Bryant, 1989) or capitalizing (Langston, 1994) is an expressive response to positive events and includes telling others about it, marking the occurrence in some way, or even thinking about the event again later on. Noting positive events is associated with increased positive affect, but capitalizing or savoring strengthens the association between positive events and positive affect (Langston, 1994).

Intentionally increasing positive life events (also called activity scheduling or behavior activation treatment) is a central part of some types of therapy for depression (Krause, 1998; Lewinsohn & Amenson, 1978; Lewinsohn, Hoberman, & Clarke, 1989; Lewinsohn, Sullivan, & Grosscup, 1980). A recent meta-analysis indicated that activity scheduling was associated with significant decreases in depression compared to control conditions (Cuijpers, van Straten, & Warmerdam, 2007), but an effect on positive affect has not been reported.

Although creating or noting positive events has not been extensively tested in experimental designs, several studies have tested closely related interventions such as positive writing. Positive writing interventions combine positive life events (writing about the "most wonderful experience or experiences in your life") and savoring ("try your best to re-experience the emotions involved"). Burton and King (2004) found that participants assigned to write about their most positive life events for 20 minutes per day for 3 days had significantly higher positive affect (happy, pleased, self-confident, enjoyment/fun, joyful, sociable/friendly, and satisfied) but did not differ in negative affect (depressed/blue, worried, upset, anxious, frustrated, unhappy, and angry/hostile) compared to a control writing condition in which participants were asked to write about their plans for the rest of the day. Similarly, Wing, Schutte, and Byrne (2006) found that participants in a positive writing condition had higher life satisfaction than participants in the comparison condition.

In reminiscence therapy, which is conducted most often with elderly samples, participants are asked to reflect back over their lives and share positive life events (Haight & Burnside, 1993). Reminiscence therapy focuses on simply reporting the past events, not evaluating or analyzing them, and can be conducted in group or individual formats. A meta-analysis of six controlled trials of reminiscence therapy (ranging from 8 to 20 sessions) indicated that participants in reminiscence therapy conditions reported significant increases in positive affect (as assessed by several different scales) compared to participants in control conditions. Reminiscence therapy was also associated with significant decreases in depression, but there were no differences in self-esteem or life satisfaction (Chin, 2007).

The *way* in which one thinks about and savors a positive event may influence positive affect, however. Lyubomirsky, Sousa, and Dickerhoof (2006) compared four ways of re-experiencing and savoring positive memories: thinking about a positive event by replaying it in one's mind (think-replay); thinking about a positive event and analyzing it (think-analyze); writing about an event by replaying it (write-replay); and writing and analyzing an event (write-analyze). The think-replay group had higher positive affect (PANAS over past 3 months) compared to the other three groups. Negative affect did not differ. In a replication of this finding from a study conducted in a single laboratory session, Vitterso and colleagues found that replaying a happy life moment (compared to analyzing one) was associated with a significant increase in positive affect (joyful, happy, contented) from before to immediately after the intervention (Vitterso, Overwien, & Martinsen, 2009).

In a variation of focusing on positive events or gratitude, Koo, Algoe, Wilson, and Gilbert (2008) brought participants into the laboratory and asked them to write about how a positive event might never have happened or might never have been part of their life (absence condition). Koo et al. found that participants in the absence condition experienced significantly more positive affect (happy, grateful, joyful, hopeful, appreciative, secure, optimistic) and less negative affect (distressed, upset, sad, lonely, depressed), measured immediately after the intervention, than participants in the presence condition, who were asked to write about how a positive event "happened easily or was certain to become part of your life" (Koo, personal communication, October 28, 2009). This study suggests that savoring a positive event can be enhanced by engaging in counterfactual thinking about how life would be different if the event had never occurred and presumably, then, reinforcing the positive aspects of the fact that the event did happen.

Overall, the literature on positive events indicates that interventions should guide participants to notice, recall, and re-experience positive life events but should avoid in-depth analysis of the explanation for the event. Encouraging participants to engage in counterfactual thinking may also increase the potency of a positive events intervention.

ACTS OF KINDNESS

Volunteerism, acts of kindness, and other altruistic behaviors are associated with better psychological well-being (Post, 2005), a lower risk of mortality (Musick & Wilson, 2003; Oman, Thoresen, & McMahon, 1999), and a lower risk of serious illness (Moen, Dempster-McCain, & Williams, 1993) in large representative samples. Experiencing a major life event, such as a diagnosis with a serious illness, can leave an individual feeling helpless and hopeless. In this context, doing something for someone else may be particularly empowering, helping the individual realize that he or she does have something to offer, leading to more positive affect and more adaptive coping behaviors.

Interventions in which participants are assigned to do something nice for someone else support the association between acts of kindness and psychological well-being. Dunn, Aknin, and Norton (2008) randomly assigned participants to receive either $5 or $20 and to spend the money that day on themselves or someone else. At the end of the day, participants who spent the money on someone else were higher on self-rated happiness than those who spent it on themselves, regardless of whether they had received $5 or $20. Lyubomirsky, Sheldon, and Schkade (2005) report that engaging in five acts of kindness per week for 6 weeks increased well-being (scale that combined positive affect, negative affect, and life satisfaction) in students, especially if they engaged in a five activities on a single day each week (rather than one per day). In another student sample, Otake and colleagues tested a kindness intervention in which participants were asked to keep track of their acts of kindness every day for 1 week. The control group consisted of students in another psychology class at the same university. Participants in the intervention group reported significant increases in happiness (on a subjective happiness scale) from the pre- to post-intervention

assessments, whereas the control group demonstrated no significant change in happiness (Otake, Shimai, Tanaka-Matsumi, Otsui, & Fredrickson, 2006). It appears, then, that intentionally engaging in altruism or acts of kindness, or at least noticing the acts of kindness that one is already doing, can increase positive affect.

POSITIVE REAPPRAISAL

According to stress and coping theory (Lazarus & Folkman, 1984), the extent to which an event is experienced as stressful depends on the individual's appraisal—the interpretation of the significance of the event for the individual. Positive reappraisal is a form of coping in which the significance of the event is reinterpreted in a more positive way. For example, seeing the silver lining in a stressful event is one form of positive reappraisal. In the coping literature, positive reappraisal is one of the few ways of coping that is consistently associated with increased positive affect (Carver & Scheier, 1994; Folkman, 1997; Sears, Stanton, & Danoff-Burg, 2003). In a meta-analysis of coping with HIV (Moskowitz, Hult, Bussolari, & Acree, 2009), positive reappraisal was among the ways of coping most strongly associated with increased positive affect, and there is some evidence that positive reappraisal is associated with increases in PANAS positive affect, but not decreases in PANAS negative affect (Kraaij, Garnefsky, & Schroevers, 2009).

Positive reappraisal is similar to cognitive restructuring or reframing, which is a standard part of many forms of cognitive-behavioral therapy and is included in several interventions for people coping with serious health concerns or other types of life stress (e.g., Antoni, Ironson, & Schneiderman, 2007; Ehde & Jensen, 2004). The reappraisals in these interventions, however, usually concern replacing negative thoughts with more rational ones, and do not explicitly focus on possible positive aspects of the situation. Unfortunately, even when positive reappraisal is a component of the intervention, positive affective outcomes are rarely assessed.

In one study that explicitly tested a *positive* reappraisal intervention, 55 women undergoing fertility treatment were assigned to either a positive reappraisal condition or a positive self-statement condition (Landcastle & Boivin, 2008). Participants were given a card with 10 statements and asked to repeat the statements at least twice per day during the period between embryo implantation and the pregnancy test. Positive reappraisal statements began with the stem "During this experience I will:" and included "focus on the positive aspects of the situation," "see things positively," "make the best of the situation," and "look on the bright side of things." The self-affirmation/positive mood statements began with the stem "During this experience I feel that:" and included "I really do feel positive," "I'm creative," "I feel good about the world," "I'm a great person," "life is great," and "I feel happy." The positive reappraisal group reported fewer harm emotions and significantly more positive challenge emotions (presumably higher activation positive affects) than the positive self-statements group (Lancastle & Boivin, 2007). In addition, the positive reappraisal group evaluated the intervention as more beneficial and felt that it would help them to "carry on or keep going" during the waiting period. Although preliminary, the fact that the positive self-statements were not associated with increased positive affect supports the idea that simply telling oneself to feel positive ("I feel happy") may not result in an actual experience of that positive affect.

SETTING ATTAINABLE GOALS

Goal-setting is common in health education and intervention programs (Strecher et al., 1995) and has been used in interventions for people with cancer, HIV, and other serious illnesses (e.g., Andersen, 1992, 2002, 2009; Antoni, Ironson, & Schneiderman, 2007; Sikkema, Kalichman, Kelly, & Koob, 1995). Goal-setting interventions have shown some association with positive affect. Sheldon, Kasser, Smith, and Share (2002) assigned college students to either a two-session goal-training condition or to participation in an unrelated study. Although the intervention group did not make more progress toward their stated goals over the course of the semester, mid-semester goal progress predicted an increased balance of positive to negative affect on the PANAS at the end of the semester.

MacLeod, Coates, and Hetherton (2008) tested a goal-setting intervention in which participants participated in three 1-hour sessions over 4 weeks that focused on selecting and visualizing goals, setting up plans for goals, and identifying obstacles. Those in the intervention group had significant increases in life satisfaction relative to a self-selected comparison group, but did not report a significant change in PANAS positive or negative affect. However, when the analyses were restricted to those who attended all the group sessions, the intervention group did have significant increases in positive affect relative to the comparison group. In a second study the authors tested a self-administered version of the intervention and found that the intervention was associated with significant increases in positive affect and life satisfaction and significant decreases in negative affect relative to a self-selected comparison group.

Observational research on goals indicates that perceptions of goal progress are associated with greater life satisfaction and higher levels of positive affect (Brunstein, Schultheiss, & Grassmann, 1998; Carver & Scheier, 1990; Lent et al., 2005), and pursuit of attainable goals (vs. more global distant goals) is associated with higher subjective well-being (Emmons, 1986, 1992). Disengaging from the untenable goals and re-engagement with new goals is associated with increased positive affect and subjective well-being (Kraaij, Garnefsky, & Schroevers, 2009; Wrosch, Scheier, Carver, & Schulz, 2003). Taken together, the observational and limited experimental research for an effect of goal-setting on positive affect indicates that this association merits additional study using randomized trial designs. (See also Wrosch, Chapter 16 in this volume).

SELF-AFFIRMATION/FOCUSING ON PERSONAL STRENGTHS

Self-affirmation involves focusing on one's own personal strengths, values, or positive qualities. Observational studies demonstrate that naturally occurring self-affirmation (sometimes called self-enhancing cognitions) is associated with better psychological adjustment to illness (Taylor et al., 1992; Taylor & Lobel, 1989) and healthier biological profiles (Taylor, Lerner, Sage, & McDowell, 2003).

Although positive affect has not often been measured as an outcome of self-affirmation techniques, affirmation of personal values is associated with a host of adaptive outcomes, including better physiological response to laboratory stress tasks (Creswell, Welch, Taylor, Sherman, & Gruenwald, 2005), greater attention to and retention of information about a serious illness threat (Reed & Aspinwall, 1998), and better school performance for racial minority students (Cohen, Garcia, Purdie-Vaughns, Apfel, & Brzustoski, 2009). For example, Cohen and colleagues conducted an intervention aimed at reducing the achievement gap between African American and European American students. The authors hypothesized that the possibility of performing poorly at school (and therefore confirming a negative stereotype about their group) is stressful for minority students. To test whether self-affirmation could counter the deleterious effects of this stress, sixth- and seventh-grade students were asked to focus on their three most important values, think about times when the values were important to them, and write a few sentences about why those values were important to them. The intervention took place over the course of multiple sessions over 2 years. The intervention did not have an effect for the European American students, but compared to a control condition in which students were asked to focus on values least important to them, racial minority students in the values affirmation condition had significantly higher grade-point averages at a 2-year follow-up (Cohen, Garcia, Purdie-Vaughns, Apfel, & Brzustoski, 2009). Although it is conjecture at this point, one possible mechanism for the effect of affirmation on GPA is increased positive affect.

Several studies have used a laboratory stress paradigm to test the effect of self-affirmation on reducing or buffering the stress response. For example, in a single experimental session, Koole and colleagues first gave subjects negative feedback about their IQ, then randomly assigned some participants to engage in self-affirmation of a highly ranked personal value. They found that those in the self-affirmation condition were less likely to ruminate on the negative information about their IQ and had higher levels of positive affect than the participants who were not asked to engage in self-affirmation (Koole, Smeets, van Knippenberg, & Dijksterhuis, 1999).

In an early test of a self-affirmation intervention, Lichter, Haye, and Kammann (1980) assigned students to engage in 2 weeks of daily rehearsal of positive self-statements (i.e., "I've got a lot of fine qualities," "I accept the fact that I have my weaknesses, but I can do something about them," and "I love being alive!"). Compared to a waitlist control group, those in the self-affirmation condition had significantly greater increases in positive affect (on a scale of general happiness and well-being) over the 2-week study period. However, the Lancastle and Boivin (2008) positive reappraisal study (reviewed above) indicated that positive self-statements were not associated with increased positive affect. These differences my be due to different samples (students compared to adults going through *in vitro* fertilization), the actual self-statements (focusing on personal strengths "I've got a lot of fine qualities" vs. explicitly stating that "I feel happy"), or differences in the measurement of affect.

In an experimental test of an Internet-delivered self-affirmation intervention, Mitchell, Stanimirovic, Klein, and Vella-Brodrick (2009) randomly assigned 160 participants to either a personal strengths (self-affirmation)-focused condition, a problem-solving condition, or a no treatment control condition. In the personal strengths condition, participants were first asked to select their perceived strengths from a list. Their homework task the following week was to share what they had learned from the exercise with a friend. In session 2, participants were asked to select 3 of their top 10 strengths and then, for their homework, to develop these strengths in their daily life. Session 3 consisted of review and a follow-up questionnaire. Results indicated that there were no group-by-time interactions on PANAS positive or negative affect, although there was a significant effect on personal well-being (satisfaction with various life domains, including health, achievements, relationships, and spirituality) such that the strengths group had a significant increase in well-being from before to after the intervention and from before the intervention to a 3-month follow-up.

The discrepant findings for the effect of self-affirmation interventions on positive affect may be due to differences in the self-affirmation manipulation (writing about personal values vs. noting personal strengths vs. noting previous acts of kindness), differences in the timing of the intervention (one time in a laboratory stress context, weekly for 3 weeks, multiple times over the course of several years), differences in the delivery of the intervention (via Internet, in laboratory study, in class), or differences in the measurement of positive affect. Future work should give careful consideration to each of these design issues.

MEDITATION

The practice of meditation is commonly considered a way to reduce stress. Recently, interest is increasing in meditation as a way to increase positive affect as well. Meditation has been defined as "the family of techniques which have in common a conscious attempt to focus attention in a non-analytical way, and an attempt not to dwell on discursive, ruminating thought" (Shapiro, 1980, p. 14). A number of different types of meditation, including mindfulness, Transcendental Meditation (TM; a form of mantram meditation), loving-kindness, and mantram, have been studied in various clinical populations such as people living with cancer (Ledesma & Kumano, 2009), pain (Teixeira, 2008), coronary artery disease (Williams, Kolar, Reger, & Pearson, 2001), HIV (Bormann et al., 2006; Cresswell, Myers, Cole, & Irwin, 2009; Hecht et al., 2010), fibromyalgia (Grossman, Tiefenthaler-Gilmer, Raysz, &

Kesper, 2007), schizophrenia (D. P. Johnson et al., 2009), and anxiety (Raskin, Bali, & Peeke, 1980).

Mindfulness is the most commonly studied form of meditation, likely due to the popularity and rapid growth of mindfulness-based stress reduction (MBSR) programs across the country (Kabat-Zinn, 2003). Mindfulness is defined as the ability to intentionally pay attention to and maintain non-judgmental awareness of one's experience (thoughts, feelings, physical sensations) in the present moment (Kabat-Zinn, 2003). Trait and state mindfulness are associated with higher positive affect and lower negative affect (Brown & Ryan, 2003), and mindfulness interventions have been shown to increase positive affect (Grossman, Tiefenthaler-Gilmer, Raysz, & Kesper, 2007; Shapiro, Brown, & Biegel, 2007). In a group of patients with fibromyalgia (*n* = 58), Grossman and colleagues found that MBSR was associated with increases in positive affect (as measured by a positive affect subscale of a German quality-of-life measure) and decreases in negative affect from before to after the intervention compared to a control condition (Grossman, Tiefenthaler-Gilmer, Raysz, & Kesper, 2007). The effects appeared to be sustained out to a 3-year follow-up assessment. Hecht et al. (2010) found that MBSR was associated with significant increases in positive affect (as measured by the PANAS) in people with HIV who were not on antiretroviral medication, although the increase was not significantly greater than the change in an attention-matched education control group. In a test of a slightly shortened MBSR intervention (four sessions instead of eight), students in the intervention showed increases in the positive affective states of focused attention, productivity, and sensuous non-sexual pleasure (the Positive States of Mind scale; Horowitz, Adler, & Kegeles, 1988). However, the increases did not differ from those in a relaxation group (Jain et al., 2007).

Loving-kindness meditation is a form of concentration meditation that focuses on positive or compassionate feelings for oneself and others. In a study designed explicitly to test meditation as a positive affect intervention, Fredrickson Cohn, Coffey, Pek, and Finkel (2008) demonstrated that a 7-week loving-kindness meditation intervention increased daily experience of positive affect (as measured by a modified Differential Emotions Scale; Fredrickson, Tugade, Waugh, & Larkin, 2003) compared to a waitlist control condition. Positive affect in turn was associated with increased life satisfaction, decreased

levels of depression, and better physical health approximately 3 months after the baseline assessment. Of note, the intervention did not have a significant effect on negative affect.

Even a single session of a loving-kindness intervention can increase positive affect and positive feelings towards others. Hutcherson, Seppala, and Gross (2008) randomly assigned students to a loving-kindness condition in which they were asked to imagine two loved ones directing love toward them, then to concentrate on a picture of a stranger and direct feelings of love and compassion to the picture. In the control condition, participants were asked to imagine two acquaintances standing next to them and concentrate on details of the appearance of a stranger. Participants in the loving-kindness condition reported significantly more positive affect (as assessed by three items: proud, happy, loving) immediately after the test than those in the control condition.

The effects of other types of meditation on positive affect have been studied as well. For example, Nidich et al. (2009) randomized 130 women with breast cancer to either a TM group or standard care. The TM condition consisted of seven approximately hour-long classes, and participants were asked to practice on their own for 20 minutes twice per day. The TM group improved significantly in quality of life and emotional well-being (as measured by a frequently used cancer quality of life instrument, the FACT-B; Cella et al., 1993) compared to the control group over the intervention period. Bormann et al. (2005) found that veterans assigned to a 5-week mantram intervention had decreased symptoms of post-traumatic stress disorder and improved quality of life compared to participants in a waitlist control condition. In a comparison of spiritual to secular mantrams, Wachholtz and Pargament (2008) randomly assigned 83 people who experienced frequent migraines to spiritual meditation (meditation on phrases like "God is peace" or "God is joy"), internally focused secular meditation ("I am content," "I am joyful"), externally focused secular meditation ("grass is green," "sand is soft"), or relaxation training. Participants were instructed to meditate 20 minutes per day for 30 days. Results indicated that the spiritual meditation group had a significant decrease in negative affect and the number of headaches compared to the other groups. Although inspection of the before/after changes indicated that scores on positive affect (as measured by the PANAS) increased somewhat in the spiritual meditation, internally focused secular meditation, and relaxation groups, the differences were not statistically significant.

PHYSICAL ACTIVITY: EXERCISE AND YOGA INTERVENTIONS

The published evidence consistently indicates that exercise is associated with a reduction in depressive symptoms. In fact, recent meta-analyses suggest that physical activity may be as effective for decreasing depressive symptoms as cognitive-behavioral therapy or antidepressants (Lawlor & Hopker, 2001; Mead et al., 2009). In general, physical activity interventions tend to increase positive affect as well (Elavsky & McAuley, 2007; Mutrie et al., 2007; Pinto, Goldstein, Ashba, Sciamanna, & Jette, 2005; West, Otte, Geher, Johnson, & Mohr, 2004).

Following on evidence that exercise is associated with better physical outcomes in women with breast cancer (Sternfeld et al., 2009) a number of exercise interventions have been conducted in women with breast cancer (Kolden et al., 2002; Mutrie et al., 2007; Pinto, Goldstein, Ashba, Sciamanna, & Jette, 2005). For example, Kolden et al. (2002) tested the effects of group exercise training for women with breast cancer within 12 months of diagnosis. The hour-long groups met 3 days per week for 16 weeks and included aerobic and resistance training. There was no control group. Participants reported significant increases in positive affect as measured by the PANAS as well as decreases in PANAS negative affect and depression. Mutrie et al. (2007) conducted a randomized trial of a 12-week group exercise program compared to usual care for women in treatment for early-stage breast cancer. The intervention was associated with significant increases in PANAS positive affect after the intervention, and the effect persisted at the 6-month follow-up. There was no effect of the intervention on PANAS negative affect, and reductions in Beck Depression Inventory depression were only marginally significant. The authors note that it wasn't clear whether it was the exercise or the group experience that drove the effect.

In another physical activity intervention with breast cancer patients, Pinto and colleagues tested a 12-week home-based exercise program in which the intervention group received instruction and weekly encouraging phone calls with suggestions for increasing their physical activity at home. The control group also received weekly phone calls but did not receive the encouragement or suggestions for exercise. The exercise group had significant increases in POMS vigor scores compared to the control group (Pinto, Goldstein, Ashba, Sciamanna, & Jette, 2005).

A study of an aerobic exercise intervention for patients with lymphoma provided additional evidence for the effect of exercise on positive affect (Courneya et al., 2009). One hundred twenty-two patients with lymphoma were randomly assigned to an aerobic exercise or treatment-as-usual condition. The aerobic exercise group was conducted three times per week for 12 weeks. Participants in the exercise group reported significantly greater increases in happiness (Fordyce, 1988) compared to the control group and the effect remained significant even when stage of disease, current treatment, age, sex, and baseline exercise levels were statistically controlled.

Beyond cancer patients and survivors, other samples also appear to reap positive psychological benefits from physical activity interventions. In a sample of healthy college students, West and colleagues examined before-and-after changes in affect among participants in a single class of yoga, African dance, or a comparison academic class (biology). Both the dance and yoga classes showed significant decreases in PANAS negative affect. There was a group-by-time interaction for PANAS positive affect such that there was a significant decline in positive affect in the biology class group, a significant increase in the dance class group, and no change in the yoga class group (West, Otte, Geher, Johnson, & Mohr, 2004). These results suggest that aerobic activities like dance may have an immediate effect on positive affect, whereas lower-intensity exercise like yoga may require a bigger "dose" to influence positive affect.

Elavsky and McAuley (2007) compared the effect of yoga to the effect of walking for menopausal symptoms. They randomly assigned 164 middle-aged women experiencing menopausal symptoms to 4 months of group walking (three times per week), group yoga (twice per week), or waitlist control. The walking and yoga groups both had significant increases in positive affect (on a scale that samples cognitive and affective terms including optimistic, enthusiastic, and loved and trusted) compared to the control condition. In addition, the walking group had a significant decrease in negative affect (e.g., hopeless, withdrawn, and confused). The yoga and control groups did not change on negative affect, and the groups did not differ on changes in menopausal symptoms.

Rather than using yoga as the comparison condition, a number of studies have examined the effects of yoga itself on psychological well-being. Yoga interventions have shown efficacy for decreasing depression (Pilkington, Kirkwood, Rampes, & Richardson, 2005) but may also increase positive affect. Danhauer and colleagues conducted two studies of yoga for women with breast or ovarian cancer (Danhauer et al., 2008, 2009). In a sample of 44 women with breast cancer, 10 weekly classes of restorative yoga, which includes poses focused on relaxation, was found to be associated with significant increases in PANAS positive affect compared to a waitlist control group. Participants with higher negative affect at baseline appeared to benefit the most from the intervention (Danhauer et al., 2009). In contrast, in an uncontrolled pilot study of 51 women with ovarian or breast cancer, Danhauer et al. (2008) found that participants who engaged in 10 restorative yoga classes did not have significant increases in PANAS positive affect. There were, however, significant decreases in PANAS negative affect that were maintained at a 2-month follow-up.

In a sample of 17 people with partially remitted depression who attended a 20-session Iyengar yoga class (which emphasizes posture, balance, and alignment), depression scores decreased significantly from before to after the intervention (Shapiro et al., 2007). Participants were also asked to report on five positive emotions and nine negative emotions at the beginning and end of each class. All the individual emotions showed the expected change from before to after the class: negative emotions decreased and positive emotions increased and, with one exception, the magnitude of these changes remained stable over the duration of the course. The exception was in reports of "happy": Over the course of the sessions, average levels of "happy" increased and the increases in "happy" from before to after class became greater as the course progressed.

Wood (1993) compared within-individual changes from before to after a single session of either pranayama yoga (focusing on the breath), progressive muscle relaxation, or visualization of energetic states. Participants were 71 community volunteers who reported their levels of alertness, enthusiasm, contentment, calmness, sluggishness, sleepiness, upset, and nervousness before and after each session. Participants reported significantly greater increases in alertness, enthusiasm, and contentment following the yoga session compared to the relaxation and visualization sessions. The yoga sessions were also associated with significant decreases in sluggishness and sleepiness compared to the relaxation and visualization sessions.

This brief overview of physical activity interventions provides just a sampling of the huge number of exercise interventions that have been conducted. I decided to include yoga under the heading of physical activity because of the number of studies that compared yoga to other types of exercise. However, it is important to note that yoga interventions often include meditation and breathing components that may be independently related to positive affect (see section on meditation). Other mindful movement practices such as tai chi (Brown et al., 1995) also hold promise for increasing positive affect, but these were not included because of a lack of empirical studies. Further, it wasn't clear whether they should be classified as a meditation, as exercise, or in another category altogether.

LAUGHTER/HUMOR

It is generally believed that laughter is associated with better physical health, although the empirical evidence is somewhat sparse (Martin, 2001, 2002). Humor is often used in clinical contexts (Gelkopf, 2009; Hunt, 1993) and humorous film clips are sometimes used as a positive affect manipulation in laboratory studies (Fredrickson, Mancuso, Branigan, & Tugade, 2000; Isen, Daubman, & Nowicki, 1987; Isen, Johnson, Mertz, & Robinson, 1985). There aren't many published studies on laughter or humor as an intervention for psychological or physical health. Recently, however, laughter yoga groups have gained popularity in the United States and around the world, and empirical studies are under way. Laughter yoga combines feigned laughter (based on the premise that the body cannot differentiate between true and feigned laughter) and some yogic breathing and gentle stretching. Although to this point no studies have been published, in a presentation at the American Society of Hypertension in 2008, Chaya and colleagues reported that participants who engaged in seven 20- to 30-minute laughter yoga sessions over 3 weeks had significantly lower post-treatment systolic and diastolic blood pressure, lower cortisol levels, and reductions in perceived stress in comparison to a control group (Chaya, Kataria, Nagendra, et al., 2008). No data were presented on changes in positive affect, and given that the laughter is initially feigned, it may be that positive affect is not significantly influenced by laughter yoga. Well-designed empirical studies of laughter yoga and other laughter/humor interventions are warranted.

CREATIVE ART ACTIVITIES

Qualitative research suggests that engaging in creative art activities is associated with positive affect in older adults with depression (McCaffrey, 2007) and children in foster care (Coholic, Lougheed, & Cadell, 2009). In a quantitative study of creative arts therapy for women with stage I and II breast cancer, 39 women were randomized to four sessions of art therapy or a waitlist control condition. The art therapy group reported significant decreases in distress but no change in positive affect (POMS Vigor) compared to a waitlist control (Puig, Lee, Goodwin, & Sherrard, 2006). In a laboratory stress study (Dalebroux, Goldstein, & Winner, 2008) participants watched a distressing film and then were randomly assigned to one of three conditions: to draw a picture of something that made them happy, to draw something expressing their current mood (venting), or to a distraction control condition. People in the happy drawing condition had significant improvements in positive affect (pleasant valence on an affect grid) than the other conditions. The group that drew something that reflected their current negative mood did not show the same increase in positive affect. Thus, the study showed that it was focusing on something that made participants happy rather than drawing *per se* that increased positive affect. Further research is needed to determine whether the beneficial effects of creative art activities are due to the artistic activity itself, due to engagement in a pleasurable activity or focus on a positive event, due to effect of engagement with a group, or perhaps due to some combination of the three.

FORGIVENESS

Forgiveness is "the willful giving up of resentment in the face of another's…considerable injustice and responding with beneficence to the offender even though that offender has no right to the forgiver's moral goodness" (Baskin & Enright, 2004, p. 80). Forgiveness interventions focus on reducing negative feelings toward the offender and fostering positive feelings such as compassion, empathy, and love. In this sense, forgiveness interventions aim to increase particular positive emotions. Interventions designed to foster forgiveness range from a single session (Christensen, Benotxch, Wiebe, & Lawton, 1995) to weekly sessions for over a year (Freedman & Enright, 1996). The widely varying length reflects two different approaches to forgiveness: the decision-based and process-based (Baskin & Enright, 2004). The process-based approach includes 20 steps within four phases (confrontation of anger, willingness to consider forgiveness, empathy toward the offender, and finding meaning for self and others) with the goal of arriving at forgiveness, whereas the decision-based approach is generally a single session with the goal of coming to the decision to forgive (McCullough & Worthington, 1995).

Recent meta-analyses indicate that forgiveness interventions are associated with significant increases in positive affect and significant decreases in negative affect (Lundahl, Taylor, Stevenson, & Roberts, 2008) compared to control groups. Individual interventions were more effective than group ones and interventions with more hours were more effective than those with fewer hours (Baskin & Enright, 2004; Lundahl, Taylor, Stevenson, & Roberts, 2008). Process-based interventions appear to be more effective in producing forgiveness than decision-based ones (Baskin & Enright, 2004), and samples that were more distressed seemed to benefit more from forgiveness interventions than those with lower levels of distress (Lundahl, Taylor, Stevenson, & Roberts, 2008).

Multiple-component interventions

Although not as widely tested as programs to decrease depression and negative affect, there have been a number of multiple-component interventions designed explicitly to increase positive affect (Fava, Rafanelli, Cazzaro, Conti, & Grandi, 1998; Fava & Ruini, 2003; Fordyce, 1981, 1983). Thirty years ago, Fordyce reported a program of research testing an intervention that consisted of "14 fundamentals" of happiness that included many of the strategies discussed above (e.g., engaging in pleasurable activities, spend more time socializing, become present-oriented, get organized and plan things out) and several additional ones that have not been specifically tested individually as predictors of positive affect (lower your expectations and aspirations, work on a healthy personality). Happiness levels in the intervention group were compared to levels in control groups that were given the expectation that participation in a class on psychological adjustment would increase their happiness. In a series of six studies, Fordyce (1981, 1983) demonstrated that students who engaged in the happiness intervention had significant increases in happiness compared to the controls. A seventh study (Fordyce, 1983) showed that the intervention groups continued to have elevated happiness 9 to 18 months after the intervention. Smith, Compton, and West (1995) tested whether adding a concentration meditation component to Fordyce's fundamentals program increased the effect of the intervention. Students who completed the program and meditated at least three times a week ($n = 7$) had significantly greater increases in happiness than those who did not meditate ($n = 17$) and an assessment-only control condition ($n = 12$).

Well-being therapy was initially developed as a form of psychotherapy aimed at increasing psychological well-being to prevent relapse of clinical disorders (Fava & Ruini, 2003) but has since been applied in nonclinical samples. Ruini and colleagues tested a version of well-being therapy in middle-school (Ruini, Belaise, Brombin, Caffo, & Fava, 2006) and high-school (Ruini et al., 2009) students. In middle-school students the intervention consisted of four 2-hour class sessions over 8 weeks and included versions of personal strengths, savoring, and positive events activities. The control condition consisted of the same number and length of classes that focused on more traditional cognitive-behavioral techniques such as cognitive restructuring. The well-being group had a significantly larger increase in physical well-being compared to the control group, but other outcome variables (anxiety, depression, contentment) did not differ between the groups. In the test of the intervention in high-school students, nine classes of ninth- or tenth-graders were randomized to either well-being therapy (consisting of six 2-hour weekly sessions addressing skills like positive reappraisal, personal strengths, positive life events, and savoring) or a comparison group (consisting of six 2-hour weekly sessions of group exercises, role-playing, games, and some relaxation exercises but no explicit focus on well-being). Although the investigators did not assess positive affect *per se,* the well-being therapy group had greater increases in positive well-being than the placebo group. The beneficial effects of well-being therapy appeared to be longer-lasting than those of the control group.

Seligman and colleagues have tested a treatment for depression called positive psychotherapy that focuses on increasing positive emotion, engagement, and meaning (Seligman, Rashid, & Parks, 2006). In group positive psychotherapy, clients participate in six weekly sessions with home exercises. Sessions focus on several of the components mentioned above: personal strengths, daily positive events, gratitude, savoring, and forgiveness. Additional components include writing one's own obituary/biography, a gratitude visit, active/constructive responding, and "satisficing" instead of maximizing.

In an initial study of the intervention, students with mild to moderate depression were randomly assigned to group positive psychotherapy or a no-treatment control group. Although there were no significant differences between the two groups immediately after the intervention, depression scores in the positive psychotherapy group were marginally ($p = .06$) lower at 3 months after the intervention and significantly lower at 6 and 12 months after the intervention. Similarly, the differences in satisfaction with life were not significant at the post-test but became significant at 3-, 6-, and 12-month follow-up assessments. Individual positive psychotherapy consists of approximately 12 weekly sessions that cover the same topics as group positive psychotherapy in an expanded format. In a pilot test, 46 clients seeking treatment at a university health center were randomly assigned to positive psychotherapy or treatment as usual. Clients who were seeking treatment for depression and were being treated with antidepressants served as a second control group (they were not randomized but were matched on several characteristics to the positive psychotherapy group). At the post-intervention assessment, both the positive psychotherapy and the medication groups improved on depressive symptoms and overall functioning compared to the treatment-as-usual (no medication) group. Participants in the positive psychotherapy condition had significantly higher scores on a measure of happiness than both the treatment-as-usual and the medication groups.

Building on their observational work on the associations of positive and negative affect among patients with rheumatoid arthritis and fibromyalgia (Zautra, Berkhof, & Nicolson, 2002; Zautra et al., 1995; Zautra et al., 2005; Zautra, Johnson, & Davis, 2005), Zautra and colleagues compared three groups of participants living with rheumatoid arthritis: an emotion regulation group that included mindfulness, positive reappraisal, and pleasant event scheduling, among other skills; cognitive-behavioral group therapy for pain; and an education-only group. Both the emotion regulation and the cognitive-behavioral groups reported a greater increase in PANAS positive affect compared to the education-only group. However, for those participants with a history of recurrent depression, the emotion regulation group reported a greater increase in positive affect than the cognitive-behavioral or education groups (Zautra et al., 2008).

Charlson and colleagues are conducting a randomized trial of an intervention for people living with asthma (n = 246) or hypertension (n = 262) or who have recently had angioplasty (n = 246), with the goal of improving health behaviors via increases in positive affect. The intervention consists of educational material plus self-affirmation and focusing on and savoring positive events, "the small things in your life that make you feel good. Things that bring a smile to your face" (p. 753). In addition, participants in the intervention condition receive some small gifts, which are also hypothesized to increase positive affect. The intervention participants receive the positive affect and self-affirmation inductions every 2 months for a year. The control group consists of educational material. Both intervention and control sessions are delivered in person and over the telephone. The primary outcomes are behavioral (physical activity for the asthma and angioplasty groups, medication adherence for the hypertension group). Positive and negative affect will be assessed with the PANAS (Charlson et al., 2007). Results are not yet available for this trial.

We are conducting a randomized trial of a positive affect intervention for people newly diagnosed with HIV (Moskowitz, 2010; Moskowitz et al., under review). The intervention consists of five weekly individual sessions with a facilitator that cover eight behaviors/skills aimed at increasing positive affect. The skills, selected based on our previous work and a review of the literature, are as follows: noting positive events, savoring them, gratitude, mindfulness, positive reappraisal, self-affirmation/personal strengths, attainable goals, and acts of kindness. Two hundred participants newly diagnosed with HIV will be recruited and randomly assigned to the intervention or the time- and attention-matched control condition, which consists of five weekly personal interview sessions.

Data collection is ongoing, so results from the full randomized trial are not yet available. However, our pilot data were encouraging (described in detail in Moskowitz, 2010, and Moskowitz et al., under review). In the pilot study, we recruited 11 participants who had received an HIV diagnosis an average of 8.5 weeks prior to the intervention. We conducted pre- and post-intervention assessments of positive and negative affect as measured with the modified Differential Emotions Scale (Fredrickson, Tugade, Waugh, & Larkin, 2003). Participants completed a second follow-up 30 days after the end of the intervention. Over the 6 weeks of the study, there were significant increases in positive affect and significant decreases in negative affect (Moskowitz et al., under review). The effect sizes obtained in this pilot study were comparable to the effects reported in the meta-analysis of interventions targeting positive affect (Sin & Lyubomirsky, 2009).

Discussion, Conclusions, and Recommendations for Positive Affect Interventions

It is still considered fairly innovative to target positive affect in interventions with people experiencing serious life stress. However, the research supporting positive affect interventions actually spans decades and is now substantial. Taken together, the studies summarized above provide useful direction.

First, the research shows that positive affect interventions are feasible, acceptable to most participants, and in many cases efficacious. Although a minority of the approaches reviewed above were designed explicitly to foster positive affect, the inclusion of outcome measures that tapped positive affective constructs provides essential data to build the case for the importance of these interventions. In addition, a number of the interventions appear to influence positive but not negative affect (Burton & King, 2004; Fredrickson, Cohn, Coffey, Pek, & Finkel, 2008; Lyubomirsky, Sousa, & Dickerhoof, 2006; Mutrie et al., 2007).

Second, many different approaches hold promise; no one approach appears to be obviously superior. As the field progresses, we will likely see more direct comparisons between multiple approaches that have demonstrated efficacy.

Third, it appears that a number of different groups, including those who are living with serious life stress such as a chronic illness, benefit from positive affect interventions. It is important to note, however, that many of the studies reviewed above were essentially proof-of-concept, conducted under tightly controlled laboratory conditions. Future work should test these approaches in more applied settings to determine whether the approach can be translated into the "real world" with all the attendant constraints, challenges, and complexities.

Fourth, as with other types of coping interventions, positive affect interventions can be self-administered or delivered by a facilitator, delivered individually or in a group format, delivered in person, over the telephone, or over the Internet. In addition, the number of sessions can vary from a single brief contact to multiple contacts over years. Scientific, financial, logistical, and practical considerations will drive the delivery format of the interventions. There is much work to be done to determine which forms of delivery work for which samples under which conditions.

Fifth, although the measurement of positive affect was somewhat limited in the studies reviewed above, it appears that both higher activation positive affects (like excitement, joy, and challenge) and lower activation (like contentment, satisfaction, and happiness) are amenable to change through these interventions.

The review also reveals a number of limitations in the existing research and points to areas for future investigation. To my mind, one of the biggest weaknesses is the limited assessment of both positive and negative affect. Many of the studies reviewed above relied on the PANAS (Watson, Clark, & Tellegen, 1988) or the Vigor subscale of the POMS (McNair, Lorr, & Droppleman, 1971). The PANAS and the POMS are well-validated, widely used measures of positive and negative affect, and it is understandable that many investigators choose them as primary outcome measures. However, both scales focus on high activation and attention positive affects (for the PANAS: active, alert, attentive, determined, enthusiastic, excited, inspired, interested, proud, and strong; for the POMS Vigor: energetic, full of pep, lively, vigorous, cheerful, carefree). Although the PANAS has been revised (Watson & Clark, 1994) to include lower activation affect (e.g., happy, calm, at ease), none of the studies reviewed above use this expanded measure. The reliance on measures of higher activation positive affect provides a possible explanation for some of the discrepant effects of positive affect interventions. For example, aerobic exercise interventions tend to influence higher activation positive affects (e.g., Mutrie et al., 2007) more than do meditation or gratitude interventions (e.g., Froh, Sefick, & Emmons, 2008; Wachholtz & Pargament, 2008).

Thus, a critical consideration for future studies of positive affect interventions is the selection of the primary affective outcome measure. The loving-kindness intervention by Fredrickson, Cohn, and colleagues is an example of careful linkage between the goals of the intervention and the measurement of affective outcome. The investigators chose a modified version of the Differential Emotions Scale (Fredrickson, Tugade, Waugh, & Larkin, 2003) to tap into the full range of positive and negative affective states (amusement, anger, awe, compassion, contempt, contentment, disgust, embarrassment, gratitude, hope, joy, interest, love, pride, guilt, sadness, shame, fear, and surprise). Analyses of positive affect as a whole revealed a significant increase in response to the meditation intervention. In a secondary analysis, the investigators explored the effect of the intervention on the individual affect of compassion—hypothesized to be particularly influenced by loving-kindness meditation. The finding was interesting: The pattern of change in compassion was the same as for the other positive affects, but the change in compassion was not significantly greater in the meditation group compared to the control condition (Fredrickson, Cohn, Coffey, Pek, & Finkel, 2008). The investigators' careful consideration of the affective outcome measure allowed the test of this theoretically derived hypothesis and should be used as a model for future studies of positive affect interventions.

We also know little about the moderating effects of stress: Does someone have to be significantly distressed or depressed to benefit from a positive affect intervention? There is some evidence that samples that were more distressed benefited more from some of the interventions (e.g., Lundahl, Taylor, Stevenson, & Roberts, 2008; Zautra et al., 2008). My hypothesis is that positive affect interventions can benefit anyone experiencing any type of stress—from major life stress such as caregiving, bereavement, or diagnosis of a serious illness to the daily hassles that everyone encounters. The effects may be stronger, however, among those experiencing severe stress. Future research will address these important questions.

Finally, because most studies report little if any follow-up, we know little about how long intervention effects may last, nor, as noted above, do we know how to determine which intervention or combination of interventions is most effective for given individuals.

Recommendations for researchers and clinicians

Given the evidence that many of these interventions are likely to have a beneficial impact on positive affect, where does a researcher or clinician start with designing an intervention? In addition to the logistical and financial considerations that inevitably influence these decisions, there are several other things to take into consideration. First, consider the sample: their cognitive and physical capabilities, and other life stress they might be experiencing. The studies reviewed above were conducted in a range of samples, including adolescents (Froh, Sefick, & Emmons, 2008; Ruini, Belaise, Brombin, Caffo, & Fava, 2006), elderly persons (Haight & Burnside, 1993), people coping with serious illness (Kolden et al., 2002;

Moskowitz et al., under review; Zautra et al., 2008), and, of course, college students (Otake, Shimai, Tanaka-Matsumi, Otsui, & Fredrickson, 2006; Sheldon, Kasser, Smith, & Share, 2002). Ideally, a given approach should be modified, through pilot testing, to fit the needs and cognitive, physical, and emotional characteristics of the sample.

Another important consideration is the type of positive affect the clinician or researcher is interested in affecting. If the goal is to increase calmness and serenity, then meditation, yoga, or gratitude may be most appropriate. If the aim is to influence excitement, enthusiasm, and other motivational affects, goal-setting or aerobic exercise may be a better fit. In addition to the importance of fit of the intervention to the targeted positive affects, another consideration is the fit of the approach to the individual (Lyubomirsky, Sheldon, & Schkade, 2005). For an intervention to be effective, the individual needs to make the targeted behaviors a habit. If the activity is a good fit, he or she is more likely to enjoy it, and more likely to continue to engage in the behavior that will support positive affect. Not all activities will appeal to all individuals. For example, meditation may have a large body of research supporting its beneficial effects, but there are some people for whom meditation is not a good fit, and these individuals are unlikely to engage in meditation to an extent that it increases their positive affect. Multiple-component interventions that offer a variety of strategies may be more effective in that individuals can emphasize the components that work best for their particular circumstances and inclinations.

In addition, over time a behavior that initially "worked" for a given participant may lose its potency. There is evidence for a genetically determined set point of positive affect (Braungart, Plomin, DeFries, & Fulker, 1992; Tellegen et al., 1988), and although life events and interventions can influence positive affect temporarily, without continued effort, individuals tend to adapt back to their set point over time (Lyubomirsky, Chapter 11 in this volume). This is the "hedonic treadmill" argument (Diener, Lucas, & Scollon, 2006). Lyubomirsky and colleagues note that having a variety of skills to choose from may help to avoid the hedonic treadmill—when one type of skill starts to lose its impact, the participant can try another one (Lyubomirsky, King, & Diener, 2005). The possibility for a variety of skills or behaviors from which to choose is another advantage of multiple-component interventions.

Conclusions

The shelves of the local bookstore are full of books for the general public arguing for the benefits of happiness, positive thinking, and positive affect and suggesting myriad way to help you become a happier, more positive person (Baker & Stout, 2003; Fredrickson, 2009; Horowitz, 2008; Lyubomirsky, 2007). A growing number of books also point out the downside of excessive reliance on positive affect and positive thinking for the individual and for society (Ehrenreich, 2009; Norem, 2001; Wilson, 2008). My focus on interventions to increase positive affect should not be interpreted as a call to deny, minimize, or otherwise ignore the potential severity of stress and the deleterious impact that it has on people's psychological and physical health. Nor should it be interpreted as advocating a simplistic "don't worry, be happy" approach to dealing with life's problems. Indeed, negative affects serve an important function that should be kept in mind (Forgas, 2007; Klinger, 1975). Rather, my point is that by expanding our focus and making room in the stress-and-coping arena for the inclusion of positive affect interventions, we will add to the coping arsenal and will be better equipped to combat the deleterious effects of stress.

References

Andersen, B. L. (1992). Psychological interventions for cancer patients to enhance the quality of life. *Journal of Consulting & Clinical Psychology, 60*(4), 552–68.

Andersen, B. L. (2002). Biobehavioral outcomes following psychological interventions for cancer patients. *Journal of Consulting & Clinical Psychology, 70*(3), 590–610.

Andersen, B. L. (2009). Biobehavioral intervention for cancer stress: Conceptualization, components, and intervention strategies. *Cognitive and Behavioral Practice, 16*, 253–65.

Antoni, M. H. (2000). Effects of cognitive behavioral stress management intervention on depressed mood, distress levels, and immune status in HIV infection. In S. L. Johnson, A. M. Hayes, T. M. Field, N. Schneiderman, & P. M. McCabe (Eds.), *Stress, coping, and depression* (pp. 241–63). Mahwah, MJ: Erlbaum.

Antoni, M. H., Ironson, G., & Schneiderman, N. (2007). *Cognitive-behavioral stress management for individuals living with HIV.* New York: Oxford University Press.

Antoni, M. H., Lehman, J. M., Klibourn, K. M., Boyers, A. E., Culver, J. L., Alferi, S. M., et al. (2001). Cognitive-behavioral stress management intervention decreases the prevalence of depression and enhances benefit finding among women under treatment for early-stage breast cancer. *Health Psychology, 20*(1), 20–32.

Arias, A. J., Steinberg, K., Banga, A., & Trestman, R. L. (2006). Systematic review of the efficacy of meditation techniques as treatments for medical illness. *Journal of Alternative and Complementary Medicine, 12*, 817–32.

Baker, D., & Stauth, C. (2003). *What happy people know*. New York: St. Martin's Press.

Baskin, T. W., & Enright, R. D. (2004). Intervention studies on forgiveness: A meta-analysis. *Journal of Counseling and Development, 82*, 79–90.

Blumenthal, J. A., Sherwood, A., Babyak, M. A., Watkins, L. L., Waugh, R., Georgiades, A., et al. (2005). Effects of exercise and stress management training on markers of cardiovascular risk in patients with ischemic heart disease: a randomized controlled trial. *Journal of the American Medical Association, 293*(13), 1626–34.

Bormann, J. E., Gifford, A. L., Sively, M., Smith, T. L., Redwine, L., Kelly, A., et al. (2006). Effects of spiritual mantram repetition on HIV outcomes: A randomized controlled trial. *Journal of Behavioral Medicine, 29*, 359–76.

Bormann, J. E., Smith, T. L., Becker, S., Gershwin, M., Pada, L., Grudzinski, A. H., et al. (2005). Efficacy of frequent mantram repetition on stress, quality of life, and spiritual well being in veterans. *Journal of Holistic Nursing, 23*, 395–414.

Braungart, J. M., Plomin, R., DeFries, J. C., & Fulker, D. W. (1992). Genetic influence on tester-rated infant temperament as assessed by Bayley's Infant Behavior Record: Nonadoptive and adoptive siblings and twins. *Developmental Psychology, 28*, 40–7.

Brickman, P., Coates, D., & Janoff-Bulman, R. (1978). Lottery winners and accident victims: Is happiness relative? *Journal of Personality and Social Psychology, 36*, 917–27.

Brown, D. R., Wang, Y., Ward, A., Ebbeling, C. B., Fortlage, L., Puleo, E., et al. (1995). Chronic psychological effects of exercise and exercise plus cognitive strategies. *Medicine & Science in Sports & Exercise, 27*(5), 765–75.

Brown, G. W., & Harris, T. O. (1989). Depression. In G. W. Brown & T. O. Harris (Eds.), *Life events and illness* (pp. 49–93). New York: Guilford.

Brown, K. W., & Ryan, R. M. (2003). The benefits of being present: mindfulness and its role in psychological well-being. *Journal of Personality and Social Psychology, 84*, 822–48.

Brunstein, J. C., Schultheiss, O. C., & Grassmann, R. (1998). Personal goals and emotional well-being: The moderating role of motive dispositions. *Journal of Personality and Social Psychology, 75*(2), 494–508.

Bryant, F. B. (1989). A four-factor model of perceived control: Avoiding, coping, obtaining, and savoring. *Journal of Personality, 57*, 773–97.

Burton, C. M., & King, L. A. (2004). The health benefits of writing about intensely positive experiences. *Journal of Research in Personality, 38*, 150–63.

Carver, C. S., & Scheier, M. F. (1990). Origins and functions of positive and negative affect: A control process view. *Psychological Review, 97*, 19–35.

Carver, C. S., & Scheier, M. F. (1994). Situational coping and coping dispositions in a stressful transaction. *Journal of Personality and Social Psychology, 66*, 184–95.

Cella, D. F., Tulsky, D. S., Gray, G., Sarafian, B., Linn, E., Bonomi, A., et al. (1993). The Functional Assessment of Cancer Therapy scale: development and validation of the general measure. *Journal of Clinical Oncology, 11*(3), 570–9.

Charlson, M. E., Boutin-Foster, C., Mancuso, C. A., Peterson, J. C., Ogedegbe, G., Briggs, W. M., et al. (2007). Randomized controlled trials of positive affect and self-affirmation to facilitate healthy behaviors in patients with cardiopulmonary diseases: rationale, trial design, and methods. *Contemporary Clinical Trials, 28*(6), 748–62.

Chaya, M. S., Kataria, M., Nagendra, R., et al. (2008, May 14, 2008). *The effects of hearty extended unconditions (HEU) laughter using laughter yoga techniques on physiological, psychological, and immunological parameters in the workplace: a randomized control trial.* Paper presented at the American Society of Hypertension, New Orleans.

Chen, E., Hanson, M. D., Paterson, L. Q., Griffin, M. J., Walker, H. A., & Miller, G. E. (2006). Socioeconomic status and inflammatory processes in childhood asthma: the role of psychological stress. *Journal of Allergy & Clinical Immunology, 117*(5), 1014–20.

Chesney, M., Chambers, D., Taylor, J. M., Johnson, L. M., & Folkman, S. (2003). Coping effectiveness training for men living with HIV: Results from a randomized clinical trial testing a group-based intervention. *Psychosomatic Medicine, 65*, 1038–46.

Chesney, M. A., Folkman, S., & Chambers, D. (1996). Coping effectiveness training. *International Journal of STD and AIDS, 7* (Suppl. 2), 75–82.

Chida, Y., & Hamer, M. (2008). Chronic psychosocial factors and acute physiological responses to laboratory-induced stress in healthy populations: a quantitative review of 30 years of investigations. *Psychological Bulletin, 134*(6), 829–85.

Chida, Y., & Steptoe, A. (2008). Positive psychological well-being and mortality: A quantitative review of prospective observational studies. *Psychosomatic Medicine, 70*, 741–56.

Chin, A. M. H. (2007). Clinical effects of reminiscence therapy in older adults: A meta-analysis of controlled trials. *Hong Kong Journal of Occupational Therapy, 17*, 10–22.

Christensen, A. J., Benotxch, E. G., Wiebe, J. S., & Lawton, W. J. (1995). Coping with treatment-related stress: effects on patient adherence in hemodialysis. *Journal of Consulting and Clinical Psychology, 63*, 454–9.

Cohen, G. L., Garcia, J., Purdie-Vaughns, V., Apfel, N., & Brzustoski, P. (2009). Recursive processes in self-affirmation: intervening to close the minority achievement gap. *Science, 324*(5925), 400–3.

Cohen, S., Janicki-Deverts, D., & Miller, G. E. (2007). Psychological stress and disease. *Journal of the American Medical Association, 298*(14), 1685–7.

Cohn, M. A., Fredrickson, B. L., Brown, S. L., Mikels, J. A., & Conway, A. M. (2009). Happiness unpacked: positive emotions increase life satisfaction by building resilience. *Emotion, 9*(3), 361–8.

Coholic, D., Lougheed, S., & Cadell, S. (2009). Exploring the helpfulness of arts-based methods with children living in foster care. *Traumatology, 15*, 64–71.

Courneya, K. S., Sellar, C. M., Stevinson, C., McNeely, M. L., Peddle, C. J., Friedenreich, C. M., et al. (2009). Randomized controlled trial of the effects of aerobic exercise on physical functioning and quality of life in lymphoma patients. *Journal of Clinical Oncology, 27*(27), 4605–12.

Cresswell, J. D., Myers, H. F., Cole, S. W., & Irwin, M. R. (2009). Mindfulness meditation training effects on CD4+ T lymphocytes in HIV-1 infected adults: A small randomized controlled trial. *Brain Behavior and Immunity, 23*, 184–8.

Creswell, J. D., Welch, W. T., Taylor, S. E., Sherman, D. K., & Gruenwald, T. L. (2005). Affirmation of personal values buffers neuroendocrine and psychological stress responses. *Psychological Science, 16*, 846–51.

Cuijpers, P., van Straten, A., & Warmerdam, L. (2007). Behavioral activation treatments of depression: a meta-analysis. *Clinical Psychology Review, 27*(3), 318–26.

Cunningham, M. R. (1988). What do you do when you're happy or blue? Mood, expectancies, and behavioral interest. *Motivation and Emotion, 12*, 309–31.

Dalebroux, A., Goldstein, T. R., & Winner, E. (2008). Short-term mood repair through art-making: Positive emotion is more effective than venting. *Motivation and Emotion, 32*, 288–95.

Danhauer, S. C., Mihalko, S. L., Russell, G. B., Campbell, C. R., Felder, L., Daley, K., et al. (2009). Restorative yoga for women with breast cancer: findings from a randomized pilot study. *Psycho-Oncology, 18*(4), 360–8.

Danhauer, S. C., Tooze, J. A., Farmer, D. F., Campbell, C. R., McQuellon, R. P., Barrett, R., et al. (2008). Restorative yoga for women with ovarian or breast cancer: findings from a pilot study. *Journal of the Society for Integrative Oncology, 6*(2), 47–58.

Danner, D. D., Snowdon, D. A., & Friesen, W. V. (2001). Positive emotions in early life and longevity: Findings from the nun study. *Journal of Personality & Social Psychology, 80*, 804–13.

Diener, E., Lucas, R. E., & Scollon, C. N. (2006). Beyond the hedonic treadmill: Revising the adaptation theory of well-being. *American Psychologist, 61*, 305–14.

Dimsdale, J. E. (2008). Psychological stress and cardiovascular disease. *Journal of the American College of Cardiology, 51*(13), 1237–46.

Dohrenwend, B. P. (2000). The role of adversity and stress in psychopathology: some evidence and its implications for theory and research. *Journal of Health & Social Behavior, 41*(1), 1–19.

Dunn, E. W., Aknin, L. B., & Norton, M. I. (2008). Spending money on others promotes happiness. *Science, 319*(5870), 1687–8.

Ehde, D. M., & Jensen, M. P. (2004). Feasibility of a cognitive restructuring intervention for treatment of chronic pain in persons with disabilities. *Rehabilitation Psychology, 49*, 254–8.

Ehrenreich, B. (2009). *Bright-sided: How the relentless promotion of positive thinking has undermined America*. New York: Metropolitan Books.

Elavsky, S., & McAuley, E. (2007). Physical activity and mental health outcomes during menopause: a randomized controlled trial. *Annals of Behavioral Medicine, 33*(2), 132–42.

Emmons, R. A. (1986). *The dual nature of happiness: Independence of positive and negative moods*. Paper presented at the American Psychological Association, Washington, DC.

Emmons, R. A. (1992). Abstract versus concrete goals: Personal striving level, physical illness, and psychological well-being. *Journal of Personality and Social Psychology, 62*, 292–300.

Emmons, R. A. (2007). *Thanks! How the new science of gratitude can make you happier*. New York: Houghton Mifflin.

Emmons, R. A., & McCullough, M. E. (2003). Counting blessings versus burdens: An experimental investigation of gratitude and subjective well-being in daily life. *Journal of Personality and Social Psychology, 84*, 377–89.

Endicott, J., Nee, J., Harrison, W., & Blumenthal, R. (1993). Quality of life enjoyment and satisfaction questionnaire: A new measure. *Psychopharmacology Bulletin, 29*(2), 321–6.

Fava, G. A., Rafanelli, C., Cazzaro, M., Conti, S., & Grandi, S. (1998). Well-being therapy. A novel psychotherapeutic approach for residual symptoms of affective disorders. *Psychological Medicine, 28*, 475–80.

Fava, G. A., & Ruini, C. (2003). Development and characteristics of a well-being enhancing psychotherapeutic strategy:

well-being therapy. *Journal of Behavior Therapy and Experimental Psychiatry, 34*, 45–63.

Fawzy, F. I., Cousins, N., Fawzy, N. W., Kemeny, M. E., Elashoff, R., & Morton, D. (1990). A structured psychiatric intervention for cancer patients. *Archives of General Psychiatry, 47*, 720–5.

Folkman, S. (1997). Positive psychological states and coping with severe stress. *Social Science and Medicine, 45*, 1207–21.

Folkman, S. (2008). The case for positive emotions in the stress process. *Anxiety, Stress & Coping, 21*, 3–14.

Folkman, S., & Moskowitz, J. T. (2000). Positive affect and the other side of coping. *American Psychologist, 55*, 647–54.

Folkman, S., Moskowitz, J. T., Ozer, E. M., & Park, C. L. (1997). Positive meaningful events and coping in the context of HIV/AIDS. In B. H. Gottlieb (Ed.), *Coping with chronic stress* (pp. 293–314). New York: Plenum.

Fordyce, M. W. (1981). *The psychology of happiness: Fourteen fundamentals*. Fort Meyers, FL: Cypress Lake Media.

Fordyce, M. W. (1983). A program to increase happiness: Further studies. *Journal of Counseling Psychology, 30*, 483–98.

Fordyce, M. W. (1988). A review of research on The Happiness Measures: A sixty-second index of happiness and mental health. *Social Indicators Research, 20*, 355–81.

Forgas, J. P. (2007). When sad is better than happy: negative affect can improve the quality and effectiveness of persuasive messages and social influence strategies. *Journal of Experimental Social Psychology, 43*, 513–28.

Frasure-Smith, N., & Prince, R. (1985). The ischemic heart disease life stress monitoring program: impact on mortality. *Psychosomatic Medicine, 47*(5), 431–45.

Fredrickson, B. L. (1998). What good are positive emotions? *Review of General Psychology, 2*, 300–19.

Fredrickson, B. L. (2009). *Positivity*. New York: Crown.

Fredrickson, B. L., & Branigan, C. (2005). Positive emotions broaden the scope of attention and thought-action repertoire. *Cognition & Emotion, 19*, 313–32.

Fredrickson, B. L., Cohn, M. A., Coffey, K. A., Pek, J., & Finkel, S. M. (2008). Open hearts build lives: Positive emotions, induced through meditation, build consequential personal resources. *Journal of Personality and Social Psychology, 95*, 1045–62.

Fredrickson, B. L., & Joiner, T. (2002). Positive emotions trigger upward spirals toward emotional well-being. *Psychological Science, 13*(2), 172–5.

Fredrickson, B. L., Mancuso, R. A., Branigan, C., & Tugade, M. M. (2000). The undoing effect of positive emotions. *Motivation and Emotion, 24*, 237–58.

Fredrickson, B. L., Tugade, M. M., Waugh, C. E., & Larkin, G. R. (2003). What good are positive emotions in crises? A prospective study of resilience and emotions following the terrorist attacks on the United States on September 11th, 2001. *Journal of Personality and Social Psychology, 84*, 365–76.

Freedman, S. R., & Enright, R. D. (1996). Forgiveness as an intervention goal with incest survivors. *Journal of Consulting & Clinical Psychology, 64*(5), 983–992.

Froh, J. J., Sefick, W. J., & Emmons, R. A. (2008). Counting blessings in early adolescents: an experimental study of gratitude and subjective well-being. *Journal of School Psychology, 46*(2), 213–33.

Gable, S. L., Gonzaga, G. C., & Strachman, A. (2006). Will you be there for me when things go right? Supportive responses to positive event disclosures. *Journal of Personality and Social Psychology, 91*, 904–17.

Gable, S. L., Reis, H. T., Impett, E. A., & Asher, E. R. (2004). What do you do when things go right? The intrapersonal and interpersonal benefits of sharing positive events. *Journal of Personality and Social Psychology, 87*, 228–45.

Gelkopf, M. (2009). The use of humor in serious mental illness: A review. *Evidence-Based Complementary & Alternative Medicine* [published online Aug. 17].

Grossman, P., Tiefenthaler-Gilmer, U., Raysz, A., & Kesper, U. (2007). Mindfulness training as an intervention for fibromyalgia: Evidence of postintervention and 3-year follow-up benefits in well-being. *Psychotherapy and Psychosomatics, 76*, 226–33.

Haight, B. K., & Burnside, I. (1993). Reminiscence and life review: Explaining the differences. *Archives of Psychiatric Nursing, 7*, 91–8.

Hammen, C. (2005). Stress and depression. *Annual Review of Clinical Psychology, 1*, 293–319.

Hecht, F. M., Moran, P., Moskowitz, J. T., Acree, M., Barrows, K., Epel, E., et al. (2010). *A randomized controlled trial of mindfulness-based stress reduction (MBSR) in HIV.* Paper presented at the American Psychosomatic Society.

Horowitz, M. (2008). *A course in happiness.* New York: Penguin.

Horowitz, M. J., Adler, N., & Kegeles, S. (1988). A scale for measuring the occurrence of positive states of mind: A preliminary report. *Psychosomatic Medicine, 50*(5), 477–83.

Hunt, A. H. (1993). Humor as a nursing intervention. *Cancer Nursing, 16*(1), 34–9.

Hutcherson, C. A., Seppala, E. M., & Gross, J. J. (2008). Loving-kindness meditation increases social connectedness. *Emotion, 8*, 720–4.

Isen, A. M., Daubman, K. A., & Nowicki, G. P. (1987). Positive affect facilitates creative problem solving. *Journal of Personality and Social Psychology, 52*, 1122–31.

Isen, A. M., Johnson, M. M. S., Mertz, E., & Robinson, G. F. (1985). The influence of positive affect on the unusualness of word associations. *Journal of Personality and Social Psychology, 48*, 1413–26.

Ismail, K., Winkley, K., & Rabe-Hesketh, S. (2004). Systematic review and meta-analysis of randomised controlled trials of psychological interventions to improve glycaemic control in patients with type 2 diabetes. *Lancet, 363*(9421), 1589–97.

Jain, S., Shapiro, S. L., Swanick, S., Roesch, S. C., Mills, P. J., Bell, I., et al. (2007). A randomized controlled trial of mindfulness meditation versus relaxation training: Effects on distress, positive states of mind, rumination, and distraction. *Annals of Behavioral Medicine, 33*, 11–21.

Johnson, D. J., Penn, D. L., Fredrickson, B. L., Meyer, P. S., Kring, A. M., & Brantley, M. (2009). Loving-kindness meditation to enhance recovery from negative symptoms of schizophrenia. *Journal of Clinical Psychology, 65*, 499–509.

Johnson, S. L., & Roberts, J. E. (1995). Life events and bipolar disorder: implications from biological theories. *Psychological Bulletin, 117*(3), 434–49.

Kabat-Zinn, J. (2003). Mindfulness-based interventions in context: Past, present, and future. *Clinical Psychology: Science and Practice, 10*, 144–56.

Kashdan, T. B., Uswatte, G., & Julian, T. (2006). Gratitude and hedonic and eudaimonic well-being in Vietnam war veterans. *Behaviour Research and Therapy, 44*, 177–99.

Klinger, E. (1975). Consequences of commitment to and disengagement from incentives. *Psychological Review, 82*(1), 1–25.

Knight, B. G., Lutzky, S. M., & Macofsky-Urban, F. (1993). A meta-analytic review of interventions for caregiver distress:

recommendations for future research. *Gerontologist, 33*(2), 240–8.

Kolden, G. G., Strauman, T. J., Ward, A., Kuta, J., Woods, T. E., Schneider, K. L., et al. (2002). A pilot study of group exercise training (GET) for women with primary breast cancer: feasibility and health benefits. *Psycho-Oncology, 11*(5), 447–56.

Koo, M., Algoe, S. B., Wilson, T. D., & Gilbert, D. T. (2008). It's a wonderful life: Mentally subtracting positive events improves people's affective states, contrary to their affective forecasts. *Journal of Personality and Social Psychology, 95*, 1217–24.

Koole, S. L., Smeets, K., van Knippenberg, A., & Dijksterhuis, A. (1999). The cessation of rumination through self-affirmation. *Journal of Personality and Social Psychology, 77*, 111–25.

Kraaij, V., Garnefsky, N., & Schroevers, M. J. (2009). Coping, goal adjustment, and positive and negative affect in definitive infertility. *Journal of Health Psychology, 14*, 18–26.

Krause, N. (1998). Positive life events and depressive symptoms in older adults. *Behavioral Medicine, 14,* 101–12.

Lancastle, D., & Boivin, J. (2007, December). *Feasibility, acceptability and usefulness of a self-administered positive reappraisal coping intervention (PRCI) card for stressful medical situations.* Paper presented at the 3rd Annual Meeting of the United Kingdom Society for Behavioural Medicine.

Landcastle, D., & Boivin, J. (2008). A feasibility study of a brief coping intervention (PRCI) for the waiting period before a pregnancy test during fertility treatment. *Human Reproduction, 23*, 2299–307.

Langston, C. A. (1994). Capitalizing on and coping with daily-life events: Expressive responses to positive events. *Journal of Personality and Social Psychology, 67*, 1112–25.

Lawlor, D. A., & Hopker, S. W. (2001). The effectiveness of exercise as an intervention in the management of depression: systematic review and meta-regression analysis of randomised controlled trials. *British Medical Journal, 322*(7289), 763–7.

Lazarus, R. S., & Folkman, S. (1984). *Stress, appraisal, and coping.* New York: Springer.

Lazarus, R. S., Kanner, A. D., & Folkman, S. (1980). Emotions: A cognitive-phenomenological analysis. In R. Plutchik & H. Kellerman (Eds.), *Theories of emotion* (pp. 189–217). New York: Academic Press.

Ledesma, D., & Kumano, H. (2009). Mindfulness-based stress reduction and cancer: a meta-analysis. *Psycho-Oncology, 18*, 571–9.

Lent, R. W., Singley, D., Sheu, H.-B., Gainor, K. A., Brenner, B. R., Treistman, D., et al. (2005). Social cognitive predictors of domain and life satisfaction: Exploring the theoretical precursors of subjective well-being. *Journal of Consulting and Clinical Psychology, 52*, 429–42.

Lewinsohn, P. M., & Amenson, C. S. (1978). Some relations between pleasant and unpleasant mood-related events and depression. *Journal of Abnormal Psychology, 87*, 644–54.

Lewinsohn, P. M., Hoberman, H. M., & Clarke, G. N. (1989). The coping with depression course: Review and future directions. *Canadian Journal of Behavioral Science, 21*, 470–93.

Lewinsohn, P. M., Sullivan, M., & Grosscup, S. J. (1980). Changing reinforcing events: An approach to the treatment of depression. *Psychotherapy: Theory, Research, and Practice, 17*, 322–34.

Lichter, S., Haye, K., & Kammann, R. (1980). Increasing happiness through cognitive retraining. *New Zealand Psychologist, 9*, 57–64.

Lundahl, B. W., Taylor, M. J., Stevenson, R., & Roberts, K. D. (2008). Process-based forgiveness interventions: A meta-analytic review. *Research on Social Work Practice, 18*, 465–78.

Lyubomirsky, S. (2007). *The how of happiness.* New York: Penguin.

Lyubomirsky, S., King, L., & Diener, E. (2005). The benefits of frequent positive affect: Does happiness lead to success? *Psychological Bulletin, 131*, 803–55.

Lyubomirsky, S., Sheldon, K., & Schkade, D. (2005). Pursuing happiness: The architecture of sustainable change. *Review of General Psychology, 9*, 111–31.

Lyubomirsky, S., Sousa, L., & Dickerhoof, R. (2006). The costs and benefits of writing, talking, and thinking about life's triumphs and defeats. *Journal of Personality and Social Psychology, 90*, 692–708.

MacLeod, A. K., Coates, E., & Hetherton, J. (2008). Increasing well-being through teaching goal-setting and planning skills: results of a brief intervention. *Journal of Happiness Studies, 9,* 185–96.

Martin, R. A. (2001). Humor, laughter, and physical health: methodological issues and research findings. *Psychological Bulletin, 127*(4), 504–19.

Martin, R. A. (2002). Is laughter the best medicine? Humor, laughter, and physical health. *Current Directions in Psychological Science, 11*, 216–20.

Matthews, K. A., & Gump, B. B. (2002). Chronic work stress and marital dissolution increase risk of posttrial mortality in men from the Multiple Risk Factor Intervention Trial. *Archives of Internal Medicine, 162*(3), 309–15.

Mausbach, B. T., Coon, D. W., Patterson, T. L., & Grant, I. (2008). Engagement in activities is associated with affective arousal in Alzheimer's caregivers: A preliminary examination of the temporal relations between activity and affect. *Behavior Therapy, 39*, 366–74.

Mausbach, B. T., Roepke, S. K., Depp, C. A., Patterson, T. L., & Grant, I. (2009). Specificity of cognitive and behavioral variables to positive and negative affect. *Behaviour Research and Therapy, 47*, 608–15.

McCaffrey, R. (2007). The effect of healing gardens and art therapy on older adults with mild to moderate depression. *Holistic Nursing Practice, 21*, 79–84.

McCullough, M. E., & Worthington, E. L. J. (1995). Promoting forgiveness: The comparison of two brief psychoeducational interventions with a waiting-list control. *Counseling and Values, 46*, 92–8.

McNair, D. M., Lorr, M., & Droppleman, L. F. (1971). *Manual for the Profile of Mood States (POMS).* San Diego, CA: Educational and Industrial Testing Service.

Mead, G. E., Morley, W., Campbell, P., Greig, C. A., McMurdo, M., & Lawlor, D. A. (2009). Exercise for depression. *Cochrane Database Systematic Reviews* (3), CD004366.

Mitchell, J., Stanimirovic, R., Klein, B., & Vella-Brodrick, D. (2009). A randomised controlled trial of a self-guided Internet intervention promoting well-being. *Computers in Human Behavior, 25*, 749–60.

Moen, P., Dempster-McCain, D., & Williams, R. M. (1993). Successful aging. *American Journal of Sociology, 97*, 1612–32.

Moskowitz, J. T. (2003). Positive affect predicts lower risk of AIDS mortality. *Psychosomatic Medicine, 65*, 620–6.

Moskowitz, J. T. (2010). Positive affect at the onset of chronic illness: Planting the seeds of resilience. In J. W. Reich, A. J. Zautra, & J. Hall (Eds.), *Handbook of adult resilience.* New York: Guilford. 465–483.

Moskowitz, J. T., Epel, E. S., & Acree, M. (2008). Positive affect uniquely predicts lower risk of mortality in people with diabetes. *Health Psychology, 27*, S73–S82.

Moskowitz, J. T., Folkman, S., Collette, L., & Vittinghoff, E. (1996). Coping and mood during AIDS-related caregiving and bereavement. *Annals of Behavioral Medicine, 18*(1), 49–57.

Moskowitz, J. T., Hult, J. R., Bussolari, C., & Acree, M. (2009). What works in coping with HIV? A meta-analysis with implications for coping with serious illness. *Psychological Bulletin, 135*, 121–41.

Moskowitz, J. T., Hult, J. R., Duncan, L. G., Cohn, M. A., Maurer, S., Bussolari, C., et al. (under review). A positive affect intervention for people experiencing health-related stress: Development and pilot testing.

Murrell, S. A., & Norris, F. H. (1984). Resources, life events, and changes in positive affect and depression in older adults. *American Journal of Community Psychology, 12*(4), 445–64.

Musick, M. A., & Wilson, J. (2003). Volunteering and depression: the role of psychological and social resources in different age groups. *Social Science & Medicine, 56*, 259–69.

Mutrie, N., Campbell, A. M., Whyte, F., McConnachie, A., Emslie, C., Lee, L., et al. (2007). Benefits of supervised group exercise programme for women being treated for early stage breast cancer: pragmatic randomised controlled trial. *British Medical Journal, 334*(7592), 517.

Nidich, S. I., Fields, J. Z., Rainforth, M. V., Pomerantz, R., Cella, D. F., Kristellar, J., et al. (2009). A randomized controlled trial of the effects of Transcendental Meditation on quality of life in older breast cancer patients. *Integrative Cancer Therapies, 8*, 228–34.

Nielsen, N. R., Kristensen, T. S., Schnohr, P., & Gronbaek, M. (2008). Perceived stress and cause-specific mortality among men and women: results from a prospective cohort study. *American Journal of Epidemiology, 168*(5), 481–496.

Norcross, J. C., Guadagnoli, E., & Porochaska, J. O. (1984). Factor structure of the profile of mood states (POMS): Two partial replications. *Journal of Clinical Psychology, 40*, 1270–7.

Norem, J. K. (2001). *The positive power of negative thinking.* Cambridge, MA: Basic Books.

Oman, D., Thoresen, C. E., & McMahon, K. (1999). Volunteerism and mortality among the community-dwelling elderly. *Journal of Health Psychology, 4*, 301–16.

Orth-Gomer, K., Schneiderman, N., Wang, H.-X., Walldin, C., Blom, M., & Jernberg, T. (2009). Stress reduction prolongs life in women with coronary disease: The Stockholm Women's Intervention Trial for Coronary Heart Disease (SWITCHD). *Circulation Cardiovascular Quality and Outcomes, 2*, 25–32.

Ostir, G. V., Markides, K. S., Black, S. A., & Goodwin, J. S. (2000). Emotional well-being predicts subsequent functional independence and survival. *Journal of the American Geriatrics Society, 48*, 473–8.

Otake, K., Shimai, S., Tanaka-Matsumi, J., Otsui, K., & Fredrickson, B. L. (2006). Happy people become happier through kindness: A counting kindnesses intervention. *Journal of Happiness Studies, 7*, 361–75.

Pilkington, K., Kirkwood, G., Rampes, H., & Richardson, J. (2005). Yoga for depression: The research evidence. *Journal of Affective Disorders, 89*, 13–24.

Pinto, B. M., Goldstein, M. G., Ashba, J., Sciamanna, C. N., & Jette, A. (2005). Randomized controlled trial of physical activity counseling for older primary care patients. *American Journal of Preventive Medicine, 29*(4), 247–55.

Post, S. G. (2005). Altruism, happiness, and health: It's good to be good. *International Journal of Behavioral Medicine, 12,* 66–77.

Pressman, S. D., & Cohen, S. (2005). Does positive affect influence health? *Psychological Bulletin, 131*(6), 925–71.

Puig, A., Lee, S. M., Goodwin, L., & Sherrard, P. A. D. (2006). The efficacy of creative arts therapies to enhance emotional expression, spirituality, and psychological well-being of newly diagnosed Stage I and Stage II breast cancer patients: A preliminary study. *The Arts in Psychotherapy, 33,* 218–28.

Raskin, M., Bali, L. R., & Peeke, H. V. (1980). Muscle biofeedback and transcendental meditation. A controlled evaluation of efficacy in the treatment of chronic anxiety. *Archives of General Psychiatry, 37,* 93–7.

Reed, M. B., & Aspinwall, L. G. (1998). Self-affirmation reduces biased processing of health-risk information. *Motivation and Emotion, 22,* 99–132.

Rethorst, C. D., Wipfli, B. M., & Landers, D. M. (2009). The antidepressive effects of exercise: a meta-analysis of randomized trials. *Sports Medicine, 39*(6), 491–511.

Rosengren, A., Orth-Gomer, K., Wedel, H., & Wilhelmsen, L. (1993). Stressful life events, social support, and mortality in men born in 1933. *British Medical Journal, 307*(6912), 1102–5.

Rowe, G., Hirsh, J. B., & Anderson, A. K. (2007). Positive affect increases the breadth of attentional selection. *Proceedings of the National Academy of Sciences of the United States of America, 104,* 383–8.

Ruini, C., Belaise, C., Brombin, C., Caffo, E., & Fava, G. A. (2006). Well-being therapy in school settings: a pilot study. *Psychotherapy & Psychosomatics, 75*(6), 331–6.

Ruini, C., Ottolini, F., Tomba, E., Belaise, C., Albieri, E., Visani, D., et al. (2009). School intervention for promoting psychological well-being in adolescence. *Journal of Behavior Therapy & Experimental Psychiatry, 40*(4), 522–32.

Schulz, R., & Beach, S. R. (1999). Caregiving as a risk factor for mortality. *Journal of the American Medical Association, 282,* 2215–9.

Sears, S. R., Stanton, A. L., & Danoff-Burg, S. (2003). The yellow brick road and the emerald city: Benefit finding, positive reappraisal coping and posttraumatic growth in women with early-stage breast cancer. *Health Psychology, 22*(5), 487–97.

Segerstrom, S. C., & Miller, G. E. (2004). Psychological stress and the human immune system: a meta-analytic study of 30 years of inquiry. *Psychological Bulletin, 130*(4), 601–30.

Seligman, M. E. P., Rashid, T., & Parks, A. C. (2006). Positive psychotherapy. *American Psychologist, 61,* 772–88.

Shapiro, D., Cook, I. A., Dvydov, D. M., Ottaviani, C., Leuchter, A. F., & Abrams, M. (2007). Yoga as a complementary treatment of depression: Effects of traits and moods on treatment outcome. *Evidence-Based Complementary and Alternative Medicine, 4,* 493–502.

Shapiro, D. H. (1980). *Meditation: Self-regulation strategy and altered state of consciousness.* New York: Aldine.

Shapiro, M., Brown, K. W., & Biegel, G. M. (2007). Teaching self-care to caregivers: Effects of mindfulness-based stress reduction on the mental health of therapists in training. *Training and Education in Professional Psychology, 1,* 105–15.

Sheldon, K. M., Kasser, T., Smith, K., & Share, T. (2002). Personal goals and psychological growth: Testing an intervention to enhance goal attainment and personality integration. *Journal of Personality, 70,* 5–29.

Sikkema, K. J., Kalichman, S. C., Kelly, J.A., & Koob, J. J. (1995). Group intervention to improve coping with AIDS-related bereavement: Model development and an illustrative clinical example. *AIDS Care, 7,* 463–75.

Sin, N. L., & Lyubomirsky, S. (2009). Enhancing well-being and alleviating depressive symptoms with positive psychology intervention: A practice-friendly meta-analysis. *Journal of Clinical Psychology, 65,* 467–87.

Smith, W. P., Compton, W. C., & West, W. B. (1995). Meditation as an adjunct to a happiness enhancement program. *Journal of Clinical Psychology, 51,* 269–73.

Sternfeld, B., Weltzien, E., Quesenberry, C. P., Jr., Castillo, A. L., Kwan, M., Slattery, M. L., et al. (2009). Physical activity and risk of recurrence and mortality in breast cancer survivors: findings from the LACE study. *Cancer Epidemiology Biomarkers & Prevention, 18*(1), 87–95.

Strecher, V. J., Seijts, G., Kok, G. J., Latham, G. P., Glasgow, R., DeVellis, B. M., et al. (1995). Goal setting as a strategy for health behavior change. *Health Education Quarterly, 22,* 190–200.

Surwit, R. S., van Tilburg, M. A., Zucker, N., McCaskill, C. C., Parekh, P., Feinglos, M. N., et al. (2002). Stress management improves long-term glycemic control in type 2 diabetes. *Diabetes Care, 25*(1), 30–4.

Taylor, S. E., Kemeny, M. E., Aspinwall, L. G., Schneider, S. G., Rodriguez, R., & Herbert, M. (1992). Optimism, coping, psychological distress, and high-risk sexual behavior among men at risk for Acquired Immunodeficiency Syndrome (AIDS). *Journal of Personality and Social Psychology, 63,* 460–73.

Taylor, S. E., Lerner, J. S. S., D.K., Sage, R. M., & McDowell, N. K. I. (2003). Are self-enhancing cognitions associated with healthy or unhealthy biological profiles? *Journal of Personality and Social Psychology, 85,* 605–15.

Taylor, S. E., & Lobel, M. (1989). Social comparison activity under threat: Downward evaluation and upward contacts. *Psychological Review, 96,* 569–75.

Teixeira, M. E. (2008). Meditation as an intervention for chronic pain. *Holistic Nursing Practice, 22,* 225–34.

Tellegen, A., Lykken, D. T., Bouchard, t. J., Wilcox, K. J., Segal, N. L., & Rich, S. (1988). Personality similarity in twins reared apart and together. *Journal of Personality and Social Psychology, 54,* 1031–9.

Turrell, G., Lynch, J. W., Leite, C., Raghunathan, T., & Kaplan, G. A. (2007). Socioeconomic disadvantage in childhood and across the life course and all-cause mortality and physical function in adulthood: evidence from the Alameda County Study. *Journal of Epidemiology & Community Health, 61*(8), 723–30.

van der Klink, J. J., Blonk, R. W., Schene, A. H., & van Dijk, F. J. (2001). The benefits of interventions for work-related stress. *American Journal of Public Health, 91*(2), 270–6.

Vittersø, J., Overwien, P., & Martinsen, E. (2009). Pleasure and interest are differentially affected by replaying versus analyzing a happy life moment. *Journal of Positive Psychology, 4,* 14–20.

Wachholtz, A. B., & Pargament, K. I. (2008). Migraines and meditation: does spirituality matter? *Journal of Behavioral Medicine, 31,* 351–66.

Wadlinger, H. A., & Isaacowitz, D. M. (2006). Positive mood broadens visual attention to positive stimuli. *Motivation and Emotion, 30,* 89–101.

Watson, D., & Clark, L. A. (1994). *The PANAS-X: Manual for the Positive and Negative Affect Schedule, Expanded Form.* University of Iowa.

Watson, D., Clark, L. A., & Tellegen, A. (1988). Development and validation of brief measures of positive and negative affect: The PANAS scales. *Journal of Personality and Social Psychology, 54*, 1063–70.

Waugh, C. E., & Fredrickson, B. L. (2006). Nice to know you: Positive emotions, self-other overlap, and complex understanding in the formation of new relationships. *Journal of Positive Psychology, 1*, 93–106.

West, J., Otte, C., Geher, K., Johnson, J., & Mohr, D. C. (2004). Effects of hatha yoga and African dance on perceived stress, affect, and salivary cortisol. *Annals of Behavioral Medicine, 28*(2), 114–8.

Williams, K. A., Kolar, M. M., Reger, B. E., & Pearson, J. C. (2001). Evaluation of a wellness-based mindfulness stress reduction intervention: A controlled trial. *American Journal of Health Promotion, 15*, 422–32.

Wilson, E. G. (2008). *Against happiness*. New York: Sarah Crichton Books.

Wing, J. F., Schutte, N. S., & Byrne, B. (2006). The effect of positive writing on emotional intelligence and life satisfaction. *Journal of Clinical Psychology, 62*(10), 1291–302.

Wood, C. (1993). Mood change and perceptions of vitality: A comparison of the effects of relaxation, visualization, and yoga. *Journal of the Royal Society of Medicine, 86*, 254–8.

Wrosch, C., Scheier, M. F., Carver, C. S., & Schulz, R. (2003). The importance of goal disengagement in adaptive self-regulation: when giving up is beneficial. *Self and Identity, 2*, 1–20.

Zautra, A. J., Berkhof, J., & Nicolson, N. A. (2002). Changes in affect interrelations as a function of stressful events. *Cognition & Emotion, 16*(2), 309–18.

Zautra, A. J., Burleson, M. H., Blalock, S. J., DeVellis, R. F., et al. (1995). Arthritis and perceptions of quality of life: An examination of positive and negative affect in rheumatoid arthritis patients. *Health Psychology, 14*(5), 399–408.

Zautra, A. J., Davis, M. C., Reich, J. W., Nicassario, P., Tennen, H., Finan, P., et al. (2008). Comparison of cognitive behavioral and mindfulness meditation interventions on adaptation to rheumatoid arthritis for patients with and without history of recurrent depression. *Journal of Consulting & Clinical Psychology, 76*(3), 408–21.

Zautra, A. J., Fasman, R., Reich, J. W., Harakas, P., Johnson, L. M., Olmsted, M. E., et al. (2005). Fibromyalgia: evidence for deficits in positive affect regulation. *Psychosomatic Medicine, 67*(1), 147–55.

Zautra, A. J., Johnson, L. M., & Davis, M. C. (2005). Positive affect as a source of resilience for women in chronic pain. *Journal of Consulting and Clinical Psychology, 73*, 212–20.

Zautra, A. J., & Reich, J. W. (1983). Life events and perceptions of life quality: developments in a two-factor approach. *Journal of Community Psychology, 11*, 121–32.

Stress, Coping, and Health in HIV/AIDS

Michael H. Antoni

Abstract

This chapter summarizes the role of psychological, social/interpersonal, and behavioral processes associated with psychosocial adjustment and health status in HIV-infected individuals. The chapter begins by presenting the nature of HIV infection in terms of physical and mental health challenges. Next we review the evidence that life stressors, coping strategies, social resources, and health behaviors influence mental (mood and quality of life) and physical (immune status, progression to AIDS) health status in persons with HIV. The chapter culminates in a summary of the rationale for the use of psychosocial interventions in HIV/AIDS. We present some of the more well-researched intervention approaches designed to modify stress and coping processes, summarize the evidence for the efficacy of these interventions in effecting optimal mental and physical health outcomes in persons living with HIV, and outline the putative mechanisms underlying these effects in support of a biobehavioral model.

Keywords: cognitive-behavioral stress management, HIV/AIDS, psychoneuroimmunology, highly active antiretroviral therapy, hypothalamic-pituitary-adrenal axis, sympathetic nervous system

Introduction

This chapter focuses on the application of stress and coping theory in the context of human immunodeficiency virus and acquired immune deficiency syndrome (HIV/AIDS). Over the past two decades health psychology researchers have drawn upon stress and coping theory and research to develop interventions that are aimed at enhancing the capacity of individuals to manage the ongoing challenges of HIV/AIDS. Health psychology research in the context of HIV/AIDS during this period has (1) identified the physical and mental health challenges of persons living with HIV, (2) examined the role of psychosocial (stress, coping, interpersonal) processes and biobehavioral (neuroimmune, health

behavior) processes in the physical and mental health of HIV-infected persons, and (3) designed and empirically demonstrated the efficacy of psychosocial interventions designed to modify psychosocial and biobehavioral processes to facilitate adjustment to this chronic disease and possibly modify its physical course.

In this chapter, we first summarize the physical and mental health challenges in HIV/AIDS. We then present work that uses stress and coping theory and psychobiological models of stress and disease to identify psychosocial and biobehavioral processes that may explain individual differences in psychological adjustment and disease management in persons with HIV. Next, we present some of the psychosocial interventions that have been designed to promote mental and physical health in HIV-infected persons. We highlight the underlying rationale for the use of cognitive-behavioral interventions focused on stress and coping processes, summarize the efficacy of these interventions for optimizing psychosocial adjustment and physical health, and propose some of the psychosocial and biobehavioral mediators of these effects. We conclude by identifying the limitations of this body of work and provide suggestions for future studies of stress and coping interventions for the growing population of persons living with HIV/AIDS.

Health Challenges in HIV/AIDS
Physical health challenges in HIV/AIDS

Persons with HIV/AIDS live with a chronic disease that causes a progressive loss of their immune repertoire against a wide range of infectious pathogens, leading in many cases to repeated bouts of outbreaks due to opportunistic infections and neoplasias. The disease is caused by HIV, a retrovirus that selectively targets a subset of lymphocytes defined by the expression of a surface T4 glycoprotein, also referred to as CD4+ T-helper cells (Klatzmann et al., 1984; Varmus, 1988). HIV makes use of CD4+ T cells for viral transcription of HIV RNA and protein synthesis, which begins the process of creating new HIV virions that can go on to target other host cells. An enzyme called protease ultimately cleaves the HIV RNA into segments that bud out of the infected cell. Through these well-orchestrated processes the infected person undergoes a progressive loss of CD4+ T cells while HIV virus concentration in the circulation (i.e., viral load) is increasing. Due to the rapid replication rate and mutation rate of HIV, the arrangement of glycoproteins on its capsid is constantly changing, which impairs the effectiveness of immune mechanisms in controlling the infection (Gaines et al., 1990).

Many persons infected with HIV develop an acute mononucleosis-like syndrome about a month after seroconversion (Tindall & Cooper, 1991). After the initial acute period of infection with HIV (Clerici et al., 1991; Tindall & Cooper, 1991), a period of clinical latency lasting for a number of years follows. This period is marked by increasing viral load, decreasing CD4+ cell count, and an increasing proportion of HIV-infected lymphoid cells (Pantaleo et al., 1993). Following this period of clinical latency, individuals may develop full-blown AIDS, defined as a decline in the number of CD4+ cells to critically low levels (<200 cell/mm^3)

or clinical signs of AIDS-defining opportunistic infections or neoplasias (Centers for Disease Control, 1992).

Despite the progressive decline in CD4+ cells and increases in HIV viral load in HIV-infected persons, not all individuals manifest clinical symptoms over a given time period. These individual differences may be due to differences in the ability to preserve certain key immune system components in spite of the HIV infection. We know that individuals with AIDS who remain healthy despite having critically low CD4+ cell counts display a relative preservation of natural killer (NK) cells and natural killer cell cytotoxicity (NKCC), innate immune parameters that are important for viral and neoplastic surveillance (Ironson et al., 2001). T-cytotoxic/suppressor (CD8+) cells are responsible for the destruction of cells that have been infected by viral pathogens and also play a role in suppression of neoplastic cell growth. The preservation of NK cells and certain subsets of CD8+ cells (e.g., memory CD8+) may be associated with enhanced immunosurveillance in persons with HIV, which may affect progression to clinically defined AIDS.

Individual differences in other immune parameters reflecting a person's ability to respond to infectious pathogens and cellular neoplastic changes may explain individual differences in the development of opportunistic disease symptoms. Importantly, for this chapter, variability in some of the immune parameters has been shown to relate to stress, coping, and related psychosocial processes in persons with HIV. Thus, studies examining these diverse immune parameters may provide insight into the possible pathways whereby psychological factors influence HIV disease progression.

Mental health challenges in HIV/AIDS

In addition to the physical burdens of HIV infections, there are mental health sequelae of HIV that are prevalent and that in turn may affect health outcomes through multiple pathways (Antoni & Carrico, in press). One of the most widely studied mental health challenges in HIV/AIDS is the elevated risk of affective and anxiety disorders (Carrico, Antoni, Young, & Gorman, 2008). From the point of notification of a positive HIV antibody test through the emergence of the first symptoms of disease, and on to the burdens of complex antiretroviral therapy (ART) regimens, a life with HIV is one filled with a multitude of psychosocial stressors. This does not come without mental health costs: Approximately half of a sample of 2,864 HIV-positive patients screened positive for a psychiatric disorder over a 1-year period, including major depression, dysthymia, and generalized anxiety disorder (Bing et al., 2001). In persons with HIV the risk of developing major depressive disorder is two times higher than in persons without HIV (Ciesla & Roberts, 2001). Depression and other mental health challenges may have an impact on the disease course in HIV via difficulties with health behaviors (increased substance use and poorer HIV medication adherence) and/or via psychoneuroimmunological processes.

There is now good evidence that elevated depressed mood and depressive symptoms may result in poorer immune status, faster HIV disease progression, and a greater risk of mortality (Leserman, 2008). It is plausible that the relationship between depression and disease progression is bidirectional. Knowledge of a declining HIV viral load has been shown to predict decreased distress (Kalichman, Difonzo, Austin, Luke, & Rompa, 2002). However, longitudinal investigations with repeated measurements of psychological and immunological data provide more clarity with regard to the temporal associations between distress/depression and disease progression. For example, depressive symptoms were associated with reductions in CD8+ and NK cell counts over a 2-year period (Leserman et al., 1997). Other work shows that depressive symptoms are associated with a more rapid CD4+ cell count decline in cohorts of HIV-positive men (Burack et al., 1993; Vedhara et al., 1997) and women (Ickovics et al., 2001). HIV-infected women whose major depression resolved over time showed concurrent increases in NKCC up to 2 years later (Cruess et al., 2005). Finally, cumulative depressive symptoms, hopelessness, and avoidant coping scores were associated with decreased CD4+ cell counts and higher HIV viral load over a 2-year period in a diverse sample of HIV-positive men and women, even after controlling for ART adherence (Ironson et al., 2005).

Do the associations between depression and immune parameters translate into poorer clinical disease outcomes in HIV-infected persons? The cumulative burden of depressive symptoms over time has been related to faster progression to AIDS (Leserman et al., 1999; Page-Shafer et al., 1996), and development of an AIDS-related clinical condition (Leserman et al., 2002) in men with HIV, and with hastened mortality in HIV-positive men (Mayne et al., 1996) and women (Ickovics et al., 2001). While discrepant findings have been reported

(Burack et al., 1993; Lyketsos et al., 1993; Page-Shafer et al., 1996), it appears that depressive symptoms may be an important predictor of HIV disease progression. In particular, investigations using longitudinal designs examining the accumulation of depressive symptoms over time have yielded the most consistent findings. Other mood states, including anger, have been associated with faster progression to AIDS (Leserman et al., 2002). Anxiety symptoms have also been related to greater CD8+38+ cell counts and higher HIV viral load—both indicators of elevated disease activity (Evans et al., 2002).

Conversely, there is some evidence that "positive" psychological states may relate to slowed HIV disease progression (Ironson & Hayward, 2008). Ickovics and colleagues (2006) observed that a composite factor of positive psychological resources (positive affect, positive HIV outcome expectancies, and benefit finding) predicted less rapid CD4+ cell decline and greater longevity over the subsequent 5 years in a cohort of women with HIV. These findings were significant over and above baseline depression and ART use over the 5-year investigation period. In other work greater positive affect predicted greater longevity in a longitudinal cohort of HIV-infected men who have sex with men (MSM; Moskowitz, 2003). Taken together, it appears that both positive and negative affective states may have implications for HIV disease progression.

There are a number of biobehavioral mechanisms that could explain the effects of affective states and disorders on HIV disease progression. These include health behaviors such as substance use and poor medication adherence, and neuroimmune pathways tied to sympathetic nervous system (SNS) and hypothalamic pituitary adrenal (HPA) neuroendocrine regulation (Antoni & Carrico, in press; Carrico, Johnson, Morin, et al., 2008). There is good evidence that each of these sets of variables is related to affective states on the one hand and HIV disease progression on the other. In the subsequent sections, we address three major questions that follow from this literature: (1) How do individual differences in stress and coping processes relate to mental and physical health in persons dealing with HIV? (2) Based on these associations, do interventions designed to modify stress and coping processes improve mental and physical health status in HIV-infected persons? (3) If so, how do these interventions have their effects? The major focus of this chapter will be on examining the evidence for psychosocial and biobehavioral mechanisms that can explain the effects of stress and coping interventions on health outcomes in persons with HIV. For a thorough review of health behavior pathways (substance use, medication adherence, sexual behaviors) that might also explain the effects of behavioral interventions on health outcomes in HIV, the reader is referred to several excellent and recently published reviews (DesJarlais & Semaan, 2008; Gore-Felton & Koopman, 2008; Kalichman, 2008; Safren et al., 2006).

Stress and Coping Processes in HIV/AIDS
Stressors and stress responses

Despite the encouraging clinical benefits of ART, HIV-positive persons must continue to cope with a number of chronic, uncontrollable stressors that may hinder optimal management of their illness. This has led investigators to ask whether stressful life experiences and the ways individuals respond to stressful challenges may affect the health burdens of HIV (Leserman, 2008). The impact of stress in persons with HIV has been widely studied over the past two decades. This research can be separated into field studies of cumulative stressful life events, high-impact stressors, and laboratory-based studies of stress responsivity.

STRESSFUL LIFE EVENTS

Investigations that employ interview-based, contextual methods and that conceptualize life event accumulation have observed the most consistent effects of negative life events on HIV disease progression (Leserman, 2003). For instance, cumulative negative life events have been associated with reduced NK and cytotoxic/suppressor (CD8+) T-cell counts over a 2-year period in HIV-positive gay men (Leserman et al., 1997). As noted previously, these immune cell subsets may play a key role in suppressing HIV replication and could therefore enhance the effectiveness of antiretroviral medication regimens (Cruess et al., 2003; Ironson et al., 2001).

Leserman and colleagues have also demonstrated that cumulative negative life events are associated with faster disease progression through 5- to 9-year follow-ups (Leserman et al., 1999, 2000, 2002). For instance, each cumulative stressor unit (based on cumulative negative life events) doubled the risk of progression to AIDS over 7.5 years (Leserman et al., 1999, 2000). In these investigations, AIDS was defined as CD4+ T-cell counts less than 200

cells/mm^3 and/or the development of an AIDS-defining clinical condition. In a subsequent investigation, greater cumulative negative life events (equivalent to one severe stressor) increased the risk of developing an AIDS clinical condition by three-fold at 9-year follow-up (Leserman et al., 2002). Interestingly, elevations in serum cortisol measured cumulatively were independently associated with faster progression to AIDS, development of an AIDS-related condition, and mortality over the same period (Leserman et al., 2002).

Because many of these prior studies were drawn from cohorts monitored in the late 1980s and early 1990s, the differences in medication regimens in that era may make it difficult to generalize the effects of stressful events for populations under active treatment today. However, cumulative negative life events have also been associated with increases in HIV viral load in cohorts of HIV-positive men and women treated with highly active antiretroviral therapy (HAART), the treatment of choice in contemporary clinical care since the late 1990s (Ironson et al., 2005). Individuals classified as experiencing a high rate (>75th percentile) of cumulative negative life events displayed a twofold increase in HIV viral load over 2 years when compared to those with lower rates (<25th percentile), even after controlling for antiretroviral medication adherence. Taken together, results of these investigations provide support for the relevance of chronic, possibly cumulative, stress in HIV disease progression. Caution is in order when interpreting these findings, as most of these studies had fairly small samples. Future investigations should examine the prospective association between negative life events and health outcomes in larger, diverse, HAART-treated cohorts of HIV-positive persons.

HIGH-IMPACT LIFE EVENTS

Rather than focusing on cumulative life stress, other investigations have examined the association between specific, poignant stressors and immune status in persons dealing with HIV. The stress of learning that one is HIV seropositive has been related to increases in distress (depressed mood and anxiety) that parallel reductions in CD4+ and NK cell counts (Antoni et al., 1991), and depressed T-lymphocyte proliferative responses (LPR) to mitogenic challenge (Ironson et al., 1990). These results suggest that stressful experiences early in HIV infection can have negative effects on immune status. One of the most common and recurring stressors for HIV-positive persons is bereavement (Martin & Dean, 1993). Importantly, bereavement has been related to more rapid declines in CD4+ T-cell counts over time (Kemeny & Dean, 1995) as well as with increases in serum neopterin (an HIV disease activity marker) and impaired LPR and NKCC (Goodkin et al., 1996; Kemeny et al., 1995). Other types of traumatic stressors have been associated with faster HIV disease progression (Leserman, 2008). One study observed a high rate of exposure to traumatic events in HIV-positive African American women (Kimmerling et al., 1999), and exposure to a traumatic stressor related to lower CD4+/CD8+ ratio at 1-year follow-up. This literature suggests that both an accumulation of negative life events and experiencing high-impact stressors may be associated with faster clinical disease progression or disease-related biological changes in persons with HIV. Gaining insight into the processes that transduce these stressful stimuli into such biological changes has motivated research relating individual differences in stress responsivity to disease progression in HIV-infected populations.

STRESS RESPONSIVITY STUDIES
Since physiological changes occurring during stress responses in the laboratory are often observable over a much shorter time frame than periods represented by chronic stressors or cumulative stressor burden, researchers have used laboratory reactivity paradigms to pinpoint endocrine and immune changes that may parallel the experience of field stressors in HIV-positive persons. In asymptomatic HIV-positive men, previous investigations have observed blunted adrenocorticotropin hormone (ACTH) responsiveness to a variety of behavioral challenges (Kumar, Kumar, Morgan, Szapocznik, & Eisdorfer, 1993; Starr et al., 1996), but no differences in cortisol increases when compared to HIV-negative men (Starr et al., 1996). This dissociation between stress-induced ACTH and cortisol responses suggests a possible dysregulation within the HPA axis due possibly to primary HIV disease, or to the cumulative stressor burden accompanying the disease. Subsequent investigations have demonstrated that compared to HIV-negative participants, HIV-positive persons showed abnormalities in immune cell trafficking that may be due, in part, to alterations in sympathoimmune communication (Hurwitz et al., 2005).

What is the health relevance of alterations in nervous–immune system communication in HIV infection? Since lymphoid organs are a primary site of HIV replication, SNS innervation of these regions might modulate HIV disease progression (Cole & Kemeny, 2001). There is evidence that norepinephrine (NE) at nerve terminals can downregulate proliferation of naïve T cells—a key component in responding to novel antigens in the lymphoid organs like the lymph nodes (Felten, 1996). The interaction of NE with β_2 adrenergic receptors on the lymphocyte membrane activates the G protein-linked adenylyl cyclase-cAMP-protein kinase A signaling cascade (Kobilka, 1992). These cellular processes are associated with decrements in interferon-gamma and interleukin-10 production, which are associated with elevations in HIV viral load over an 8-day period (Cole, Korin, Fahey, & Zack, 1998).

Other *in vivo* work has examined the role of autonomic nervous system (ANS) activity in HIV-positive persons initiating a HAART regimen. Those showing greater ANS activity at rest prior to beginning HAART subsequently demonstrated poorer suppression of HIV viral load and decreased CD4+ T-cell reconstitution over the next 3 to 11 months (Cole et al., 2001). Furthermore, other work by this laboratory showed that more socially inhibited HIV-infected men displayed an eightfold increase in plasma HIV viral load set point and poorer responses to HAART (Cole, Kemeny, Fahey, Zack, & Naliboff, 2003); these effects were mediated by elevated ANS activity levels in the more socially inhibited men. Thus, stress-related alterations in HPA- and SNS-related neuroendocrine functioning influence immune status in persons infected with HIV. These data suggest that individual differences in stress responsivity may influence the effectiveness of HAART and the course of HIV disease. If so, then interventions capable of changing stress responses (e.g., cognitive-behavioral therapy) may have implications not only for mental health (reducing anxiety and depressed mood) but also affecting immune and viral processes driving HIV disease progression. Central to the therapeutic actions of many of these psychosocial interventions is the ability to modify cognitive appraisals of stressors or other external stimuli.

Stressor appraisals
Individual differences in cognitive appraisals of stressors may moderate the association between stressful life events and health status in HIV-positive persons. Some work suggests that positive illusions and unrealistically optimistic appraisals may confer health-protective benefits in HIV (Taylor, Kemeny, Reed, Bower, & Gruenewald, 2000). In terms of the

stress of bereavement, HIV-positive men who engaged in cognitive processing about the death of a close friend or partner were more likely to report finding meaning or personal benefit following the loss (Bower, Kemeny, Taylor, & Fahey, 1998). Finding meaning/benefit was related to a slower CD4+ T-cell decline and greater longevity over a 2- to 3-year follow-up (Bower, Kemeny, Taylor, & Fahey, 1998). The idea that finding benefits through adversity might promote better health outcomes in medical disease is attracting growing interest among health psychologists (Park, Lechner, Stanton, Antoni, 2008). More recent research shows that benefit-finding uniquely predicted lower 24-hour urinary-free cortisol output in a diverse cohort of HAART-treated HIV-positive persons, even after accounting for the effects of depressive symptoms (Carrico, Ironson, Antoni, et al., 2006). In other research with HIV-positive gay men following Hurricane Andrew, dispositional optimism was associated with lower Epstein-Barr virus (EBV) and human herpes virus type-6 (HHV-6) IgG antibody titers, suggesting better immunological control over these viruses (Cruess, Antoni, Kilbourn, et al., 2000b). Taken together, this work suggests that maintaining a positive outlook toward the future or finding benefits in one's experiences with HIV may predict better health outcomes.

There is also work suggesting that negative appraisals may be related to poorer health in HIV infection. Having negative HIV-specific expectancies (e.g., fatalism) may increase the risk for initial symptom onset in asymptomatic HIV-positive men dealing with bereavement (Reed, Kemeny, Taylor, & Visscher, 1999) and may also increase the risk for mortality in men who already have AIDS (Reed, Kemeny, Taylor, Wang, & Visscher, 1994). Among HIV-positive women, pessimism was associated with lower CD8+ T-cell percentages and lower NKCC after controlling for negative life events (Byrnes et al., 1998). Thus, negative or pessimistic appraisals about stressors or one's efficacy in coping with them are associated with poorer immune status and greater risk for disease progression. On the other hand, maintaining optimism and finding benefits in the challenges of HIV/AIDS are associated with lower levels of adrenal stress hormones, better immunological control over herpesviruses, and possibly better health outcomes. As noted previously, interventions such as cognitive-behavioral therapy and various stress-management strategies can be used to reduce stress/distress by modulating cognitive appraisal processes and teaching new

cognitive and behavioral coping strategies in HIV-positive persons (Antoni, Ironson & Schneiderman, 2007; Carrico, Antoni, Pereira et al., 2005; Lutgendorf et al., 1998).

Coping strategies

One of the sequelae of cognitive appraisals is the coping strategies that individuals decide to employ in dealing with stressors (Folkman, Lazarus, Dunkel-Schetter, Delongis, & Gruen, 1986). In general, mostly cross-sectional and retrospective research conducted in the 1980s held the view that coping strategies characterized by avoidance are associated with increased distress in medical patients dealing with stressors (Holohan & Moos, 1986; Taylor & Aspinwall, 1990). Subsequent longitudinal research revealed that medical patients using denial and avoidance as a coping strategy after a medical diagnosis of breast cancer (Carver et al., 1993) or HIV infection (Antoni, Goldstein, Ironson, et al., 1995) have greater levels of distress over the subsequent year. More recent work suggests that cognitive coping strategies (positive refocusing, positive reappraisal, putting things into perspective) may be more closely associated with anxiety and depression than are behavioral coping strategies among HIV-positive MSM (Kraaij et al., 2008).

There are a number of studies suggesting that patients with HIV who use certain coping strategies for dealing with the demands of their disease may also show better physical health outcomes (Antoni & Scheiderman, 1998). For instance, in the 1990s it was shown that greater denial coping at the time of a diagnosis of HIV infection predicted greater impairments in immune status 1 year later (Antoni, Goldstein, et al., 1995) and a greater likelihood of progression to AIDS several years later (Ironson et al., 1994; Leserman, Pettito, Golden et al., 2000). Other studies have related coping strategies such as active confrontation (Mulder, Antoni, Duivenvoorden, et al., 1995) and realistic acceptance (Reed, Kemeny, Taylor, Wang, & Visseher, 1994) to differences in disease progression for HIV-infected individuals. These findings have largely held in research conducted to date. One recently published meta-analysis concluded that coping strategies that involve direct action (e.g., active coping, planning) and positive reappraisal (e.g., acceptance, positive reframing) are consistently associated with better mental and physical health and well-being, while coping that involves disengagement (behavioral disengagement, denial, substance use) is related to poorer mental and physical health outcomes (Moskowitz, Hult, Bussolari, &

Acree, 2009). There is evidence that more complex coping personality "patterns" comprising emotional non-expression and alexithymia (impaired ability to discern emotional experiences) are associated with immunological indicators that are linked to HIV disease progression (Temoshok, Waldstein, Wald, et al., 2008).

Emerging models of coping suggest the importance of studying coping strategies that not only mitigate distress but actually promote positive affect (Folkman, 2008) and positive adaptation to medical illness (Park, Lechner, Antoni, & Stanton, 2008). Coping processes that may facilitate positive emotions include benefit-finding, reordering priorities, and finding positive meaning in life experiences (Folkman, 2008). Some of these processes have been associated with more positive physical health outcomes in persons with HIV (Bower, Kemeny, & Taylor 1998; Ironson & Hayward, 2008; Moskowitz, 2003). Whether these associations are accounted for by neuroimmune mechanisms or improvements in health behaviors such as medication adherence remains to be demonstrated. Interestingly, among HIV-positive methamphetamine users, positive affect was independently associated with better self-reported medication adherence (Carrico, Johnson, Colfax, & Moskowitz, 2009).

Interpersonal processes: social support, disclosure, and conflict

A final set of stress-related process that has been the focus of much health psychology research concerns the association of mental and physical health outcomes with interpersonal processes. One psychosocial factor that has been related to medical patients' ability to adjust to the stressors of their disease is social support (House, 1981; Cohen & Willls, 1985). Social support can be grouped into one of several categories such as tangible aid, information, emotional assistance, nurturance, social integration, and sense of belonging (Cutrona & Russell, 1987; Schaefer, Coyne, & Lazarus, 1981). Medical patients who have rewarding personal relationships have shown better psychological adjustment to conditions such as cancer (Alferi, Carver, Weiss, et al., 2001; Helgeson & Cohen, 1996; Siegal, Calsyn, & Cuddihee, 1987; Taylor et al., 1984), end-stage renal disease (Siegel et al., 1987), and arthritis (Fitzpatrick, Newman, Lamb, & Shipley, 1988) as well as in HIV/AIDS (Zuckerman & Antoni, 1995). Social support may affect patients' psychological adjustment to a chronic illness by way of multiple pathways, including as a stress buffer (Cohen &

Wills, 1985; Zich & Temoshok, 1987), facilitating use of adaptive coping strategies (Dunkel-Schetter, Folkman, & Lazarus, 1987; Leserman et al., 1992; Thoits, 1987), decreasing HIV stigma (Galvan, Davis, Banks & Bing, 2008), and enhancing medication adherence (Gonzalez, Penedo, Antoni et al., 2004; Wallston et al., 1983).

It is also possible that patients' adverse emotional reactions to the stressors of their disease may act to drive away potential sources of social support (Wortman & Conway, 1985; Zuckerman & Antoni, 1995). Social isolation (Turner, Hays, & Coates, 1993) and social conflict (Leserman et al., 1995) may in turn forestall a person's ability to manage the demands of chronic HIV disease, resulting in greater distress, depression, and withdrawal, thereby creating a vicious circle. Animal research using a simian immunodeficiency virus (SIV) model in rhesus macaques suggests that sustained social conflict may promote the progression of disease (Capitano et al., 2008) This suggests that the chronic stress of social conflict may contribute to disease progression in humans with HIV infection.

One very tangible example of interpersonal processes operating in the context of HIV infection involves personal disclosure. This may involve disclosure of one's sexual orientation or one's serostatus. Prior work has shown that non-disclosure of sexual identity among gay men with HIV predicted faster progression to AIDS (Cole, Kemeny, Taylor, & Visscher, 1996). Other work has shown that serostatus disclosure is associated with emotional and physiological status in men and women dealing with HIV and that this may vary as a function of perceived social support received (Fekete, Antoni, Lopez et al., 2009; Fekete, Antoni, Duran et al., 2009). Specifically, among lower-income women with HIV, serostatus disclosure to their mothers was associated with lower depression and urinary cortisol under conditions of high family social support yet was associated with greater depression and cortisol when family support was low (Fekete, Antoni, Duran et al.,2009). In men with HIV, serostatus disclosure to their mothers was related to lower HIV viral load, but only in non-Hispanic White men with high family support (Fekete, Antoni, Lopez et al., 2009). It is plausible that individuals who were able to discern the best situations in which to disclose their status may have fared better. This literature suggests that the mere presence of social network members in the lives of persons with HIV is not sufficient to confer mental and physical health benefits, and that having the skills to identify, select, and communicate one's needs to others may be the key to deriving the benefits of social support in the context of HIV infection.

Psychosocial Interventions in HIV/AIDS
Rationale for psychosocial intervention in HIV/AIDS

The use of psychosocial interventions to help individuals with HIV cope with their illness and associated stressors has been extensively researched in the past 20 years. One model for the development of a stress management intervention in HIV/AIDS was proposed initially in the early 1990s and has since been refined (Antoni et al., 1990; Antoni, 2003a). The basic rationale for the use of a specific type of stress management—cognitive-behavioral stress management (CBSM)—follows directly from the longitudinal observations that have been summarized in this chapter. Since variations in stressors experienced, stress responses, cognitive appraisals of stress, coping strategies, and interpersonal processes may be related to poorer mental and physical health status in persons dealing with HIV, then it follows that multimodal interventions that attempt to modify stressor perceptions and affective, behavioral, and interpersonal responses using cognitive-behavioral techniques may improve mental and physical health. It is also plausible that stress-management interventions have their effects on mental health status by teaching anxiety-reduction behavioral skills such as relaxation, imagery, deep breathing, and meditation. The cognitive-behavioral elements of CBSM may reduce negative mood states such as depression, anxiety, and anger by changing cognitive appraisals to improve outlook and attitudes, teaching new coping strategies to increase a sense of self-efficacy, and providing interpersonal skills to better attract and maintain positive social support (Antoni, 2003a; Antoni, Schneiderman, & Ironson, 2007).

How might intervention-associated psychosocial changes translate into biological changes relevant to HIV/AIDS? It has been hypothesized that changes in affective status might be accompanied by an improved regulation of SNS and HPA axis functioning as reflected in changes in output of peripheral catecholamines and cortisol, since it is well established that changes in distress and mood states are associated with alterations in neuroendocrine regulation (Chrousos & Gold, 1992; McKewen, 1998). Accordingly, it has been proposed that improvements in neuroendocrine regulation with distress reduction would relate to a partial "normalization"

of immune system functions in HIV-infected persons to the extent that stress-related processes had added to the immunological impairments primary to HIV infections (Antoni et al., 1990). Several adrenal hormones—including cortisol and catecholamines (norepinephrine and epinephrine)—are known to be altered as a function of an individual's appraisals of and coping responses to stressors (McEwen, 1998; Sapolsky, Romero, & Munck, 2000).

In HIV-positive persons, elevations in neuroendocrine hormones have also been associated with alterations in multiple indices of immune status (Antoni & Schneiderman, 1998). Elevated levels of cortisol inhibit cellular-immune responses via changes in DNA and RNA synthesis (Cupps & Fauci, 1982) and enhance *in vitro* HIV p24 antigen production (Swanson, Zeller, & Spear, 1998). By synergizing with gp120, cortisol may enhance rates of CD4+ cell decline (Nair et al., 2000) and apoptosis (programmed cell death) (Amendola et al., 1996). In HIV-positive men, greater serum cortisol is associated with progression to AIDS, development of an AIDS-related complex symptom, and increased mortality over a 9-year period (Leserman et al., 2002). SNS neurohormones such as NE also affect immune system functions that are relevant to HIV disease. The sympathetic branch of the ANS innervates lymphoid tissue in the thymus, spleen, lymph nodes, and gut-associated lymphoid tissue (Nance & Sanders, 2007). We know that SIV replication is nearly quadrupled near catecholaminergic varicosities in macaques (Sloan et al., 2006). Moreover, persons with elevated ANS activity at rest prior to beginning ART demonstrated poorer suppression of HIV viral load and decreased CD4+ cell reconstitution (Cole et al., 2001).

If such changes in stress physiology influence the status of specific immune parameters (likely via cytokine regulation and other aspects of immune system communication), then HIV-infected persons undergoing stress-reduction intervention might derive immunological benefits. These improvements in immune function might include more efficient surveillance of opportunistic pathogens (e.g., reactivated latent herpesvirus infections) that might contribute directly to increased HIV replication through "transactivation" of HIV-infected CD4+ T cells (Antoni et al., 1995) and direct surveillance over life-threatening opportunistic infections or neoplastic cell changes due to oncogenic viruses (e.g., Jensen, Lehman, Antoni, & Pereira, 2007). Thus, stress management may help normalize immune surveillance, which may, in turn, forestall increases in viral load and the manifestation of other clinical symptoms in HIV/AIDS.

Efficacy of cognitive-behavioral interventions in HIV/AIDS

Over the past 20 years there have been a small collection of studies demonstrating the effects of CBSM and other cognitive-behavioral interventions that have been tested in different populations of persons dealing with HIV infection. Over this period a number of reviews have been published documenting the effects of these interventions on mental health indicators such as anxiety and depressed mood, as well as physiological parameters such as neuroendocrine and immune variables that may have health implications in HIV-infected persons (Antoni, 2003b; Carrico & Antoni, 2008; Crepaz, Passin, Herst et al., 2008). However, there is no study to date showing that these interventions have an impact on progression to AIDS or on mortality rates. The remainder of this chapter focuses on research that has attempted to test the efficacy of these interventions in different populations of persons with HIV.

A number of excellent reviews addressing the efficacy of cognitive-behavioral interventions for HIV-infected persons have been published in the past few years. The target outcomes of these reviews have included assorted health behaviors such as sexual risk behaviors (Kalichmen, 2008), drug use (DesJarlais & Semaan, 2008), HIV medication adherence (Simoni, Pearson, Pantalone, et al., 2006), and mental health variables such as mood and quality of life (Antoni, 2003a). In support of the model put forth in this chapter we will focus here on research on cognitive-behavioral interventions targeting stress and coping processes that have demonstrated parallel effects on psychosocial and physiological parameters that have implications for both mental and physical health in persons with HIV.

Many of the studies in this area have been summarized in two recent reviews (Carrico & Antoni, 2008; Crepaz, Passin, Herst et al., 2008). Some broad conclusions have emerged. Crepaz et al. (2008) conducted a meta-analytic review of cognitive-behavioral interventions on mental health and immune status outcomes in persons with HIV. Using a formal search of the literature from 1988 to 2005, they included 15 studies that met entry criteria in the meta-analysis and focused on selected mental health (depression, anxiety, anger, and stress) and immune (CD4+ T-cell counts) outcomes.

The majority of the studies used interventions delivered over 3 to 17 sessions (median 10), in a group format, and covered content areas including cognitive reappraisal/cognitive restructuring (n = 15), coping skills training (n = 14), stress-management skills training (n = 11), and social support (n = 7). They concluded that there was sufficient evidence for cognitive-behavioral intervention effects on all mental health outcomes, with effects sizes ranging from .30 to 1.00, but noted nonsignificant effects on CD4+ cells. Findings varied as a function of the techniques used in the interventions, with significant effects on depression and anxiety found only in studies providing stress management and in those having at least 10 intervention sessions (Crepaz et al., 2008). The authors recommended that future work identify other relevant factors associated with intervention effects.

According to the literature reviewed in prior sections of this chapter, some of intervention factors capable of mediating mental and physical health effects might include stress and coping processes (appraisals, coping strategies, and social support) on the one hand, and neuroendocrine and immune system regulation on the other. The absence of intervention effects on overall CD4+ cell counts in the review by Crepaz et al. (2008) may be due to the fact that stress-response processes may not relate directly (especially over short follow-up periods) to the numbers of immune cells, but rather to their functions (LPR and antiviral mechanisms, including NKCC) and the regulation of signaling molecules (cytokines) that orchestrate these functions. This is not surprising, as there is much stronger evidence in the psychoneuroimmunology literature for associations between field stress variables (chronic stress, mood) and immune functional indices than immune cell counts (Herbert & Cohen, 1993a,b).

If one proposes neuroendocrine (via HPA and SNS hormones) mediation of the association between stress and disease progression in HIV, the evidence linking cortisol and catecholamines to the immune system is strongest for neuroimmune associations with cellular immune functional parameters (Antoni, Penedo, & Schneiderman, 2007). An emerging body of research demonstrates that neuroendocrine factors may mediate stress effects on HIV disease progression through direct effects on dysregulation of Th1 cytokines, chemokines, and HIV transcription factors that favor increased HIV replication rate, which predates increased viral load in the circulation and ultimately clinical disease progression (Cole, 2008).

A second review published in 2008 focused exclusively on the effects of psychological interventions on neuroendocrine regulation and immune status in persons with HIV (Carrico & Antoni, 2008). This review was restricted to 14 randomized controlled trials published between 1987 and 2007 as identified using PubMed and PsycINFO. Most of the intervention studies in this analysis were group-based and ranged from 4 days to 16 weeks, with a mode of 10 weeks in duration. The studies were grouped into those that were cognitive-behavioral (mixture of cognitive-behavioral and relaxation-related strategies), those using relaxation and meditation only, and those focused on emotional expression.

The majority of the studies that showed effects on neuroendocrine hormones cortisol and catecholamines, and immune and viral parameters (lymphocyte proliferation, herpesvirus antibody titers, HIV viral load) involved 10 weeks of group-based CBSM. A second major finding of this review was that while not all interventions had significant effects on neuroendocrine and immune outcomes, it was clear that those interventions that were most successful in improving psychological adjustment (reducing depressed mood, anxiety, distress) were more likely to have beneficial effects on neuroendocrine regulation and immune status. This pattern suggests that interventions capable of modulating health-relevant physiological parameters must modulate distress or mood states, and that these sets of effects may have a common mediator related to a successful modification of stress and coping processes. Review articles cannot shed light on the mechanism analyses that are required to support these hypotheses. To illuminate and test these possible pathways it is necessary to unpack some of the research that has combined the use of randomized controlled trial designs with biobehavioral mechanisms analyses by testing the effects of psychosocial interventions on parallel measurements of psychosocial, neuroendocrine, and immunological parameters over time in HIV-positive samples (Antoni, 2003b). This chapter will next focus on one form of psychosocial intervention that has shown such parallel effects on stress and coping processes on the one hand and physiological processes (neuroendocrine, immune, and virologic) on the other in persons living with HIV.

CBSM intervention for persons with HIV

In the late 1980s research using cognitive-behavioral intervention to target stressful experiences, stress responses, and coping efforts relevant for persons infected with HIV was initiated (Antoni et al., 1990; Antoni, Ironson, & Schneiderman, 2007). Over the next 20 years randomized controlled trials of stress-management interventions demonstrated effects on a range of psychosocial and physiological indicators in different populations of persons infected with HIV along the continuum from antibody testing and diagnosis notification, the early symptomatic period, and on to chronic disease management in the era of HAART.

CBSM INTERVENTION COMPONENTS

The most widely tested stress-management approach in HIV/AIDS uses a 10-week group-based CBSM intervention that blends anxiety-reduction techniques (progressive muscle relaxation, guided imagery, autogenics, deep breathing, and mindfulness meditation) with cognitive-behavioral techniques (raising awareness of stress responses and cognitive appraisals, cognitive restructuring, coping skills training, assertiveness training, anger management, and social support-building strategies) (Antoni, Ironson, & Schneiderman, 2007) (Table 21.1). Each CBSM session begins with a training exercise in one of several anxiety-reduction techniques and then proceeds to an introductory didactic and experiential exercise focused on one of assorted cognitive-behavioral techniques. Sessions end with a short review, and homework is assigned, which typically involves participants practicing newly learned anxiety-reduction techniques and monitoring stress and coping processes on a daily basis between weekly sessions.

Each CBSM session begins with a new anxiety-reduction exercise, beginning with progressive muscle relaxation. It was reasoned that placing the relaxation and other anxiety-reduction exercises at the beginning of each session would allow participants to habituate to the group setting and would help them be more open, focused, and accepting of the cognitive-behavioral techniques that they learned later in the sessions (Antoni, 1997). Techniques presented across sessions were designed to build on one another—anxiety-reduction techniques began with those that were easiest to learn (muscle relaxation) and moved on to more complex exercises (mindfulness meditation) across the 10-week period (see Table 21.1).

Similarly, cognitive-behavioral techniques introduced over the first few weeks focus on building awareness of stress response cues and different moods, and then move on to awareness of cognitive

Table 21.1 Components of cognitive-behavioral stress management intervention

I. Relaxation Component
  a. Progressive muscle relaxation
  b. Guided imagery
  c. Autogenic training
  d. Mindfulness meditation
  e. Breathing

II. Cognitive-Behavioral Therapy Component
  a. Raising awareness of stress response
    i. Physical responses
    ii. Emotional responses
    iii. Cognitive responses
    iv. Social responses
  b. Changing stressor appraisals
    i. Automatic thoughts
    ii. Cognitive restructuring
  c. Coping skills training
    i. Coping repertoire
    ii. Coping effectiveness training
    iii. Executing coping responses
  d. Interpersonal skills training
    i. Assertiveness skills
    ii. Anger management
    iii. Social support building steps

appraisals and cognitive distortions. The intervention modules then focus on methods of challenging appraisals (cognitive restructuring) before moving on to coping skills training. The middle weeks of the intervention period address coping theory and the enactment of specific coping strategies. To reach more efficient use of coping to deal with ongoing stressors, the framework of Coping Effectiveness Training (CET; Chesney, Folkman, & Chambers, 1996) was used. Here, participants first identify their coping repertoire and distinguish direct from indirect and emotion-focused versus problem-focused strategies. They then learn to separate stressors into changeable and unchangeable components and to match direct, problem-focused coping strategies to situations/stressor features that are changeable, and direct, emotion-focused strategies to unchangeable aspects of stress. The final 3 weeks focus on a set of interpersonal skills designed to improve the acquisition, utility, and maintenance of social support resources. Participants learn to map out their social support networks and distinguish persons who might offer emotional supports versus those who were better able to offer tangible/instrumental support. Following from their CET training, participants learn to use emotionally

supportive persons for unchangeable stressful experiences (e.g., loss of loved one or friends) and those offering instrumental support for changeable aspects of stressors (e.g., needing transportation, advice on doctors or treatments). Subsequent sessions teach participants cognitive-behavioral techniques for communicating with their social support network members (assertiveness, anger management, and conflict resolution). Individuals are taught to use these techniques together in responding to stressors. For a possible sequence of responses to a stressful encounter, see Figure 21.1.

EFFECTS OF CBSM INTERVENTION IN HIV/AIDS

Over the past two decades a series of studies have tested the effects of the CBSM intervention on psychosocial and physiological variables relevant to mental and physical health in mostly middle-income, well-educated MSM as well as lower-income minority women who are at various points in the disease experience. In the initial work in this area CBSM was shown to buffer the negative mood and immunological changes that occurred after MSM were notified of a seropositive antibody test result (Antoni et al., 1991). Importantly, decreases in negative mood (anxiety, depressed mood) and increases in immune parameters from before to after notification were proportional to the frequency of home practice of relaxation exercises, suggesting that the effects on mood and immune parameters might be due to CBSM skills learned or a greater sense of efficacy in using these skills. This suggested that one might employ a coping intervention in anticipation of the stress of serostatus notification, a notion that may be relevant for persons preparing to undergo other stressful procedures (e.g., surgery, cancer screening, genetic testing).

Stressful event
↓
AWARENESS
(thoughts, feelings, physical sensations)
APPRAISAL
(THOUGHTS: inaccurate ⟶ Rational thought replacement)
APPRAISAL
(SITUATION: controllable or uncontrollable)
COPING
(CHOICE: problem-focused or emotion-focused)
RESOURCES
(CHOICE: use instrumental or emotional support)

Fig. 21.1 Coordinated response to stressful encounter.

Interestingly, HIV-positive men receiving CBSM have also shown significant decreases in IgG antibody titers (reflecting better immunological control) to EBV viral capsid antigen (EBV-VCA) and to HHV-6, which each moved into the normal range for age-matched healthy male laboratory control values (Esterling et al., 1992). The reductions in EBV-VCA IgG antibody titers in the CBSM group appeared to be mediated by the greater perceived social support levels maintained in this condition (Antoni, Lutgendorf, Ironson, Fletcher, & Schneiderman, 1996). These findings suggest that changes in immunological parameters did map onto some of the intervention's psychosocial targets, which may have been achieved through changes in coping effectiveness skills or other interpersonal skills (e.g., assertiveness). Finally, a 2-year follow-up of this cohort of HIV-positive men revealed that less distress at diagnosis, decreased HIV-specific denial coping after diagnosis, and better participant adherence to CBSM sessions and homework practice all predicted slower disease progression to symptoms and AIDS (Ironson et al., 1994), suggesting that intervention-associated changes may have been responsible for these longer-term outcomes.

CBSM intervention has also been used to assist HIV-positive MSM in managing the emergence of disease symptoms, where it has been shown to decrease depressive symptoms, anxiety, and mood disturbance over the 10-week intervention period (Lutgendorf et al., 1998). Importantly, parallel changes in cognitive coping strategies (acceptance, and positive reinterpretation and growth) and social support (social attachment, guidance) acted to explain the effects of CBSM on these mood variables (Lutgendorf et al., 1998). Thus, CBSM-induced changes in coping and social support (possibly via intervention modules focused on these areas) can improve mental health functioning. Men assigned to CBSM also showed decreases in IgG antibody titers to herpes simplex virus type 2 (HSV-2), reflecting better immunological control over latent genital herpesvirus infections (Lutgendorf et al., 1997). Decreases in depressive symptoms (Lutgendorf et al., 1997) and enhanced social support (Cruess, Antoni, Cruess, et al., 2000c) over the 10-week intervention period partially explained concurrent reductions in these HSV-2 antibody titers. Further analyses revealed that reductions in HSV-2 titers were proportional to increases in perceived social support and relaxation-associated distress reduction during home practice over the 10-week period (Cruess et al., 2000c). These findings

suggested that CBSM-associated changes in mood, which may have been secondary to relaxation practice, and perceived social support changes were related to the degree to which beneficial immune changes occurred during the intervention period.

The disease relevance and biobehavioral mechanisms underlying the effects of CBSM in persons with HIV were documented by monitoring concurrent changes in psychological, neuroendocrine, and immune indicators occurring during CBSM (Antoni, 2003b). In multiple instances, CBSM effects on neuroendocrine regulation (decreased urinary cortisol and norepinephrine) were associated with decreased negative mood (depressed mood and anxiety) on the one hand, and preserved or reconstituted immune parameters (cytotoxic T lymphocytes and naïve T-helper cells) on the other (Antoni, Cruess, Wagner, et al., 2000a; Antoni, Wagner, et al., 2000b; Antoni et al., 2002, 2005; Cruess et al., 2000c). Intensive analyses of week-to-week changes within the CBSM condition revealed that greater perceived skills at using relaxation exercises at home were related to greater before-to-after in-session evening decreases in salivary cortisol and negative mood (Cruess, Antoni, Kumar, & Schneiderman, 2000a) on the one hand, and greater improvements in antiviral immune function over the 10-week training period (Cruess, Antoni, Cruess, et al., 2000c) on the other. These analyses lend strong support for a psychoneuroimmunological model wherein changes in mood and cortisol regulation parallel improved immunological control over a latent herpesvirus—a potential analog for susceptibility to other opportunistic viral infections. It is plausible that these immune changes observed after the CBSM intervention may have changed secondary to other immunological changes (decreased HIV viral load, better Th1 cytokine regulation), which may be directly tied to neuroendocrine regulation (Cole, 2008). It is plausible that the recovery or preservation of cell populations observed in men receiving CBSM may have been secondary to decreases in HIV viral load occurring over the follow-up period.

In the HAART era beginning in the late 1990s, studies of stress-management interventions revealed further interesting effects on disease progression. One study noted an association between stress and coping processes on the one hand and the evolution of medication adherence and viral load on the other over time in a cohort of men and women recently initiating a HAART regimen (Weaver, Llabre, Duran, et al., 2005). Specifically, greater use of avoidant coping, lower social support, and negative mood all predicted poorer HAART adherence, which in turn predicted greater viral load over time. This suggested also that if stress-management interventions could improve negative mood by modifying coping and social support (Lutgendorf et al., 1998), then it might also facilitate the effectiveness of these then-new HAART medications by improving the ways people handled stress.

Since medication adherence is believed to be critical for HAART effectiveness (Bangsberg et al., 2001), many medication adherence training (MAT) programs have been tested and found to be useful in HIV-infected persons (Safren et al., 2006). Many of these employ cognitive-behavioral principles based on self-efficacy theory (Johnson, Catz, Remien, et al., 2003; Simoni, Frick, Pantalone, & Turner, 2003). When CBSM is used in combination with MAT it has been shown to decrease depressed mood and HIV viral load up to 15 months, even after controlling for ART adherence over this entire period (Antoni, Carrico, et al., 2006). Interestingly, decreases in depressed mood (which are tied to decreased denial coping) have been shown to explain the effects of CBSM on viral load decreases over time (Antoni, Carrico, et al., 2006). In addition, greater attendance at CBSM sessions was associated with lower HIV viral load at follow-up. Ongoing work in this area examines putative neuroendocrine (urinary cortisol and catecholamines) and health behavior changes (substance use, sleep) that may have covaried with mood and coping changes as possible explanations for these effects on viral load. Interestingly, other work has shown that elevated levels of NE (which has previously been shown to be decreased by CBSM) predicts less effectiveness of a newly initiated protease inhibitor in reducing HIV viral load over a 6-month period among persons with HIV (Ironson, Balbin, Stieren, Detz, Fletcher, Schneiderman, & Kumar, 2008).

It is important to note that none of the CBSM trials just summarized have demonstrated direct effects of the intervention on HIV clinical disease progression. Observed effects include short-term immune changes surrounding diagnosis notification, apparent improvements in immunological control of latent viral infections over longer periods, and better recovery or preservation of immune cell populations that are relevant for immune surveillance over opportunistic pathogens and neoplastic cell changes. That persons on HAART receiving CBSM appear to show decreased viral load out to 15 months of follow-up is encouraging and suggests

that a stress-management intervention used in combination with MAT may be useful for optimal disease management. It is also encouraging that in each of these cohorts of men with HIV, the effects of CBSM on mental health and immune and virologic variables appear to be tied to the neuroendocrine changes hypothesized to accompany beneficial changes in stress physiology.

One set of studies has shown that stress processes and CBSM may be associated with at least one aspect of HIV clinical disease progression: carcinogenic changes. Specifically, this work examines the effects of stress, immune parameters, and disease progression in lower-income women with HIV who are at elevated risk for developing an AIDS-defining clinical outcome—cervical cancer—because they are co-infected with different types of human papillomaviruses (HPVs). These co-infected women are at a markedly increased risk for developing cervical intraepithelial neoplasia (CIN) as well as invasive cervical carcinoma (Jensen, Pereira, Antoni et al., 2007; Maiman, Fruchter, Clark, et al., 1997). Since HIV-negative women reporting elevated negative events, pessimistic attitudes, poor coping strategies, and low social support have an elevated risk for presenting with more advanced stages of CIN (Antoni & Goodkin, 1988; Antoni & Goodkin, 1989; Goodkin, Antoni, & Blaney, 1986), it is plausible those with HIV might also be susceptible to stress effects on disease progression to CIN.

The Centers for Disease Control & Prevention declared that cervical cancer was an AIDS-defining condition and CIN was an AIDS-related complex indicator in 1993 (CDC, 1992). Psychosocial research in HIV-positive, HPV-positive women showed that greater pessimism was associated with poorer NK cell cytotoxicity (Byrnes et al., 1998) and that those reporting greater negative life events over the prior year showed a greater risk of developing CIN (Pereira et al., 2003a) as well as HSV-2 genital herpesvirus outbreaks (Pereira et al., 2003b) over a 1-year follow-up. Thus, stress processes may relate to clinical outcomes in women with HIV, and especially in women who were vulnerable to specific opportunistic cancers. Teaching this vulnerable group methods for better managing stress and coping could affect distress as well as psychoneuroimmunological processes possibly related to cervical carcinogenesis. Stress-associated neuroendocrine factors might affect multiple steps in viral oncogenesis, including HPV-associated neoplastic changes (for a review see Antoni, Lutgendorf, Cole, et al., 2006).

The majority of HIV-positive, HPV-positive women in this country are lower-income African American women. In studies using psychosocial interventions adapted to the needs of these lower-income women (Pereira, 2002), it has indeed been shown that women receiving CBSM show significant decreases in perceived stress and a decreased risk for persistent CIN over time, even after controlling for HPV type, CD4+ cell counts, HAART medications, and tobacco smoking (Antoni, Pereira, et al., 2008). One can hypothesize that these effects were due to changes in neuroendocrine (urinary cortisol and NE) or immunological (NKCC, HIV viral load) variables on the one hand or health behavior change variables (e.g., sexual behaviors, smoking, alcohol and drug use, medication adherence) on the other.

In summary, interventions based on cognitive-behavioral therapy have been shown to improve mental health outcomes such as distress and depressive symptoms in persons with HIV. In studies focused specifically on examining psychoneuroimmunological outcomes—mostly involving group-based CBSM—there is a strong trend suggesting that only those studies showing psychological effects were able to demonstrate changes in endocrine and immunological parameters (Carrico & Antoni, 2008). More recently published studies suggest that CBSM may also affect specific disease activity processes such as HIV viral load and cervical neoplasia. The effects of CBSM on psychosocial, neuroendocrine, immunological, and disease outcomes are summarized in Table 21.2.

Referring back to the theoretical model introduced previously, intervention results just reviewed suggest that (1) CBSM may help individuals manage the "stress" of HIV infection by improving psychological adjustment and physiological regulation at several points in the HIV disease experience, including serostatus testing and notification, the early symptomatic stage preceding AIDS, and throughout disease management with ART, including HAART regimens; (2) CBSM may decrease indicators of distress (anxiety and depressed mood) by increasing use of adaptive cognitive coping strategies (acceptance and positive reframing) and perceived social support (instrumental and emotional); (3) greater reductions in distress during CBSM were accompanied by greater reductions in SNS activity (urinary norepinephrine) and HPA axis output (urinary cortisol); (4) greater reductions in distress and/or neuroendocrine output during the 10-week intervention predicted more favorable immune

Table 21.2   Effects of cognitive behavioral stress management on psychosocial, neuroendocrine, immunologic, and disease activity indicators in persons with HIV

- **Psychosocial**
  - Dysphoric mood
  - Anxious mood
  - Social support
  - Adaptive coping
- **Neuroendocrine**
  - 24-hour urinary free cortisol output
  - 24-hour urinary norepinephrine output
  - Salivary cortisol output
  - Sex hormones (testosterone)
- **Immunological**
  - CD4, CD56 cells at diagnosis notification
  - Transitional naive CD4 cells and CD8 cells
  - Immune control over EBV, HHV-6, HSV-2
- **Disease activity**
  - Decreased HIV viral load
  - Decreased progression to symptoms/AIDS
  - Decreased neoplastic changes (CIN)

status (greater immune system reconstitution and cytotoxic T-cell numbers and better control of latent herpesviruses) concurrently and lower disease activity (HIV viral load) at follow-up; and (5) greater psychological and physiological changes appear to be proportional to the "dose" of CBSM received or practiced, as indicated by measures of group attendance and home practice. Taken together, these findings make a strong case for the efficacy of CBSM—an intervention designed to modify stress and coping responses as individuals manage HIV infection—for optimizing mental and physical health outcomes. However, much more work needs to be done to test whether these effects are durable and generalizable to real-life situations where HIV is taking its greatest tolls. It is also reasonable that stress-management interventions such as CBSM will serve the greatest good when used in combination with optimal ART, MAT, and risk-reduction programs that are carefully designed to be relevant and acceptable to the largest populations dealing with the disease.

Future Research

Despite the pattern of reasonably consistent results for the effects of cognitive-behavioral therapy, CBSM, and similar stress and coping interventions on mental health outcomes, and psychosocial and physiological processes in persons with HIV, not all of the research findings in the field have been consistent. For instance, not all studies of CBSM have shown improvements in disease status (HIV viral load, CD4 cell counts), even when the interventions produced positive improvements in mental health variables (Berger, Schad, VonWyl, et al., 2008; McCain, Munjas, Munro, et al., 2003). It is plausible that the specific techniques used across these studies varied in a systematic way. Accordingly, interventions that emphasize mostly cognitive restructuring and interpersonal skills training may produce large effects on psychological outcomes, whereas those emphasizing anxiety-reduction techniques such as relaxation may be associated with larger effects on neurohormones that relate more directly to immune functions. There is also evidence that alternative forms of psychosocial intervention, including tai chi, massage, and written emotional expression may produce similar effects to CBSM on certain immune parameters in persons with HIV (Diego, Field, Hernandez-Reif, Shaw, Friedman, & Ironson, 2001; McCain, Gray, Elswick, et al., 2008; Petrie, Fontanilla, Thomas, Booth, & Pennebaker, 2004). These interventions may work on alleviating unexpressed concerns, bodily tension, and physiological activation, though it is less clear how they might improve coping with future HIV-related stressors.

The great majority of studies investigating the effects of cognitive-behavioral intervention in persons with HIV have been focused on examining effects on distress, depressive symptoms, and other indicators of negative affect. Given that positive affect and an increased sense of meaning have been shown to predict better disease course in persons with HIV (Bower et al., 1998; Moskowitz, 2003), it is reasonable to test the effects of interventions such as CBSM and expressive writing on indicators of positive affect, positive states of mind, and benefit-finding. It is worth noting that a 10-week CBSM program similar to the one presented in this chapter (Antoni, Schneiderman, & Ironson, 2007) has been tailored for persons dealing with the stress of breast cancer treatment (Antoni, 2003c) and prostate cancer treatment (Penedo, Antoni, & Schneiderman, 2008). In these cancer populations CBSM has been shown to increase positive affect, positive states of mind, and benefit-finding (Antoni et al., 2001; Antoni, Lechner, Kazi, et al., 2006; Penedo, Molton, Dahn, et al., 2006).

Whether one observes significant effects of psychosocial interventions on negative or positive psychological experiences, it is important to keep in perspective that the jury is still out on whether CBSM or any of these other forms of intervention can influence the course of HIV disease over the long haul. Future work needs to follow these cohorts over longer periods, as has been done in the psycho-oncology literature, though often revealing mixed results (Andersen et al., 2008; Goodwin et al., 2001; Spiegel et al., 1989).

Another limitation of this body of work concerns the lack of studies conducted with HIV populations outside of middle-class White MSM. While some studies have shown encouraging results with CBSM (Antoni et al., 2008) and CBSM-like (Lechner et al., 2003) interventions among lower-income women with HIV, little is known about their longer-term effects on disease course or the mechanisms that could explain their effects. Research aiming to modify stress and coping processes in ethnic minority populations calls for carefully targeting the intervention material to be culturally sensitive as well as relevant to the nature of stressors that each population must deal with. As noted previously, many of the stress and coping interventions tested to date in persons with HIV have involved either individual-based or group-based approaches. More work needs to focus these interventions at the level of the romantic dyad (Fife, Scott, Fineberg, & Zwickl, 2008) and the family system (Szapocnik, Feaster, Mitrani, et al., 2004) to ensure optimal carryover to the social milieu where longer-term coping skills will be enacted. Future intervention research might benefit by using more efficient methods of intervention delivery that capitalize on community-based participatory research methods and advances in telephonic and Web-based technologies (Heckman, Barcikowski, Ogles, Suhr, Carlson, Holroyd, & Garske, 2006; Stein, Herman, Bishop, Anderson, Trisvan, Lopez, Flanigan, & Miller, 2007).

The major focus of this chapter has been on stress-related psychosocial processes surrounding stress and coping and physiological processes encompassing neuroendocrine–immune interactions. Studies of biobehavioral processes that might mediate the effects of these interventions on mental and physical health outcomes in persons with HIV would be wise to include measures of psychosocial processes and neuroimmune changes in addition to changes in health behaviors such as medication adherence, sexual risk behaviors, and substance use. There is a growing body of clinical trials research demonstrating the effects of health behavior change interventions targeting these interrelated behaviors (DeJarlis et al., 2008; Kalichman, 2008; Safren,

Knauz, O'Cleririgh, et al., 2006; Safren, O'Cleirigh, Tan, et al., 2009; Sikkema, Wilson, Hansen, Kochman, Neufeld, Ghebremichael, & Kershaw, 2008). Failing to incorporate health behavior processes such as these into stress and coping intervention explanatory models could give a very distorted picture of the mechanisms of action that are operating in interventions designed to improve the way people cope with HIV. This is turn could affect decision-making as investigators attempt to refine the content of future interventions that are submitted to effectiveness trials in the community.

References

Alferi, S., Carver, C. S., Antoni, M. H., Weiss, S., & Duran, R. (2001). An exploratory study of social support, distress, and disruption among low-income Hispanic women under treatment for early stage breast cancer. *Health Psychology, 20*, 33–41.

Amendola, A., Gougeon, M. L., Poccia, F., Bondurand, A., Fesus, L., & Piacentini, M. (1996). Induction of tissue transglutaminase in HIV pathogenesis: Evidence for high rate of apoptosis on CD4+ T lymphocytes and accessory cells in lymphoid tissues. *Proclamation of the National Academy of Sciences USA, 93*, 11057–62.

Andersen, B., Yang, H. C., Farrar, W., Golden-Kreutz, D., Emery, C., Thornton, L., et al. (2008). Psychologic intervention improves survival for breast cancer patients. *Cancer, 113*, 3450–8.

Antoni, M. H. (1997). Cognitive behavioral stress management for gay men learning of their HIV-1 antibody test results. In J. Spira (Ed.), *Group therapy for patients with chronic medical diseases* (pp. 55–91). New York: Guilford Press.

Antoni, M. H. (2003a). Stress management and psychoneuroimmunology in HIV infection. *CNS Spectrums, 8*, 40–51.

Antoni, M. H. (2003b). Stress management effects on psychological, endocrinological and immune function in men with HIV: Empirical support for a psychoneuroimmunological model. *Stress, 6*, 173–88.

Antoni, M. H. (2003c). *Stress management intervention for women with breast cancer.* Washington DC: American Psychological Association Press.

Antoni, M. H., Baggett, L., Ironson, G., August, S., LaPerriere, A., Klimas, N., et al. (1991). Cognitive–behavioral stress management intervention buffers distress responses and immunologic changes following notification of HIV-1 seropositivity. *Journal of Consulting and Clinical Psychology, 59*(6), 906–15.

Antoni, M. H., & Carrico, A. (in press). Psychological and biobehavioral processes in HIV disease. In A. Baum & T. Revenson (Eds.), *Handbook of clinical health psychology.*

Antoni, M. H., Carrico, A. W., Durán, R. E., Spitzer, S., Penedo, F., Ironson, G., et al. (2006). Randomized clinical trial of cognitive behavioral stress management on human immunodeficiency virus viral load in gay men treated with highly active antiretroviral therapy. *Psychosomatic Medicine, 68*, 143–51.

Antoni, M. H., Cruess, D., Klimas, N., Carrico, A.W., Maher, K., Cruess, S., et al. (2005). Increases in a marker of immune system reconstitution are predated by decreases in 24-hour urinary cortisol output and depressed mood during a 10-week stress management intervention in symptomatic HIV-infected gay men. *Journal of Psychosomatic Research, 58*, 3–13.

Antoni, M. H., Cruess, D., Klimas, N., Maher, K., Cruess, S., Kumar, M., et al. (2002). Stress management and immune system reconstitution in symptomatic HIV-infected gay men over time: Effects on transitional naïve T-cells (CD4+CD45RA+CD29+). *American Journal of Psychiatry, 159*, 143–5.

Antoni, M. H., Cruess, D., Wagner, S., Lutgendorf, S., Kumar, M., Ironson, G., et al. (2000a). Cognitive behavioral stress management effects on anxiety, 24-hour urinary catecholamine output, and T-Cytotoxic/suppressor cells over time among symptomatic HIV-infected gay men. *Journal of Consulting and Clinical Psychology, 68*, 31–45.

Antoni, M. H., Esterling, B., Lutgendorf, S., Fletcher, M. A., & Schneiderman, N. (1995). Psychosocial stressors, herpes virus reactivation and HIV-1 infection. In M. Stein & A. Baum (Eds.), *AIDS and oncology: Perspectives in behavioral medicine.* Hillsdale, NJ: Erlbaum.

Antoni, M. H., Goldstein, D., Ironson, G., LaPerriere, A., Fletcher, M. A., & Schneiderman, N. (1995). Coping responses to HIV-1 serostatus notification predict concurrent and prospective immunologic status. *Clinical Psychology and Psychotherapy, 2*(4), 234–48.

Antoni, M. H., & Goodkin, K. (1988). Life stress and moderator variables in the promotion of cervical neoplasia. I: Personality facets. *Journal of Psychosomatic Research, 32*(3), 327–38.

Antoni, M. H., & Goodkin, K. (1989). Life stress and moderator variables in the promotion of cervical neoplasia. II: Life event dimensions. *Journal of Psychosomatic Research, 33*(4), 457–67.

Antoni, M. H., Ironson, G., & Schneiderman, N. (2007). *Stress management for persons with HIV infection.* New York: Oxford University Press.

Antoni, M. H., Lechner, S., Kazi, A., Wimberly, S., Sifre, T., Urcuyo, K., et al. (2006). How stress management improves quality of life after treatment for breast cancer. *Journal of Consulting and Clinical Psychology, 74*, 1143–52.

Antoni, M. H., Lehman, J., Kilbourn, K., Boyers, A., Yount, S., Culver, J., et al. (2001). Cognitive-behavioral stress management intervention decreases the prevalence of depression and enhances benefit finding among women under treatment for early-stage breast cancer. *Health Psychology, 20*, 20–32.

Antoni, M. H., Lutgendorf, S., Cole, S., Dhabhar, F., Sephton, S., McDonald, P., et al. (2006). The influence of biobehavioral factors on tumor biology, pathways and mechanisms. *Nature Reviews Cancer, 6*, 240–8. (b)

Antoni, M. H., Lutgendorf, S., Ironson, G., Fletcher, M.A., & Schneiderman, N. (March, 1996). *CBSM intervention effects on social support, coping, depression and immune function in symptomatic HIV-infected men.* Paper presented at the American Psychosomatic Society, Williamsburg, VA.

Antoni, M. H., Pereira, D. B., Buscher, I., Ennis, N., Peake-Andrasik, M. Rose, R., et al. (2008). Stress management effects on perceived stress and cervical intraepithelial neoplasia in low-income HIV-infected women. *Journal of Psychosomatic Research, 65*, 389–401.

Antoni, M. H., & Schneiderman, N. (1998). HIV/AIDS. In A. Bellack & M. Hersen (Eds.), *Comprehensive clinical psychology* (pp. 237–75). New York: Elsevier Science.

Antoni, M. H., Schneiderman, N., Fletcher, M., Goldstein, D., Laperriere, A., & Ironson, G. (1990). Psychoneuroimmunology and HIV-1. *Journal of Consulting and Clinical Psychology, 58*(1), 38–49.

Antoni, M. H., Wagner, S., Cruess, D., Kumar, M., Lutgendorf, S., Ironson, G., et al. (2000b). Cognitive behavioral stress management reduces distress and 24-hour urinary free cortisol among symptomatic HIV-infected gay men. *Annals of Behavioral Medicine, 22*, 29–37.

Bangsberg, D. R., Perry, S., Charlebois, E. D., Clark, R. A., Roberston, M., Zolopa, A. R., et al. (2001). Non-adherence to highly active antiretroviral therapy predicts progression to AIDS. *AIDS, 15(9)*, 1181–3.

Berger, S., Schad, T., VonWyl, V., Ehlert, U., Zellweger, C., Furrer, H., et al. (2008). Effects of cognitive behavioral stress management on HIV-1 RNA, CD4 cell counts and psychosocial parameters of HIV-infected persons. *AIDS, 22*, 767–75.

Bing, E. G., Burnam, M. A., Longshore, D., Fleishman, J.A., Sherbourne, C.D., London, A.S., et al. (2001). Psychiatric disorders and drug use among human immunodeficiency virus-infected adults in the United States. *Archives of General Psychiatry, 58*, 721–8.

Bower, J., Kemeny, M., Taylor, S., & Fahey, JL. (1998). Cognitive processing, discovery of meaning, CD4 decline and AIDS-related mortality among bereaved HIV-positive seropositive men. *Journal of Consulting and Clinical Psychology, 66*, 979–86.

Burack, J. H., Barrett, D. C., Stall, R. D., Chesney, M. A., Ekstrand, M. L., & Coates, T. J. (1993). Depressive symptoms and CD4 lymphocyte decline among HIV-infected men. *Journal of the American Medical Association, 270*, 2568–73.

Byrnes, D., Antoni, M. H., Goodkin, K., Efantis-Potter, J., Simon, T., Munajj, J., et al. (1998). Stressful events, pessimism, natural killer cell cytotoxicity, and cytotoxic/suppressor T-cells in HIV+ Black women at risk for cervical cancer. *Psychosomatic Medicine, 60*, 714–22.

Capitano, J., Abel, K., Mendoza, S., Blozis, S., McChesney, M., Cole, S., & Mason, W. (2008). Personality and serotonin transporter genotype interact with social context to affect immunity and viral set-point in simian immunodeficiency virus disease. *Brain, Behavior and Immunity, 22*, 676–89.

Carrico, A. W., Antoni, M. H., Pereira, D. B., Fletcher, M. A., Klimas, N., Lechner, S. C, & Schneiderman, N. (2005). Cognitive behavioral stress management effects on mood, social support, and a marker of anti-viral immunity are maintained up to one year in HIV-infected gay men. *International Journal of Behavioral Medicine, 12*, 218–26.

Carrico, A., Ironson, G., Antoni, M. H., Lechner, S., Durán, R., Kumar, M., & Schneiderman, N. (2006). A path model of the effects of spirituality on depressive symptoms and 24-hour urinary-free cortisol in HIV-positive persons. *Journal of Psychosomatic Research, 61*, 51–8.

Carrico, A. W., & Antoni, M. H. (2008). The effects of psychological interventions on neuroendocrine hormone regulation and immune status in HIV-positive persons: A review of randomized controlled trials. *Psychosomatic Medicine, 70*, 575–84.

Carrico, A. W., Antoni, M. H., Young, L., & Gorman, J. M. (2008). Psychoneuroimmunology and HIV. In M. A. Cohen & J. M. Gorman (Eds.), *Comprehensive textbook of AIDS psychiatry* (pp. 27–38). Oxford, UK: Oxford University Press.

Carrico, A. W., Johnson, M. O., Colfax, G. N., & Moskowitz, J. T. (2009). Affective correlates of stimulant use and adherence to anti-retroviral therapy among HIV-positive methamphetamine users. *AIDS and Behavior*. DOI 10.1007/s10461-008-9513-y.

Carrico, A. W., Johnson, M. O., Morin, S. F., Remien, R. H., Riley, E. D., Hecht, F. M., et al. (2008). Stimulant use is associated with immune activation and depleted tryptophan among HIV-positive persons on anti-retroviral therapy. *Brain, Behavior, and Immunity, 22,* 1257–62.

Carrico, A. W., & Moskowitz, J. T. (2008). *Positive affect promotes decreases in stimulant use following a HIV seropositive diagnosis.* Poster presented at the 10th International Congress of Behavioral Medicine, Tokyo, Japan.

Carver, C. S., Pozo, C., Harris, S. D., Noriega, V., Scheier, M. F., Robinson, D. S., et al. (1993). How coping mediates the effect of optimism on distress: A study of women with early stage breast cancer. *Journal of Personality and Social Psychology, 65*, 375–90.

Centers for Disease Control (CDC). (1992). 1993 revised classification system for HIV infection and expanded surveillance case definition for AIDS among adolescents and adults. *Morbidity and Mortality Weekly Report*, 41, RR-171–19.

Chesney, M., Folkman, S., & Chambers, D. (1996). Coping effectiveness training for men living with HIV: preliminary findings. *International Journal of STD and AIDS 7 Suppl, 2*, 75–82.

Chrousos, G. P., & Gold, P. W. (1992). The concepts of stress and stress system disorders. Overview of physical and behavioral homeostasis. *Journal of the American Medical Association, 267*, 1244–52.

Cielsa, J. A., & Roberts, J. E. (2001). Meta-analysis of the relationship between HIV infection and the risk for depressive disorders. *American Journal of Psychiatry, 158*, 725–30.

Clerici, M., Berzofsky, J. A., Shearer, G. M., & Tacket, C. O. (1991). Exposure to human immunodeficiency virus type 1-specific T helper cell responses before detection of infection by polymerase chain reaction and serum antibodies. *Journal of Infectious Diseases, 164*, 178–84.

Cohen, S., & Wills, T. A. (1985). Stress social support, and the buffering hypothesis. *Psychological Bulletin, 98*, 310–57.

Cole, S. W., Kemeny, M. E., Fahey, J. L., Zack, J. A., & Naliboff, B. D. (2003). Psychological risk factors for HIV pathogenesis: Mediation by the autonomic nervous system. *Biological Psychiatry, 54*, 1444–56.

Cole, S. W., Kemeny, M. E., Taylor, S. E., & Visscher, B. R. (1996). Accelerated course of human immunodeficiency virus infection in gay men who conceal their homosexual identity. *Psychosomatic Medicine, 58*, 219–31.

Cole, S. W. (2008). Psychosocial influences on HIV-1 disease progression: Neural, endocrine, and virologic mechanisms. *Psychosomatic Medicine, 70*, 562–8.

Cole, S. W., Korin, Y. D., Fahey, J. L., & Zack, J. A. (1998). Norepinephrine accelerates HIV replication via protein kinase A-dependent effects on cytokine production. *Journal of Immunology, 161*, 610–6.

Cole, S. W., & Kemeny, M. E. (2001). Psychosocial influences on the progression of HIV infection. In R. Ader, D. L. Felten, & S. Cohen (Eds.), *Psychoneuroimmunology* (3rd ed.). San Diego, CA: Academic Press.

Cole, S. W., Naliboff, B. D., Kemeny, M. E., Griswold, M. P., Fahey, J. L., & Zack, J. A. (2001). Impaired response to HAART in HIV-infected individuals with high autonomic nervous system activity. *Proceedings of the National Academy of Sciences USA, 98,* 12695–700.

Corley, P. A. (1996). Acquired immune deficiency syndrome: The glucocorticoid solution. *Medical Hypotheses, 47,* 49–54.

Crepaz, N., Passin, W., Herbst, J., Rama, S., Malow, R., Purcell, D., & Wolitski, R. (2008). Meta-analysis of cognitive behavioral interventions on HIV-positive person's mental health and immune functioning. *Health Psychology, 27,* 4–14.

Cruess, S., Antoni, M. H., Cruess, D., Fletcher, M. A., Ironson, G., Kumar, M., et al. (2000c). Reductions in HSV-2 antibody titers after cognitive behavioral stress management and relationships with neuroendocrine function, relaxation skills, and social support in HIV+ gay men. *Psychosomatic Medicine, 62,* 828–37.

Cruess, S., Antoni, M., Kilbourn, K., Ironson, G., Klimas, N., Fletcher, M. A., et al. (2000b). Optimism, distress, and immunologic status in HIV-infected gay men following Hurricane Andrew. *International Journal of Behavioral Medicine, 7,* 160–82.

Cruess, D., Antoni, M. H., Kumar, M., & Schneiderman, N. (2000a). Reductions in salivary cortisol are associated with mood improvement during relaxation training among HIV-1 seropositive men. *Journal of Behavioral Medicine, 23,* 107–22.

Cruess, D. G., Douglas, S. D., Petitto, J. M., Have, T. T., Gettes, D., Dube, B., et al. (2005). Association of resolution of major depression with increased natural killer cell activity among HIV-seropositive women. *American Journal of Psychiatry, 162,* 2125–30.

Cupps, T., & Fauci, A. (1982). Corticosteroid-mediated immunoregulation in man. *Immunology Review, 65,* 694–7.

Cutrona, C., & Russell, D. (1987). The provision of social relationships, adaptation to stress. In W. H. Jones & D. Perlman (Eds.), *Advances in personal relationships* (Vol. 1, pp. 37–67). Greenwich, CT: JAI Press.

DesJarlais, D., & Semaan, S. (2008). HIV prevention and injecting drug users: The first 25 years and counting. *Psychosomatic Medicine, 70,* 606–11.

Delahanty, D. L., Bogart, L. M., & Figler, J. L. (2004). Posttraumatic stress disorder symptoms, salivary cortisol, medication adherence, and CD4 levels in HIV-positive individuals. *AIDS Care, 16*(2), 247–60.

Diego, M. A., Field, T., Hernandez-Reif, M., Shaw, K., Friedman, L., & Ironson, G. (2001). HIV adolescents show improved immune function following massage therapy. *International Journal of Neuroscience, 106,* 35–45.

Dunkel-Schetter, C., Folkman, S., & Lazarus, R. S. (1987). Correlates of social support receipt. *Journal of Personality and Social Psychology, 53,* 71–80.

Dybul, M., Fauci, A. S., Bartlett, J. G., Kaplan, J. E., & Pau, A. K. (2002). Guidelines for using antiretroviral agents among HIV-infected adults and adolescents. *Annals of Internal Medicine, 137,* 381–433.

Esterling, B., Antoni, M., Schneiderman, N., Ironson, G., LaPerriere, A., Klimas, N., & Fletcher, M. A. (1992). Psychosocial modulation of antibody to Epstein-Barr viral capsid antigen and herpes virus type-6 in HIV-1 infected and at-risk gay men. *Psychosomatic Medicine, 54,* 354–71.

Evans, D. L., Ten Have, T. R., Douglas, S. D., Gettes, D., Morrison, C. H., et al. (2002). Association of depression with viral load, CD8 T lymphocytes, and natural killer cells in women with HIV infection. *American Journal of Psychiatry, 159,* 1752–9.

Fekete, E. M., Antoni, M. H., Lopez, C. R., Duran, R. E., Penedo, F. J., Bandiera, F.C., Fletcher, M.A., Klimas, N., Kumar, M. & Schneiderman, N. (2009). Men's serostatus disclosure to parents: Associations among social support, ethnicity, and disease status in men living with HIV. *Brain, Behavior & Immunity, 23*(5), 693–696.

Fekete, E., Antoni, M.H., Duran, R., Stoelb, B., Kumar, M. & Schneiderman, N. (2009). The Moderating Effects of Social Support on Serostatus Disclosure to Family Members and Distress in HIV+ Women. *International Journal of Behavioral Medicine, 16,* 367 – 376.

Felten, D. (1996). Changes in neural innervation of the lymphoid tissues with age. In N. Hall, F. Altman, & S. Blumenthal (Eds.), *Mind-body interactions and disease and psychoneuroimmunological aspects of health and disease.* Washington, DC: Health Dateline Press.

Fife, B., Scott, L., Fineberg, N., & Zwickil, B. (2008). Promoting adaptive coping by persons with HIV disease: Evaluation of a patient/partner intervention model. *Journal of the Association of Nurses in AIDS Care, 19,* 75–84.

Fitzpatrick, R., Newman, S., Lamb, R., & Shipley, M. (1988). Social relationships and psychological well-being in rheumatoid arthritis. *Social Science and Medicine, 27,* 399–403.

Folkman, S., Lazarus, R., Dunkel-Schetter, C., DeLongis, A., & Gruen, J. (1986). Dynamics of a stress encounter: Cognitive appraisals, coping and encounter outcomes. *Journal of Personality and Social Psychology, 50,* 992–1003.

Folkman, S. (2008). The case for positive emotions in the stress process. *Anxiety, Stress, and Coping, 21,* 3–14.

Folkman, S., & Moskowitz, J. T. (2000). Positive affect and the other side of coping. *American Psychologist, 55,* 647–54.

Friedland, G. H., & Williams, A. (1999). Attaining higher goals in HIV treatment: the central importance of adherence. *AIDS, 13,* S61–72.

Gaines, H., von Sydow, M. A., von Stedingk, L. V., Biberfeld, G., Bottiger, B., Hansson, et al. (1990). Immunological changes in primary HIV-1 infection. *AIDS, (4),* 995–99.

Galvan, F., Davis, E., Banks, D., & Bing, E. (2008). HIV stigma and social support among African Americans. *AIDS Patient Care and STDs, 22,* 423–36.

Gan, X., Zhang, L., Newton, T., Chang, S. L., Ling, W., Kermani, V., et al. (1998). Cocaine infusion increases interferon-gamma and decreases interleukin-10 in cocaine-dependent subjects. *Clinical Immunology and Immunopathology, 89,* 181–90.

Giorgi, J.V., Hultin, L. E., McKeating, J. A., Johnson, T. D., Owens, B., Jacobson, L. P., et al. (1999). Shorter survival in advanced human immunodeficiency virus type 1 infection is more closely associated with T lymphocyte activation than with plasma virus burden or virus chemokine coreceptor usage. *Journal of Infectious Diseases, 179,* 859–70.

Gonzalez, J. S., Penedo, F. J., Antoni, M. H., Duran, R. E., McPherson-Baker, S., Ironson, G., et al. (2004). Social support, positive states of mind, and HIV treatment adherence in men and women living with HIV/AIDS. *Health Psychology, 23*(4), 413–8.

Goodkin, K., Antoni, M., & Blaney, P. (1986). Stress and hopelessness in the promotion of cervical intraepithelial neoplasia to invasive squamous cell carcinoma of the cervix. *Journal of Psychosomatic Research, 30,* 67–76.

Goodkin, K., Tuttle, R., Blaney, N., Feaster, D., Shapshak, P., Burhalter, J., et al. (1996). A bereavement support group intervention is associated with immunological changes in

HIV-1+ and HIV-1– homosexual men. *Psychosomatic Medicine, 58*, 83.

Goodwin, P. J., Leszcz, M., & Ennix, M. et al. (2001). The effect of group psychosocial support on survival in metastatic breast cancer. *New England Journal of Medicine, 345*, 1719–26.

Gore-Felton, C., & Koopman, C. (2008). Behavioral mediation of the relationship between psychosocial factors and HIV disease progression. *Psychosomatic Medicine, 70*, 569–74.

Heckman, T. G., Barcikowski, R., Ogles, B., Suhr, J., Carlson, B., Holroyd, K., & Garske, J. (2006). A telephone-delivered coping improvement group intervention for middle-aged and older adults living with HIV/AIDS. *Annals of Behavioral Medicine, 32*, 27–38.

Helgeson, V., & Cohen, S. (1996). Social support and adjustment to cancer: Reconciling descriptive, correlational, and intervention research. *Health Psychology, 15*, 135–48.

Herberman, R., & Holden, H. (1978). Natural cell-mediated immunity. *Advances in Cancer Research, 27*, 305–77.

Herbert, T., & Cohen, S. (1993a). Stress and immunity in humans: A meta-analytic review. *Psychosomatic Medicine, 55*, 364–79.

Herbert, T., & Cohen, S. (1993b). Depression and immunity: A meta-analytic review. *Psychological Bulletin, 113*, 472–486.

Holahan, C. J., & Moos, R. H. (1986). Personality, coping, and family resources in stress resistance: A longitudinal analysis. *Journal of Personality and Social Psychology, 51*, 389–95.

House, J. A. (1981). *Work stress and social support.* Reading, MA: Addison-Wesley.

Hunt, P. W., Deeks, S. G., Bangsberg, D. R., Moss, A., Sinclair, E., Liegler, T., et al. (2006). The independent effect of drug resistance on T cell activation in HIV infection. *AIDS, 20*, 691–9.

Hurwitz, B. E., Brownley, K. A., Motivala, S. J., Milanovich, J. R., Kibler, J. L., Fillion, L., et al. (2005). Sympathoimmune anomalies underlying the response to stressful challenge in human immunodeficiency virus spectrum disease. *Psychosomatic Medicine, 67*, 798–806.

Ickovics, J. R., Hamburger, M. E., Vlahov, D., Schoenbaum, E. E., Schuman, P., Boland, R.J., et al. (2001). Mortality, CD4 cell count decline, and depressive symptoms among HIV-seropositive women: Longitudinal analysis from the HIV Epidemiology Research Study. *Journal of the American Medical Association, 285*, 1460–5.

Ickovics, J. R., Milan, S., Boland R., Schoenbaum, E., Schuman, P., Vlahov, D., et al. (2006). Psychological resources protect health: 5-year survival and immune function among HIV-infected women from four U.S. cities. *AIDS, 20*, 1851–60.

Ironson, G., LaPerriere, A., Antoni, M. H., O'Hearn, P., Schneiderman, N., Klimas, N., & Fletcher, M. A. (1990). Changes in immune and psychological measures as a function of anticipation and reaction to news of HIV-1 antibody status. *Psychosomatic Medicine, 52*, 247–70.

Ironson, G., Balbin, G., Solomon, G., Fahey, J., Klimas, N., Schneiderman, N., et al. (2001). Relative preservation of natural killer cell cytotoxicity and number in healthy AIDS patients with low CD4 cell counts. *AIDS, 15*, 2065–73.

Ironson, G., & Hayward, H. (2008). Do positive psychological factors predict disease progression in HIV-1? A review of the evidence. *Psychosomatic Medicine, 70*, 546–54.

Ironson, G., Balbin, E., Stieren, E., Detz, K., Fletcher, M. A., Schneiderman, N., & Kumar. M. (2008). Perceived stress and norepinephrine predict effectiveness of response to protease inhibitors in HIV. *International Journal of Behavioral Medicine, 15*, 221–6.

Ironson, G., O'Cleirigh, C., Fletcher, M. A., Laurenceau, J. P., Balbin, E., Klimas, N., et al. (2005). Psychosocial factors predict CD4 and viral load change in men and women with human immunodeficiency virus in the era of highly active antiretroviral therapy. *Psychosomatic Medicine, 67,* 1013–21.

Ironson, G., Friedman, A., Klimas, N., Antoni, M. H., Fletcher, M. A., LaPerriere, A., et al. (1994). Distress, denial and low adherence to behavioral intervention predict faster disease progression in gay men infected with human immunodeficiency virus. *International Journal of Behavioral Medicine, 1*, 90–105.

Irwin, M. R., Olmos, L., Wang, M., Valladares, E. M., Motivala, S. J., Fong, T., et al. (2007). Cocaine dependence and acute cocaine induce decreases of monocyte proinflammatory cytokine expression across the diurnal period: autonomic mechanisms. *Journal of Pharmacology and Experimental Therapeutics, 320,* 507–15.

Jensen, S., Lehman, B., Antoni, M. H., & Pereira, D. (2007). Psychoneuroimmunologic applications to human papillomavirus mediated cervical neoplasia research among the iatrogenically immunocompromised. *Brain, Behavior and Immunity, 21*, 758–66.

Johnson, M. O., Charlebois, E., Morin, S. F., Catz, S. L., Goldstein, R. B., Remien, R. H., et al. (2005). Perceived adverse effects of antiretroviral therapy. *Journal of Pain and Symptom Management, 29*, 193–205.

Johnson, M. O., Catz, S. L., Remien, R. H., Rotheram-Borus, M. J., Morin, S. F., Charlebois, E., et al. (2003). Theory-guided, empirically supported avenues for intervention on HIV medication nonadherence: findings from the Healthy Living Project. *AIDS Patient Care STDS, 17*(12), 645–56.

Johnson, M. O., Gamarel, K. E., & Dawson-Rose, C. (2006). Changing HIV treatment expectancies: A pilot study. *AIDS Care, 18*, 550–3.

Kalichman, S. (2008). Co-occurrence of treatment nonadherence and continued HIV transmission risk behaviors: Implications for positive prevention interventions. *Psychosomatic Medicine, 70*, 593–7.

Kalichman, S. C., Difonzo, K., Austin, J., Luke, W., & Rompa, D. (2002). Prospective study of emotional reactions to changes in HIV viral load. *AIDS Patient Care and STDs, 16*(3), 113–20.

Kaplan, L. D., Wofsky, C. B., & Volberding, P. A. (1987). Treatment of patients with acquired immunodeficiency syndrome and associated manifestations. *Journal of the American Medical Association, 257*, 1367–76.

Kemeny, M. E., & Dean, L. (1995). Effects of AIDS-related bereavement on HIV progression among New York City gay men. *AIDS Education and Prevention, 7*, 36–47.

Kemeny, M. E., Weiner, H., Durán, R., Taylor, S. E., Visscher, B., & Fahey, J. L. (1995). Immune system changes after the death of a partner in HIV-positive gay men. *Psychosomatic Medicine, 57*, 547–54.

Keruly, J. C., & Moore, R. D. (2007). Immune status at presentation to care did not improve among antiretroviral-naïve persons from 1990 to 2006. *Clinical Infectious Diseases, 45*, 1369–74.

Kiecolt-Glaser, J. K., McGuire, L., Robles, T. F., & Glaser, R. (2002). Psychoneuroimmunology: Psychological influences on immune function and health. *Journal of Consulting and Clinical Psychology, 70*, 537–47.

Kimmerling, R., Ouimette, P., Cronkite, R., & Moos, R. (1999). Depression and outpatient medical utilization: A naturalistic

10-year follow-up. *Annals of Behavioral Medicine, 21,* 317–21.

Klatzmann, D., Champagne, E., Chamaret, S., Gruest, J., Guetard, D., Hercend, T., et al. (1984). T-lymphocyte T4 molecule behaves as the receptor for human retrovirus LAV. *Nature, 312,* 767–8.

Kraaij, V., Van Der Veek, S., Garnefski, N., Schoevers, M., Witlox, R., & Maes, S. (2008). Coping, goal adjustment and psychological well-being in HIV-infected men who have sex with men. *AIDS Patient Care and STDs, 22,* 395–402.

Kumar, M., Kumar, A. M., Morgan, R., Szapocznik, J., & Eisdorfer, C. (1993). Abnormal pituitary-adrenocortical response in early HIV-1 infection. *Journal of Acquired Immune Deficiency Syndrome & Human Retrovirology, 6,* 61–5.

Lechner, S., Antoni, M. H., Lydston, D., LaPerriere, A., Ishii, M., Stanley, H., et al. (2003). Cognitive-behavioral interventions improve quality of life in women with AIDS. *Journal of Psychosomatic Research, 54,* 253–61.

Lederman, M. M., & Valdez, H. (2000). Immune restoration with antiretroviral therapies: Implications for clinical management. *Journal of the American Medical Association, 284*(2), 223–8.

Leserman, J. (2008). Role of depression, stress, and trauma in HIV disease progression. *Psychosomatic Medicine, 70,* 539–45.

Leserman, J., Jackson, E. D., Petitto, J. M., Golden, R. N., Silva, S. G., Perkins, D. O., et al. (1999). Progression to AIDS: The effects of stress, depressive symptoms and social support. *Psychosomatic Medicine, 61,* 397–406.

Leserman, J., Petitto, J. M., Perkins, D. O., Folds, J. D., Golden, R. N., & Evans, D. L. (1997). Severe stress and depressive symptoms, and changes in lymphocyte subsets in human immunodeficiency virus infected men. *Archives of General Psychiatry, 54,* 279–85.

Leserman, J., Petitto, J. M, Golden, R. N, Gaynes, B. N., Gu, H., Perkins, D. O., et al. (2000). Impact of stressful life events, depression, social support, coping, and cortisol on progression to AIDS. *American Journal of Psychiatry, 157,* 1221–8.

Leserman, J., Petitto, J. M., Gu, H., Gaynes, B. N., Barroso, J., Golden, R. N., et al. (2002). Progression to AIDS, a clinical AIDS condition and mortality: Psychosocial and physiological predictors. *Psychological Medicine, 32,* 1059–73.

Leserman, J., DiSantostefano, R., Perkins, D., Murphy, C., Golden, R., & Evans, D. (1995). Longitudinal study of social support and social conflict as predictors of depression and dysphoria among HIV-positive and HIV-negative gay men. *Depression, 2,* 189–99.

Lucas, G. M., Griswold, M., Gebo, K. A., Keruly, J., Chaisson, R. E., & Moore, R. D. (2006). Illicit drug use and HIV-1 disease progression: a longitudinal study in the era of highly active antiretroviral therapy. *American Journal of Epidemiology, 163,* 412–20.

Lutgendorf, S., Antoni, M. H., Ironson, G., Starr, K., Costello, N., Zuckerman, M., et al. (1998). Changes in cognitive coping skills and social support mediate distress outcomes in symptomatic HIV-seropositive gay men during a cognitive behavioral stress management intervention. *Psychosomatic Medicine, 60,* 204–14.

Lutgendorf, S. K., Antoni, M. H., Ironson, G., Klimas, N., Kumar, M., Starr, K., et al. (1997). Cognitive behavioral stress management intervention decreases dysphoria and herpes simplex virus-type 2 titers in symptomatic HIV-seropositive gay men. *Journal of Consulting and Clinical Psychology, 65,* 23–31.

Lyketsos, C. G., Hoover, D. R., Guccione, M., Senterfitt, W., Dew, M. A., Wesch, J., et al. (1993). Depressive symptoms as predictors of medical outcomes in HIV infection. *Journal of the American Medical Association, 270,* 2563–7.

Lyketsos, C. G., Hoover, D. R., Guccione, M., Dew, M. A., Wesch, J. E., Bing, E. G., et al. (1996). Changes in depressive symptoms as AIDS develops. The Multicenter AIDS Cohort Study. *American Journal of Psychiatry, 153,* 1430–7.

Makisumi, T., Yoshida, K., Watanabe, T., Tan, N., Murakami, N., & Morimoto, A. (1998). Sympatho-adrenal involvement in methamphetamine-induced hyperthermia through skeletal muscle hypermetabolism. *European Journal of Pharmacology, 363,* 107–12.

Maiman, M., Fruchter, R., Clark, M., Arrastia, C., Matthews, R., & Gates, E. J. (1997). Cervical cancer as an AIDS-defining illness. *Obstetrics and Gynecology, 89,* 76–80.

Martin, J. L., & Dean, L. (1993). Effects of AIDS-related bereavement and HIV-related illness on psychological distress among gay men: A 7-year longitudinal study, 1985-1991. *Journal of Consulting and Clinical Psychology, 61,* 94–103.

Mayne, T. J., Vittinghoff, E., Chesney, M. A., Barrett, D. C., & Coates, T. J. (1996). Depressive affect and survival among gay and bisexual men infected with HIV. *Archives of Internal Medicine, 156,* 2233–8.

McCain, N., Munjas, B., Munro, C., Elswick, R., Robins, J., Ferreira-Gonzalez, A., et al. (2003). Effects of stress management on PNI-based outcomes in persons with HIV disease. *Research in Nursing and Health, 26,* 102–17.

McCain, N., Gray, D., Elswick, R., Robins, J., Tuck, I., Walter, J., et al. (2008). A randomized clinical trial of alternative stress management interventions in persons with HIV infection. *Journal of Consulting and Clinical Psychology, 76,* 431–41.

McEwen, B. (1998). Protective and damaging effects of stress mediators. *New England Journal of Medicine, 338,* 171–9.

Mildvan, D., Spritzler, J., Grossberg, S. E., Fahey, J. L., Johnston, D. M., Schock, B. R., et al. (2005). Serum neopterin, an immune activation marker, independently predicts disease progression in advanced HIV-1 infection. *Clinical Infectious Diseases, 40,* 853–8.

Morin, S. F., Sengupta, S., Cozen, M., Richards, T. A., Shriver, M. D., & Palacio, H. (2002). Responding to racial and ethnic disparities in the use of HIV drugs: Analysis of state policies. *Public Health Reports, 117,* 263–72.

Moskowitz, J. T., Hult, J., Bussolari, C., & Acree, M. (2009). What works in coping with HIV? A meta-analysis with implications for coping with serious illness. *Psychological Bulletin, 135,* 121–41.

Moskowitz, J. T. (2003). Positive affect predicts lower risk of AIDS mortality. *Psychosomatic Medicine, 65,* 620–6.

Motivala, S. J., Hurwitz, B. E., Llabre, M. M., Klimas, N., Fletcher, M. A., Antoni, M. H., et al. (2003). Psychological distress is associated with decreased memory helper T-cell and B-cell counts in pre-AIDS HIV seropositive men and women but only in those with low viral load. *Psychosomatic Medicine, 65,* 627–35.

Mulder, C. L., Antoni, M. H., Duivenvoorden, H. J., Kauffman, R. H., & Goodkin, K. (1995). Active confrontational coping predicts decreased clinical progression over a one year period in HIV-infected homosexual men. *Journal of Psychosomatic Research, 39,* 957–65.

Nair, M. P. N., Mahajan, S., Hou, J., Sweet, A. M., & Schwartz, S. A. (2000). The stress hormone, cortisol, synergizes with

HIV-1 gp120 to induce apoptosis of normal human periph-eral blood mononuclear cells. *Cellular and Molecular Biology, 46(7)*, 1227–38.

Nance, D. W., & Sanders, V. M. (2007). Autonomic innervation and regulation of the immune system (1987–2007). *Brain, Behavior, and Immunity, 21*, 736–45.

Page-Shafer, K., Delorenze, G. N., Satariano, W., & Winkelstein, W. (1996). Comorbidity and survival in HIV-infected men in the San Francisco Men's Health Survey. *Annals of Epidemiology, 6*, 420–30.

Pantaleo, G., Graziosi, C., & Fauci, A. S. (1993). The immunop-athogenesis of human immunodeficiency virus infection. *New England Journal of Medicine, 328*, 327–35.

Park, C., Lechner, S., Antoni, M. H., & Stanton, A. (Eds.). (2008). *Medical illness and positive life change: Can crisis lead to personal transformation?* Washington, EC: American Psychological Association.

Park, W., Laura, Y., Scalera, A., Tseng, A., & Rourke, S. (2002). High rate of discontinuations of highly active antiretroviral therapy as a result of antiretroviral intolerance in clinical practice: Missed opportunities for support? *AIDS, 16*(7), 1084–6.

Patterson, T. L., Williams, S. S., Semple, S. J., Cherner, M., McCutchman, A., Atkinson, J. H., et al. (1996). Relationship of psychosocial factors to HIV disease progression. *Annals of Behavioral Medicine, 18*, 30–9.

Pavlidis, N., & Chirigos, M. (1980). Stress-induced impairment of macrophage tumoricidal function. *Psychosomatic Medicine, 42*, 47–54.

Penedo, F. J., Molton, I., Dahn, J. R., Shen, B. J., Kinsinger, D., Schneiderman, N., & Antoni, M. (2006). A randomized clinical trial of group-based cognitive-behavioral stress man-agement (CBSM). in localized prostate cancer: Development of stress management skills improves quality of life and benefit finding. *Annals of Behavioral Medicine, 31*(3), 261–70.

Penedo, F., Antoni, M. H., & Schneiderman, N. (2008). *Stress management for prostate cancer recovery.* New York: Oxford University Press.

Pereira, D., Antoni, M. H., Simon, T., Efantis-Potter, J., Carver, C.S., Durán, R., et al. (2003a). Stress and squamous intra-epithelial lesions in women with human papillomavirus and human immunodeficiency virus. *Psychosomatic Medicine, 65*, 427–34.

Pereira, D., Antoni, M. H., Simon, T., Efantis-Potter, J., Carver, C.S., Durán, R., et al. (2003b). Stress as a predictor of symp-tomatic genital herpes virus recurrence in women with human immunodeficiency virus. *Journal of Psychosomatic Research, 54*, 237–44.

Pereira, D. B. (2002). Interventions for mothers during preg-nancy and postpartum: Behavioral and pharmacological approaches. In M. Chesney & M. H. Antoni (Eds.), *Innovative approaches to health psychology: Prevention and treatment: Lessons learned from AIDS.* Washington, DC: American Psychological Association Press.

Petrie, K. J., Fontanilla, I., Thomas, M. G, Booth, R. J., & Pennebaker, J. W. (2004). Effect of written emotional expres-sion on immune function in patients with human immuno-deficiency virus infection: a randomized trial. *Psychosomatic Medicine, 66*, 272–5.

Pinkerton, S. D. (2008). Probability of HIV transmission during acute infection in Rakai, Uganda. *AIDS and Behavior, 12*, 677–84.

Rabkin, J. G., Ferrando, S. J., Lin, S. H., Sewell, M., & McElhiney, M. (2000). Psychological effects of HAART: A 2-year study. *Psychosomatic Medicine, 62*, 413–22.

Reed, G. M., Kemeny, M. E., Taylor, S. E., & Visscher, B. R. (1999). Negative HIV-specific expectancies and AIDS-related bereavement as predictors of symptoms onset in asymptomatic HIV-positive gay men. *Health Psychology, 18*, 354–63.

Reed, G. M., Kemeny, M. E., Taylor, S. E., Wang, H. J., & Visscher, B. R. (1994). Realistic acceptance as a predictor of decreased survival time in gay men with AIDS. *Health Psychology, 13*(4), 299–307.

Riley, E. D., Bangsberg, D. R., Guzman, D., Perry, S., & Moss, A. R. (2005). Antiretroviral therapy, hepatitis C virus, and AIDS mortality among San Francisco's homeless and mar-ginally housed. *Journal of Acquired Immune Deficiency Syndromes, 38*, 191–5.

Rutherford, G. W., Lifson, A. R., & Hessol, N. A. (1990). Course of HIV-1 infection in a cohort of homosexual and bisexual men: An 11-year follow-up study. *British Medical Journal, 301*, 1183–91.

Safren, S., Knauz, R. O., O'Cleirigh, C., Lerner, J., Greer, J., Harwood, M., et al. (2006). CBT for HIV medication adherence and depression: Process and outcome at post-treatment and three-month cross over. *Annals of Behavioral Medicine, 31*, S006.

Safren, S., O'Cleirigh, C., Tan, J., Raminani, S., Reilly, L.,Otto, M., & Mayer, K. (2009). Cognitive behavioral therapy for adherence and depression (CBT-AD) in HIV-infected indi-viduals. *Health Psychology, 28*, 1–10.

Sapolsky, R. M, Romero, L. M., & Munck, A. U. (2000). How do glucocorticoids influence stress responses? Integrating permissive, suppressive, stimulatory, and preparative actions. *Endocrine Reviews, 21*, 55–89.

Schaefer, C., Coyne, J. C., & Lazarus, R. S. (1981). The health-related functions of social support. *Journal of Behavioral Medicine, 4*, 381–406.

Schneiderman, N., Antoni, M. H., Ironson, G., Fletcher, M.A., Klimas, N., & LaPerriere, A. (1994). HIV-1, immunity and behavior. In R. Glaser (Ed.), *Handbook of human stress and immunity.* New York: Academic Press.

Siegal, B. R., Calsyn, R. J., & Cuddihee, R. M. (1987). The rela-tionship of social support to psychological adjustment in end-stage renal disease patients. *Journal of Chronic Disease, 40*, 337–44.

Sikkema, K., Wilson, P., Hansen, N., Kochman, A., Neufeld, S., Ghebremichael, M., & Kershaw, T. (2008). Effects of a coping intervention on transmission risk behavior among people living with HIV/AIDS and a history of childhood sexual abuse. *Journal of Acquired Immune Deficiency Syndrome, 47*, 506–13.

Simoni, J. M., Pearson, C. R., Pantalone, D. W., Marks, G., & Crepaz, N. (2006). Efficacy of interventions in improving highly active antiretroviral therapy adherence and HIV-1 RNA viral load. A meta-analytic review of randomized con-trolled trials. *Journal of Acquired Immune Deficiency Syndromes, 43 Suppl 1*, S23–S35.

Sledjeski, E. M., Delahanty, D. L., & Bogart, L. M. (2005). Incidence and impact of posttraumatic stress disorder and comorbid depression on adherence to HAART and CD4+ counts in people living with HIV. *AIDS Patient Care STDS, 19*(11), 728–36.

Sloan, E. K., Tarara, R. P., Capitanio, J. P., & Cole, S. W. (2006). Enhanced replication of simian immunodeficiency virus adjacent to catecholaminergic varicosities in primate lymph nodes. *Journal of Virology, 80,* 4326–35.

Spiegel, D., Kraemer, H. C., Bloom, J. R., & Gottheil, E. (1989). Effect of psychosocial treatment on survival of patients with metastatic breast cancer. *Lancet, 2,* 888–91.

Starr, K. R., Antoni, M. H., Hurwitz, B. E., Rodriguez, M. S., Ironsong, G., Fletcher, M. A., et al. (1996). Patterns of immune, neuroendocrine, and cardiovascular stress responses in asymptomatic HIV serpositive and seronegative men. *International Journal of Behavioral Medicine, 3,* 135–62.

Starace, F., Ammassari, A., Trotta, M. P., Murri, R., De Longis, P., Izzo, C., et al. (2002). Depression is a risk factor for suboptimal adherence to highly active antiretroviral therapy. *Journal of Acquired Immune Deficiency Syndromes, 31 Suppl 3,* S136–9.

Stein, M. D, Herman, D. S, Bishop, D., Anderson, B. J., Trisvan, E., Lopez, R., et al. (2007). A telephone-based intervention for depression in HIV patients: negative results from a randomized clinical trial. *AIDS Behavior, 11,* 15–23.

Swanson, B., Zeller, J. M., & Spear, G.T. (1998). Cortisol upregulates HIV p24 antigen production in cultured human monocyte-derived macrophages. *Journal of the Association of Nurses in AIDS Care, 9*(4), 78–84.

Szapocznik, J., Feaster, D. J., Mitrani, V. B., Prado, G., Smith, L., Robinson-Batista, C., et al. (2004). Structural ecosystems therapy for HIV-seropositive African American women: effects on psychological distress, family hassles, and family support. *Journal of Consulting Clinical Psychology, 72,* 288–303.

Tamalet, C., Fantini, J., Tourres, C., & Yashi, N. (2003). Resistance of HIV-1 to multiple antiretroviral drugs in France: A 6-year survey (1997–2002) based on an analysis of over 7000 genotypes. *AIDS, 17,* 2383–8.

Taylor, S. E., Lichtman, R. R., & Wood, J. V. (1984). Attributions, beliefs about control, and adjustment to breast cancer. *Journal of Personality and Social Psychology, 46,* 489–502.

Taylor, S. E., & Aspinwall, L. G. (1990). Psychosocial aspects of chronic illness. In P. Costa & G. van den Bos (Eds.), *Psychological aspects of serious illness: Chronic conditions, fatal diseases, and clinical care* (pp. 7–60). Washington, DC: American Psychiatric Association Press.

Taylor, S. E, Kemeny, M. E, Reed, G. M, Bower, J. E., & Gruenewald, T. L. (2000). Psychological resources, positive illusions, and health. *American Psychologist, 55,* 99–109.

Temoshok, L., Waldstein, S., Wald, R., Garzino-Demo, S, Synowski, S., Sun, L., & Wiley, J. (2008). Type C coping, alexithymia, and heart rate reactivity are associated independently and differentially with specific immune mechanisms linked to HIV progression. *Brain, Behavior and Immunity, 22,* 781–92.

Thoits, P. A. (1987). Gender and marital status differences in control and distress: Common stress versus unique stress explanations. *Journal of Health and Social Behavior, 28,* 7–22.

Tindall, B., & Cooper, D. A. (1991). Primary HIV infection: Host responses and intervention strategies. *AIDS, 5,* 1–15.

Turner, H. A., Hays, R. B., & Coates, T. J. (1993). Determinants of social support among gay men: The context of AIDS. *Journal of Health and Social Behavior, 34,* 37–53.

Varmus, H. (1988). Retroviruses. *Science, 240,* 1427–34.

Vedhara, K., Nott, K. H., Bradbeer, C. S., Davidson, E. A. F., Ong, E. L. C., Snow, M. H., et al. (1997). Greater emotional distress is associated with accelerated CD4+ cell decline in HIV infection. *Journal of Psychosomatic Research, 42,* 379–90.

Vranceanu, A. M., Safren, S. A., Lu, M., Coady, W. M., Skolnik, P. R., Rogers, W. H., et al. (2008). The relationship of posttraumatic stress disorder and depression to antiretroviral medication adherence in persons with HIV. *AIDS Patient Care STDS, 22,* 313–21.

Wallston, B. S., Alagna, S. W., De Vellis, B., & DeVellis, R. F. (1983). Social support and physical health. *Health Psychology, 2,* 367–91.

Weaver, K. E., Llabre, M. M., Duran, R. E., Antoni, M. H., Ironson, G., Penedo, F. J., et al. (2005). A stress and coping model of medication adherence and viral load in HIV-positive men and women on highly active antiretroviral therapy (HAART). *Health Psychology, 24*(4), 385–92.

Wortman, C., & Conway, T. (1985). The role of social support in adaptation, recovery from physical illness. In S. Cohen & S. Syme (Eds.), *Social support and health* (pp. 281–302). New York: Academic Press.

Zich, J., & Temoshok, L. (1987). Perceptions of social support in men with AIDS and ARC: Relationships with distress and hardiness. *Journal of Applied Social Psychology, 17,* 193–215.

Zuckerman, M., & Antoni, M. H. (1995). Social support and its relationship to psychological physical and immune variables in HIV infection. *Clinical Psychology and Psychotherapy, 2*(4), 210–9.

PART 8

Conclusions and Future Directions

CHAPTER
22

Stress, Health, and Coping: Synthesis, Commentary, and Future Directions

Susan Folkman

Abstract

This chapter summarizes the major developments in stress and coping research that are presented in this volume. Lazarus and Folkman's (1984) theory of stress and coping provides a framework for organizing the central themes of the discussion, including problems associated with aspects of the model, gaps in the original model, and new directions in research that have emerged in the intervening years. Advances in understanding antecedents of the appraisal process are noted, as are problems with the original formulation of emotion-focused coping. Future-oriented coping, interpersonal coping, and religious and spiritual coping are introduced into the stress and coping model. The scope of coping has been broadened to include the regulation of positive as well as negative emotion states. Meaning-focused kinds of coping that help motivate and sustain positive well-being in the face of stress are introduced. Strategies for examining cause-and-effect relationships between coping and health are discussed.

Keywords: stress, coping, emotion regulation, positive emotion, meaning-focused coping

Stress and coping research has undergone 30 years of vigorous growth. Earlier ideas are now more fully developed and, as the chapters in this volume demonstrate beautifully, there is a wealth of exciting new ideas to pursue. The emphasis in this volume is on coping. Aside from the fact that coping is an inherently fascinating topic that provides insights into the human capacity to survive both the ordinary and extraordinary challenges of daily living, it is one of the few variables in the stress process that lends itself to intervention. As several authors point out, a portion of our response to stress is influenced by aspects of our biological heritage and characteristics of the social and physical environment over which we have little or no control. But our coping responses—what we think and what we do

in response to stress, and to a certain extent the emotions we feel—are at least potentially under our control. Coping is thus a critical point of entry for protecting mental and physical health from the harmful effects of stress and worthy of the time and effort the authors of these chapters have invested over the years.

In this chapter I attempt to synthesize the major ideas in this volume, summarizing what we have learned and how we might continue moving the field forward. I have chosen to organize these comments within a theoretical framework. As Stroebe notes in her thoughtful review of theories related to coping and bereavement (Chapter 8), theories offer the opportunity to test assumptions that guide stress and coping research, and theories also provide guidelines regarding practicalities of research design and measure development. I find that theoretical frameworks have an additional practical advantage: they provide a structure for connecting findings from diverse studies, thereby helping to create a coherent data-based explanatory narrative.

Several important theories are presented in this volume, including Hobfoll's (Chapter 7) theory of conservation of resources, Stroebe and Schut's (1999) dual process model of coping with bereavement (Chapter 8), Taylor's (Chapter 5) tend-and-befriend theory, Zautra and Reich's (Chapter 9) resilience model, and Lyubomirsky's (Chapter 11) theory of hedonic adaptation. However, Lazarus and Folkman's (1984) cognitive theory of stress, appraisal, and coping appears to have had the major influence on research on psychological stress and coping over the past three decades. Conveniently, it is also the model with which I have the greatest familiarity, and so I shall use it to frame my comments.

Although the Lazarus and Folkman (1984) model has stood the test of time as a useful framework, it was not free of problems and limitations, many of which are addressed by chapters in this volume. The chapters also highlight ways in which the model has evolved in the intervening years and introduce new ideas that broaden the model further. In accord with this framework, I begin with comments about appraisal and then move on to coping.

Antecedents of Appraisal

The coping process is initiated in response to a cognitive appraisal of a situation as stressful, which means it is personally significant and it taxes or exceeds the person's resources for coping. A major strength of this definition is that it allows for individual differences in the stressfulness of a given event (e.g., the departure of the last child may be a relief to one parent and a great sadness to the other). The definition also allows for changes in meaning of a given event for a given individual (e.g., a job loss that is experienced once when a person is single vs. again when he or she is supporting a family).

The appraisal is made by a person with a particular psychosocial and biological heritage at a particular developmental stage in a particular setting, with particular personal, social, and material resources for coping, and with other demands competing for those resources. Important theory and research has developed our understanding of the influence of some of these variables since Lazarus and Folkman outlined the antecedents of appraisal in their 1984 book.

Others have received less attention. Personality variables such as optimism, pessimism, and resilience have been included in many studies, but less often linked to the appraisal process are a number of variables brought forward in the chapters of this volume, such as:

- "Wired-in" responses of the autonomic nervous system and the genome (e.g., Tugade, Chapter 10; Taylor, Chapter 5)
- The person's global belief system (Park, Chapter 12)
- Developmental stages of control processes, and appraisal and coping skills (Aldwin, Chapter 2; Skinner & Zimmer-Gembeck, Chapter 3)
- Gender roles (Helgeson, Chapter 4)
- Environmental, social, and material resources (Hobfoll, Chapter 7)

Specific recommendations for incorporating these variables in research are offered in the respective chapters. It is important that these dimensions be considered as they are likely to increase our understanding of variability in both the appraisal and coping process.

Challenges of Coping

Lazarus and Folkman (1984) approached coping in terms of thoughts and actions that people used in stressful situations. As noted in Aldwin's (Chapter 2) review, this was a departure from earlier approaches in which coping was defined in terms of personality styles or defense mechanisms derived from ego psychology. Lazarus and Folkman defined two major coping categories: (1) emotion-focused coping, which refers to the regulation of emotions that are generated by the appraisal process, such as anger or sadness in response to the appraisal of loss, anxiety, or fear in the case of the appraisal of threat, and eagerness and excitement, mixed with some worry, in the case of the appraisal of challenge; and (2) problem-focused coping, which refers to the management of the problem itself. That formulation was the jumping-off point for many of the chapters in this volume. Here I highlight issues with emotion-focused coping and three major gaps in the original formulation pertaining to future orientation, religious and spiritual coping, and interpersonal coping.

Coping with emotion-focused coping

Problems with the formulation of emotion-focused coping became evident when self-report measures were developed to measure it. These problems are discussed in detail by Stanton (Chapter 18). Briefly, one problem was caused by the heterogeneity of questionnaire items asking about emotion-focused coping. This problem had its origin in a major tenet of stress and coping theory: The evaluation of the appropriateness of a given coping strategy should be made in the context of the stressful encounter. Distancing, for example, is appropriate in a situation where there is nothing that can be done (as when waiting for the outcome of an exam), but it is inappropriate when action is called for (as when preparing for the exam). This tenet resulted in measures of emotion-focused coping that combined what on face value appeared to be maladaptive (e.g., escape-avoidance) and adaptive (e.g., positive reappraisal) strategies. Our first version of the Ways of Coping (Folkman & Lazarus, 1980), which had just the two scales for problem- and emotion-focused coping, illustrates this problem. In subsequent revisions of the Ways of Coping (Folkman, Lazarus, Dunkel-Schetter, DeLongis, & Gruen, 1986), we distinguished among types of emotion-focused coping, as did other measures of coping that followed, including the COPE (Carver, Scheier, & Weintraub, 1989) and the Coping Inventory for Stressful Situations (Endler & Parker, 1990). Nevertheless, many researchers still collapse diverse categories into one emotion-focused scale and one problem-focused scale, so the problem persists.

Another major tenet of stress and coping theory held (and still holds) that coping, both in its definition and its measurement, had to be independent of outcomes. Nevertheless, as Stanton (Chapter 18) points out, self-report questionnaire items assessing the regulation of emotion were often confounded with outcomes, especially mood outcomes.

Stanton's Emotion Approach Coping (EAC) scale addressed both problems by directing attention to emotion processing (EP) and emotion expression (EE), without reference to outcomes. Work with this measure has led to important contributions about the regulation and expression of emotions during stressful encounters, as summarized by Stanton in her chapter. The care with which the EAC was developed is exemplary, and it is a valuable addition to the assessment of emotion regulation under conditions of stress.

Although I agree with Stanton about the problems with emotion-focused coping, I do not think those problems negate the importance of assessing the regulation of emotion along established dimensions such as distancing, cognitive reframing, or seeking emotional support. What is needed is a careful review of questionnaire items to assure they are not confounded with outcomes, and careful classification processes that meet both empirical and theoretical standards for coherence.

Future-oriented coping

Although the major forms of stress appraisal set forth by Lazarus and Folkman (1984)—harm/loss, threat, and challenge—are oriented to the past, present, and future, most measures of coping tend to be past- or present-oriented; the future gets short shrift. Fortunately, this situation is improved substantially with the contributions of Wrosch (Chapter 16) and Aspinwall (Chapter 17).

The pursuit of meaningful goals is by definition future-oriented; it is also central to well-being. However, not all goals are feasible, nor do all goals retain their value over time. Adaptive coping requires that people recognize when goals are no longer tenable or valuable and then disengage from those goals and re-engage in alternative goals that are realistic and meaningful. Although Lazarus and Folkman (1984) discuss goals, they did not elaborate the process of goal revision. Wrosch (Chapter 16) provides an excellent review of theory and research on goal revision with very helpful discussion of the details of the disengagement process, including withdrawing both effort and commitment, and the re-engagement process, including identifying, committing to, and pursuing alternative goals.

A major question, however, still needs explication: How do we decide when to give up a goal? We tend to value persistence in pursuit of socially approved goals. Our heroes are athletes who overcome physical handicaps in pursuit of gold medals, entrepreneurs who invest all their resources in a zany new concept, scientists who pursue a hypothesis that is judged by peers to be absurd. When does persistence turn into counterproductive obstinacy? How do we know when to quit? I hope that Wrosch and others who are studying goal processes pursue this perplexing question.

Another form of future-oriented coping is proactive coping, which is based on the assumption that one can proactively minimize or prevent future stress and promote favorable outcomes. Aspinwall (Chapter 17), who has done a great deal to develop the theory and research in this area, provides an excellent overview. Some might question whether it is possible to have coping in the absence of stress. I think of proactive coping as preventive coping, and consider it an important addition to the stress and coping model.

What is particularly appealing about proactive coping is that it lends itself beautifully to prospective research designs. It is theoretically sensible to ask whether proactive coping at Time 1 affects the frequency of unwanted events or states that are the object of the proactive coping at Time 2. The proactive coping research related to health outcomes reviewed by Aspinwall is a case in point. Below I comment on the challenges involved in establishing causal links between coping with ongoing stress and future outcomes.

Religious and spiritual coping
Although Lazarus and Folkman (1984) mention religious and spiritual beliefs in relation to coping resources, very little is said about the use of religion and spirituality for coping. The original Ways of Coping (Folkman & Lazarus, 1980), for example, did not contain any items pertaining to religious coping.

Pargament's 1997 book, *The Psychology of Religion and Coping: Theory, Research, Practice*, changed this pattern. Pargament not only provided a framework for research on religious coping, but he also seems to have legitimized the study of religious coping for many psychologists who had previously been squeamish about researching this topic. In the intervening years research on religious and spiritual coping has burgeoned, as summarized by Pargament (Chapter 14) and Ironson and Kremer (Chapter 15). Religious coping appears to be distinct from secular coping, adding an important dimension to the coping process. The effects of religious coping cannot be fully explained by more basic social, physiological, and psychological variables, although Ironson and Kremer suggest a process through which spirituality can confer benefits, especially in the case of serious illness. However, like its secular counterpart, religious coping can have both beneficial and harmful effects on mental well-being and physical health. Clearly, assessments of religious and spiritual coping should be included along with assessments of secular coping.

Interpersonal coping
Any recommendation that is offered independently by multiple authors in this volume deserves close attention. One such recommendation concerns interpersonal coping processes, an area that was not fully addressed in Lazarus and Folkman's (1984) model. Helgeson (Chapter 4) discusses co-rumination; Skinner and Zimmer-Gembeck (Chapter 3)

talk about social processes involved in the acquisition of mastery coping. Aspinwall (Chapter 17) offers compelling reasons for exploring interpersonal aspects of proactive coping, as does Park (Chapter 12) with respect to meaning-making. Stroebe (Chapter 8) points to the importance of clarifying features of pre-bereavement relationships in explaining the subsequent adjustment of the surviving partner, presumably including the ways in which they coped with their shared stressors. Pargament (Chapter 14) recommends that we turn to interpersonal religious coping.

Revenson and DeLongis (Chapter 6) have developed special expertise in dyadic coping, a topic to which they devote their chapter. In dyadic coping, the members of the couple participate in an interactive coping process that plays out in a context of psychological interdependence, or mutual influences. Revenson and DeLongis review a bevy of theoretical models of dyadic processes, and it does not take long to realize that the study of these processes confronts the researcher with formidable challenges. Fortunately, Revenson and DeLongis and others who conducted research in this area were not daunted, and Revenson and DeLongis' review of research in this area is very engaging. Questions raised by Revenson and DeLongis, such as what are the roles of empathy, engagement, and congruence in dyadic coping, point both to the complexity of the interactive coping process and to the rich insights it can provide regarding the ways in which the couple as a dyadic unit confront stressors in their lives. Revenson and DeLongis also provide very helpful direction regarding measurement and analysis. The work on dyadic coping is an important contribution to the field.

Broadening the Scope of the Stress and Coping Model: Beyond Negative Emotions
A dramatic shift in thinking about the stress process began to appear in the mid-1990s. Zautra and Reich (Chapter 9) refer to the shift as "a sea change" that "has now opened up new horizons by bringing to the fore conceptualizations and measurement of the strengths of people and their societies rather than attending solely to their weaknesses." I agree with Zautra and Reich regarding the significance of this sea change; it has had implications for virtually every aspect of the stress process, especially coping and outcomes.

The sea change had a number of sources: interest in the adaptive functions of positive emotions with respect to broadening resources for coping and "undoing" the sympathetic arousal created by negative emotions (Fredrickson, 1998; Fredrickson & Joiner, 2002; Tugade, Chapter 10); observations that positive emotions co-occurred with negative ones even in the most dire of circumstances (Folkman, 1997; Folkman & Moskowitz, 2000; Moskowitz, Chapter 20) and contribute independently to adaptational outcomes (Moskowitz, Chapter 20; Tugade, Chapter 10); and observations that many people find positive meaning and perceive growth and benefit as a result of their stress (Helgeson, Reynolds, & Tomich, 2006; Tennen & Affleck, 1998; Pakenham, Chapter 13; Park, Chapter 12).

Zautra and Reich (Chapter 9) place the concept of resilience at the vortex of this swirl of observations. Resilience is another of those ideas touched upon independently by several authors, including Litt, Tennen, and Affleck (Chapter 19), Lyubomirsky (Chapter 11), Park (Chapter 12), Skinner and Zimmer-Gembeck (Chapter 3), and Tugade (Chapter 10), reflecting the widespread interest in this response to stress. Despite the number of different discussions about resilience, Zautra and Reich point out that there is widespread agreement that resilience includes recovery, sustainability, and growth.

Until recently, resilience has been studied primarily in terms of stable aspects of personality and social network, with reference also to genetic and neural underpinnings (Lyubomirsky, Chapter 11; Tugade, Chapter 10; Zautra and Reich, Chapter 9). Tugade, for example, reviews evidence of neural and autonomic correlates of resilience, and there is substantial support for the notion of resilience as a trait.

Now researchers are turning their attention to *actual coping processes* that sustain positive well-being, promote recovery, and provide opportunity for growth. The developments in this area are leading to a fuller understanding of the scope of coping, especially in relation to chronic stress that persists over time, with the potential for exhausting the person's coping resources.

Finding positive meaning in the stress
The past 10 years have seen a surge of interest in meaning-making coping strategies for wresting something good from something bad. Meaning-making coping typically draws on values, goals, and beliefs, both global and situational (Park, Chapter 12). This coping category is explored in chapters on meaning-making and made meaning (Park,

Chapter 12), benefit-finding and sense-making (Pakenham, Chapter 13; Tugade, Chapter 10), religious coping (Pargament, Chapter 14), and goal processes (Wrosch, Chapter 16). Hobfoll's (Chapter 7) discussion of engagement, defined by Schaufeli (2002) as "a persistent, pervasive and positive affective-motivational state of fulfillment in individuals who are reacting to challenging circumstances," is an interesting complement to this list. Not all meaning-making processes support positive emotions, but many do, such as finding resolution, reappraising the meaning of the stressor, perceiving growth or positive life changes, and pursuing meaningful goals.

Elsewhere, I have stated that the meaning-making coping described above, which I call "meaning-focused coping," is a third function of coping that is distinct from problem- and emotion-focused coping (Folkman, 1997; Folkman & Moskowitz, 2000; Park & Folkman, 1997) and is an important addition to the original stress and coping framework. I have hypothesized that meaning-focused coping becomes especially important in stressful situations that are prolonged or chronic, where problem- and emotion-focused coping fail to make things better. Under these conditions, meaning-focused coping reminds the person of his or her values, goals, beliefs, and commitments, and this connection helps sustain coping efforts (Folkman, 1997; Park & Folkman, 1997). Moskowitz (Chapter 20), for example, notes that the more distressed the person is, the more meaning-focused interventions boost positive affect. This boost can in turn motivate subsequent coping.

These ideas have been incorporated into the stress and coping model (Folkman, 1997; Folkman & Moskowitz, 2000), and evidence in their support is beginning to accumulate (Folkman, 2008). The timing of meaning-focused coping efforts may be a key to understanding an individual's ability to generate and sustain positive well-being during prolonged periods of stress, as well as his or her ability to recover once it is in the past. This is another feature of the coping process that should be taken into account, especially when studying coping with chronic stress.

Attending to the positive while dealing with the negative
Lyubomirsky (Chapter 11) comments that there is a natural process through which people adapt to both positive and negative life changes with fading of the

associated positive and negative emotions, the positive emotions fading more quickly than negative ones. In short, positive emotions, or for that matter negative emotions, do not sustain themselves.

These observations lead directly to the question of how to keep positive emotions alive while dealing with a stressor. Tugade (Chapter 10) comments that resilient people may actively cultivate positive emotions to downregulate distress and describes several practices for this purpose. One general strategy Lyuobmirsky recommends is to actively try to generate, or be open to, unexpected and variable experiences. Another is to engage in practices that delay adaptation to positive emotions once they occur. Examples of such practices include gratitude meditations; appreciative attention, as in savoring a positive moment; and positive thinking. Moskowitz (Chapter 20) reviews the rapidly expanding literature on these and other practices, including acts of kindness, forgiveness, reminiscence therapy, positive reappraisal, positive affirmations, goal-setting, yoga, meditation, and exercise, in her comprehensive review of interventions to boost positive affect. This literature is still young, but as Moskowitz's review indicates, it is growing rapidly with some promising implications for health.

What is significant about the strategies for maintaining positive states described by Lyubomirsky, Tugade, and Moskowitz is that often these strategies are not directed at the immediate stressors, but elsewhere at positive events, conditions, or changes in the person's life—past, present, or anticipated. This approach is entirely consistent with the idea that positive events and emotions can co-occur with negative ones, and that the positive emotions can help sustain the individual's efforts to cope with ongoing stress.

Studies of coping should routinely include questions about positive events or changes happening elsewhere in people's lives (Moskowitz, Chapter 20). Such questions may go far in helping us understand how people are able to persist in stressful situations, such as caregiving for a spouse with Alzheimer's disease, that do not improve over time.

Coping, Health, and Well-Being

An important reason for studying coping is its hypothesized role as a mediator of the effects of stress on mental and physical health. The case for a relationship between coping and psychological outcomes is substantial. Virtually every chapter in this volume provides evidence of this robust connection.

The connection between coping and physical health is less well documented, except in the instances described earlier in which coping is directly health-related.

Lazarus and Folkman's (1984) model discussed health outcomes in general terms. The model did not specify causal mechanisms. Investigations of this question tend to be formulated *ad hoc*, without much attention to approaches that can help forge links among studies.

How do we know when coping has an effect?

The ultimate demonstration of a cause-and-effect relationship is a randomized controlled clinical trial. Such a trial has the advantages of randomization and a control condition to help rule out alternative hypotheses regarding cause-and-effect relationships. Fortunately, coping lends itself to intervention. Coping skills can be taught along the lines of cognitive-behavioral therapy, and the chapters in this volume provide many examples (e.g., cognitive-behavioral stress management [Antoni, Chapter 21], proactive coping interventions [Aspinwall, Chapter 17], spiritual and religious coping interventions [Ironson & Kremer, Chapter 15; Pargament, Chapter 14], and positive meaning coping interventions [Lyubomirsky, Chapter 11; Moskowitz, Chapter 20; Pakenham, Chapter 13]).

Two tasks must be addressed to determine whether coping affects outcomes: (1) There needs to be a way to determine whether coping has changed, and (2) There needs to be a plausible map showing pathways through which coping can affect outcomes.

DETERMINING CHANGES IN COPING

Litt et al. (Chapter 19) comment that the best way to show that coping influences outcomes is to show that changes in coping are related to changes in outcomes. This objective is best achieved by assessing coping that pertains substantively to both the stressful context and the outcome of interest. Litt et al., for example, review a number of intervention studies in the fields of pain and addiction that failed to produce evidence that changes in coping were associated with changes in outcome. Based on their review, they developed coping measures tailored to the nature of the stressor and the outcome of interest, such as thoughts and actions related to drinking in response to the offer of a drink in the case of alcohol addiction. By tailoring the assessment of coping to the context and a specific outcome (in the case of alcohol addiction, did the person draw on the preferred cognitive coping strategies and refuse the drink), it was possible to determine that in fact changes in coping *were* related to changes in the outcome.

The design described by Litt et al. (Chapter 19), however, is often not feasible. Many studies have samples dealing with stressors that are complex and dynamic, such as those associated with bereavement (Stroebe, Chapter 8), chronic illness (Antoni, Chapter 21; Ironson and Kremer, Chapter 15; Pakenham, Chapter 13), and existential uncertainty (Pargament, Chapter 14). Under such circumstances it is difficult to measure changes in coping in a way that is meaningful, because what the person is coping with is also changing. How do you interpret the change in coping? Is the change due to the intervention, or to change in the stressor, or to both? For example, Chesney and I and our colleagues (Chesney, Neilands, Chambers, Taylor, & Folkman, 2006) originally tried to measure changes in coping by holding constant what people were coping with, such as a chronic interpersonal problem. But we found that there was no such thing as holding a stressor constant. Situations change, and even a transaction that involves the same people in contention over the same issue (i.e., one member of a dyad is always late), the situation at Time 1 does not remain frozen in time; the dynamics will differ at Time 2, even if only minutely.

A way around this problem is to identify surrogate markers of the coping process (variables in which change must occur if there is to be change in coping) and to examine their shifts over time. For example, in the study mentioned above (Chesney et al., 2006), we assessed changes in coping self-efficacy regarding the coping principles we were teaching rather than actual coping processes. These changes were associated with the intervention and mediated psychological outcomes. In a study of a program for pain coping, Litt et al. (Chapter 19) note that self-efficacy expectancies explained more pain outcome variance than did coping. Thus, coping self-efficacy may serve as a surrogate in studies that aim to measure changes in coping. Another example is provided by Wrosch (Chapter 16), who assesses *capacity* for goal engagement and disengagement rather than the engagement and disengagement processes themselves.

MAPPING CAUSAL PATHWAYS

The second task is to identify plausible pathways of effect from stress through coping to health outcomes. In some instances, the path from coping is direct and unambiguous. For example, Aspinwall (Chapter 17) describes proactive coping in the form of health behaviors, such as being screened for risk factors. Goal-setting processes described by Wrosch (Chapter 16) can also affect health directly when the goal is health-related, as when a person commits to eating a healthier diet with the goal of reducing cholesterol.

In most studies, however, the most common pathway of effect seems to be indirect, through psychological or spiritual well-being. To be credible this pathway needs to show that there is stress to begin with, and that there is reason to believe that stress can harm the health outcome of interest. A case in point is HIV disease. As Antoni (Chapter 21) and Ironson and Kremer (Chapter 15) point out, HIV carries many stressful burdens, and physiological stress reactivity has been found to be associated with HIV disease progression. These features of HIV create a plausible pathway in which the ways people cope with the stress of HIV can influence the effects of stress on HIV progression. Ironson and Kremer summarize the results of longitudinal studies that show effects of five categories of coping on a range of HIV-related health outcomes, especially CD4 cell levels. They found support for the notion that avoidant coping predicts faster disease progression. They also found support for effects between other kinds of coping and HIV-related outcomes. Antoni's (Chapter 21) review concurs. Antoni also provides a detailed description of plausible and testable pathways through which his cognitive-behavioral stress management program can proceed from psychological adjustment through psychoneuroimmunological pathways to affect clinically relevant HIV disease markers.

Until recently, most research focused on a negative affect pathway on the assumption that its regulation would reduce the harmful effects of stress emotions such as hostility, depression, despair, anger, or guilt on the body's defenses. Now attention is turning to a positive affect pathway to determine how it may protect, restore, and sustain the body's physical health during periods of stress. Given evidence that positive affect is beneficial to health (Lyubormisky, Chapter 11; Moskowitz, Chapter 20; Tugade, Chapter 10), this pathway is an exciting new direction in stress and coping theory and research. The full picture requires that we pay attention to both positive and negative affect, as noted throughout this volume.

Methodological Issues

As noted in virtually every chapter of this volume, there are the inevitable methodological issues to consider. I highlight three here: capturing the dynamic quality of coping, a few comments about measures, and a concluding observation regarding specificity versus generalizability.

Capturing the dynamic quality of coping

Litt, Tennen, and Affleck (Chapter 19) make the important point that most research treats coping in "a unidirectional, static and deterministic way." Their concern is that "There is little recognition that changes in coping lead to changes in adaptational outcomes, which in turn may lead to changes in subsequent appraisals, coping, or external contingencies on behavior. The transactional nature of coping is not captured." They review daily process and momentary assessment technologies and multilevel statistical techniques that capture the dynamic, mutually reciprocal nature of appraisal and coping outcomes. These methods might also be useful for capturing the interplay between members of a dyad, or between types of coping processes such as Wrosch's (Chapter 16) goal-engagement and goal-disengagement processes, Tugade's automatic and controlled coping processes (Chapter 10), and Stroebe and Schut's (1999) loss and restoration orientation within their Dual Process Model of coping.

Measures

The measurement of multidimensional, dynamic subjective phenomena is always complicated and imperfect. Within this volume, for example, Stanton's (Chapter 18) discussion of emotion-focused coping highlights common shortcomings in the assessment of this form of coping and offers a psychometrically sound alternative. Stroebe (Chapter 8) reviews the shortcomings of measures of bereavement coping. Pakenham (Chapter 13) reviews issues in the measurement of benefit-finding and sense-making, Pargament (Chapter 14) discusses measures of religious coping, and Moskowitz (Chapter 20) offers clear direction for improving measures of positive emotions.

Overall, measures need to be appropriate for the question addressed by the research. Aldwin (Chapter 2) points out that more immediate measures of daily stressors may be better for assessing very variable health outcomes such as blood pressure or noradrenaline, but it is unlikely that a daily stressor by itself is of sufficient magnitude to affect long-term health outcomes. Measures of life events and trauma may be more relevant for studies of morbidity and mortality. Another volume could easily be dedicated to this topic. For now, researchers contemplating assessing variables related to the stress process should consult the reviews contained in these chapters.

Creating the stress and coping narrative: Generalizability of findings

Most stress and coping research is conducted in specific contexts such as chronic illness, divorce, natural disasters, or terrorism. The introduction to any context-specific research report usually contains highly elaborated description of the context, especially the nature of the stressor and its trajectory over time, context-specific resources for coping, and context-specific constraints that might impede coping efforts.

Many people assume that context specificity limits the generalizability of findings, and indeed caveats to this effect are included in most articles. Ironically, in my experience, just the opposite is more often the case: Well-characterized contexts allow greater precision in defining correlative or predictive relationships that turn out to be relevant in diverse contexts. We have many examples. The Dual Process Model that was developed by Stroebe (Chapter 8) and her colleagues specifically to characterize the ways people cope with bereavement contains an important general principle that should apply to any chronic stressor: The person is likely to oscillate between dual coping orientations to deal with loss and restoration, or to deal with the stressor while also maintaining well-being. Pakenham (Chapter 13) refers to the adaptive tasks associated with chronic illness. Adaptive tasks can be defined in almost any stressful context and, in fact, should be defined so that there is a way to determine whether coping has been effective (Folkman, 2001). Ironson and Kremer's (Chapter 15) research on stress and coping in the context of HIV led to the observation that confronting a stressor and managing it well can lead to increased self-efficacy. This observation happens to converge with and add to the general benefit-finding literature discussed by Park (Chapter 12), Pakenham (Chapter 13), and Moskowitz (Chapter 20). The discovery of positive emotions in the reports of the gay caregiving partners of men dying of AIDS turned out to echo findings from a range diverse of settings (Folkman, 1997; Moskowitz, Chapter 20) and led to the principle that positive and negative emotion co-occur in the stress process (Folkman & Moskowitz, 2000).

Researchers should thus not assume the contextual nature of their research necessarily limits the generalizability of their findings; instead, we should look for underlying principles in context-specific findings. These principles can be added to the framework for other researchers to test in their own studies and make research on the links among stress, health, and coping ever more fruitful.

Conclusion

Stress and coping research is like the stress process: It is dynamic, multidimensional, complex, and fascinating. There can be little doubt that we have learned a great deal, but each increment of progress seems to spawn multiple new questions. So, although we know more than we did in previous years, we have many new questions enumerated in the chapters that we must now address, especially those linking coping to health. These questions need to be considered from many different perspectives and examined with carefully designed studies.

Earlier, I mentioned how the stress and coping narrative evolves with the accumulation of research findings. We can see this process at work in this volume: Virtually every author draws on work of other authors to inform the discussion at hand. For example, Pargament cites Ironson, and Ironson cites Moskowitz, who cites Lyubomirsky, who in turn cites Skinner and Taylor. Skinner and Zimmer-Gembeck cite Stroebe, who in turn cites Moskowitz, Aldwin, and Skinner. The pattern continues throughout the volume. This cross-talk solidifies links among findings and also helps pinpoint work that still needs to be done.

However, stress and coping research requires more than cross-talk among psychologists: The research requires truly multidisciplinary approaches. Genetics, and now epigenetics, cognitive and affective neuroscience, and specialties such as psychoneuroimmunology and psychoneuroendocrinology are all relevant to the initial response to a stress appraisal and how it plays itself out at every level: biological, psychological, and social. Taylor's Tend-and-Befriend theory (Chapter 5) illustrates the interplay among biological, psychological, and social responses to threats. We must also cross boundaries within the social and behavioral sciences: Hobfoll's (Chapter 7) research, for example, on the communal or societal level of analysis illustrates the importance of resources at these levels for understanding responses at the individual level. Helgeson's (Chapter 4) research on gender differences in stress exposure and vulnerability is another example of the importance of multi-level models.

We also must learn to take advantage of new technologies for data acquisition and analysis. The new techniques should allow us to arrive at greater understanding of the momentary flow of stress and coping processes, which in turn should allow us to derive additional underlying principles that can be used to think about stress and coping processes at meta-levels.

Multidisciplinary approaches, new methods, and the new ideas and recommendations offered in this volume constitute a powerful formula for advancing this exciting field of research. I would urge us all to approach the work with open minds, giving special attention to the design of the research and to its unexpected findings.

References

Carver, C. S., Scheier, M. F., & Weintraub, J. K. (1989). Assessing coping strategies: A theoretically based approach. *Journal of Personality and Social Psychology, 56*, 267–83.

Chesney, M. A., Neilands, T. B., Chambers, D. B., Taylor, J. M., & Folkman, S. (2006). A validity and reliability study of the coping self-efficacy scale. *British Journal of Health Psychology, 11*, 421–37.

Endler, N. S., & Parker, J. D. A. (1990). *Coping Inventory for Stressful Situations*. Toronto: Multi Health Systems.

Folkman, S. (1997). Positive psychological states and coping with severe stress. *Social Science and Medicine, 45*, 1207–21.

Folkman, S. (2001). Revised coping theory and the process of bereavement. In M. Stroebe, W. Stroebe, R. Hansson, & H. Schut (Eds.), *New handbook of bereavement: Consequences, coping, and care* (pp. 563–84). Washington, DC: American Psychological Association.

Folkman, S. (2008). The case for positive emotions in the stress process. *Anxiety, Stress & Coping: An International Journal, 21*, 3–14.

Folkman, S., & Lazarus, R. S. (1980). An analysis of coping in a middle-aged community sample. *Journal of Health and Social Behavior, 21*, 219–39.

Folkman, S., Lazarus, R. S., Dunkel-Schetter, C., DeLongis, A., & Gruen, R. (1986). The dynamics of a stressful encounter: cognitive appraisal, coping and encounter outcomes. *Journal of Personality and Social Psychology, 50*, 992–1003.

Folkman, S., & Moskowitz, J. T. (2000). Positive affect and the other side of coping. *American Psychologist, 55*, 647–54.

Fredrickson, B. L. (1998). What good are positive emotions? *Review of General Psychology, 2*, 300–19.

Fredrickson, B. L., & Joiner, T. (2002). Positive emotions trigger upward spirals toward emotional well-being. *Psychological Science, 13*(2), 172–5.

Helgeson, V. S., Reynolds, K. A., & Tomich, P. L (2006). A meta-analytic review of benefit finding and growth. *Journal of Consulting & Clinical Psychology, 74*, 797–816.

Lazarus, R. S., & Folkman, S. (1984). *Stress, appraisal, and coping*. New York: Springer.

Pargament, K. I. (1997). *The psychology of religion and coping*. New York: Guilford.

Park, C. L., & Folkman, S. (1997). Meaning in the context of stress and coping. *Review of General Psychology, 1*, 115–44.

Schaufeli, W. B., Salanova, M., Gonzalez-Roma, V., & Bakker, A. B. (2002). The measurement of engagement and burnout: A two sample confirmatory factor analytic approach. *Journal of Happiness Studies, 3*, 71–92.

Stroebe, M., & Schut, H. (1999). The dual process model of coping with bereavement: rationale and description. In R. A. Neimeyer (Ed.), *Meaning reconstruction and the experience of loss.* Washington, DC: American Psychological Association.

Tennen, H., & Affleck, G. (1998). Three compulsions of stress and coping research: A systems framework cure? *Psychological Inquiry, 9*(2), 164–8.

INDEX

Note: Page numbers followed by "*f*" and "*t*" denote figures and tables, respectively.